FRAGMENTS FOR A HISTORY OF THE HUMAN BODY    PART THREE

# Fragments for a History of the Human Body

## Part Three

**Edited by Michel Feher**

**with Ramona Naddaff and Nadia Tazi**

**Editors:** Jonathan Crary, Michel Feher, Hal Foster, Sanford Kwinter

**Special Editor of this Issue:** Michel Feher

**Associate Editors of this Issue:** Ramona Naddaff, Nadia Tazi

**Managing Editor:** Ramona Naddaff

**Designer:** Bruce Mau

**Translation Editor:** Siri Hustvedt

**Translations:** Lydia Davis, Leigh Hafrey, Martha Houle, Astrid Hustvedt, Tina Jolas, Janet Lloyd, Brian Massumi, Patricia Ranum, Shelley Temchin.

**Editorial Assistance:** Judith Aminoff, Ted Byfield, Reynolds Childress, Barbara Czarnecki, Deborah Drier, Meighan Gale, Freya Godard, Astrid Hustvedt, Mike Taylor, Nancy Worman.

**Production:** Steven Bock, John Calvelli, Alison Hahn, Anita Matusevics, Damian McShane, Susan Meggs-Becker, Greg Van Alstyne, Dorothy Vreeker.

**Picture Research:** CLAM! (Christine de Coninck, Anne Mensior) and Marie-Hélène Agueros.

**Special thanks to:** Archie, Ron Date, Mark Elvin, Madeleine Feher, Albert Fuss, Marvin Green, Judith Gurewich, Krista Hinds, Jonathan Joaquin, Barbara Kerr, Gus Kiley, Kerri Kwinter, Rick Lambert, G.E.R. Lloyd, Janet Lloyd, Sandra Naddaff, Mary Picone, John Scinocco, Alice Sindzingre, Mike Tibre.

Typesetting by Canadian Composition.

Film Preparation by P.B.C. Lithoprep.

Printed in Canada by Provincial Graphics.

Distributed by The MIT Press, Cambridge, Massachussetts and London, England.

We gratefully acknowledge translation assistance provided for this volume by the French Ministry of Culture and Communication.

ISBN: 0-942299-27-2 (cloth)      0-942299-28-0 (paper)

Library of Congress Catalog Card Number: 88-051439

# ZONE 5

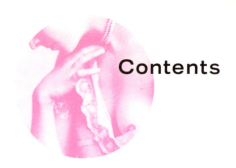

# Contents

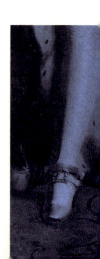

FRAGMENTS FOR A HISTORY OF THE HUMAN BODY    PART TWO

# Foreword

The present volume forms the third part of *Fragments for a History of the Human Body*. As the notion of fragment implies, the texts collected here do not pretend either to form a complete survey or to define a compact portion of the history of the body. The fact that so many problems are addressed only indicates the extent of the field to be explored and marks the several approaches of the ongoing investigation. These fragments, therefore, find their consistency in a cross section in which the connections among different themes and disciplines — history, anthropology, philosophy, etc. — are highlighted rather than in a general overview or a strictly delimited schema. Each of the three volumes of this project corresponds to a specific research approach — though the articles in it complement and connect with one another in more than one way.

The first approach can be called vertical since what is explored here is the human body's relationship to the divine, to the bestial and to the machines that imitate or simulate it. The second approach covers the various junctures between the body's "outside" and "inside": it can therefore be called a "psychosomatic" approach, studying the manifestation — or production — of the soul and the expression of the emotions through the body's attitudes, and, on another level, the speculations inspired by cenesthesia, pain and death. Finally, the third approach, represented by the present volume, brings into play the classical opposition between organ and function by showing how a certain organ or bodily substance can be used to justify or challenge the way human society functions and, reciprocally, how a certain political or social function tends to make the body of the person filling that function the organ of a larger body — the social body or the universe as a whole.

*Michel Feher*

11

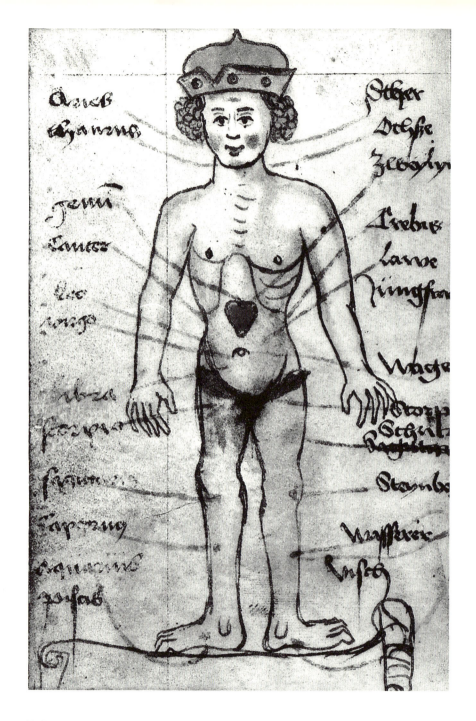

Zodiac man; names of the signs of the zodiac in Latin on
the right and in German on the left. From a 15th-century German
manuscript (Paris, Bibliothèque nationale).

# Head or Heart?
# The Political Use of Body Metaphors
# in the Middle Ages

*Jacques Le Goff*

Organicist conceptions of society based on bodily metaphors, and referring both to the parts of the body and to the functioning of the human (or animal) body as a whole, seem to go back to early Antiquity.

The apologue of the belly and the limbs, which prompted one of the most famous fables published by Jean de La Fontaine in 1668 ("Les Membres et l'Estomac," *Fables* 3.2), goes back at least to Aesop (fables 206 and 286) and was set in a traditional episode from Roman history: the secession of the plebeians to the Sacred Mount in 494 B.C. (Later accounts set the event on the Aventine Hill.) According to Livy (2.32-33), Consul Menenius Agrippa put an end to the incident by telling this fable, in which he reminded the people that cooperation between the head (the Roman Senate) and the limbs (the plebeians) is a necessity, and that the limbs are obligatorily subordinate to the head.

The head (*caput*), seat of the brain, was for the Romans — and for most peoples — the organ that contains the soul (that is, a person's vital force) and that exerts the directing function within the body. Paul-Henri Stahl has recently demonstrated how decapitation practices, which were very common in archaic, antique and medieval societies, bear witness to these beliefs about the power of the head. Head-hunting was motivated by the desire to destroy and often to appropriate for oneself the personality and the power of an outsider, a victim or an enemy, by possessing his head or skull.[1]

Without making an in-depth study, I would like to emphasize in these pages the potential contribution to be made by research into the application of bodily metaphors to politics and to suggest several lines of investigation.[2]

Medieval Christianity probably inherited the political use of bodily metaphors from Greco-Roman Antiquity. Here, I believe, we can discern one of those reworkings of the configurations of symbolic values that marks the replacement of ancient value systems by new Christian ones. Pagan beliefs remained in force, but their meaning was modified through a shift in emphasis, through the substitution of certain values for others, and through the devaluation or the valorization of commonly used metaphors.

It seems to me that the bodily metaphors of Antiquity hinged primarily on a system head/intestines/limbs (*caput/venter/membra*), despite the fact that the chest (*pectus*) and the heart (*cor*), as seats of thought and feeling, obviously lent themselves to metaphorical use. Among the intestines, the liver (sometimes *hepar*, a term borrowed from the Greeks, or more often *iecur* or *iocur*) played an especially important symbolic role. First of all, it was used for the auguries inherited from the Etruscans, who considered the liver as a sort of sacred organ. In addition, it was believed to be the seat of the passions. In Menenius Agrippa's apologue, the belly (*venter*) — in other words, the intestines as a whole — plays the coordinating role within the body, and the limbs (*membra*) obey its orders, for the belly transforms food into blood, which is then sent through the veins to the entire body.

The Christian system of bodily metaphors is based chiefly upon the pair *head/heart*. But within this system, the impact of these metaphors stems from the fact that the Church, as a community of the faithful, is considered to be a *body* of which Christ is the Head. This conception, which is strongly marked by Hellenistic influences and which holds that believers are like multiple limbs connected, through Christ, to the unity of a single body, was established by Saint Paul.[3] Along with the conception of the mystic body of Christ, it dominates medieval ecclesiology.[4] It found its way into political ideology during the Carolingian period when the empire, which was for them an embodiment of the Church, formed a single body of which Christ was the head, and which Christ directed on earth through two intermediaries, "the sacerdotal person and the royal person," that is, the pope and the emperor (or the king).[5]

The symbolic value of the head became unusually strong in the Christian system. It was enriched by the increased value given to that which was *high* within the fundamental subsystem *high/low*, an expression of the Christian principle of the *hierarchy*, and by the fact that not only is Christ the Head of the Church, that is of soci-

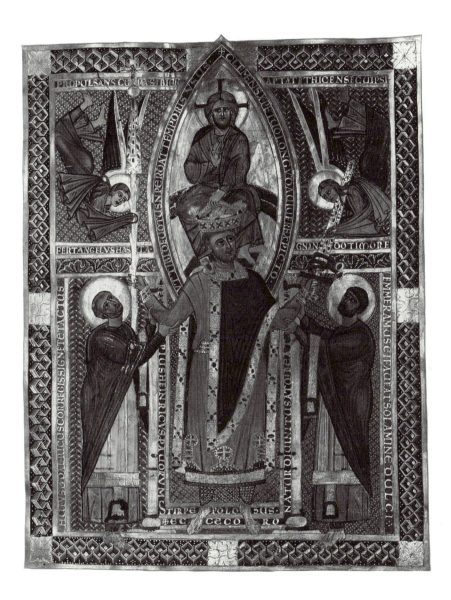

God crowning the Emperor Henry II. From Abbess Uta
of Niedermunster, *The Book of Pericopes*, beginning of the 17th
century (Munich, Staatsbibliothek).

ety, but also that God is Christ's head.[6] Echoing ancient physiology, Paul states, in Colossians 2.19, that the head is the principle of cohesion and growth.

The metaphorical strengthening of the *heart* is even greater in Christianity. Xavier-Léon Dufour has observed that, in the New Testament, the heart is not only the "seat of vital forces," but that it also designates the affective life and interiority, usually in a metaphorical sense. "The source of intellectual thoughts, of faith, of comprehension," it is the "center of decisive things, of the moral conscience, of unwritten law, of encounters with God."[7]

On the other hand, there is a "loser" in this metaphorical configuration: the liver. Christianity's rejection of all forms of pagan divination had completely effaced the prestige given the liver in augury, which was already an archaic practice and which the Romans had always considered "foreign." The liver had, in addition, acquired a markedly pejorative physiologico-symbolic status. In the bodily metaphors used by medieval Christianity, and in particular Isidore of Seville, who represented basic "scientific" knowledge which mingled physiology and moral symbolism, it had become the "seat of voluptuousness and concupiscence."[8] The liver/belly, or intestines, had been cast *down*, below the belt, to the region occupied by the shameful parts of the body, where it became the seat of lewdness, of the concupiscence that Christianity had been persecuting and repressing ever since Paul and Augustine.

It seems that the metaphorical use of bodily parts took shape during the early Middle Ages, in the writings of Gregory the Great, in Bede's *Commentary on the Song of Songs*, and in Beatus's *Commentary on the Apocalypse*. In successive phases, these metaphors became politicized during the Carolingian period, then during the Gregorian reform, and finally during the twelfth century, which was particularly enamored of this comparison.[9]

An especially interesting text can be found in the treatise *Against the Simoniacs* (1057) written by Humbert de Moyenmoutier, a monk from Lorraine who became a cardinal and who was one of the promoters of the so-called Gregorian reform. Indeed, this text combines an organicist imagery with the famous trifunctional scheme of society, which was experiencing its first period of success in the medieval West.[10] In conformity with the ideology of the reforming clergy of the day, it emphasizes the subordination of the popular masses to the clergy and to the lay nobility:

The clerical order is first in the Church as the eyes are first in the head. It was of the clergy that the Lord was speaking when He said, "Whoever touches you, touches the apple of my eye." [Zachariah 2.12]. Lay power is like the chest and the arm whose might is accustomed to obeying the Church and to defending it. As for the masses, which resemble the lower limbs and the extremities of the body, they are subject to ecclesiastical and secular power, but are at the same time indispensable to that power.[11]

The political use of the organicist metaphor reached its classic definition in the *Policraticus* of John of Salisbury (1159):

> The state [*res publica*] is a body [*corpus quoddam*].... Within that state, the prince [*princeps*] occupies the place of the head; he is subject to the unique God and to those who are his lieutenants on earth, for in the human body the head is also governed by the soul. The senate occupies the place of the heart, which gives good and bad deeds their impulses. The function of the eyes, the ears and the tongue is asssured by the judges and the provincial governors [*judices et praesides provinciarum*]. The "officers" and "soldiers" [*officales et milites*] can be compared to the hands. The prince's regular assistants are the flanks. The quaestors [*quaestous* or stewards] and the registrars [*commentarienses* or secretary-registrars; I am not referring to prison directors but to the "earls" of the private treasury] evoke the image of the belly and the intestines which, if they have been stuffed through excessive greed and if they hold in their contents too obstinately, give rise to countless and incurable illnesses and, through their vices, can bring about the ruin of the body as a whole. The feet that always touch the soil are the peasants [*agricolae*]. Being governed by the head is especially necessary for them, because they are faced by numerous detours as they walk upon the earth in the service of the body, and because they need the firmest support in order to keep the mass of the entire body erect, to support it and to move it about. Deprive the most robust body of the support given by its feet, and it will not advance under its own strength but will either crawl shamefully, painfully and unsuccessfully on its hands, or will move about like brute beasts.

These lines surprise us with their archaism, which is poorly adapted to the institutional and political realities of the Middle Ages. For example, the senate and the quaestors are anachronisms. Indeed, John of Salisbury presents this text as part of a treatise on political education that Plutarch was said to have written for Emperor Trajan. This was, of course, a false attribution. Exegetes of this text generally think that it is a posterior Greek text subsequently translated into Latin and inserted into his treatise by John of Salisbury, who credited Plutarch on the basis of a false attribution being circulated in the learned circles of the twelfth century. But commentators tend increasingly to think that this is a pastiche of an ancient text written by John of Salisbury himself, and I am inclined to agree with them. In any event, the so-called *Institutio Traiani* text both expresses the political thought of a humanist current that was characteristic of the period known as the twelfth-century renaissance, and also exposes a theme that was frequently borrowed by the "mirror of princes" literature of the thirteenth-century and the later Middle Ages.[12]

I am less concerned with the attribution of this text than with the evidence it provides about how the organicist metaphor functioned in the medieval political realm, on which I will now comment very briefly. You will have noticed that the superior functions are distributed among the head, that is, the prince (or, to be more precise, the king during the twelfth and thirteenth centuries) and the heart, that is, a hypothetical senate. In the head reside the honorable representatives of society, that is, the judges and the head's representatives to the provinces, symbolized by the eyes, the ears and the tongue — expressive symbols of what has been called the administrative or bureaucratic monarchy.[13] All the other socioprofessional categories are represented by less noble parts of the body. Civil servants and warriors (*officiales et milites*) are likened to the hands, a portion of the body whose status is ambiguous, for the hands partake of both the low esteem of manual work and the honorable role played by secular power (le bras séculier). The peasants do not escape being compared to the feet, that is to say, with the lowest part of the human body. Yet, in emphasizing the properly fundamental role played by this foundation of the social body, the text adheres to the position taken by eleventh- and twelfth-century ecclesiastical writers who emphasized the dramatic situation of the rural masses that fed the higher orders of society but that were, at the same time, subjected to their scorn and extortion. The members of the social body occupying the least desirable position are the specific representatives of the third function, those who embody the economy and, more precisely, money handling. Ancient thought and Christian thought unite here in their scorn for the accumulation of wealth, which takes place within the ignoble convolutions of the belly and the intestines, organs which are definitively degraded, which contain a ferment of illnesses and vices, and which are the seat of an obscene constipation that holds onto the supplies collected by a parsimonious, miserly state which shows no generosity and no largess.

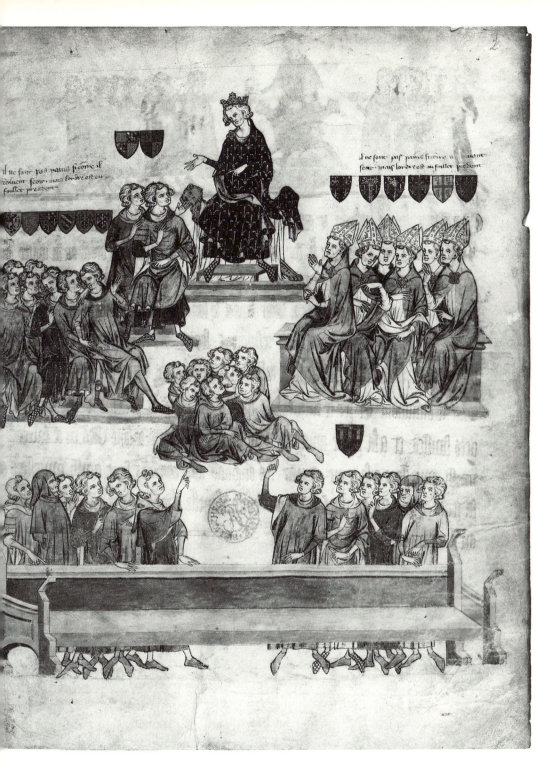

The Trial of Robert III of Artois, Count of Beaumont,
with Philip VI presiding over the court of peers. Manuscript from
the 14th century (Paris, Bibliothèque nationale).

From the thirteenth to the fifteenth century, the ideology about the heart grew and proliferated with the help of an imagery that sometimes bordered on delirium. Take, for example, the theme of the devoured heart that found its way into thirteenth-century French literature – from the *Lai d'Ignauré* (which recounts how twelve ladies, having been seduced by Ignauré, kill their twelve cuckolded husbands, who had avenged themselves by castrating Ignauré, ripping out his heart and feeding it, along with his phallus, to twelve infidels), to the *Roman du châtelain de Couci et de la dame de Favel* (which likewise tells of a cruel meal in which the lady in question must eat her lover's heart).[14] In the saturnine melancholy of the waning Middle Ages, that is, the fifteenth century, the allegory of the heart inspired King René's book, the *Coeur d'amour épris*.[15]

A slow evolution in the metaphor would eventually lead to the veneration of the Sacred Heart of Jesus during the late sixteenth century and especially during the seventeenth century, a baroque avatar of the mystique surrounding the heart that had been prepared from the Middle Ages on by Saint Bernard's twelfth-century *Cor Jesu dulcissinuem* ("very sweet heart of Jesus"), and by the transfer of the crucified Christ's wound from the right side to the left, the heart's side. During the same period, that is, in the fifteenth century, the Virgin's heart was portrayed as pierced by the swords of the seven sorrows.[16]

From the sixteenth century on, the importance and the multiple meanings of the word "heart" are manifest in the mystical spirituality of the Franciscan Johannes Vitrarius and the Carthusian Johannes Justus Lanspergius, while the veneration of the Sacred Heart of Jesus developed from the Middle Ages to the Baroque period in the writings of Saint Gertrude the Great of Helfta (who died in 1301 or 1302) and of Lanspergius, master of the novices at the Cologne Charterhouse between 1523 and 1530.[17]

It is striking to note that the pair *body/soul* never appears in the instructions that Louis IX, commonly known as Saint Louis, left for his son and successor Philip III, and for his daughter Isabel, and that the antithetical metaphor that expresses the structure and functioning of the Christian individual is the pair *body/heart*. This pair of images has absorbed everything that is spiritual in man.[18]

But, for me, the most interesting episode involving the political use of bodily metaphors occurred at the end of the thirteenth century, within the context of a violent conflict that pitted Philip the Fair, king of France, against Pope Boniface VIII. Just as the Investiture Quarrel of the eleventh and twelfth centuries gave birth to the writings known as the *Libelli de lite*, so the polemic between king and pope gave rise to a swarm of treatises, libels and pamphlets, albeit of a more modern sort since they involved public opinion and not just the great laymen and ecclesiastics. An anonymous treatise, *Rex pacificus*, written in 1302 by one of the king's supporters, used the metaphor of the man–microcosm in a particularly interesting way.

According to this treatise, man, the microcosm of society, has two principal organs: the head and the heart. The pope is the head, which gives the members, that is to say, the faithful, the true doctrine and which persuades them to do good deeds. From the head emanate the nerves, that is, the ecclesiastical hierarchy, which binds the limbs to one another and to their head, Christ, represented by the pope, who sees to the unity of belief. The prince is the heart from which emanate the veins that distribute the blood. In like manner, from the king emanate ordinances, laws and customs that have the force of law, all of which carry the nourishing substance, that is to say, justice, into every part of the social organism. Since blood is the vital element par excellence, indeed the most important element of the whole human body, it follows that the veins are more precious than the nerves, and that the heart wins out over the head. The king is, therefore, superior to the pope.

Three other arguments complete this demonstration. The first, borrowed from embryology, carries these bodily symbols a step farther. In the fetus, the heart appears before the head. Royalty, therefore, precedes priesthood. In addition, authorities confirm the superiority of the heart over the head. Thus, the author of the treatise proceeds to enroll Aristotle, Saint Augustine, Saint Jerome and Isidore of Seville in his camp. The Greek word for king is *basileus*, which derives from *basis*; and so the king is the base upon which society rests. The author of *Rex pacificus* is not troubled by this sleight of hand, which moves the prince from the head to the heart, and from the heart to the base. Wherever there is power, there is the prince (or the state), by priority. This anonymous author's conclusion is, however, a compromise in which the hierarchy involving the heart and the head cedes in favor of an autonomous cohabition:

As a result of all this, it is evident that, just as there are two principal parts in the human body, the head and the heart, each with distinct functions, so that the one does not encroach upon the duties of the other, so there are in the universe two separate jurisdictions, the spiritual and the temporal, with very clear-cut attributes.

Princes and popes must consequently remain in their places. The unity of the human body is sacrificed in the name of the separation of the spiritual and the temporal. The organicist metaphor became blurred.[19]

The conception of a double circuit enclosed within the human body, a circuit of nerves emanating from the head and a circuit of veins and arteries branching out from the heart — in other words, a conception that authorizes the metaphorical use of these two parts of the body to explain the structure and the functioning of the social body — corresponds closely to the medieval physiological knowledge inherited from Isodore of Seville and strengthened by the symbolic and metaphorical promotion of the heart during the Middle Ages.

This is what Isodore writes about the head:

The first part of the body is the head, and it received this name, *caput*, because all the feelings and nerves [*sensus omnes et nervi*] have their origin there [*initium capiunt*] and because all the wellsprings of strength emanate from it.[20]

And about the heart:

The heart [*cor*] comes from the Greek term *kardian*, or from *cura* [care, concern]. Indeed, in it resides all solicitude and the cause of knowledge. From it two arteries emanate, the one on the left having more blood, and the one on the right having more spirit [*spiritus*]. This is why we take the pulse on the right arm.[21]

Henry of Mondeville, Philip the Fair's surgeon and hence the approximate contemporary of the anonymous author of *Rex pacificus*, wrote a treatise on surgery between 1306 and 1320. In this treatise, which is the focus of Marie-Christine Pouchelle's fine book *Corps et chirurgie à l'apogée du Moyen Age*, Mondeville attributed a primordial importance to the heart. It had become the *center*, the metaphorical center of the body politic. The centrality attributed to the heart expresses the evolution of the monarchical state in which the most important thing is the *centralization* that is taking place around the prince, not the vertical hierarchy expressed by the head, and even less the idea of unity — the union between the spiritual and the temporal characteristic of an outmoded Christianity that is breaking into a thousand pieces.

Surgeon Henry of Mondeville's expertise about the human body shores up this new political physiology. Building upon Isidore, the surgeon bends his knowledge in favor of the heart and, thus, makes possible this metaphorical thought about the nascent state:

> The heart is the principal organ par excellence [*membrum principalissimum*] which gives vital blood, heat and spirit to all other members of the entire body. It is located in the very middle of the chest, as befits its role *as the king in the midst of his kingdom*.[22]

Pouchelle asks Henry of Mondeville a cogent question: Who is the Sovereign of the body? He replies unequivocally: the heart, that is, the king.

But, generally speaking, the head remains, or once again becomes, chief of the body politic. In the early fifteenth century, John of Terrevermeille, a jurist from Nîmes and a theorist on the monarchy, penned three treatises during 1418 and 1419, to support the legitimacy of Dauphin Charles, the future Charles VII. (In the late sixteenth century, these writings would in turn serve the cause of Henry of Navarre, the future Henry IV.) The author holds that the "mystical or political body of the kingdom [*corpus mysticum sive politicum regni*]" must obey the head, which represents the essential unifying principle and assures order within society and the state. It is the principal member (*membrum principalium*) that the other members must obey. And, since a two-headed society would be monstrous and anarchic, the pope is merely a secondary head, a *caput secundarium*, as John Gerson would likewise call him.[23]

This brief sketch has no greater ambition that to prompt research that will attempt to fit medical conceptions and medical treatises into the corpus of documents indispensable to the historian who wishes to understand the values, ideology and imagery of an epoch.[24]

NOTES

1. Paul-Henri Stahl, *Histoire de la décapitation* (Paris: Presses Universitaires de France, 1986).

2. As far as I know, one of the few studies addressing this question is Marie-Christine Pouchelle's remarkable pioneering book, *Corps et chirurgie à l'apogée du Moyen Age: Savoir et imaginaire du corps chez Henri de Mondeville, chirurgien de Philippe le Bel* (Paris: Flammarion, 1983). For more general remarks on bodily metaphors, see Judith Schlanger, *Les métaphores de l'organisme* (Paris: Vrin, 1971).

3. Cf. Xavier-Léon Dufour, *Dictionnaire du Nouveau Testament* (Paris: Seuil, 1975), s.v. "corps," "corps du Christ," "tête." For example, Paul asserts in Rom. 12.4-5: "For as in one body we have

many members, and all the members do not have the same function, so we, though many, are one body in Christ, and individually members one of another [*Sicut enim in uno corpore multa membra habemus, omnia autem membra non eundem actum habent, ita multi unum corpus sumus in Christo, singuli autem alter alterius membra*]." And in Eph. 5.23-24: "For the husband is head of the wife as Christ is the head of the church, his body, and is himself its savior. As the Church is subject to Christ, so let wives be subject in everything to their husbands [*Quoniam vir caput est mulieris, sicut Christus caput est ecclesiae, iste salvator corporis eius. Sed sicut ecclesia subjecta est Christo, ita et mulieres viris suis in omni-bus*]." Here it is a question of domination and subjection, we are in the realm of *power*, even if it is only a question of marital power. (All biblical references taken from *The New Oxford Annotated Bible*, Revised Standard Version, 2d ed. (New York: Oxford University Press, 1971.)

4. Henri de Lubac, *Corpus mysticum: L'Eucharistie et l'Eglise au Moyen Age*, 2d ed. (Paris, 1949); Yves Congar, *L'ecclésiologie du haut Moyen Age* (Paris: Cerf, 1968); Yves Congar, *L'Eglise de Saint Augustin à l'époque moderne* (Paris: Seuil, 1970).

5. For example, canon 3 of the Council of Paris of 829: *Quod eiusdem ecclesiae corpus in duabus principaliter dividatur personis* ("That the body of the same Church is principally divided into two persons") a text drawn up by bishop Jonas of Orléans and echoed by him in his treatise *De institutione regia* — one of the most ancient political treatises in the so-called "mirror of princes" literature. Cf. Congar, *L'écclésiologie du haut Moyen Age*, pp. 81-82.

6. According to Paul, "the head [*caput*] of every man is Christ, the head of a woman is her husband, and the head of Christ is God [*caput vero Christi Deus*]," 1 Cor. 11:3.

7. Dufour, *Dictionnaire*, p. 171.

8. "*In jecore autem consistit voluptas et concupiscentia,*" Isidore of Seville, *Etymologiae* 11.127, *Patrilogiae cursus completus: Series Latina*, ed. Jacques-Paul Migne (Paris, 1844-64) p. 82, col. 413. This statement concludes the definition of the physiological function of the liver (*jecur*): "The liver gets its name from the fact that it is the seat of the fire that rises to the head [an etymology based on *jacio, jeci*: to throw, to launch, to send]. From there it spreads to the eyes and to the other senses and limbs and, thanks to its heat, transforms the sap sucked from food into blood, which it offers each member so that it can be nourished."

9. Cf. Congar, *L'ecclésiologie du haut Moyen Age*, p. 83.

10. On the trifunctional scheme during the Middle Ages, which Georges Dumézil defined as an Indo-European cultural heritage, see especially Georges Duby, *Les trois ordres ou l'imaginaire du féodalisme* (Paris: Gallimard, 1978); Jacques Le Goff, "Les trois fonctions indo-européennes, l'historien et l'Europe féodale," *Annales E.S.C.* 34 (1979), pp. 1187-1215; and Dominique Iogna-Prat, "Le 'baptême'

du schéma des trois ordres fonctionnels: l'apport de l'École d'Auxerre dans la seconde moitié du IXe siècle," *Annales E.S.C.* 41 (1986), pp. 101-26. The three functions are, schematically, the sacred, the warring and the laborious.

11. Humbert of Moyenmoutier, cardinal of Silva Candida, *Adversus simoniacos (Patrilogia latina*, p. 143, col. 1005ff.; *Monumenta germaniae historica: Libelli de tite*, vol. 1); trans. André Vauchez, "Les laïcs dans l'Eglise à l'époque féodale," *Notre Histoire* 32 (1987), p. 35, reprinted in *Les laïcs au Moyen Age* (Paris: Cerf, 1987), p. 52.

12. The text that appears in Chapter 5.2 of John of Salisbury's *Policraticus*, ed. C.C.J. Webb (Oxford, 1909); and in the English translation by John Dickinson, *The Statesman's Book of John of Salisbury* (New York, 1927), with its introduction to the author's political thought, was edited in part from dubious fragments of Plutarch's works in the Teubner edition procured by G.N. Bernardakis, *Plutarchi Moralia* (Leipzig, 1896), vol. 7: pp. 183-93.

13. C. Warren Hollister and John W. Baldwin, "The Rise of Administrative Kingship: Henri I and Philip Augustus," *American Historical Review* 83 (1978), pp. 867-905.

14. *Le coeur mangé: récits érotiques et courtois — XIIe et XIIIe siècles*, translated into modern French by Danielle Régnier-Bohler with a preface by Claude Gaignebet and a postface by Régier-Bohler (Paris: Stock, 1979).

15. Marie-Thérèse Gousset, Daniel Poirion and Franz Unterkircher, *Le coeur d'amour épris* (Paris: Philippe Lebaud, 1981).

16. Louis Réau, *Iconographie de l'art chrétien* (Paris: Presses Universitaires de France, 1957), vol. 2, pp. 47-49, 108-10.

17. Carl Richstatter, *Die Herz-Jesu-Verehrung des deutschen Mittelalters*, 2d ed. (Munich, 1924); Pierre Debongnie, "Commencement et recommencement de la dévotion au Coeur de Jésus," *Etudes carmélitaines* 29 (1950), pp. 146-92; André Godin, *Spiritualité franciscaine en Flandre au XVIe siècle: l'Homéliaire de Jean Vitrier* (Geneva: Droz, 1971); Gérald Chaix, "La place et la fonction du coeur chez le Chartreux Jean Lansperge," in *Acta conventus neolatini Turonensis*, ed. Jean-Claude Margolin (Paris: Vrin, 1980), pp. 869-87.

18. Preferable to the arranged text given by Joinville in his *Life of St. Louis*, is the version of the *Enseignements* that St. Louis wrote for his son and daughter, published in its original form by David O'Connell, *The Teachings of St. Louis: A Critical Text* (Chapel Hill, 1972) and, in a modern French translation by David O'Connell, *Les propos de saint Louis* (Paris: Gallimard, 1974), with a preface by Jacques Le Goff.

19. Victor Martin, *Les origines du gallicanisme* (Paris: Bloud et Gay, 1939), vol. 1, pp. 216-17.

20. Isidore, *Etymologiae* 11.25, *Patrilogia latina*, p. 82: col. 400.

21. *Ibid.*, col. 411.

22. Pouchelle, *Corps et chirurgie*, pp. 198-99.

23. Jean Barbey, *La fonction royale: essence et légitimité d'après les Tractatus de Jean de Terrevermeille* (Paris: Nouvelles Éditions Latines, 1983), pt. 2, ch. 1; *Corpus mysticum sive politicum regni*, pp. 157-268. The justifiably famous book by Ernest Kantorowicz, *The King's Two Bodies: A Study in Medieval Political Theology* (Princeton, 1957), presents a thesis that serves as a backdrop to my reflections on this subject.

24. Let us remember the pioneering work done, for Antiquity, by Paul Veyne; Michel Foucault; and Aline Rousselle, *Porneia: On Desire and the Body in Antiquity*, trans. Felicia Pheasant (New York: Basil Blackwell, 1988); by Danielle Jacquard and Claude Thomasset, *Sexualité et savoir médical au Moyen Age* (Paris: Presses Universitaires de France, 1985); and, for a philosophical legitimation of the body as a means of expressing thoughts about the origins of the State, the fine book by José Gil, *Metamorphoses du corps* (Paris: La Différence, 1985). The cover illustration of Gil's book, a fourteenth-century image of the zodiac–man, shows the adaptability of the human body to the evolution of symbolism. We are familiar with the success of astrology and of its applications to fourteenth-century politics. Cf. Maxime Préaud, *Les astrologues à la fin du Moyen Age* (Paris: J.-Cl. Lattès, 1984).

**Translated by Patricia Ranum.**

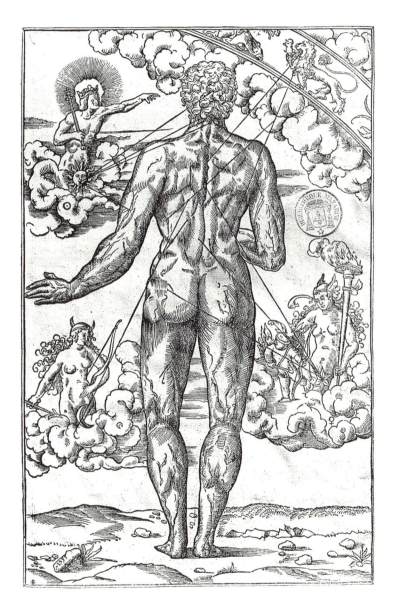

The influence of the stars on the human body, 1533
(Paris, Bibliothèque Mazarine).

zone

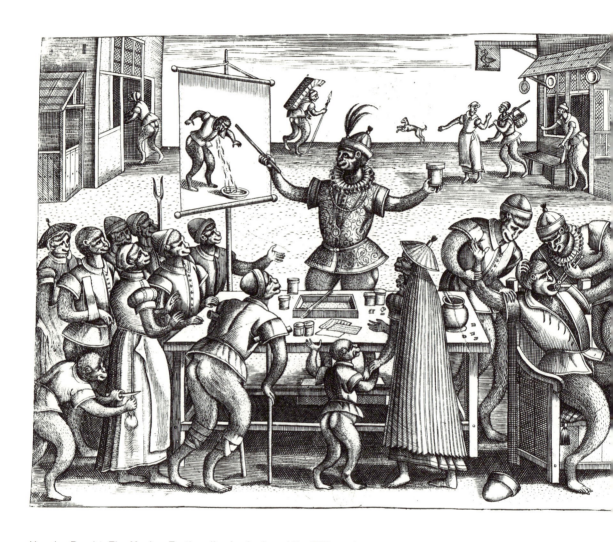

Van der Borcht, The Monkey Tooth-puller, beginning of the 17th century.

# The Art of Pulling Teeth in the Seventeenth and Nineteenth Centuries: From Public Martyrdom to Private Nightmare and Political Struggle?

*David Kunzle*

This much has not changed in centuries: for most healthy people the teeth are the only part of our body requiring regular surgery. The dentist is the only medical practitioner that we regularly visit. The tooth is the only part of the sentient body we fear and consider it normal to lose. While fear of tooth loss, toothache and the pain of dental treatment should have diminished radically, the dentist himself retains the aura of torturer – witness the scene in the recent film *Brazil*, by Terry Gilliam, where the torture chamber in the modern terror state is accoutred like the dentist's.

While modern dentistry bids fair to prevent them, toothache and tooth loss remain with us as a nightmare, an atavism, a psychic archetype of pain, a metaphor of impotence and fear of death. We are thankful for anesthetics and very sophisticated, painless conservation techniques; but it is as if our consciousness were still overlaid with inherited fear and guilt from pre-anesthetic martyrdoms. In the past, toothache was regarded as a punishment of sexual guilt; and today, medical science warns us that tooth decay is the result of our excessive indulgence in the sweet things of life.

The theme of teeth-pulling plays such an inordinate role in art – greater, surely, than any other single medical operation – that one is driven to seek a broader, metaphorical meaning for it. The two-part essay that follows is based primarily on (a) pictures from the seventeenth century, a sampling from over fifty extant drawings, prints and paintings from the Netherlands, where the theme acquired something of the status of a subgenre in itself; and (b) comic strips and related cartoons from the nineteenth century, some of them hitherto unknown, drawn from an extensive survey I have just completed.[1] My evidence is inevitably selected somewhat at random, and I combine concrete data with speculations on deeper metaphorical

29

meanings which could, I am sure, be more fully substantiated from literary sources. These must surely exist, and in abundance from the nineteenth century, but have yet to be gathered into that *social* history of dentist, tooth and toothache which remains to be written.

The tooth has always been accorded a special, magical role among all peoples and at all times, and has stood for power, and its loss for loss of power. In ancient folk belief, and in our nightmares today, every tooth that falls, naturally or forcibly extracted, is a more or less symbolic little death. Even — especially — the mutilation of teeth for aesthetic, totemistic, apotropaic and sacrificial purposes, which is so foreign to the Western tradition, has its roots in their power symbolism. Toothache, wrote Ambroise Paré, an ancient authority, in the sixteenth century, is the greatest and most eternal of all pains, excepting death.[2] Toothache was the fiery torture of the damned in hell; the tooth-worm consumed the body whole and alive, like the diabolical serpent.[3] The toothache was caused by the devil, "her Dreadfulness Satania Infernalis."[4]

My starting point for the "deep structure" of tooth-pulling in the modern age is, appropriately enough, an essay from Petrarch's prolix mid-fourteenth-century hodgepodge *On the Remedies to Both Kinds of Luck, Good and Bad*, where toothache and the pulling of teeth, with all their pain and inconvenience, are to be welcomed as reminders of death, which itself promises eternal life. Toothlessness, notes Petrarch with a touch of humor, has the advantage of discouraging licentiousness: eating, laughing, adultery and taking bites out of other people's reputations. The loss of worldly power and pleasure occasioned by loss of teeth encourages the ideal ascetic, inward, solitary life.[5] This sounds thoroughly medieval, in one hailed as the "first modern man," but Petrarch's attitude survived deep into the modern age, certainly into the nineteenth century, when the comic strips also experience tooth extraction as a dreadful expiation from which sexual guilt is not absent.

The explicit equation of dental with moral corruption — or sin — while it is not apparent from the iconography, was still commonplace in late seventeenth-century texts. In a German illustrated "sociology" of trades and professions, we read under "Dentist" the epigraph "Sin will not come out without pain and suffering," and the verse "Evil lust clings like a tooth in the vein-roots, and causes pain in the conscience. Out with it [the lust], or the pain will grow. Flesh must be crucified for the heart to rest in peace."[6] The popular preacher Abraham a Sancta Clara, using the same engraving and verse, was even more explicit in seeking the root of rotten teeth in original sin: "We unfortunate humans! We all have toothache and suffer ever and always from the teeth with which Adam bit the forbidden apple." Freedom from toothache must be primeval bliss, pre-Adamite innocence. God punishes us in our post-Edenic corruption by sending us bodily ills; the corruption of the teeth is both "shameful and damaging." In the German of a Sancta Clara, ever one to play with words, a single letter separates the shameful: "schändlich" from the damaging: "schädlich." God rewarded Moses by letting him die, at 120 years, with all his teeth intact.[7] These were, of course, the teeth of godly power. But "bad teeth" were, unfortunately, not only weak teeth; they could also be strong, aggressive, evil-intentioned teeth which (as in the Petrarch passage cited) "leave almost no decent people unbitten."

Teeth, like power, could be used for good and evil purposes. It was of course good that evil people should lose their teeth (power to oppress), as in the nineteenth-century cartoons we shall discuss; and it was necessary that a bad tooth be sacrificed by a good person for better health. The question that arises with the seventeenth-century iconography is whether that tooth and that health are moralized as spiritual as well as physical. The degree of implied moralization in "innocent" genre scenes is a matter that currently vexes much historiography of Dutch seventeenth-century art. My starting point, however, is a social one: the evidence that tooth-pulling is shown *exclusively* as inflicted on the poor – a disempowering and humiliation of those already powerless, humble and ipso facto innocent. This is also, to a degree, true of the nineteenth-century sample where it is a relatively poor and powerless lower-middle class which sits in the dentist's chair. These were classes which felt themselves to be voiceless. Surgical intervention into a part of the body, the mouth, which is the source and instrument of vocal expression and resistance is a literal as well as metaphorical suppression and silencing, quite apart from the disempowerment of tooth loss.

The process of disempowerment, with strong connotations of spiritual purification and expiation of sin, was dramatized in various iconographic formulae from the sixteenth century onward. Beyond and in some sense contradictory to the sin symbolism, the pictures encode increasingly, by the seventeenth century, a social transaction, a struggle fought out in more or less realistic milieus between unequal social forces, a class struggle: that of the well-armed dentist, representing power and wealth, and the patient, representing powerlessness and poverty. Later, if the patient is still punished for his/her sins, they are of a nonspecific, existential kind; he/she is, increasingly, innocent, and therefrom flows pathos, comedy and drama. In a world where the rich were as prone to sin as the poor, and where the rich suffered as much from their teeth as the poor, it was invariably the poor who were depicted as suffering, in that classic oxymoron, the "tender cruelties " of the dentist. With not even Saint Apollonia, patron saint of toothache much depicted in the Middle Ages, visibly present to comfort them.

Up to the nineteenth century tooth-pulling was for the great majority of Europeans a public event, performed in public, outdoors, attended by an audience; it was part sacrificial drama, part street or fairground entertainment, part judicial execution. Already in the seventeenth century, however, we find among the Dutch, that precociously burgher society, signs of the ceremony's withdrawal indoors, into the more private environment of the lonely duel characteristic of the nineteenth century. Whether it is – or was – easier to bear physical suffering publicly or privately is a weighty and subtle question. Martyrs by temperament or vocation need an audience to magnify the significance of their sacrifice. Great criminals, those found guilty of some socially or politically resonant crime, may have welcomed a public expiation. Lesser mortals, however, suffering from an all too common ailment, may have preferred not to bare before the public that innermost humiliation of tooth extraction and its innermost pain (literally: the tooth was believed to rot from within by the action of a caries worm). But they had no choice. Dental operations, to be sure, did not lend themselves to heroics, like that of Duke Christian of Brunswick who had his arm – injured in battle in 1622, en route to relieve the Dutch town of Bergen op Zoom – amputated before his whole army to a fanfare of trumpets.[8] His pain, and loss, thus dramatized to the world, became literally exemplary, and surely more bearable thereby.

I have no literary documentation on the matter, but many seventeeth-century paintings seem to show bystanders who are evidently sympathizers, friends and/or relatives, sometimes openly distressed, offering support, comfort and courage. At the same time, in street or fairground one risked the idle curiosity of strangers, even

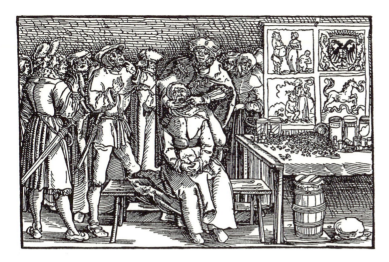

Figure 1: Petrarch Master, On Toothache. From Petrarch, *On the Remedies to Both Kinds of Luck, Good and Bad*, 1532 (Augsburg, Private Collection).

the heartless laughter of the unfeeling. Those who could afford to visit the barber-surgeon in his shop and those rich enough to be attended in their homes were exempt from such intrusive indifference and mockery. The rich were exempt, too, from the public gaze of posterity, for art has passed them by. Literary sources tell us how that perennial sufferer from toothache, Queen Elizabeth I, fearful of having a rotten tooth pulled, was prevailed upon and lent courage to do so by the heroic Bishop of London, who first had a tooth extracted in her presence. There is not — nor could there be — any picture of this episcopal heroism and royal indignity.

To repeat our leitmotiv: the patient is always depicted poorly dressed, especially vis-à-vis the better, sometimes opulently or exotically, attired dentist. This is apparent in our first example, a woodcut for the Petrarch essay cited above, from the first illustrated edition of 1532 (figure 1). The woman patient seated on the bench and the peasant standing to the left pointing to his rotten tooth are in contrast both to the operator and the wealthy bystander with the sword on the far left. (We know from other illustrations for the same book that the Petrarch Master, as the anonymous artist is called, was an unusually class-conscious man.) The table is laden with "miraculous" potions and a great pile of extracted teeth, trophies of long experience and successful practice. These teeth, which were also worn in the form of a necklace (Rombouts: figure 14), constituted a macabre charnel treasure which enhanced the dentist's power aura.

The banner, an indispensable prop in such scenes, also serves to reinforce the itinerant quack's authority, by depicting his cures, dental and otherwise, and his remedies: typically, here, for the worms that attacked various parts of the body including, supposedly, the teeth. The upper left quarter of the banner shows bodily deformities, the lower two giant snakelike worms emitted by humans and a horse. These worms, which rarely appear on banners of the seventeenth-century practitioners, must also have evoked sin in the popular mind:[9] Satan himself, of course, took the form of a serpent, and the worms depicted are of voracious, "satanic" proportions. To be purged of worms, then, as of bad teeth, was to be purged of sin. The quack was a miracleworker in a virtually religious sense: he often claimed to be and was believed to be. The upper right quarter of the banner displays an imperial eagle – a kind of certification that later, in the seventeenth century, will appear as a separate, often elaborate document with a seal. Certification was easy to fake; and where authorities did try to certify itinerant practitioners, they were generally ineffective.

Itinerant medical operators, tooth-pullers and purveyors of folk medicines were assumed to be quacks, with no formal training. In Italian they were called *ciarlatani*, hence our (and the French) charlatans, from "ciarlare" meaning to chat, babble or have the gift of the gab. Our "quack" comes from the early modern Dutch "quaecksalver," to quack (gabble) out salves or ointments. They drummed up their audience with gaudy promises and other theatrical tricks, to attract the gullible and the needy. "Needy" in two senses: in great pain and poor. Regular practitioners, even the lowly but qualified barber-surgeons with a fixed shop in town, cost too much money; the itinerant "quack" was cheap, maybe even free.

To some artists and most of their wealthier clients, as well as to the certified doctors and surgeons, the quack was a cheat, playing to a gullible – stupid – people who were believed, often enough, to deserve being cheated. Thus "charlatan" or "quack" became synonymous with cheat and deceiver. In order to unmask him, the artist may show him as literally a thief, or a thief twice over: once stealing by taking money for false promises, and again by having an accomplice cut the patient's purse while he or she is distracted. The best-known genre painting illustrating this charge is the famous late-fifteenth-century painting by Hieronymus Bosch of a conjurer performing a trick before a rapt public, one of whom has his purse cut. A similar message underlies the same artist's *Cure of Folly*; and in the center foreground of the famous *Haywain* triptych, Bosch has placed a dentist operating on a woman, a

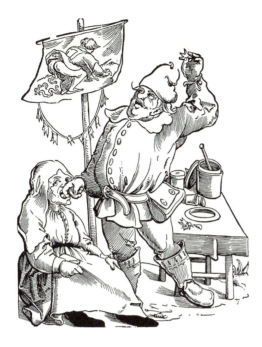

Figure 2: Leonard Beck, The Dentist, ca. 1521
(Augsburg, Private Collection).

motif that, in the context, must signify some form of depravity, probably cheating the public. The magician and surgeons in Bosch stand for public deceivers of all kinds, whose purpose is to rob; they are prestidigitators like the dentist who claims to be able to extract firmly rooted teeth "painlessly" by the skill or magic of his fingers. The attitude of a tooth-puller in Leonhard Beck's woodcut (c. 1521: figure 2) — one hand holding up the (an?) extracted tooth, the other in the patient's mouth — suggests that it was all a matter of digital skill; no instruments are visible on his table. He extracts teeth as swiftly and surely — and painlessly? — as he expels worms (see his banner).

There is no thieving accomplice here, but two of the best-known contemporary renditions, one by Lucas van Leyden, where the patient is conspicuously poor, tattered like a beggar and therefore a particularly unfair target for theft, and another, somewhat later and very probably dependent on Lucas, by the Nürnberger Hans Sebald Beham (figure 3), show the accomplice theft as a major motif, scarcely subordinate to that of the simultaneous tooth-pulling. In the Beham woodcut our attention is directed to the theft by an embracing couple to the left; but the message here is surely not "watch out you don't get robbed while you are having a tooth

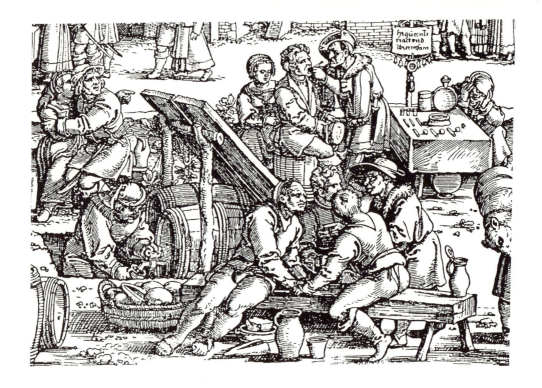

Figure 3: Hans Sebald Beham, detail of The Great Country Fair, 1539 (Nuremberg, Private Collection).

pulled" (in reality one can hardly imagine dentists crooked and cruel enough, or spectators blind enough to permit this to happen). Rather, the point must be the more general one that "charlatans will cheat you," and, more broadly still, that there are thieves, cheats, deceivers everywhere, in crowds, at fairs and in social and business relations generally, especially when your defenses are down through pain, moral or physical. The fairground thief makes his appearance more commonly not as the accomplice of the dentist-as-master-thief in the formula of Lucas van Leyden and H.S. Beham, but as a free lance taking advantage of the press and distraction among the crowd, a motif that survives into the seventeenth century but does not, I believe, necessarily implicate the morality of the quack directly. The free-lance thief occurs in a Brueghelesque (sixteenth-century) painting in Copenhagen of Jesus driving the money changers out of the Temple, where he steals a bird from the basket of a woman rapt by a "miracle extraction" – the dentist flourishes the tooth of a woman swooning before him on the ground.[10] Theft was part of the punishment for sexual sin in scenes showing the Prodigal Son of the biblical parable, as in a print by Lucas van Leyden.[11] The whore here, like Lucas's dentist, is a cheat exploiting human weakness.

The dentist–quack will gradually extricate himself from the aura of deception which surrounds the itinerant medical man. The more dangerous charlatans, more-over, were to be found not at popular fairs, but in the higher professional ranks, those of the law and religion, for instance, which came in for a crescendo of satiri-cal attack in the Reformation years. But it was not always prudent to attack them directly. Mutual suspicion and rivalry between competing classes and sectors, between town and countryside, engendered pervasive fears of being cheated; prov-erb lore is rife with it. There is, incidentally, a hint of another townsman–peasant exploitation in the foreground of the Beham print just below the dentist, where a standing figure in a fancy hat and fur collar, surely a townsman like the similarly dressed dentist, seems to be proposing some kind of deal to three seated peasants, one of whom is barefoot.

The quack doctor was a favorite butt of German carnival farce (*Fastnachtspiel*);[12] his victim was usually a peasant, which allowed middle-class audiences to laugh, as with our pictures, at both deceiver and deceived. Beham's dentist, a regular gentle-man in his fur collar, should be viewed in the context of similar prints with panora-mas of rustic life which both celebrate and mock the rude customs of village carnival or "kirmes" (church festival), and the lecherous, drunken, boorish (*boer/Bauer* = peas-ant), even murderous behavior of the peasantry, from whom the townsman, the print-makers' patron, wished to distance himself. This was an age of peasant revolts, the greatest of which culminated as recently as 1525-26. The peasant and the poor gen-erally were the victims, scapegoats at a time of rising social tensions and continu-ous warfare. The iconography of the dentist in this period, as part of the plethora of comical, satirical and realistic picture-making concentrated in Germany in the 1520s and '30s, is to be viewed in a framework of real and conscious class hostili-ties, not only between townsman and peasant, but also between and within upper and middle classes. There was much readiness to knock out someone else's tooth, literally and figuratively.

### Dutch Seventeenth-Century Dental Martyrdoms

The Dutch were pretty well continuously at war in the later sixteenth century and throughout the seventeenth century. The first half of the seventeenth century and the age of the Thirty Years War saw a renewal of social tension and political vio-lence, and a new infusion of realism into art. The prevalence of the dentist in Dutch art of the Golden Age has to do not only with the native preference for scenes of everyday life, especially those of a comic nature, but also with the relatively easy access of the population at large to some form of more or less specialized and professional medical treatment. Even the itinerant quacks come under the latter category: it was surely better to have your teeth pulled by a specialized if not guild-certified surgeon tooth-puller than by the village blacksmith, a figure entirely absent from the seventeenth-century iconography, although present, as an exotic or barbaric survival, in nineteenth-century genre painting and cartoon.

A Dutch medical historian has set up five categories of dental practitioners: first, medical doctors who, inspired by Fallopius, Eustachius and the famous Vesalius (a South Netherlander, who devoted two folio pages to the teeth in his 1543 *Fabrica*), did not consider it beneath their dignity to treat teeth; second, surgeons qualified to handle teeth (although the best left this to specialists); third, barbers; fourth, charlatans; fifth, specialized, but largely uncertified, and probably itinerant "dentatores," who may have transmitted their skills from father to son. If it is indeed this category that is represented in the iconography, they cannot have been "very few," as the Dutch writer claims.[13]

There was a natural repugnance on the part of regular surgeons against the more radical, painful and riskier kinds of operation, especially those involving bones, which often did more harm than good and were apt to injure their reputations as well as their patients. "Bone-setting," for instance, was a specialty practiced, to a degree, outside the guilds and with authorization from town authorities. These practitioners were, typically, of low birth, as we may surmise the dentists in our paintings to be; but they could, if skilled, earn a legitimate reputation, like Mr. Arnoldus Feij of Oirschot (d. 1679) who, "rude and rustic as he was [al was hij lomp en boers]," became famous all over Holland, was invited by Louis XIV to cure his mother of breast cancer, became the orthopedist to the daughters of Jan de Witt, and was ennobled by the elector Frederick William of Brandenburg.[14]

There were also reasons for dentists to have been particularly in demand in Holland. For with their relative wealth, and their world empire, the Dutch had access, as did no other European country, to sugar. Denounced in vain by the preachers, (Brazilian) sugar, in the words of Simon Schama, "poured into the Republic in adequate quantities to reduce the cost factor sufficiently to reach tables of 'the middling

sort,' " and "pandered to the already well-established Dutch hankering for confec-
tions and delicacies. By the 1640s there were already more than fifty sugar refineries
operating in Amsterdam...." Schama goes on to cite two museum-going dentists
from the United States, who determined from a professional inspection of the condition of Dutch teeth and gums inferable from contemporary Dutch seventeenth-century portraits that "the impact of all this sticky stuff on crunching molars was a
plague of cavities, an epidemic of decalcification. Rembrandt, they gloomily concluded, 'was a dental cripple' doomed [Schama glosses] to suffer torments more
excruciating than any Calvinist pastor could possibly have devised."[15] This seventeenth-century Dutch "epidemic" of edentulousness was in contrast to the sample of
hundreds of recently discovered sixteenth-century Flemish skulls, in which "cavities
were rare and surprisingly few teeth were missing."[16] While one may challenge the re-
liability on this topic of the evidence of Dutch portraiture in general and Rembrandt's
self-portraits in particular, one cannot doubt the high level of sugar consumption
among the Dutch, nor its connection with the need for dentists, and the popularity
of the pictures of dental operations. The clerical denunciations serve to remind us
of the continuing connection, in the popular mind, between (sweet) tooth and sin.

Medical science enjoyed high status in Holland. Several Netherlandish doctors of
the sixteenth century have entered the history of dentistry: Pieter Foreest, Jan van
Heurne and Volcker Coiter, who first described the tooth pulp.[17] In the seventeenth
century physicians Cornelis Solingen of the Hague and Anton Nuck, professor at
Leiden University, are remembered for new techniques in prosthesis, instrumenta-
tion and filling teeth.[18] The illustrious inventor of the microscope, microbiologist
Anthonie van Leeuwenhoek, first described the dental canaliculi (*Zahnbeinkanälchen*),
and thought he saw dental bacteria. Surgical operations on various parts of the body
are shown by Dutch painters, in compositions directed at sectors both elite (Rembrandt's famous *Anatomies*) and popular (Brouwer, Jan Steen, etc.). This argues for
the general availability of medical treatment. While elsewhere in Europe peasants
would doctor themselves and resort (for tooth-pulling) to the local blacksmith, in
the densely populated, urbanized and wealthy province of Holland, more or less
expert medical treatment (including dental) was available even in villages. In the
paintings, even the most primitive practitioners are not generally figures of fun,
although their patients may be, insofar as they are shown sometimes crying out

in pain. The quack–dentists are, rather, power-figures within the limited hierarchy of village life.[19]

The Dutch people more than other Europeans had access to specialized medical and dental practitioners. Even if a major history of dentistry notes that "on the whole, [the Dutch] made little [technical] progress during the seventeenth century,"[20] this alone would surely be progress. The pictorial evidence is far from endorsing the view of a recent history of Dutch genre painting that "a popular conception of the doctor [and dentist] was of a fraudulent quack or brutal butcher,"[21] whatever may be the (unspecified) supporting literary evidence. The situation is more nuanced. There was, to be sure, a proverb: "He lies like a tooth-puller."[22] The upper classes, who could pay for qualified doctors and surgeons, must certainly have looked askance at the street operator. The qualified practitioners, from their position of power in the guilds, had every interest in repressing free-lance competitors, and blackening their reputation. That is what guilds were for. A lawsuit brought at Louvain (Southern Netherlands) in 1658 against the Surgeon's Guild tells how one Sr. de la Rocca was refused admission to the guild because he had allegedly acted as a "quacksalver publicquelyc," shaved dogs, and played the "charletemps."[23]

The art we shall describe, however, represents a relatively benign view, that of a middle class, perhaps, which patronized the "dentatores" and recognized the value of their work, while preferring to distance themselves from the patients, who are invariably of the poorer class. This distance, however, is relative; there is no evidence of that upper-class assumption that the lower classes, being used to a rougher life, felt pain less. There is, on the contrary, a real identification: the pain of the poor was a shared pain, a universal pain.

The banner proclaiming miracle cures has now largely disappeared.[24] The hostile motif of the purse-cutting by an accomplice, as we saw it in the sixteenth century, is now the exception, not the rule. It occurs in Adriaen van de Venne,[25] who in much of his work shows a marked bias in favor of the poor and hostility to the rich, of whom the dentist is the representative. Hostility to the dentist also shows clearly in a Van de Venne print described below, and a painting by Quast where the (ill-favored, disheveled, perhaps himself toothless) village barber–surgeon treating his patient is compared to the monkey treating the owl, as pictured in a print pinned to the wall.[26] But these negative views are in the minority.

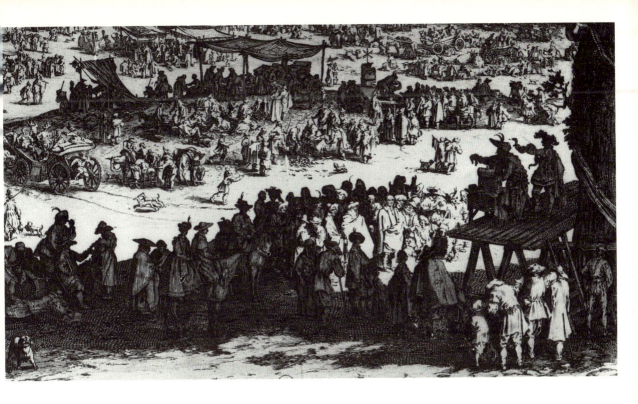

Figure 4: Jacques Callot, detail of The Fair at Impruneta, ca. 1621
(Paris, Bibliothèque nationale).

The honest dentist was increasingly distanced from the quack or charlatan. Abraham a Sancta Clara, indeed, carefully distinguished between the two: the honest dentist or *Zahnartet* (he doesn't say qualified surgeon) and the lying, cheating quack. In painting, the quack constituted a distinct and popular subgenre by the seventeeth century. The most spectacular example is probably by the foremost genre painter of Leyden, Gerard Dou, who also showed dentist–surgeons working modestly and professionally in their shop. Dou's *Quack Doctor* in Rotterdam[27] is a morally rich and complex painting in which the performer holds forth on the virtues of his remedies to a crowd and in an environment redolent of folly, gullibility and deception. Among his remedies, the dental kind are conspicuous by their absence. In another morally resonant painting by Dou, the dentist is shown operating in the background of a room in a home, the foreground of which is occupied by a woman suckling a baby; she has been interpreted as Nature giving, and the dentist as Nature taking away (or active nature and passive nature) — a complementary but not morally opposed function.[28]

We can see quack and dentist working side by side in Callot's famous, teeming *Impruneta Fair* (figure 4). The artist is from Lorraine, the scene is set near Florence, but crowd and entertainments are surely universal. The quack, a major motif silhouetted by the foreground right, conspicuous in the baggy trousers and bizarre hat of a Commedia dell'Arte actor, holds forth his wares before a large throng, like the huge tree its branches behind and above, while an associate theatrically brandishes a snake. To the left and beyond, inconspicuous, businesslike, without fanfare, barely recognizable as such (on this tiny scale), the dentist stands behind a patient seated on a small platform before a much smaller crowd; his tooth collection surmounts a chest (of potions, no doubt). Most attractive of all, in terms of crowd appeal, and profiled by Callot against a light ground in an eye-catching way, is a figure, apparently a vendor found guilty of selling false measure, being punished by the strappado on a tall frame (far left middleground; not visible in detail reproduced). Here then are three kinds of theatrical spectacle, with the dentist cast as the least sensational and the least meretricious.

Attitudes toward dentists in Holland were mixed. My aim is to show that in the art of the period a relatively favorable view predominated. We may start with such a view, a remarkable painting by the Haarlem painter Pieter Jansz Quast, which as a primary cultural document is logically preserved in the Cultural Historical Collection of the Federal Association of German Dentists in Cologne-Lindenthal (figure 5). It represents in some ways a transition to a more civilized historical moment: the scene is set indoors although the dentist is probably not working in his own premises, but is an itinerant who, perhaps so as to escape the rain, has moved his paraphernalia — a table with unguents and diploma — under the roof of a dilapidated inn. The operation is watched by a small and mixed but apparently sympathetic group, perhaps friends and family. This is no casual throng such as one sees in fairground and street scenes with dentists; all focus on the operation, lending silent dignity to a dingy locale. The dentist is perfectly businesslike, pulling (or probing, preparing) unviolently, and, as is not often the case, he is relatively poorly dressed, nearer the same class as his patient. The patient rolls his eyes upward and clasps his hands before him; this attitude and the slightly back-tilted body are redolent of prayer and painful or pained repentance. One is tempted to speak of a hushed, religious silence, appropriate to a sacrificial act, an expiation.

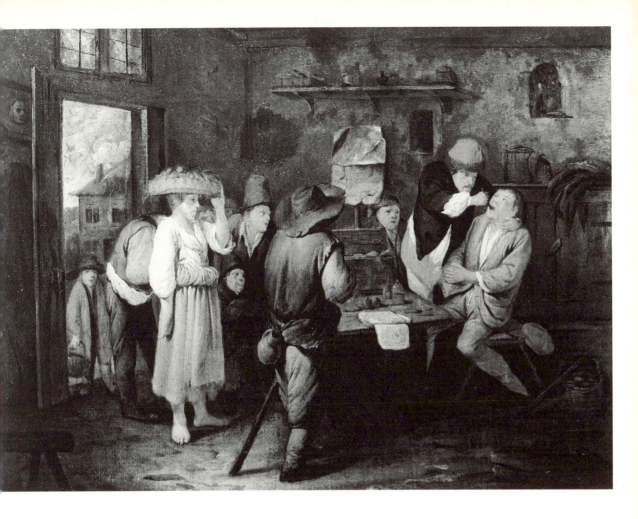

Figure 5: Pieter J. Quast, The Dentist (Cologne, Kulturhistorische Sammlung des Bundesverbandes der deutschen Zahnaerzte).

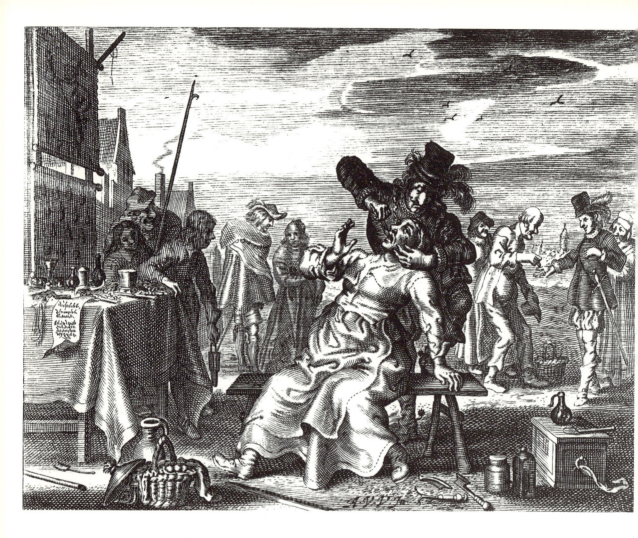

Figure 6: Adriaen van de Venne, Dentist. Illustration to Jacob Cats,
"On the sight of a person having a tooth pulled," ca. 1600.

Contrast Quast's dentist with his confrere in a markedly hostile print by Adriaen van de Venne, an artist known for his lower-class sympathies (figure 6). Here the operator in his fancy hat and curled mustache violently assaults the tooth of a woman who is flung backward against his knee, one arm raised in anguish, the other stemmed against the bench. The small ax, lying alongside more appropriate-looking dental instruments, may have been included as evidence of the dentist's recourse to clumsy violence. Conspicuous among the group of spectators positioned at the far side of the worktable, is a leering lout, apparently a bargee. In the background right an older, bald and poor man, surely a postoperative patient, humbly pays the required fee to a well-dressed gentleman, presumably an assistant, unless he is another dentist. The relationship between giver and receiver is precisely that of the beggar giving alms to the rich man, as in a "World Upside Down" print.

The payment here, an unusual feature, may represent a strictly literary input. The van de Venne print illustrates a poem by Jacob Cats, the popular Dutch poet, lawyer and statesman, which notes the paradox ("strange transaction") of paying "a good part of one's good money and with much gratitude, now and for the rest of his life, for having a great, firmly rooted tooth extracted." But, says Cats, who unlike his illustrator offers no criticism of the dentist, this is fair payment for relief of pain which robs one of all the pleasures of life. The poet concludes, in his characteristic way, with the religious view for which the Quast painting would be a more appropriate illustration of toothache and tooth extraction as divine reminders of our mortality and sinfulness, which by causing suffering, strengthen the soul.[29] In another poem[30] the poet apostrophizes his tooth: "You were my own member, part of my own sick frame, now...you lie there a rotten, hollow, worthless, lifeless bone. Part of me is dead – how can the rest last much longer?"

In the logic of Cats's religious view the dentist is cast as a priest or confessor, insofar as he is an agent of expiation; and while Cats stops short of actually praising the dentist, the preacher Abraham a Sancta Clara, in the chapter from which we quoted above, lauds the *Zahnarzt* (dentist, tooth-doctor, as opposed to deceitful charlatan) as the "very useful reliever of pain," "worthy of all praise and honor," "highly skilled in science." Moreover, "complete peasants" are aware of the advantage of being treated by such a man, which leaves open the question of how often they enjoyed it.[31]

zone

The hands clasped as if in prayer or supplication, together with eyes closed rather than upturned, but equally redolent of prayer, reappear in a work by Jan Victors, who specialized in painting dental and foot surgery. This work (figure 7) reunites typical and traditional elements of the tooth-pulling scenario: a dentist in fancier dress (old-fashioned yellow velvet, slashed jacket), street setting, a considerable, casual, well-dressed crowd, some of them smiling. An older child is offering an apple to a monkey who is perhaps the source of the woman's as well as the child's amusement, and who serves here (aside from his generalized folly symbolism) in strictly practical terms to attract future customers as well as, perhaps, to distract the present one. By his dress the patient is poor, another quite typical feature, poorer not only than the dentist, but most of the audience as well.

Assuming that the woman in the black jacket to the left is smiling at the antics of the monkey rather than at the sufferings of the patient, and that the drawn-back mouth of the dentist is indicative of his concentration rather than of his sadistic pleasure, one may derive from the scene a certain moral comfort, to which the trio to the right contribute a note of active sympathy: a richly attired woman with her hand in a box leans in evident concern toward a seated, more simply dressed girl nursing her head, obviously a sufferer from the toothache, silently awaiting her turn. Perhaps these are mistress and maid (the Dutch were known for their kindness to servants), and the older woman looking out toward us at the extreme edge of the picture could be the mother of either.

Smiles of mockery or smiles of sympathy? Although I lack literary evidence on the reaction of bystanders, my preference is for sympathy. The smiling audience seems to have been a specialty of Victors's. However idle bystanders or friends of the patient may have reacted in reality, the smiling audience serves, psychologically, to mitigate the tangibility of a torture which the purchasers and viewers of such pictures would themselves most likely have undergone or would undergo. We laugh at what we fear for ourselves. Another *Dentist* by Victors[32] (figure 8), which lacks the monkey as a possible source of the amusement, has seven of the eight bystanders, of varying social degrees, all more or less smiling; the eighth is herself suffering from the toothache, awaiting her turn or summoning up courage beforehand. Yet another rather similar composition by the same artist, again with smiling spectators, includes at the center the dentist's good-looking wife holding up an unguent

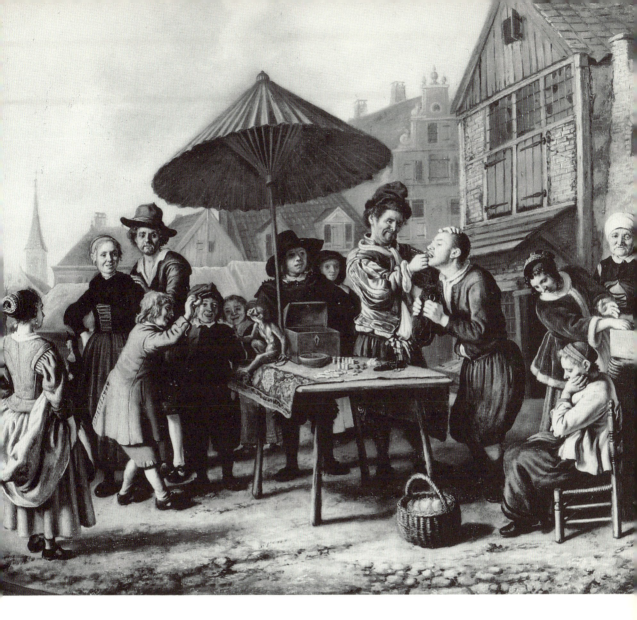

Figure 7: Jan Victors, The Dentist
(Cologne, Kulturhistorische Sammlung des
Bundesverbandes der deutschen Zahnarzte).

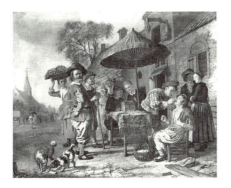

Figure 8: Jan Victors, Tooth-puller
(Amsterdam, Rijksmuseum).

with a slight, encouraging smile, and a fool (dressed as such, in the traditional manner)[33] playing the fiddle to drown the patient's screams. In all three Victors paintings the dentist is much better dressed than the patient, although in the last he has rather an ill-favored face. A woman spectator directs the attention of a small child to the operation: to the morality, the necessity of suffering?

The audience could be somber, too. In a fourth type of dentist painting by Victors, set indoors, the patient has his hands folded as in prayer, while an older couple, perhaps parents, observe sympathetically; another concerned person helps administer what may be some kind of anesthetic.[34] In a Molenaer painting of 1630 (figure 9) no fewer than three of the observers of the extraction, which takes place, perhaps not accidentally, hard by a church, have their hands clasped, one of them, a woman, with eyes cast heavenward, unambiguously prayerful. She may even be kneeling. Another has her eyes cast downward, almost closed – which is unfortunate, for she fails to see that a bird in her basket is being filched by a soldier, which can hardly be blamed on the completely preoccupied dentist. The contrast here between the elegant dentist, who is not at all "brutish,"[35] and the poor peasant lad (he was carrying eggs to market like the patient in the Quast: figure 5)[36] with his hose out at the knee, is very striking. The spectators are all decently dressed and a couple walking past, unseeing or uncaring of the foreground drama, are positively rich. Could the artist be saying: such pain, such public trial, is the lot of the poor, which they must suffer with Christian patience?

Imagery in Calvinist Holland converted, of necessity, from the religious to the secular, from the representation of sacred miracles to the comedy of everyday life. Our dentists are a case study in the argument, familiar now among scholars of Dutch art, about how much moral meaning may be contained or coded in or reasonably "read into" genre scenes. Conservatively one may say that the kinds and degrees of meanings read from genre scenes depended on the viewers' education and religious and moral sensibilities. We look for what we have learned to expect. Thus, to the religious, and those familiar with religious art, the petty dental martyrdom may have evoked greater martyrdoms.

How could the painting by Harmen Hals of Haarlem,[37] son of the famous Frans (figure 10), with the patient placed more or less frontally and filling much of the picture, his rather lifeless head cradled by the dentist behind, his one arm held by a

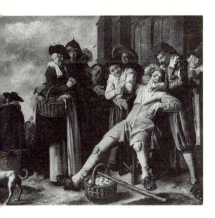

Figure 9: Jan Molenaer, The Dentist, 1630
(Brunswick, Herzog Anton Ulrich-Museum).

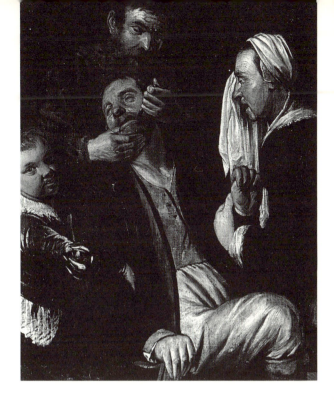

Figure 10: Harmen Hals, The Dentist
(Cologne, Kulturhistorische Sammlung des
Bundesverbandes der deutschen Zahnarzte).

child, the other by a conspicuously weeping woman, have failed to resonate with some viewers as a kind of Pietà? Which is not to say that the patient is consciously seen as a Christ figure, but rather that his sufferings, like those of all innocent, virtuous and repentent people, are to be borne publicly and contemplated with Christlike fortitude. The lamenting woman who reminds one so strongly of a weeping Mary also appears elsewhere, in prints of dentists after Andries Both,[38] in paintings by Brouwer,[39] Jan Steen,[40] and Gerard Dou,[41] as well as the Molenaer described. The cradled head appears together with another Pietà-like feature, the reclining, tortured body, in an Adriaen van Ostade drawing showing a village barber–surgeon at work in his premises (figure 11).[42]

In the Both etching (figure 12) the religious aura is enhanced by the identification of one of the principal bystanders as a pilgrim; he makes a gesture of pity. The overtly distressed woman to the right is the patient's wife; in the verse below the print he complains of the pain the dentist ("Miester Jeurian") is causing him, and she responds, "Oh Fop, I wring my hands." Fop then cries out that he is fainting and summons his wife to fetch "Doctor Lubbert" — who apparently disdained to perform such operations himself.

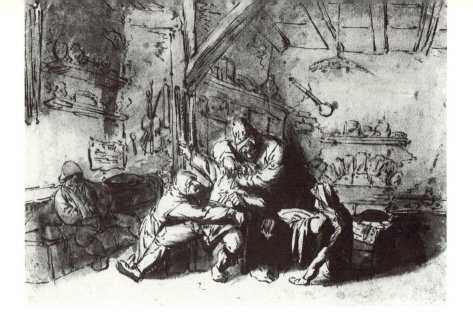

Figure 11: Adriaen van Ostade, The Dentist (Amsterdam, Rijksprentenkabinett).

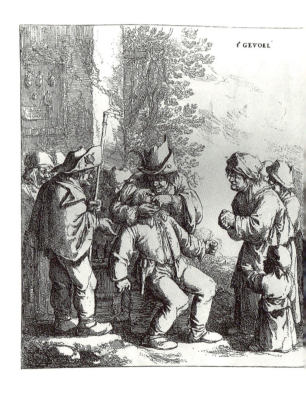

Figure 12: Tooth-puller. After A. Both, 17th century (Paris, Bibliothèque des Arts Décoratifs).

Theologically the Crucifixion confirmed both the corporeal humanness of Christ and his supreme humility, which were emphasized by the tortured and inferior position he adopts at the Deposition. Paré recommended that the dentist hold the patient seated on the ground and between his knees.[43] While this exact position is rarely depicted in art (it can have been efficient only for work on the lower jaw), the dentist is shown in the clear majority of our examples operating from behind and above, with the patient seated on a stool or bench. Whether or not this position summoned up in spectator or patient the dread image of the hangman slipping the noose over the head of the condemned, as Hillel Schwartz has suggested,[44] it established superiority and dominance in a way that reinforced the socially essential, unequal power relationship, even as it cast the patient in the role of Christlike sufferer. Occasionally the dentist is shown working from horseback,[45] a highly impractical vantage point, but one which obviously increased his power aura.

The taste for emotional scenes with violently gesturing figures in half or three-quarter length, set in a tightly enclosed and strongly illuminated space, was started by Caravaggio and developed by his followers, who included various (Catholic) artists working in Utrecht during and after the 1620s. There was a painting (now lost) of a dentist pulling the tooth of a peasant by Caravaggio in the collection of the Grand Duke of Tuscany, no less.[46] The "Caravaggist" method cast the vulgar, commonplace moment of tooth extraction in another, literal kind of religious and melodramatic light. In a typical candlelit composition by Honthorst (figure 13) the patient is struck down, as it were, in a pool of luminary pain emanating from his breast and is the center of a circle of amazement. The foremost figure left, leaning forward with rippling eyebrows to peer into the oral cavity, reminds one of a Saint Thomas verifying with astonishment Jesus' wound in his side, or the most rapt of the surgeons in Rembrandt's *Anatomy Lesson of Dr. Tulp*. Plural astonishment surrounding singular pain is also the predominant emotional mix in another large Honthorst painting of a dentist, with an outdoor setting but a comparable large-figure arrangement.[47] An older peasant type in this picture, leaning forward on a stick and with parted lips, looks very like a shepherd at an Adoration of the infant Jesus, where the rustic raptness means religious rapture. As in the Molenaer described above, a woman on the left with prayerfully clasped hands is robbed of a fowl from her basket.

In a comparable painting by the Antwerper Theodor Rombouts (figure 14), a simi-

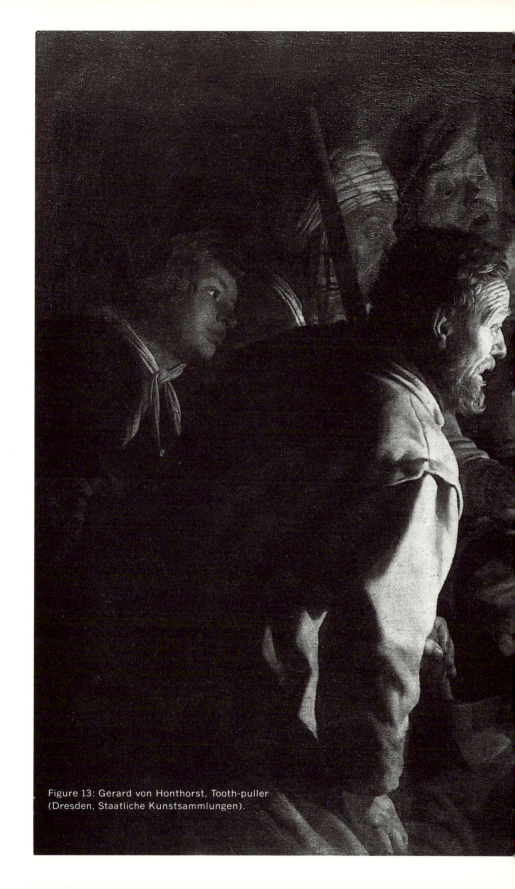

Figure 13: Gerard von Honthorst, Tooth-puller
(Dresden, Staatliche Kunstsammlungen).

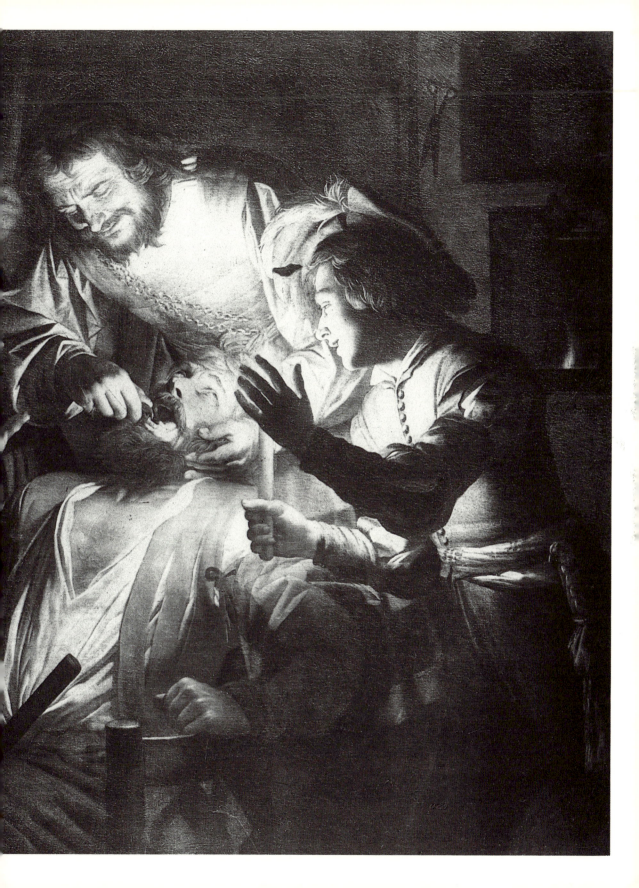

larly posed figure on the left, physically dominant and emotionally intense, is an elderly, obtuse pharisaic type, putting in place, as it were, the spectacles of disbelieving curiosity at the sight of some Christian revelation, while other onlookers stand or sit in amazement. The whole gives off a theatrical effect, especially via the armored figure at the right who leans and looks toward us, pointing rhetorically to the operation, as if in professional recognition of the patient's martial courage. Courage indeed he needs, for his head is twisted agonizingly sideways and upward, in dramatic contrast to the dentist's complacent face, smiling slightly but directly out toward us and quite averted from the tricky job in hand.

Another remarkable feature of the painting, which offsets its theatrical air, is the "still life" of surgical instruments on the table in the very center foreground, rendered with scientific precision and pointed out by one of the bystanders. The mechanical here thus predominates over the traditional pharmaceutical array (bottles, pots, etc.), and testifies to sophistication and specialized practice. These are exclusively dental instruments, identifiable by name, and similar to those we find illustrated in the medical texts; there is no razor, scissors or shaving brush visible, to identify the operator as a more lowly kind of barber–surgeon, as in the Honthorst painting (figure 13).

Of all the comparable, individually delineated faces in the group of large-figure paintings of dental operations, Rombouts's dentist has the most portraitlike particularity. Portrait-types were of course commonplace in genre painting, whether as part of a group or on their own. Gerard Dou[48] painted such a portrait-type, dignified, very much in command, in his own barber-surgical premises, demonstratively holding up a just-extracted tooth in one hand, the other placed on the head of the patient who is washing out his mouth; the dentist's gesture is one of aid, comfort and, as it were, blessing, his unusual facial expression appeals for sympathy, perhaps expresses his own relief at the outcome (figure 15). This expression varies in other versions of this obviously popular type of painting; the patient is sometimes a young girl.

David Teniers has left us a comparable but more important painting of a dentist which may be unique of its kind (figure 16). Small as it is, it has a monumental air. The subject is no longer the tooth-pulling or probing operation, as in all the pictures we have been looking at, although the patient is present, nursing his cheek sorrowfully in the background, whether before or after the extraction is unclear.

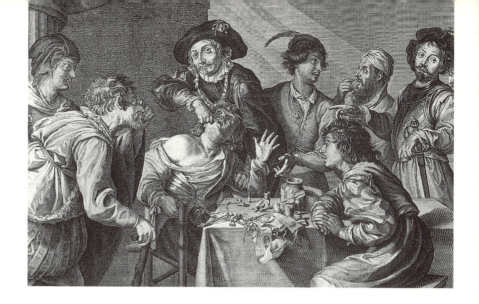

Figure 14: Tooth-puller. After Th. Rombouts, 17th century
(Paris, Musée de la Société de l'Ecole Dentaire de Paris).

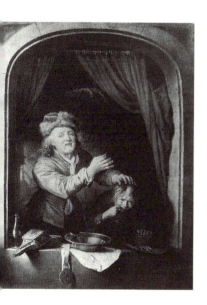

Figure 15: Gerard Dou, The Dentist, 1672
(Dresden, Staatliche Kunstsammlungen).

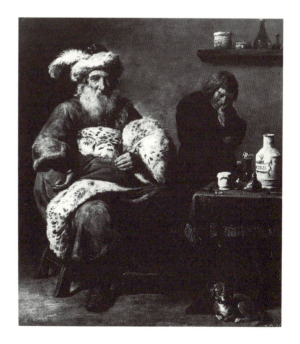

Figure 16: David Teniers, The Dentist
(Dresden, Dresden Museum).

He functions more as an attribute to the foreground figure who sits in a remarkably Michelangelesque pose, a heavily bearded, prophet-type in an impressive furry mantle and hat, discreetly holding in his lap a pointed instrument (a pincette?) tipped by a (the just-extracted?) tooth, as a writer might hold a pen. Is this the mechanical craft of dentistry raised to the level of a liberal art?

## Transition to the Nineteenth Century

In the eighteenth century, the first age of great individual practitioners and manuals which laid the foundations of modern dentistry, the iconography (summarily and internationally considered) dwells upon the fairground performance and its theatrical, charlatanlike character. This is surely more a matter of artistic selection than an objective change in the behavior of dentists. Artists and their patrons, less likely to resort to itinerant public practitioners than in previous centuries, were assuming an increasing distance. The signs of compassion, the sense of a special kind of martyrdom we detected in the Dutch seventeenth century, dissipates in an atmosphere of fairground histrionics. In one picture we are unsure if we are seeing a tooth-pulling scene from a play or merely a dentist taking advantage of scenery left up by a traveling theatrical troupe; in another the charlatan's stage looks like it was home to a violent (and obscene) farce.[49] A poster has survived in which a well-known German comic actor (calling himself a Hans Wurst type) boasts of a second professional skill, that of dentist.[50]

In the revolutionary period of the later eighteenth century, as during the age of Reformation and the Thirty Years War, we find a revival of comic and satirical art. This allows artists working for the popular market, now properly called caricaturists, to vent their social hostility upon dentists who function as scapegoats for broadly felt social resentments against authority figures. The dentist, taken now often enough out of his social context, becomes a humorous but demonic figure; his operations are seen as cruel farce or outright torture.

Among the most grotesque and socially pungent of these is a Rowlandson engraving of 1787, thus on the eve of the French Revolution (figure 17), showing how on the altar of poverty the lower classes sacrifice their teeth to the rich. This was a time when even the most reputable experts, such as the illustrious surgeon John Hunter, were recommending "live" tooth transplants (a vogue which continued deep into the nineteenth century). In the center an old hag takes smelling salts to overcome the nausea caused by the looks and smell of her prospective donor, a wretched, dark-faced young chimney sweep. To the right an aristocratic officer in regimentals gazes (in dissatisfaction?) at his new tooth or teeth; and to the left a huddled, half-naked beggar-type departs, clutching his ravaged jaw, in the company of a buxom, good-looking wench, also nursing her jaw and contemplating the paltry coins she received in exchange for her (their) tooth or teeth. She could be a portrait of Victor Hugo's Fantine (cf. below). There could be no more painful emblem of how the poor are reduced to selling for a pittance not only the labor of their bodies, but their very bodies themselves.

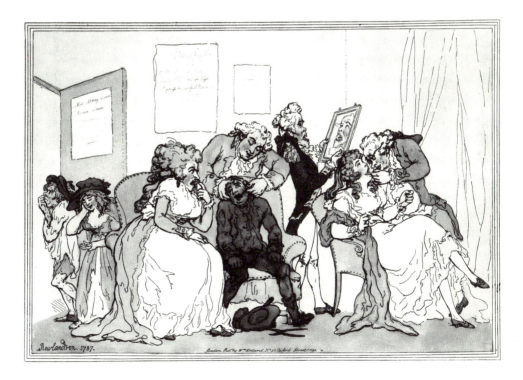

Figure 17: Rowlandson, Transplanting of Teeth, 1787
(London, British Museum).

## The Nineteenth Century —
## Private Nightmare, Political Struggle

"I mean to say," he says to me,
"The world is really a fun place to be.
I can't relate for a moment
To that silly chatter about pain and torment.
I enjoy what is given to me
With the pure nature of a child
And a heavenly spiritual serenity
Flows through my whole being."

Hardly had he uttered this, than
"Aiii," he cried in direst woe.
"That old rotten molar
Is becoming unbearable again."
     — Wilhelm Busch, *Kritik des Herzens*, 1874.[51]

Wilhelm Busch, the immensely popular German poet and caricaturist, mocks the blithe optimism that so pervaded the nineteenth century but which was at the same time so vulnerable. This optimism was based upon an enhanced sense of physical security and power, deriving from real scientific progress in which medicine played a decisive role. The nineteenth century was the period in which dentistry, belatedly and trailing far behind medical practice in general, struggled into professional respectability.

In 1819 the dentist was described as a mere "artisan"; "head surgeons in London deem this branch of their art beneath notice and generally decline interfering in it."[52] Anesthetics and more sophisticated kinds of reconstruction (filling, etc.) became available from the mid-nineteenth century, but only to the few who could afford it. Journal caricature (the equivalent, now, of the seventeenth-century popular Dutch painting and engraving) ignores these advances, still preserving a largely prescientific, preanesthetic age, which was that of the vast majority, even in urban centers. The ancient violence of clumsiness and ignorance was still rife. Patients had to be pinioned and strapped down, and became hysterical; their screams attracted police and crowds in the street outside. Specialized scientific training in dental schools, and a licensing system for the practice of dentistry, were not set up in England until the 1850s. Professional dentistry imposed itself late and erratically over a garish fog of rustic folk remedies, which survived deep into the nineteenth and even twentieth centuries. The tooth, toothache and tooth extraction continued to carry with them a cluster of ancient fears and superstitions, a central component of which, to judge by the popular comic art of the period, was that the dentist was not only a charlatan but also (what does not appear at all in seventeenth-century art) a demon, a sadist.

If in the seventeenth century tooth-pulling was a spectacle, attracting public sympathy and curiosity, in the nineteenth it was a duel undergone alone and always on the dentist's private turf. The patient in the nineteenth-century dentist's surgery room confronted the terror of pain (and possibly fear of death) as an isolated individual. In this he[53] resembled alienated twentieth-century man; and he shared the fate of the nineteenth-century criminal who likewise was no longer subject to public degradation, but was degraded and suffered nonetheless.

The nineteenth-century dentist took over some of the demonic mystique surrounding the executioner of old. He represented power of life and death, not that wielded directly by the State, of course, but a power magnified by the aura of science with which, rightfully or not, he was endowed. This power asserted itself particularly in the 1840s and early '50s, which were a key moment in the struggle for dental professionalization, accompanied by a crisis in public confidence. In an age of extravagant advertising of health products of all kinds, some dentists played a con game with an insecure, gullible, neophiliac and hypochondriac lower-middle-class audience, while other dentists sought hard to improve techniques and advance knowledge. So it was in education and in politics: charlatans cheek by jowl with and sometimes indistinguishable from sincere reformers.

This same mid-century period saw waves of comic art, from which the toothache emerged as symbolic of the painful struggle against a cruel social "nature." No longer were original sin and divinely ordained punishment a sufficient explanation of bodily ills. Evils were social and political. "Do the people love their princes? No more than fearful souls their dentist."[54] The dentist, as the more feared and contentious figure, tends in the nineteenth century to replace the doctor of the older cartoon tradition who served in political allegories to punish, "cure," "purge" the evil person. But back in the seventeenth century already the political doctor may be a dentist: Swedish king Gustavus Adolphus, for instance, cures the imperialist Catholic forces of toothache, incurred by enjoying too many illicit sweets of victory.[55]

The examples of "political dentistry" in nineteenth-century comic art must be legion and testify to the broad acceptance of the inevitability of violent and/or painful "surgical" intervention as a means of preserving or restoring the health of the body politic. The following sample from various times and places comprises two basic types of cartoon: first, where the rotten tooth represents an evil to be extirpated by a good reformer, and second, where the dentist represents the evil tyrant who pulls good teeth which oppose him. Starting with the French revolutionary period: the French Republican dentist pulls (evil) royalist and clerical teeth;[56] in Spain of the same period, by contrast, Goya shows an (evil) aristocrat pulling the teeth of common people.[57] Under Louis-Philippe, Daumier shows a representative of the old, enemy aristocracy, fitted with false teeth, which even do his chewing for him (that is, he is politically impotent).[58] In 1850, the period of reaction after the 1848 revolution, France is shown suffering the extraction of all the "molars and [political] institutions" which might give her trouble.[59] From the Risorgimento, Piedmont, the reformer, demands that bad Italian politicians be pulled;[60] Italy waits for Time, the dentist, to extract the rotten tooth who is Napoleon III.[61] The tyrant Bismarck pulls all the teeth of Prussia in order to render it helpless.[62] Uncle Sam pulls the Kaiser's teeth.[63] And so on down to the present.[64] Finally, an all-too-current example: a Nicaraguan cartoon showing the CIA offering to extract the "rotten tooth of Nicaragua" from the head of Uncle Sam.[65] In French caricature the stereotypical Englishman is shown with long protruding teeth of (political) rapacity; in an ostensibly nonpolitical variation on this stereotype, the enormous Anglo fang will not yield; rather, the whole head comes off.[66]

People may have sought comfort in the knowledge that their political masters suffered as much as common mortals from their teeth. They would have been wrong to do so: political decisions affecting them might suffer adversely under the impact of a royal or ministerial toothache, of the chronic or acute kind suffered by the likes

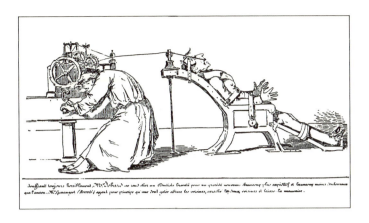

Figure 18: Cham, The Story of Mr. Jobard, 1840.

of Francis I, Henry IV and Louis XIV of France, Elizabeth I of England, General Washington, Gladstone and particularly Bismarck. Louis XIV's toothaches coincided with declining foreign policy fortunes; his having been born with teeth was regarded as an evil omen by powers which had reason to fear French aggression.

Political evils were like bad teeth which must be extracted because they caused social discomfort and might affect other, good teeth. Dentists pulled good teeth "by mistake," in recklessness[67] or cruelty, like tyrants out to disarm their opponents. Multiple or total extraction of good teeth and the substitution of dentures, even in a nonpolitical comic strip, carried overtones of total and/or collective disempowerment, class tyranny perhaps; the extraction of a single bad tooth by contrast was a necessary sacrifice, a victory in its way. The extraction of a good tooth was an outrage to be avenged. In a comic strip by Palmer Cox (1877) a furious patient counterattacks with the dentist's own instrument on the dentist's own teeth – which come flying out all too easily, for they are false.[68] Total extraction could never be imagined as justified in any way, but only as the result of incompetence, cruelty and greed. In a not uncommon and very hardy (also twentieth-century) caricatural theme, the dentist pulls all the good teeth, one by one, leaving only the bad one.[69]

In mid-century France certain dentists made great efforts to sell the idea of dentures as a "fashionable" item. Wholesale extractions increased. Cham showed the typical lower-middle-class hypochondriac undergoing this fate, inflicted on him by a complicated machine cranked by a demonic-looking dentist, according to a "new, patented, much more expeditious and much less painful procedure," on the "principle that a rotten tooth harms its neighbors" – so that these are pulled, leaving the bad one behind (figure 18). The patient is left with dentures which do not work either. The "Demon Dentist" of a later strip, thus titled, after committing

# THE DEMON DENTIST.

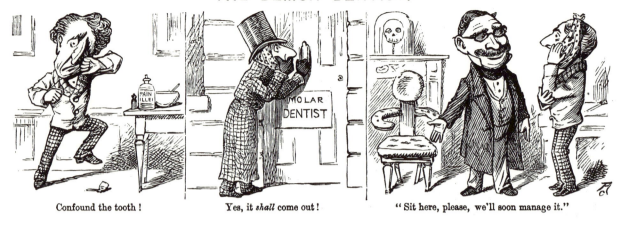

Confound the tooth !

Yes, it *shall* come out !

" Sit here, please, we'll soon manage it."

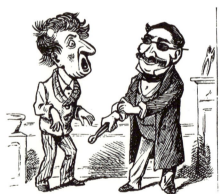

Currrrrrunch !

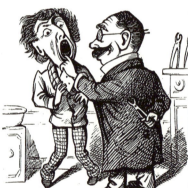

" Not the right one ! Then, my dear sir, we must try again."

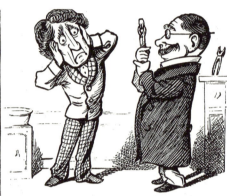

" Not it yet ! Dear, dear, they must be *all* bad. This is very far gone."

(After several trials.) " Only one left. Well, come, we are sure to be right this time."

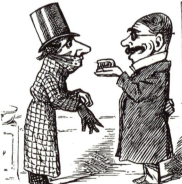

" Better have a set of our five-guinea teeth, as natural as life, and most becoming." . . . .

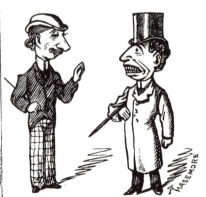

" By jove, old man, what have you been doing ! Swallowing your wife's piano, and left the keys sticking out ?"

Figure 19: A. Chasemore, The Demon Dentist.
From *Judy* (London, 1878).

the same crime, cheerfully proposes "our five-guinea teeth, as natural as life, and most becoming" (figure 19). After his seizure of absolute power, the emperor Napoleon III rooted out French democratic institutions by means of the "chloroform" of manipulated plebiscites. It is by chloroform (not otherwise alluded to in the comic strips) that the dentist Chicotard succeeds in extracting all the teeth of a patient, Isidore Coquerel, whose own diagnosis was one bad tooth. This story has a patently improbable happy ending which seems to parody some professional publicity: Coquerel's very expensive dentures, called "osanores," impress a rich English widow whom he marries, and he produces a series of children all born with "the most beautiful 'osanores.' "[70]

This "happy ending" is that of social quiescence politically imposed and "bought" by some material gains for the lower as well as upper classes. (Note that Coquerel marries a rich widow.) In 1853 the French democrats and republicans had little means of redress. Two major comic strips we shall now analyze in some depth, a British one of 1849 and a German one of 1862, bracket a period of relative peace and prosperity for the middle and skilled working classes. In both strips the patient is relieved of the one tooth troubling him, and returned to (social) health; the dentist is benign and efficient, akin to the moderate reformer who satisfied some immediate middle-class demands. Those strips where the dentist is vilified and demonized, and the patient suffers needlessly, are of a later, more combative period (cf. the vindictive Palmer Cox strip cited above).

*The Toothache*, drawn by George Cruikshank and conceived by Horace Mayhew, was first published in London in 1849 as a little "concertina" album, or "roller picture" of forty-four scenes (figure 20). It was copied in a French magazine of 1851, reprinted in another French magazine of 1856, and appeared, abbreviated, in a German magazine of 1860.[71] The dentist, whose face we do not see until the end, proves to be young and handsome. The viewer, and perhaps the patient, registers this as a happy reversal of the stereotype which saw dentists as demons, as did Heinrich Heine, according to his picturesque account of his visit to the dentist in Berlin in 1837. Fearing tooth-extraction as "something like being beheaded," Heine mistook a villainous-looking neighbor at a table in an inn for a particular "tooth executioner" (*Zahnhenker*) whom he sought, and who turned out to be a theatrical director; the dentist proved to be the most charming, handsome and gentle person.[72] Cruikshank's

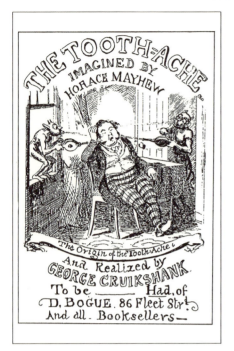

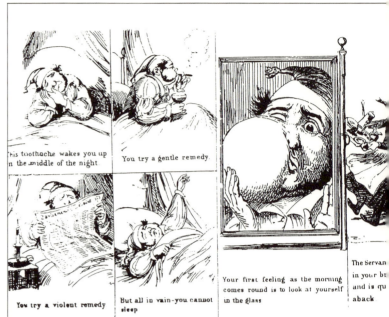

Figure 20: Horace Mayhew and George Cruikshank, *The Toothe-ache* (London, 1849).

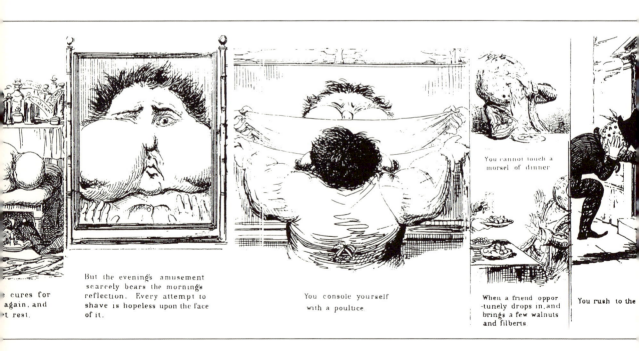

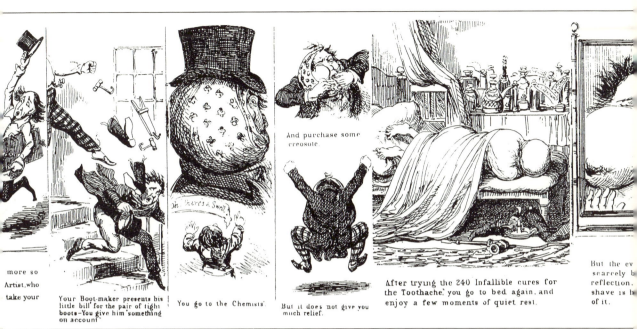

more so
Artist, who
take your

Your Boot-maker presents his little bill for the pair of tight boots—You give him 'something on account'

You go to the Chemists'

And purchase some creosote.

But it does not give you much relief.

After trying the 240 Infallible cures for the Toothache, you go to bed again, and enjoy a few moments of quiet rest.

But the ev
scarcely b
reflection,
shave is h
of it.

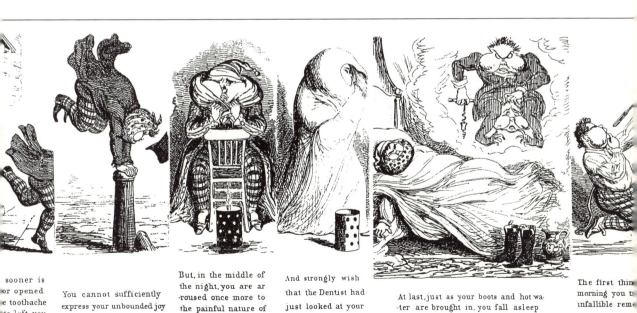

sooner is
or opened
e toothache
te left you,

You cannot sufficiently express your unbounded joy

But, in the middle of the night, you are ar-roused once more to the painful nature of your position

And strongly wish that the Dentist had just looked at your tooth.

At last, just as your boots and hot wa--ter are brought in, you fall asleep and have the most delicious dreams,

The first thin
morning you t
infallible reme

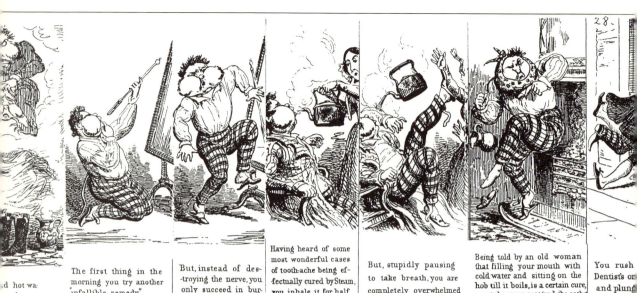

d hot wa-
asleep
dreams,

The first thing in the
morning you try another
"infallible remedy".

But, instead of des-
-troying the nerve, you
only succeed in bur-
-ning your fingers.

Having heard of some
most wonderful cases
of tooth-ache being ef-
-fectually cured by Steam,
you inhale it for half
an hour.

But, stupidly pausing
to take breath, you are
completely overwhelmed
by the consequences

Being told by an old woman
that filling your mouth with
cold water and sitting on the
hob till it boils, is a certain cure,
you take your seat (and the oaths
accordingly, but want the firm-
-ness and coolness to persevere

You rush
Dentist's or
and plung
-long in

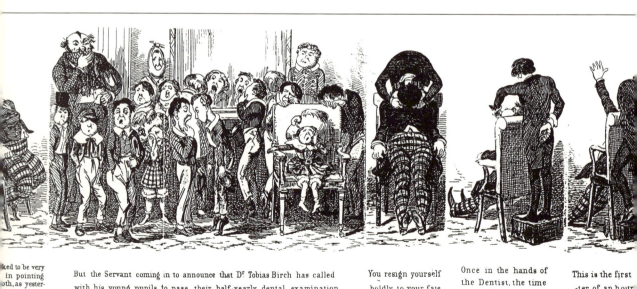

ked to be very
in pointing
oth, as yester-
ntist pulled out
ne by mistake.

But the Servant coming in to announce that Dr. Tobias Birch has called
with his young pupils to pass their half-yearly dental examination,
you are strongly requested "to be a man, and please make haste."

You resign yourself
boldly to your fate

Once in the hands of
the Dentist, the time
seems interminable.

This is the first
-ter of an hour

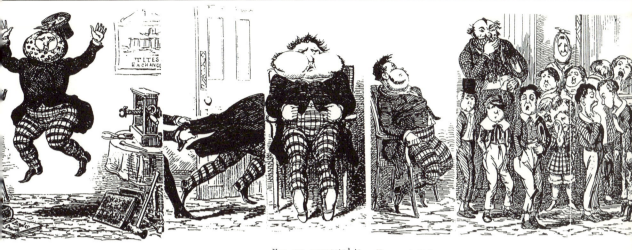

a scream in the next room
arly lifts you off your feet. You
ermine upon going home

When a strong feeling of
shame pulls you back, and

You are requested to
sit down for a few
minutes, and make
yourself comfortable

You are asked to be very
particular in pointing
out the Tooth, as yester-
day the Dentist pulled out
a wrong one by mistake

But the Servant coming in to announce th
with his young pupils to pass their ha
you are strongly requested to be a ma

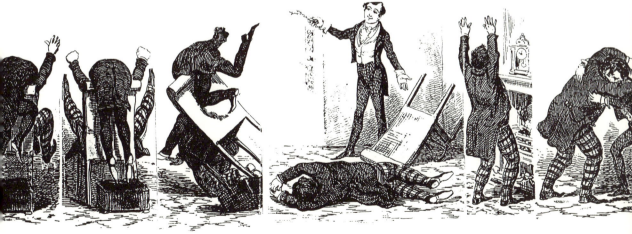

nd quarter
hour !!

The third quarter
of an hour !!!

The fourth quarter
of an hour !!!!

But, AT LAST IT IS OUT !

When you are as-
tonished to find
that the operation
has lasted less
than a minute.

You bless the Denti

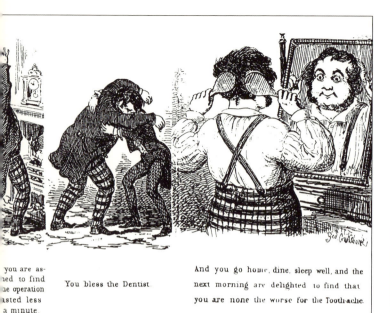

you are as-
ked to find
the operation
lasted less
a minute.

You bless the Dentist.

And you go home, dine, sleep well, and the
next morning are delighted to find that
you are none the worse for the Toothache.

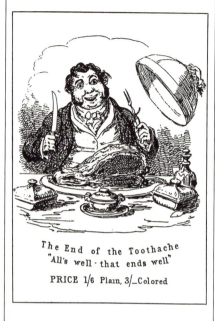

The End of the Toothache
"All's well · that ends well"
PRICE 1/6 Plain, 3/_ Colored

dentist adopts at the end an attitude of straightforward professional satisfaction, rather than personal triumph, although it is the fruit of a long and violent struggle which is discreetly veiled from us by the artist's rear view, ending with the patient thrown prostrate to the ground. Victor and victim are instantly transformed, in the next vignette, in the mutual embrace of savior and saved; the word "sauveur" actually appears in the French caption. This embrace of former "antagonists" stands in the context of our study as an emblem of the British sense of social harmony at this moment in mid-century, achieved after some bitter political struggle during the previous decades, but without the violent repression following the continental revolutions of 1848 which left Britain relatively unscathed. The former martyr to the toothache is left at the end fully restored to social and physical health (and in the French version, sexual health too: he dances that same evening at a ball).

The section in the Cruikshank print depicting the struggle and triumph at the dentist's is balanced by a somewhat longer section which accumulates a series of folk remedies ("240 infallible cures"), some of them quite dangerous and painful, all of them quite useless and apt to cause violently antisocial behavior. They fail to drive away a pain which was brought on at the opening of the story on the cover by a diabolically inspired draught (literally: "inspired" by devils blow-ing and pumping bellows at the victim's cheeks as he lies asleep by the window). The home remedy can take on a heroic cast: at one point the sufferer kneels to raise the red-hot poker to his mouth, like an ancient Roman hero the sword of suicide to his breast.

When the home remedies prove useless, he finally runs to the dentist. At the door terror overcomes pain, he flees, tries more home remedies, returns at a gallop, and from the waiting room, seeing himself surrounded by (imagined) instruments of torture and hearing (real) cries of pain from the surgery next door, attempts to flee yet again. He is physically held back by a servant in fancy livery, of the kind employed by dentists (some of whom became quite wealthy, earning up to £20,000 a year) in order to impress their clientele. (In the French version, this servant is black — definitely a status symbol.) The initial failure of nerve at the sight of the dentist's office, the return in even greater desperation and the forcible restraint by a servant form a characteristic rhythm of the dental comic strip. Servants chosen for their beefiness prevent flight and hold down the patient during the operation; on one occasion the patient himself resorts to paying burly workmen, who happen to be passing by in the street, to prevent him from fleeing.[73] In another, it is the dentist who resorts to extreme measures, fitting a steel gate which comes crashing down behind the patient once he has stepped inside.[74]

The fractured form and hectic energy of Cruikshank's *Tooth-Ache* have to do not only with the subject matter, but also with the revolutionary moment, which was marked in this early phase of English comic-strip history by comparable disjunct, pull-out strips in an obscure, short-lived magazine called *Man in the Moon* (1847-49). These too have a frenetic quality; but what is socially dispersed there is sharply, agonizingly concentrated in the *Tooth-Ache*, where the fracturing of graphic format corresponds to the fracturing of the human body, physically by the loss of a tooth, psychologically by pain.

Our second major document is German, a rather shorter (twenty-five drawings) *Bilderbogen* by Wilhelm Busch, called *The Rotten Tooth* (Der hohle Zahn) and dated 1862 (figure 21). Like Cruikshank the artist starts with a prolonged sequence of home remedies, punctuated by violent anger at an innocent person. The flight and return are however compressed into a single gesture of resistance. Spare and elegant in his

## Der hohle Zahn

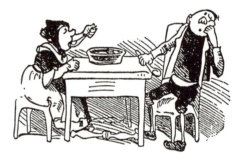

Oftmalen bringt ein harter Brocken
Des Mahles Freude sehr ins Stocken.

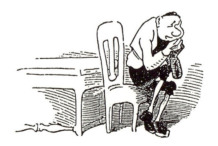

So geht's nun auch dem Friedrich Kracke;
Er sitzt ganz krumm und hält die Backe.

Figure 21: Wilhelm Busch, *Der hohle Zahn*, 1862.

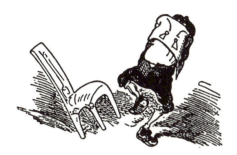

Um seine Ruhe ist's getan;
Er biß sich auf den hohlen Zahn.

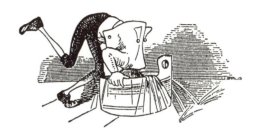

Er taucht den Kopf mitsamt dem Übel
In einen kalten Wasserkübel.

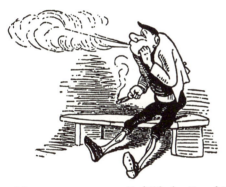

Nun sagt man zwar: Es hilft der Rauch!
Und Friedrich Kracke tut es auch;

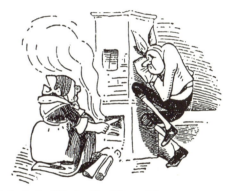

Jedoch das Übel will nicht weichen,
Auf andre Art will er's erreichen.

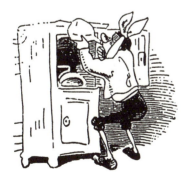

Allein schon treiben ihn die Nöten,
Mit Schnaps des Zahnes Nerv zu töten.

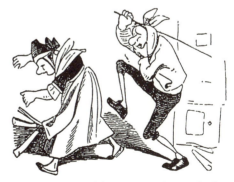

Umsonst! — Er schlägt, vom Schmerz bedrängt,
Die Frau, die einzuheizen denkt.

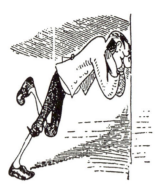

Auch zieht ein Pflaster hinterm Ohr
Die Schmerzen leider nicht hervor.

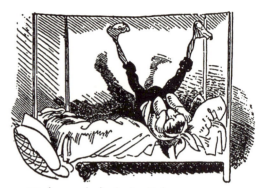

Und zappelnd mit den Beinen
Hört man ihn bitter weinen.

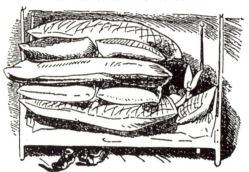

„Vielleicht" — so denkt er — „wird das Schwitzen
Möglicherweise etwas nützen."

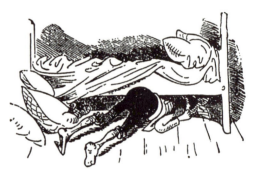

Jetzt sucht er unterm Bette
Umsonst die Ruhestätte.

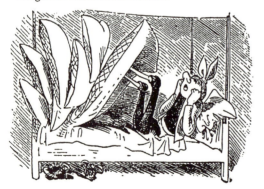

Indes die Hitze wird zu groß,
Er strampelt sich schon wieder los;

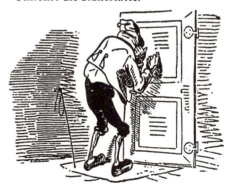

Zuletzt fällt ihm der Doktor ein.
Er klopft. — Der Doktor ruft: „Herein!"

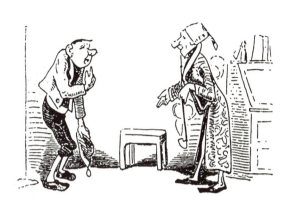

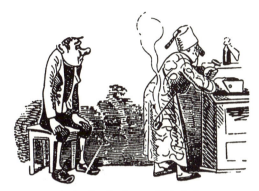

"Ei, guten Tag, mein lieber Kracke,
Nehmt Platz! Was ist's denn mit der Backe?

Nun geht der Doktor still beiseit.
Der Bauer ist nicht sehr erfreut.

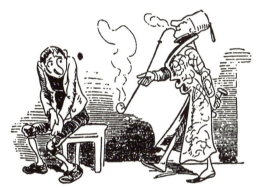

Und lächelnd kehrt der Doktor wieder.
Dem Bauern fährt es durch die Glieder.

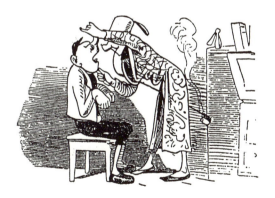

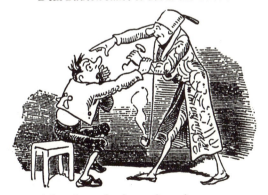

Laßt sehn! Ja, ja! Das glaub ich wohl!
Der ist ja in der Wurzel hohl!"

Ach, wie erschrak er, als er da
Den wohlbekannten Haken sah!

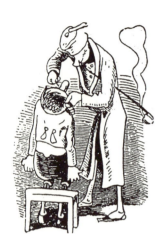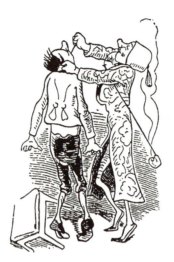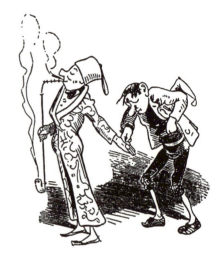

Der Doktor, ruhig und besonnen,
Hat schon bereits sein Werk begonnen.

Und unbewußt nach oben
Fühlt Kracke sich gehoben.

Und — rack! — da haben wir den Zahn,
Der so abscheulich weh getan!

Mit Staunen und voll Heiterkeit
Sieht Kracke sich vom Schmerz befreit.

Der Doktor, würdig wie er war,
Nimmt in Empfang sein Honorar.

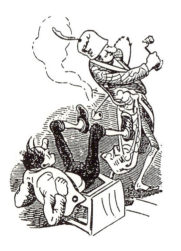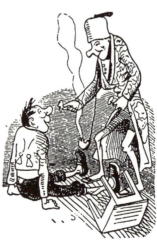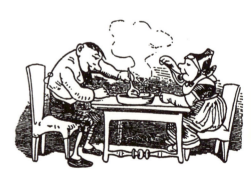

Und Friedrich Kracke setzt sich wieder
Vergnügt zum Abendessen nieder.

silk gown and tasseled fez, the doctor (as he is called) greets his patient in his surgery, smiling and smoking, quietly confident. He politely inquires after the problem of the figure cringing before him, cap in hand, and gestures to him to take a seat. The dentist then inspects the patient's mouth, with the thumb of one professional hand drawing down the lower jaw, forefinger and thumb of the other hand holding the patient's prominent nose by the tip, to raise the upper jaw. Manipulated via the nose which tilts like putty, the patient is unmanned (Busch is rife with nose-as-phallus, and indeed "nasal castration" symbolism).[75] The patient holds his hands in the posture of a begging puppy.

The dread diagnosis is made. Silently the dentist turns to select his instrument, his weapon. In a superb mimetic dialectic showing Busch at his best, first the dentist approaches, craftily, diplomatically, hiding behind his back the "familiar hook" (of a type called in English "key"), while the patient shrinks away, wringing his hands; then, as the patient stretches out his hand to fend off the hand with the weapon, the dentist stretches out his other hand, in an exactly parallel movement, over the cringing patient's head — the traditional gesture of authority and command, as well as, here, an exorcism of his fear and will to resist. There ensues a short, sharp and unequal battle (in other strips, notably the Cruikshank, the battle is more prolonged), won by the dentist without apparent effort, without even removing from his mouth the pipe that, for all its enormous length, incommodes the operation not in the least (could this pipe also be a phallic symbol here, as elsewhere in Busch?). With one pull, he lifts the patient off his stool and whisks the tooth out with the flourish of the fairground huckster dramatically flicking out a tooth with a sword, to the accompanying verbal flourish of the caption: "And Rack-rack! There goes the tooth,/ that hurt you so atrociously!"[76] The patient falls back onto the chair which has overturned as he was lifted up, and in a counter-motion, the dentist spins around in the attitude of a boxer who has delivered a knockout blow, triumphantly, as if to an invisible applauding audience. He then turns back to stand genially over his grounded patient, displaying to him the trophy he has won (he gets to keep it). The sufferer's joy at his release from pain mutes a little at the final phase of the transaction, coins paid out reluctantly (in stereotypical peasant avarice) and received with studied nonchalance. The dentist's back is turned, as if he spurned payment, but the receiving hand is well in position. (The contradiction — let us not call it hypocrisy — is still with us, for while financial rewards are certainly a major attraction of the profession, what dentist, doctor or lawyer today would demean himself by personally demanding payment?)

There remains to identify the protagonists in this little drama, who represent not only individuals, but distinct and potentially antagonistic social classes. As in comparable situations — for instance, the barber who cruelly (accidentally-on-purpose) mutilates his client, cutting off the tips of his nose and ears[77] — Busch has cast the client as peasant, in clogs, breeches and short jacket, and the doctor as bourgeois, in elegant dress. The power relations in the dentist's office are precisely those of the declining and rising classes. The peasant was embattled everywhere, especially in industrializing Europe, where he was driven off the land as agriculture was "rationalized" and landholdings were enlarged and monopolized; he became a landless laborer-for-hire and/or was drawn into the cities to find work; in either case, he was proletarianized. The work he found was paid with a small wage disproportionate to the value of his labor; as Karl Marx was at pains to show, he invariably ended up enriching his employer more than himself, just as Busch's peasant enriches the very man who "robbed" him of his tooth, which in other caricatures may even be a good one.

As he lost ears, nose or tooth, so he lost land and independence. The agrarian body politic all over Europe was mutilated in this way, cracked apart (Busch's peasant is actually named Kracke) by capitalistic economic forces. Without admitting that they have caused this crack in the first place, the bourgeoisie offer a remedy: extract the peasant from the land, as the tooth is extracted from the gum. And substitute a machine. Traditional, local (folk) remedies cannot cure the aching tooth; only urban bourgeois science can do so, offering as an extreme and brutal but all-too-common remedy the definitive, "elegant" cure, total extraction, and the ultimate in dental technology: dentures.

In Busch the battle is decided from the outset. There is little resistance, as indeed there was relatively little resistance to industrialization (after 1848-49) in Germany. In France and England in the 1870s the lower classes began to fight back. In the best French revolutionary[78] tradition, a patient (not, to be sure, a peasant, but a lower-middle-class type with his own war against authority) in a French comic strip (figure 22), which was quickly copied in the United States, on discovering that the

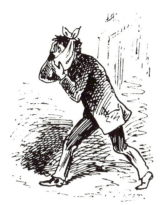

Néanmoins, la douleur l'emporte et le fait revenir chez le dentiste, qui lui arrache une dent.

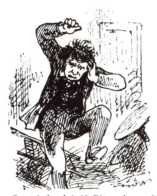

Rentré chez lui, M. Pitou s'aperçoit avec terreur que le dentiste s'est trompé et a laissé la mauvaise dent.

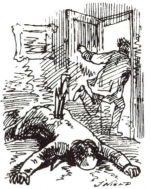

Colère de M. Pitou qui court chez le dentiste et le laisse pour mort.

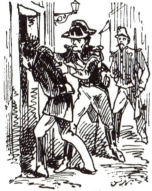

Aussitôt, appréhendé au corps, M. Pitou est conduit à la préfecture,

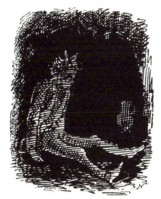

où, il pense philosophiquement qu'une mauvaise dent est quelquefois *le chemin du crime.*

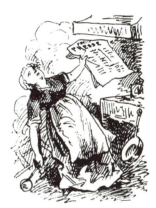

Le bruit ayant couru que *M. Ponson du Terrail* était l'auteur du crime commis sur un dentiste, une abonnée de la *Petite Presse* pense en mourir.

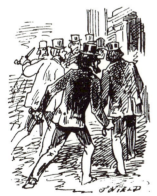

Tous les directeurs de journaux se rendent en haut lieu, pour obtenir sa grâce.

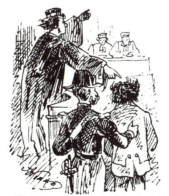

M. Pitou, cause involontaire de tant de bruit, est acquitté grâce aux circonstances atténuantes.

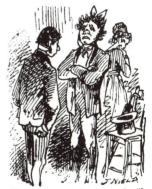

Et rentre au sein de sa famille, fraîchement augmentée d'un cousin à lui inconnu.

Figure 22: John Nield, *Histoire d'une fluxion*. From *Petit Journal Comique*, 1869-70 (Paris, Bibliothèque nationale).

wrong tooth has been pulled in a manifest *social* injustice, storms, rages and kills the dentist with that quintessentially bourgeois symbol, an umbrella. "Attenuating circumstances," and a great press campaign, another very French feature, secure the homicide's acquittal. But his problem remains (he still has the toothache), and it has metastasized into his family and sexual life. He returns home from prison to find his family "newly augmented with a cousin unknown to him" (his wife's lover). He receives a sexual punishment for what was, in origin, subliminally, a voyeuristic sexual sin: for the toothache was initially brought on by a draught of air "which at first caused M. Pitou [the hero] some pleasure," by lifting the skirts of a fair female form climbing the stairs. The characteristic French shift into the sexual realm may be observed in a different way in a French imitation of Busch's *Rotten Tooth*,[79] which substitutes a final scene of rustic courtship for Busch's typically German scene of eating — both celebrations, in their different ways, of triumphant survival and the return to basic pleasures. We have now returned to the "medieval" theme of toothache as punishment for sexual sin, to which William Rogers, one of the most famous French dentists, adverted in his *Manuel* of 1845. Rogers maintained that passions such as anger could cause toothache, and the "other passions which I need not specify [i.e. sexual] cause the total loss of teeth under terrible suffering."[80]

The sexual component is enlarged and the class referents of bourgeois triumphing over peasant are reversed twenty-one years later in Busch's *Clement Dove, or the Poet Frustrated* (Balduin Bählamm, der verhinderte Dichter), a longer story published as a separate little book. This appeared during the 1880s, when industrialization was a fait accompli in Germany, and the peasant no longer constituted a threat to it. Now it is the (petty) bourgeois city clerk with aspirations for poetic laurels who is smitten with the toothache. Unable to cultivate his muse amid the din of city and family, he repairs to a village where Nature herself should foster his imagined natural gift. Nature, alas, deals him one blow after another, weather, animals and rustics all conspiring to torment and humiliate him. His attempts at poetic composition are doomed from the start; his attempts at the sexual conquest of nature, a buxom goatherd, are punished by a symbolic castration at the hands of the goatherd and her legitimate rustic lover, who trap him in a basket, thrust a pole between his legs and dunk him in the pond (figure 23). This gives him a cold, which brings on the toothache.

Both intensely localized and overwhelming as described (in the verse) by Busch, the toothache is the negative counterpart and fitting punishment of sexual pleasure. But it is more than this, for toothache (according to a small verse digression) has the perverse virtue of expelling all triviality and mundanity from one's consciousness, and thereby laying bare the very soul itself – in Clement Dove's case, the poetic soul "which resides in the narrow socket of the molar."

The toothache, from a metaphor of the pain and terror of the social struggle, has become quite explicitly a metaphor of the pain of poetic gestation to which we know Busch was remarkably sensitive. But this is no great shift, for poetry is conceived by the little city clerk, as it was by Busch himself, the son of a petty-bourgeoisified peasant, as a means of escaping, transcending that struggle. Poetic pain, like the toothache, is transcendent.

Clement Dove resorts to the genial efforts of a dentist, Dr. Smirke (*Schmurzel* = *Schmunzel* = smirk), whose name and expression suggest untoward enjoyment of his painful art, and whose prompt demand for payment when he fails reveals his mercenary character (figure 24). The tooth will not come out; is it because poetic genius is too firmly (if narrowly) rooted to be forcibly extracted? In this particular case, probably not, for it seems that once the hero's illusions of possessing such genius fade, the pain of the tooth fades with them. It could also be that since Dove has already suffered his sexual expiation, to lose a tooth at this point would be supererogatory. At any rate, the toothache has served its purpose to drive the would-be poet out of a world where he does not belong, and which caused him so much misery. The metaphorical "tooth of poetic genius" is extracted by a hostile nature and vengeful peasants; the real tooth-as-tooth may remain.

Normally the patient pays thrice over, with pain, tooth and money, and remains subject to bourgeois science and power. His own resources – folk cures – prove both useless and ridiculous; when they fail, he must resort to the dentist. It is the supposed failure of a lower-class economy (or mode of life or character), be it peasant or urban, that allows the bourgeoisie to intervene, to apply remedies, to enact scientific and social "reforms" which may indeed bring some kind of immediate relief, but which serve ultimately to reinforce (upper) bourgeois domination. This process emerges transparently from another Busch picture story called *Buzz——buzz, or the Bees*, his first in book form (1869), where the incompetent old-fashioned peasant who suffers the loss of his bees and beehives has to be rescued by the school-

79

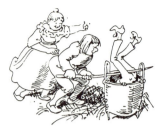

He threads it through the hamper's eyes
Between the inmate's weaving thighs;
And thus uncomfortably grooved,
Dove feels himself picked up and moved.

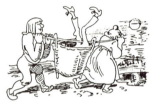

He struggles hotly, for profound
Yawns the dark query: Whither bound?

A well-spring, moonlit, deep and cool
Awaits the swaying reticule.

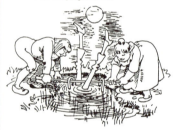

Here they proceed to dunk the basket
More frequently than Dove would ask it.

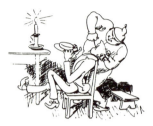

Heave-ho!!
How was it? Did you feel it shift?"
"I certainly felt something lift."

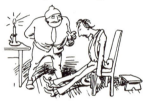

"In that case there is nothing to it!
Another little tug will do it!

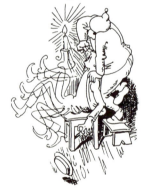

Heeaa—ve-ho!!!"
He prises with a hamlike paw.

The tooth stays rooted in the jaw.

"I thought as much," says Dr. Pocket.

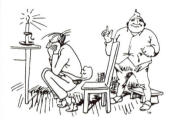

"The obstacle is in the socket.
Five dollars net is all you owe.

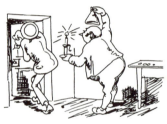

I hope it passes. Let me know!"

Figure 23: Wilhelm Busch, "Clement Dove gets dunked" in *Clement Dove or the Poet Frustrated*, ch. 7, 1883. From Walter Arndt, *The Genius of Wilhelm Busch, Comedy of Frustration* (Berkeley, 1982).

Figure 24: Wilhelm Busch, "Clement Dove at the Dentist" in *Clement Dove or the Poet Frustrated*, ch. 8, 1883. From Walter Arndt, *The Genius of Wilhelm Busch, Comedy of Frustration* (Berkeley, 1982).

master, representative of bourgeois know-how, to whom he then surrenders his own flesh and blood, his beautiful daughter, in marriage.

There is another article — a book maybe — to be written on the sexual symbolism of teeth, with which nineteenth- and twentieth-century media must surely be rife. Let some jottings suffice here. There was an old tradition that considered tooth-ache to be as acute, overwhelming and incurable as love: "I am troubled with a tooth-ache, or with love, I know not whether; there is a worm in both."[81] Our age of psychoanalysis and dream interpretation has no difficulty in seeing (fear of) loss of teeth as fear of death and castration, as well as loss of power generally. As we have shown, the idea of sexual guilt was present from Petrarch on, and figured promi-nently in our French and German nineteenth-century comic-strip sample. Tooth extraction was akin to castration. In a folk-tale motif, a lover gets the wife to have her husband's best tooth drawn and give it to him (the lover); the husband is thus symbolically castrated, or at least disempowered in favor of the lover.[82] In a French comic strip, an adulterer is punished by the husband, who happens to be a dentist, with the extraction of a healthy tooth.[83] When David Copperfield, provoked to an uncharacteristic fit of violent rage, physically attacks his sexual rival Uriah Heep, he cracks Heep's tooth, which has to be extracted. It should be possible to point to a particularly British sense of sexuality embodied in teeth as in so many other symbolic bodily arenas (hair, feet, etc.). While French dentists brazenly advertised dentures and individually became rich manufacturing them, the British were pro-foundly ashamed of this artifice. Like prostitution and venereal disease, they were a disgraceful, taboo subject, ignored by polite literature, although many men, including the famous, had them. They learned not to smile too broadly, and to chew carefully. To expose oneself publicly as the wearer of false teeth was akin to sexual self-exposure.

The tooth also figures as a symbol of sacrificial love. In an example remarkable for the fact that it was drawn by Europe's only female professional caricaturist, Marie Duval, working in the crudest and most childish style, a lover offers his own good tooth, secretly, to replace one accidentally knocked out of the mouth of his beloved, by transplanting it "warm," according to the still current belief. But the extracted tooth goes by mistake to the wrong woman. Another secret sacrifice is

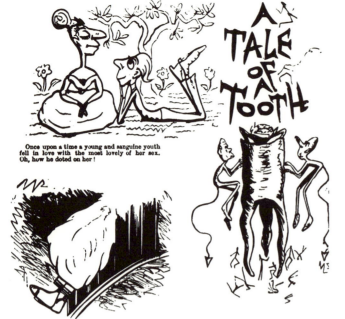

# A TALE OF A TOOTH

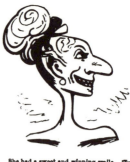

Once upon a time a young and sanguine youth fell in love with the most lovely of her sex. Oh, how he doted on her!

She had a sweet and winning smile. 'Twas that which won him.

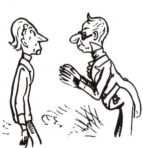

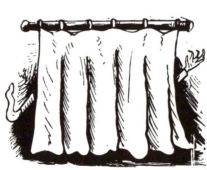

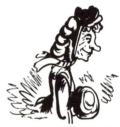

But oh, sad day of woe! a terrible accident befell this young and beauteous maiden.

She came down a most tremendous cropper, and knocked her eye-tooth out.

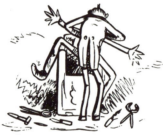

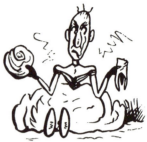

In this dire strait, whom could she seek for consolation but he who loved her? He, in his turn, sought out a cunning man, and heard a theory:—If a tooth is wrenched from one head and put warm into another head, it will take root

Do you suppose our hero hesitated? (He had never had a tooth drawn, and had no notion what the sensation was like.) He gave himself up to the cunning man, and the tooth was extrac-AC-AC-TED!

This was in secret—the loved one knew not whose tooth she was to have. But oh, bitter tale of agony and remorse, when he had strength to look out of the window, he saw another patient going away triumphantly with his tooth in her head, and it was the wrong woman!

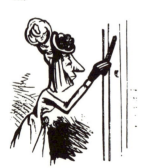

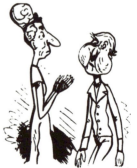

At that moment there came a knock at the door—the right woman at last.

But could he part with his other eye-tooth—could he renew the torture? What! was his affection not strong enough for that? Perish the thought, and produce the pinchers! But please let us draw the curtain on the hideous details.

Three days afterwards, when he crawled, crushed and maimed, to the loved one's presence, she simply said, "Good gracious me! what a horrid fright you have made of yourself!"

He left her at these cruel words and fled the scene, and subsequently destroyed himself. Few besides JUDY have shed a tear upon his hapless fate.

Figure 25: Mary Duval, A Tale of a Tooth. From *Judy*, 1870 (London, British Museum).

made, leaving the (literally) love-sick donor so deformed-looking that his beloved spurns him (figure 25).

Has he symbolically castrated himself? Obviously not the kind of sacrifice a prospective bride would welcome. Sacrificial love, as well as class exploitation, is the meaning of the incident in Victor Hugo's *Les Misérables*. Fantine, who had already sold her magnificent long hair, allows an unscrupulous itinerant dentist to buy her two beautiful upper front teeth, in order to pay for medicines to save her child, Cosette, whom she believes to be dangerously sick.[84] Disfigured, she becomes a common prostitute and soon dies in misery.

To a low-class institution like caricature, the power and pretentions of dentists were an irresistible target. The symbolic or substitute revenge of art served to release otherwise dangerous frustration, fear and anger, which, I have argued, were social and political as well as personal. There is a tremendous irony, and a certain logic, in the fact that dentists themselves offered the comic journals which carried all the jokes about and against them as a kind of psychological anesthetic or homoeopathic remedy in the waiting rooms of their surgeries, a role that *Punch*, the *New Yorker* and their kin still fulfill today. As van Gogh testified, "Daumier's prints are so true they almost make one forget the toothache."[85]

Almost.

NOTES

1. David Kunzle, *History of the Comic Strip II: The Nineteenth Century* (Berkeley: University of California Press, 1989).

2. Cited by Heinz Lässig and Rainer A. Muller, *Die Zahnheilkunde in Kunst und Kulturgeschicte* (Cologne, 1983), p. 60.

3. Cf. two scenes carved into the replica of a tooth, c. 1780, reproduced in Malvin E. Ring, *Dentistry: An Illustrated History* (New York, 1985), pp. 2 and 17.

4. This title was invented by Hans Christian Andersen in his "Auntie Toothache" story, cited by J.J. Pindborg and L. Marvitz, *The Dentist in Art* (Chicago, 1960), p. 112.

5. The first and only complete English translation is entitled *Phisicke against Fortune...*, trans. Thomas Twyne (London, 1579; facsimile, with an intro. by B. Kohl, New York: Delmar, 1980), 104th dialogue, pp. 284-86.

6. Christoph Weigel, *Abbildung der Germein-Nutzlichen Hauptstände* (Regensburg, 1698), pt. 4, no. 8, p. 148, reproduced in Lässig and Muller, *Die Zahnheilkunde*, fig. 89, p. 73.

7. *Deuteronomy* 34.7, which has in the Revised Standard Version "nor his natural force abated." Abraham a Sancta Clara, *Etwas für Alle* (1699; Nuremberg, 1711), ch. 13, pp. 94-98; "Der Zähn-Artzt," transcribed by H. Christian Greve, *Aphorismen zur Kulturgeschicte der Zahnheilkund und des ärtzlichen Standes* (Leipzig, 1930), pp. 41-43, cites the Latin, "nec dentes illius moti."

8. C.V. Wedgwood, *The Thirty Years War* (Harmondsworth, 1957), p. 140.

9. For an example of the worm as punishment of sexual sin, see *Admonition to Refrain from Adultery*, a print of c. 1600 by Crispin de Passe, discussed by Ilja Veldman, "Lessons for Ladies...," *Simiolus* 16.2-3 (1986), p. 119.

10. There is a good color reproduction of this detail in Lässig and Muller, *Die Zahnheilkunde*, fig. 53.

11. Jacques Lavallye, *Pieter Bruegel the Elder and Lucas van Leyden: The Complete Engravings, Etchings, and Woodcuts* (New York, n.d.), pl. 214.

12. Cf. Keith Moxey, "Sebald Beham's Church Anniversary Holidays...," *Simiolus* 12 (1981-82), p. 120.

13. C. Gysel, "Over de betekenis van Andreas Vesalius voor de tandheelkunde," *Nederlands tijdschrift voor tandheelkunde* 73 (January 1966), pp. 68-76.

14. M.A. van Andel, *Chirurgiíns, Vríje Meesters, Beunhazen en Kwaksalvers* (P.N. Van Kampen: Amsterdam, 1946; also Denttaag, 1981), pp. 172-74.

15. Simon Schama, *The Embarrassment of Riches: An Interpretation of Dutch Culture in the Golden Age* (New York, 1987), pp. 165-66, citing James Gorman, "Sweet Toothlessness," *Discover* 1 (October 1980), p. 52.

16. Gorman, "Sweet Toothlessness," p. 52.

17. H. Christian Greve, *Vom Zahnheilhandwerk zur Zahnheilkunde* (Munich, 1952), pp. 24ff.

18. Lässig and Muller, *Die Zahnheilkunde*, p. 68.

19. See H. Kümmel, *Die Ahnherren der Zahnheilkunde: Kulturgeschichtliche Essays* (Berlin, 1910), chs. 3 and 4. It is noteworthy that the least scientific and most superstition-ridden writers on dentistry tend to be German and Italian: Leonhard Thurneysser zum Thurn, for instance, who has been called the very model of the medical alchemist–villain, a man of idiotic vanity, a mass-murderer, who recommended as a remedy for toothache the tooth of a man broken on the wheel; or the otherwise reputable Dr. Hieronymus Cardanus of Milan, polymath author of 222 works, addicted to the torture of witches, with a view of teeth that was astrological and cabbalistic. These were

not "quacks," but men who had studied, learned scholars and writers, men with official positions.

20. Ring, *Dentistry*, p. 152.

21. Christopher Brown, *Scenes of Everyday Life: Dutch Genre Painting of the Seventeenth Century* (London, 1984), p. 94. Elsewhere (p. 74), he refers without justification to an operator's "clumsiness" (in a painting by Jan Steen) as "exaggerated to the point of caricature." For Otto Naumann (*Von Frans Hals bis Vermeer: Meisterwerke höllandischer Genremalerei*, exhibition catalogue (Berlin: Gemäldegalerie, 1984), pp. 331-32), dentistry is a "pseudoprofession"; itinerant medical men in literature and art are "almost always ridiculed." Cf. also *ibid.*, no. 59, p. 204, and no. 105, p. 296.

22. From Carolus Tuinman's *Oorsprong…Nederduytsche Spreckwoorden* (Middelburg, 1720), p. 92, cited in *Die Sprache des Bilder*, exhibition catalogue (Braunschweig, 1978), p. 107. The proverb is also cited by Herman Roers in his study of tooth and dentistry in Netherlandish proverb-lore, without any further evidence that dentists were generally ill-regarded by the common people: see *Ärtliches in Sprichwörtern und Redensarten der Holländer und Flamen unter besonderer Berucksichtigung der Zahnheilkunde* (Dissertation; Abel: Greifswald, 1938).

23. René Boisson, *Chroniques chirurgicales* (Brussels, 1970), bk. 1, p. 480.

24. It figures in a drawing by Lambert Doomer (reproduced by Brown, *Scenes of Everyday Life*, p. 99) of an operator who wears a sword and is obviously a quack. The banner shows, apparently, the rectal and oral expulsion of worms. The conspicuous presence of a defecating dog in the foreground of the scene adds an appropriate note of disgust.

25. Painting in Frankfurt, 1631, reproduced in Maria Elisabeth Wasserfuhr, *Der Zahnarzt in der niederländenischen Malerei des 170 Jhdts* (Diss. 1970), 2d ed. (Cologne: Arbeiten der Forschungsstelle des Instituts für Geschichte der Universität Köln, 1977), vol. 1, fig. 10. "Accomplice-theft" occurs also in a picture by G. van Vliet and another by Justus van der Nypoort, where the dentist is also an alchemist. Both are reproduced in Georges Dagen, *Le dentiste d'autrefois* (Paris, 1923), n.p.

26. Lässig and Muller, *Die Zahnheilkunde*, fig. 34.

27. Boymans-van Beuningen Museum; reproduced in *Tot Lering en Vermaak*, exhibition catalogue (Amsterdam, 1976), p. 11; and Brown, *Scenes of Everyday Life*, p. 24.

28. Surviving in an eighteenth-century copy, and (now) called *Nature, Teaching and Practice*, this triptych of c. 1660 is analyzed in *Tot Lering en Vermaak*, no. 17, pp. 191-93, with reproduction; good color reproduction also in Brown, *Scenes of Everyday Life*, p. 165.

29. Jacob Cats, "On the Sight of a Person Having a Tooth Pulled," in his *Invallende gedachten* (1657), 14, pp. 9-10, in *Alle de wercken* (Amsterdam: Jan Jacobsz. Schipper, 1658, 1659). A German translation appears in H. Hofmeier, "Zwei Gedichten des niederländischen Schriftstellers Jakob

Cats...," *Zahnärztliche Mitteilungen* 12 (1967), pp. 621-22, and in Wasserfuhr, *Der Zahnarzt*, pp. 42-45.

30. Contributed to the popular medical moralist Johan van Beverwyck's *Schat der ongesontheyt* (Compendium of Ill-health), 2d ed. (1644), reprinted in Cats, *Invallende gedachten*, 15, p. 10; and translated by Hofmeier, "Zwei Gedichten," and in Wasserfuhr, *Der Zahnarzt*. My citation is a paraphrase.

31. Abraham a Sancta Clara, *Etwas für Alle*, p. 42.

32. In Amsterdam; reproduced in Lässig and Muller, *Die Zahnheilkunde*, fig. 72.

33. His presence immediately raises the question: could this and other pictures of dental operations represent theatrical performances? While this remains a possibility, it is certain that they do not do so to the extent of the pictures of another kind of operation on the head, the Operation for the Stone, which was not performed in reality (see William Schupbach, "A New Look at *The Cure of Folly*," *Medical History* 22.3 (July 1978), pp. 267-81). My thanks go to Dr. Schupbach for bibliographical and other help pertaining to the present article.

34. Lepke auction, Berlin, November 28, 1911, no. 114; photograph in the Rijksbureau voor Kunsthistorische Documentatie, the Hague.

35. As described by Brown, *Scenes of Everyday Life*, p. 52. Nor can I agree that the smile on the face of old woman on crutches watching in the Jan Steen painting (p. 70) is one necessarily of "ghoulish pleasure." His female companion is positively anxious.

36. The eggs may carry sexual associations as enhancers of male potency, in which case the positioning of the stick in the Quast is not accidental. The same configuration occurs in a painting of a dentist by Gerard Dou in the Louvre. Cf. also a painting by Adriaen van de Venne, *Wat maeck men al om gelt*, reproduced in *Tot Lering en Vermaak*, no. 66. p. 252. If tooth-pulling is a form of sexual expiation, there would be an obvious irony in its infliction upon lusty youths peddling eggs-as-aphrodisiacs.

37. Identical composition reproduced as "Jordaens (?), formerly Milan," in Wasserfuhr, *Der Zahnarzt*, fig. 16a.

38. "Touch," in a series of the Five Senses, reproduced in Brown, *Scenes of Everyday Life*, p. 39.

39. Painting engraved by C. Allard, reproduced in *Prints Related to Dentistry* (Bethesda, Md.: National Library of Medicine, n.d.), fig. 43 (the Both is fig. 42).

40. Brown, *Scenes of Everyday Life*, p. 70.

41. Rijksmuseum, Amsterdam.

42. The painting by the same artist reproduced in Lässig and Muller, *Die Zahnheilkunde*, on the same page (fig. 77) is another good representation of the locale for an operation more commonly depicted outdoors and as conducted by an itinerant dentist.

43. Wasserfuhr, *Der Zahnarzt*, pp. 6ff.

44. Private communication. He adds the following points of similarity: "the head in both cases is at issue; the body in both cases flails to no avail; and the pain of tooth/sin/crime is insufficient punishment – the tooth must come out, the life must end."

45. Painting by Johannes Lingelbach of 1651 (large color reproduction in Ring, *Dentistry*, pp. 10-11). Although mounted, the dentist is not well dressed. He constitutes the major incident in a street at the outskirts of an imaginary Italianate city. Beside and behind him stands a huge classic pedestal, in the shape of an urn, which is oddly missing its monument. Urns usually had sacrificial associations.

46. *Die Sprache der Bilder*, exhibition catalogue (Braunschweig, 1978), no. 21, p. 107.

47. Louvre, 1628; reproduced in Brown, *Scenes of Everyday Life*, p. 68.

48. By Peter Argillis, 1685-1736; reproduced in Curt Proskauer and Fritz Witt, *A Pictorial History of Dentistry* (Cologne, 1962), fig. 114.

49. By Franz Anton Maulpertsch, 1724-96; reproduced in Proskauer and Witt, *Pictorial History*, fig. 115.

50. Reproduced in Proskauer and Witt, *Pictorial History*, fig. 79.

51. Translated from the standard edition, ed. Friedrich Bohne, *Wilhelm Busch Werke* (Hamburg, 1959), vol. 2, p. 500.

52. J. Menzies Campbell, *Dentistry Then and Now* (Glasgow, 1963).

53. "He": all the patients in the nineteenth-century comic strips known to me are men. In earlier pictures women were often depicted. Van Beverwyck (cf. n.30) believed women to be superior in this capacity to endure pain. Was nineteenth-century tooth extraction experienced as so terrifying that only male heroism could survive it?

54. The musician André Grétry (1741-1813), cited by Greve, *Aphorismen*, p. 32.

55. *Der Alte Deutsche Zahnbrecher*, 1632; reproduced in Lässig and Muller, *Die Zahnheilkunde*, fig. 88.

56. Reproduced in J.J. Pindborg and L. Marvitz, *The Dentist in Art* (Chicago, 1960), pp. 102-03.

57. *Capricho* no. 33.

58. *Le charivari*, September 12, 1845.

59. By Vernier, Lässig and Muller, *Die Zahnheilkunde*, fig. 333.

60. *Il fischietto*, November 16, 1854.

61. *Il fischietto*, 1858.

62. *Frankfurter Laterne*, June 30, 1863.

63. Pindborg and Marvitz, *Dentist in Art*, pp. 116-17.

64. For twentieth-century examples, see Erich Heinrich, *Der Zahnarzt in der Karikatur* (Munich, 1963), figs. 102-14.

65. *La semana comica*, Managua, Edicion Especial, July 19, 1986.

66. Döes, "A Traveller's Tribulations: The French Dentist and the English Tooth," pirated in *Pick-Me-Up*, August 11, 1894, p. 291; reproduced in Kunzle, *History of the Comic Strip II*, figs. 15-69.

67. It was common practice, in order to extract a rotten tooth, to use as a base of support a good neighboring tooth which cracked under the pressure.

68. Palmer Cox, "Dr. Denz und sein Patient," *Schnedderedengg* (New York), March 20, 1877.

69. For instance in *La caricature*, June 12, 1880, an issue dedicated wholly to the dentist.

70. Ragut, "Histoire véridique de M. Isidore Coquerel et de sa dent," *Le charivari*, May 19, 1853.

71. Nadar, "Le Mal de Dents: Molaire arrachée à Cruickshank" [sic], *Journal pour Rire*, February 14, 1851, and *Petit journal pour rire* 4 (1856); "Zahnschmerzen," *Illustrirte Welt* 2 (1860), reduced to 28 scenes.

72. "Über Frankreich und die französiche Bühne," 1837. Passage transcribed by Greve, *Aphorismen*, pp. 50-53, and in Heinrich Heine, *Historischkritische Gesamtausgabe der Werke*, ed. Manfred Windfuhr (Hamburg, 1980), 5, 12/1, pp. 233-34.

73. F.M. Howarth, "Toothache and Terror," *Puck*, November 2, 1892, p. 172.

74. F.M. Howarth, "Dr. Twister's Device . . . ," *Puck*, October 31, 1894, p. 176.

75. Cf. Kunzle, *History of the Comic Strip II*, ch. 11.

76. The captions were added in the 1868 and subsequent editions.

77. "Der gewandte, kunstreiche Barbier . . . ," in *Wilhem Busch Werke*, vol. 1, pp. 390ff.

78. The strip appeared in 1869-70, the year preceding the 1870-71 revolutions, in the *Petit journal comique* 34, and in *Paris comique* 44, with a large additional scene of a nightmare that further demonizes the dentist. The American copy was entitled "The Tragic Story of a Toothache," *Wild Oats* (November 1870).

79. G. Randon, "La dent creuse," *Le journal amusant*, May 30, 1874, no. 926.

80. William Rogers, *Manuel de l'hygiène dentaire* (Paris, 1845), p. 57. The author must be referring to the effects of venereal disease.

81. Philip Massinger, *Parliament of Love* (1624), quoted in Leo Kanner, *Folklore of the Teeth* (New York, 1928), p. 110.

82. Thomas F. Crane, ed., *The Exempla . . . of Jacques de Vitry* (1890; New York, 1971), 247, p. 238. The motif also appears in Boccaccio, *Decameron*, 7.9, where the wife draws her husband's tooth with her own hand.

83. Cham (pseud. Amédée de Noé), *Les aventures de Monsieur Beaucoq* (Paris: Arnauld de Vresse, 1856). The same motif in Gavarni, *Les maris vengés* series, no. 10.

84. Victor Hugo, *Les Misérables*, trans. and with an intro. by Norman Denny (1862; Harmondsworth, 1980), pt. 1, bk. 5, ch. 10, p. 177.

85. Howard Vincent, *Daumier and His World* (Evanston, Ill., 1968), p. 162.

BIBLIOGRAPHY

Brown, Christopher, *Scenes of Everyday Life: Dutch Genre Painting in the Seventeenth Century*. London, 1984.

Greve, H. Christian, *Aphorismen zur Kulturgeschichte der Zahnheilkund und des ärtzlichen Standes*. Leipzig, 1930.

Kunzle, David, *History of the Comic Strip II: The Nineteenth Century*. Berkeley: University of California Press, 1989.

Lässig, Heinz and Rainer A. Muller, *Die Zahnheilkunde in Kunst und Kulturgeschichte*. Cologne, 1983.

Proskauer, Curt and Fritz Witt, *A Pictorial History of Dentistry*. Cologne, 1962.

Ring, Malvin E., *Dentistry: An Illustrated History*. New York, 1985.

*Tot lering en vermaak*. Exhibition catalogue. Amsterdam, 1976.

Wasserfuhr, Maria Elisabeth, *Der Zahnarzt in der niederländenischen Malerei des 17. Jhdts* (Dissertation 1970). 2d ed. Cologne: Arbeiten der Forschungsstelle des Instituts fur Geschichte der Universität Köln), vol. 1, 1977.

zone

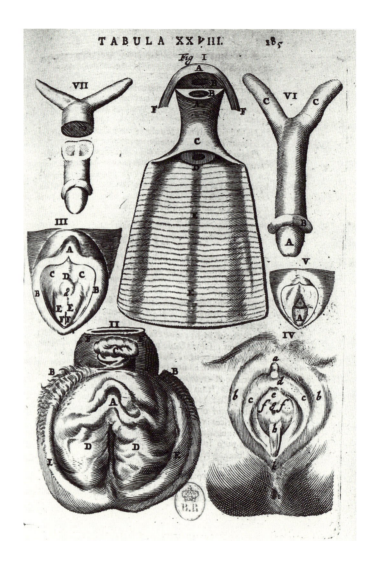

From Thomas Bartholinus, *Anatomia ex Caspari Bartholini parentis institionibus*, Lyon, 1651 (Paris, Bibliothèque nationale).

# "Amor Veneris, vel Dulcedo Appeletur"

*Thomas W. Laqueur*

"If it is permissible to give names to things discovered by me, it should be called the love or sweetness of Venus," urged one of the great and immodest anatomical explorers of the Renaissance. Like Adam, he claimed the privilege of naming what he had been the first to see: that which was "preeminently the seat of women's delight."[1] This Columbus, not Christopher but Renaldus, announced with much fanfare in 1559 that he had discovered the clitoris. ("O my America, my new found land!")

In 1905 Sigmund Freud rediscovered the clitoris, or in any case the clitoral orgasm, by inventing its vaginal counterpart. After four hundred, perhaps even two thousand years, there was all of a sudden a second place postulated from which women derived sexual pleasure. In 1905, for the first time, a doctor claimed that there were two kinds of orgasm and that the vaginal sort was the expected norm among adult women.

Both discoveries were and are controversial. Columbus's colleagues disputed his claim to precedence, arguing that the organ about which he made such a fuss either had been discovered by someone else or had been common knowledge since Antiquity. Freud's discovery generated an immense polemical and clinical literature. More ink has been spilled, I suspect, about the clitoris than about any other organ, or at least about any organ its size.[2]

I shall not enter directly into these controversies. Instead I want to sketch the history of the clitoris in Western, predominantly medical, literature in order to make two points. In the first place, prior to 1905 no one thought that there was any other kind of female orgasm than the clitoral sort. It is well and accurately described in hundreds of learned and more popular medical texts as well as in a burgeoning pornographic literature. Thus, it simply is not true that, as Robert Scholes has argued,

91

there has been "a semiotic coding that operates to purge both texts and language of things [the clitoris as the primary organ of woman's sexual delight] that are unwelcome to men." The clitoris, like the penis, was for two millennia both "precious jewel" and sexual organ, a connection not "lost or mislaid" through the ages, as Scholes would have it, but only — if then — since Freud.[3] To put it differently, Masters and Johnson's revelation that female orgasm is almost entirely clitoral would have been a commonplace to every seventeenth-century midwife and had been anticipated in considerable detail by nineteenth-century investigators. For some reason, a great amnesia in this matter descended on scientific circles around 1900 so that hoary truths could be hailed as earth-shatteringly new in the second half of the twentieth century.

My second point is that there is nothing natural about how the clitoris is construed. It is not self-evidently the female penis nor is it self-evidently opposed to the vagina. Nor have men always regarded clitoral orgasm as absent, threatening or unspeakable because of some primordial male fear of, or fascination with, female sexual pleasure. The history of the clitoris is part of the history of sexual difference generally and of the socialization of the body's pleasures. Like the history of masturbation, it is a story as much about sociability as about sex.

### Freud and History's Clitoris

"If we are to understand how a little girl turns into a woman," Freud writes in the third of his epochal *Three Essays on the Theory of Sexuality*, "we must follow the further vicissitudes of [the] excitability of the clitoris." During puberty, so the story goes, there occurs in boys "an accession of libido," while in girls there is "a fresh wave of repression in which it is precisely clitoroidal sexuality that is effected." The development of women as cultural beings is thus marked by what seems to be a physiological process: "what is overtaken by repression is a piece of masculine machinery."[4]

Like a Bahktiari tribesman in search of fresh pastures, female sexuality is said to migrate from one place to another, from the "male-like" clitoris to the unmistakably female vagina. The clitoris, according to Freud, does not, however, entirely lose its functions as a result of pleasure's short but significant journey. Rather, it becomes the organ *through which* excitement is transmitted to the "adjacent female sexual parts," to its permanent home, to the true locus of a woman's erotic life, to the vagina. The clitoris, in Freud's less than illuminating simile, becomes "like pine shavings," used "in order to set a log of harder wood on fire."[5]

This unlikely and strangely inappropriate identification of the cavity of the vagina with a hot log is not my concern here. Stranger still is the tension between the biological and the cultural claims of Freud's famous essay. A little girl's realization that she does not have a penis and that her sexuality resides in its supposed opposite, in the cavity of the vagina, elevates a "biological fact" into the cornerstone of culture. He writes as if he has discovered the basis in anatomy for the entire nineteenth-century world of gender. In an age obsessed with being able to justify and distinguish the social roles of women and men, science seems to have found in the radical difference of the penis and vagina not just a sign of sexual difference but its very foundation. "When erotogenic susceptibility to stimulation has been successfully transferred by a woman from the clitoris to the vaginal orifice, it implies that she has adopted a new leading zone for the purposes of her later sexual activity."[6]

In fact, Freud goes even further by suggesting that the repression of female sexuality in puberty, marked by its abandonment of the clitoris, heightens male desire and thus tightens the web of heterosexual union on which reproduction, the family and, indeed, civilization itself appear to rest: "The intensification of the brake upon sexuality brought about by pubertal repression in women serves as a stimulus to the libido of men and causes an increase in its activity."[7] When everything has settled down, the "masculine machinery" of the clitoris is abandoned, the vagina is erotically charged, and the body is set for reproductive intercourse. Freud seems to be taking a stab at universal historical bio-anthropology, to be making the claim that female modesty incites male desire while female acquiescence, in eventually allowing it to be gratified, lies at the very foundation of humanity's journey from the savage's cave.

Perhaps this is pushing one paragraph too hard, but in the passages I have quoted Freud is very much in the imaginative footsteps of Diderot, for example, who argues that civilization, and with it the family, began when women began to discriminate, to limit their availability. Possessing them, being the preferred one, loomed up as supreme happiness; monogamy and marriage became the price paid by men to once again gain access:

> Then, when the veils that modesty cast over the charms of women allowed an inflamed
> imagination the power to dispose of them at will, the most delicate illusions competed

zone

with the most exquisite of senses to exaggerate the happiness of the moment; the soul was possessed with an almost divine enthusiasm; two hearts lost in love vowed themselves to each other forever, and heaven heard the first indiscreet oaths.[8]

Freud is not quite so explicit in the *Three Essays* but he does appear to be arguing that femininity, and thus the place of women in society, is grounded in the developmental neurology of the female genitals.

He cannot, however, really have meant this. In the first place, history would have shown him that the vagina fails miserably as a "natural symbol" of interior sexuality, of passivity, of the private against the public, of a critical stage in the ontogeny of woman. In the one-sex model that dominated anatomical thinking for two millennia, woman was understood as man inverted. The uterus was the female scrotum, the ovaries were testicles, the vulva a foreskin, and *the vagina was a penis*. This account of sexual difference, though as phallocentric as Freud's, offered no real female interior, only the displacement inward to a more sheltered space of the male organs, as if the scrotum and penis in the form of uterus and vagina had taken cover from the cold.[9]

Freud may not have been aware of this arcane history. But he must have known that there was absolutely no anatomical or physiological evidence for the claim that "erotogenic susceptibility to stimulation" is successfully transferred during the maturation of women "from the clitoris to the vaginal orifice." The abundance of specialized nerve endings in the clitoris and the relative impoverishment of the vagina had been demonstrated half a century before Freud wrote and had been known in outline for hundreds of years. Common medical knowledge available in any nineteenth-century handbook thus makes a farce of Freud's story if it is construed as a narrative of biology. And, finally, if the advent of the vaginal orgasm was the consequence of neurological processes, then Freud's question of "how a woman develops out of a child with bisexual dispositions" could be resolved by physiology without any help from psychoanalysis.

Freud's answer, therefore, must be a narrative of culture in anatomical disguise. The story of the clitoris is a parable of culture, of how the body is forged into a shape usable by civilization despite, not because of, itself. The language of biology gives this tale its rhetorical authority but does not describe a deeper reality in nerves and flesh.

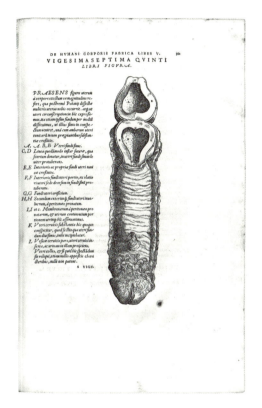

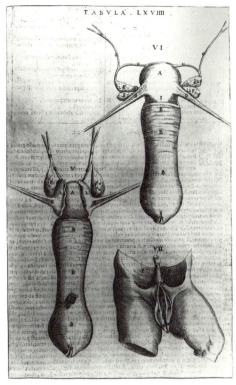

From Vesalius, *De humani corporis fabrica*,
Bâle, 1543 (Paris, Bibliothèque nationale).

From Vidus Vidius, *Artis medicinalis*, bk. 7,
"De anatome," Venice, 1611
(Paris, Bibliothèque nationale).

Freud, in short, must have known that he was inventing vaginal orgasm and that he was at the same time giving a radical new meaning to the clitoris. Richard von Krafft-Ebing may have anticipated him a bit when in the 1890s he wrote that "the erogenous zones in women are, while she is a virgin, the clitoris, and, after defloration, the vagina and cervix uteri." But this is in the context of a discussion of a variety of erogenous zones; immediately following is the observation that "the nipple particularly seems to possess this [erogenous] quality." Krafft-Ebing, like many of his contemporaries, believed that the "normally developed mentally and well-bred" woman's sexual desires were small. He also regarded woman's supposed sexual passivity (a synecdoche for her passivity in public life) as embedded in "her sexual organization."[10]

But neither he, nor anyone else, drew social consequences from the distinction between vaginal and clitoral eroticism. There was, in fact, no evidence in any of the contemporary literature for the sort of vaginal sexuality Freud postulates. On the other hand, there was also no interest in denying it. The stark contrasts that appear below are the result of a historical juxtaposition of texts. Authorities in France, Germany and England during Freud's time and stretching back to the early seventeenth century were unanimous in holding that female sexual pleasure originated in the structures of the vulva generally and in the clitoris specifically. No alternative sites were canvassed.

The major English language medical encyclopedia of Freud's day begins the "Clitoris" subheading of a lengthy and up-to-date entry on "Sexual Organs, Female" by citing the Viennese anatomist and philologist Joseph Hyrtl's derivation of the word "clitoris" from a Greek verb meaning "to titillate" and his observation that these etymological roots are reflected in the German colloquial term *kitzler* ("tickler").[11] Its anatomy is presented as the homologue of the penis, although the clitoris's nervous supply is "far greater, in proportion to its size." Indeed,

> its cutaneous investment is supplied with special nerve endings, which give it remarkable and special sensitivity.... At the base of the papillae are the endings which Krause believes to be related to the peculiar sensibility of the organ and has named corpuscles of sexual pleasure [*Wollustkörperchen*]. They are usually called genital corpuscles.[12]

On the other hand, the upper and middle portions of the vagina are enervated by "the same sources as the uterus." It is "not very sensitive"; indeed, the anterior wall is so *insensitive* that it "can be operated on without much pain to the patient."[13] This may be hyperbole but it suggests that to nineteenth-century authorities the vagina was an unlikely candidate for the primary locus of sexual pleasure in women.

No one took it to be such. Freud's contemporary, the gynecologist E.H. Kisch, for example, cites Victor Hensen's article on the physiology of reproduction in Hermann's authoritative *Handbuch der Physiologie* (1881) to the effect that direct stimulation of sexual feeling is via the dorsal nerve of the penis and the clitoris. Kisch then notes that sexual pleasure in women is due chiefly to friction on the clitoris through the intromitted penis that stimulates the nerve fibers connected to Krause's genital corpuscles (the *Wollustkörperchen*).[14]

The major French medical reference work of the late nineteenth century describes the clitoris as an erectile organ situated at the upper end of the vulva which has the same structure as the corpus cavernosum of the penis, the same erotic functions, but lacks a urethra.[15] The vagina, on the other hand, is defined simply as the passage from the vulva to the uterus which serves to evacuate the menses, contain the male organ during copulation and expel the product of fecundation. Most of the article is devoted to its pathologies.[16]

As early as 1844, with the publication of Georg Ludwig Kobelt's massively documented *The Male and Female Organs of Sexual Arousal in Man and Some Other Mammals*,[17] the anatomy of genital pleasure was firmly established. Kobelt, first of all, devised a technique for injecting the vasculature of the clitoris so that an organ notoriously difficult to study in postmortem material could be readily examined. He then proceeded to describe its structure and function in exquisite detail and concluded, based on the clitoris's erectile tissues, blood and nerve supply, that the *glans cliteroides* was the primary locus of sexual arousal in both humans and other mammals and the precise homologue of the male organ, the glans of the penis. (Kobelt distinguished the passive male and female organs, i.e., the glans of the penis and clitoris, from the active organs, i.e., the shafts of these structures.)

Kobelt's work is based on great learning in human and comparative anatomy. In marsupials, for example, where the glans of the penis is divided in two, so is the glans of the clitoris. The two knobs and the distinct coronal rim of the stallion's *glans penis* is also repeated in the mare's *glans cliteroides*, etc. The glans of the clitoris

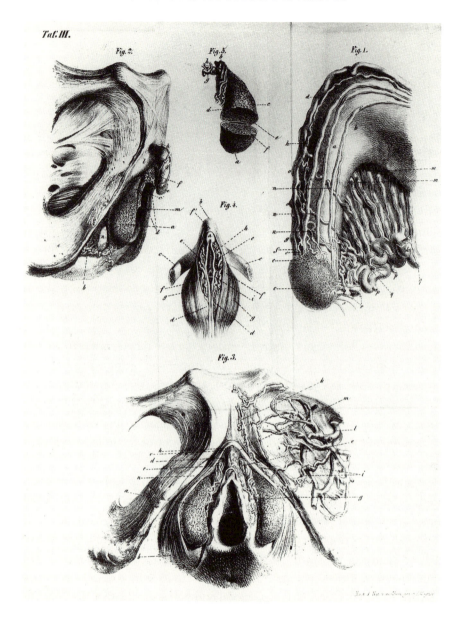

From G.L. Kobelt, *Die Männlichen und Weiblichen*
*Wollusts-Organe des Menschen und verschiedene Saugetiere*, 1844
(Paris, Bibliothèque nationale).

Figure 1: The human clitoris, enlarged, seen from the left.
Figure 2: The passive female sex organs seen from the right, with
superficial structures dissected away.
Figure 3: The pelvis and vestibular bulbs, viewed from the front.
Figure 4: The vestibular bulbs.
Figure 5: The vestibular bulb, seen from the left.

of humans is, however, comparatively much more densely innervated than the glans
of the penis, because the two branches of the dorsal nerve are relatively three to
four times larger there.[18]

The function of all this machinery is of course to make possible sexual pleasure, which in the case of women will make them want to have intercourse despite
the dangers of pregnancy and trials of motherhood. Its physiology is described in
clinical detail:

> When outside stimuli come into contact with the glans of the clitoris, then the blood
> which is causing the *bulbus* to swell, by way of the reflex spasms of the *musculus con-*
> *strictor cunni*, is propelled through the exposed *pars intermedia* into the glans, now ready
> for the stimulus; and thereby the purpose of the entire passive apparatus (the sensation
> of sexual pleasure) is achieved. The sexually pleasurable titillation increases with con-
> tinuing stimulation up to its final transformation into indifference [i.e., orgasm], and
> return to the usual quiescent state of the affected parts. The process is further supported
> by the same sort of auxiliary means as in the male.[19]

The vagina, Kobelt thinks, is so well known that it warrants no extended description.
But he nevertheless pauses to point out that it plays a minimal role in genital orgasm:

> The small number of nerves which, singly, make their way down into the voluminous
> vaginal tube puts the vagina so far behind the glans — small but very rich in nerves — that
> we can grant the vagina no part in the creation of the specific pleasurable sex feeling in
> the female body.[20]

Kobelt's book was by far the most detailed account of the clitoris ever published
but it did not radically revise established views. The major early nineteenth-century
French medical encyclopedia came to roughly the same conclusions. "Clitoris," it
says, derives from the Greek verb *kleitoriazein*, meaning to touch or titillate lasciviously, to be inclined to pleasure. A synonym is *oestrus veneris*, a sort of frenzy of sexual passion. The clitoris is like the penis in form and structure and "enjoys an
exquisite sensibility," which makes it highly susceptible to "abuse." For example,
the author of this entry disapproves strongly of titillating the clitoris, as some colleagues recommend, to cure certain nervous disorders like catalepsy. Although unac-
knowledged, it was a therapy derived from a famous case of Galen's in which a widow,
laboring under a purported backup of "semen," suffered from backaches and other
pains until the pressure was relieved by a midwife who rubbed her genitals. A sub-

sequent entry on "Clitorisme," the female equivalent of masturbation, discusses further abuses which this site of pleasure invites.[21]

In the "Vagine" entry, on the other hand, its subject is defined as the "cylindrical and elastic passage from the uterus to the external parts." There follows a short discussion of nomenclature which warns against confusing the vagina with the cervix, that is, the part which used to be called "the neck of the womb," but includes no discussion of its innervation or erotic functions.[22]

These articles from the early nineteenth century refer in turn to a seventeenth-century text by François Mauriceau, one of the luminaries of French obstetrics. He notes that the clitoris is

> where the Author of Nature has placed the seat of voluptuousness — as He has in the glans of the penis — where the most exquisite sensibility is located, and where he placed the origins of lasciviousness in women.[23]

Indeed the pudendum more generally has the capacity to engender extraordinary delight because the nerves that supply the clitoris supply it too.[24]

Mauriceau, after describing for almost six pages the clitoris's muscles, nerves and vasculature, concludes that it functions just like the penis. Like the penis, it becomes erect from the retention of "blood and spirits"; its glans, like the glans of the penis, is the site of the "pleasures [douceurs] of Venus and the agreeable sensitivity one encounters in sexual congress." Like the penis, the clitoris gives pleasure when rubbed.[25]

The vagina is a far duller organ. It is the tube leading from the uterus to the outside, "a slack canal [mol et lâche] which during coition embraces the penis." Only the glands near its outer end are relevant to sexual pleasure, because they pour out great quantities of a saline liquor during coition which increases the heat and enjoyment of women. These are the substances, Mauriceau suggests, to which Galen was referring when he spoke of needing to use other means to cause their release when the caresses of a man were not available.[26]

The history of the clitoris can be pushed back. In 1612, three years before "clitoris" was first used in English, a French doctor discusses the organ and the word in great detail. "Cleitoris," he says, is known by many Latin names, including Columbus's neologism. As for the vernaculars,

> In French it is called temptation, the spur to sensual pleasure, the female rod and the scorner of men: and women who will admit their lewdness call it their great joy [En

François elle dite tentation, aiguillon de volupté, verge feminine, le mespris des hommes: et les femmes qui font profession d'impudicité la nomment leur *gaude mihi*].[27]

Duval echoes the certainties and tensions of both later and also earlier accounts. On the one hand, the clitoris is the organ of sexual pleasure in women. On the other, its easy responsiveness to touch makes it difficult to domesticate for reproductive, heterosexual intercourse. This was Freud's problem, and I will return to it in the last section of this essay.

Freud may not have been aware of the detailed history of genital anatomy I have just recounted but it is impossible that he would not have known what was in the standard reference books of his day. He was, after all, especially interested in zoology during his medical student days and was an expert neurologist. Furthermore, one did not have to be a scientist to know about clitoral sexuality. Walter, the protagonist of *My Secret Life*, notes in his review of the copulative organs that the clitoris is an erectile organ which is "the chief seat of pleasure in a woman."[28] Nicholas Venette's *Tableau de l'amour conjugal*, first published in the late seventeenth century, translated and republished in many languages and in innumerable editions and still popular in the nineteenth century (the pharmacist's son in *Madame Bovary* consults it), remarks that in the clitoris "nature has placed the seat of pleasure and lust, as it has on the other hand in the glans of a man...; there is lechery and lasciviousness established."[29] And, of course, Freud himself points out that biology has been "obliged to recognize the female clitoris as a true substitute for the penis," though it does not follow from this, as Freud seems to think, that children recognize that "all human beings have the same (male) form of genital," or that little girls therefore suffer penis envy because their genital is so small.[30]

Freud, in short, must have known that what he wrote in the language of biology regarding the shift of erotogenic sensibility from the clitoris to the vagina had no basis in the facts of anatomy or physiology. Both the migration of female sexuality and the opposition between the vagina and penis must therefore be understood as representations, namely, something made to present a social ideal in another form. On a formal level the opposition of the vagina and penis represents an ideal of parity. The social thuggery which takes a polymorphously perverse infant and bullies it into a heterosexual man or woman finds an organic correlative in the body, in the opposition of the sexes and their organs. Perhaps because Freud is the great theorist of sexual ambiguity he is also the inventor of a dramatic sexual antithesis: that between the embarrassing clitoris that girls abandon and the vagina whose erotogenic powers they embrace as the mark of the mature woman.[31]

More generally, what might loosely be called patriarchy may have appeared to Freud as the only possible way to organize the relations between the sexes, leading him to write as if its signs in the body (external active penis versus internal passive vagina) were "natural." But in Freud's question of how it is that "a woman develops out of a child with a bisexual disposition," the word "woman" clearly refers not to "natural" sex, but to "theatrical" gender, to socially defined roles.[32] As Gayle Rubin puts it, gender is "a socially imposed division of the sexes," the "product of the social relations of sexuality." The supposed opposition of men and women, "exclusive gender identity," in Rubin's terms, "far from being an expression of natural differences... is the suppression of natural similarities."[33]

Indeed, if structuralism has taught us anything, it is that humans impose their sense of opposition on a world of continuous shades of difference and similarity. In nearly all of North America, to use Lévi-Strauss's example, sage brush (Artemisia) plays "a major part in the most diverse rituals as the opposite of other plants: 'Solidaga,' 'Chrysothamnus,' 'Gutierrezia.' " It stands for the feminine in Navaho ritual while "Chrysothamnus" stands for the masculine, which does not follow from features of these plants readily detected by the outsider.[34] Their differences or similarities, like Freud's, are in the most immediate sense "man-made."

This is not the place to give and defend a structuralist reading of Freud generally. Yet *Civilization and Its Discontents* bears the most poignant reminders of the processes Lévi-Strauss describes. Civilization, like a conquering people, subjects "another one to its exploitation," proscribes "manifestations of sexual life in children," makes "heterosexual genital love" the only permitted sort, and in so doing takes the infant, "an animal organism with (like others) an unmistakably bisexual disposition," and forces it into the mold of *either* a man or a woman.[35] The power of culture thus represents itself in bodies, and forges them, as on an anvil, into the required shape.

Freud's myth of sexuality's migration, his invention of the vaginal orgasm that supplants a clitoral orgasm appropriate to an earlier developmental stage, is so powerful precisely because it is not a story of biology. What Rosalind Coward has called in another context "ideologies of appropriate desires and orientations" must struggle – one hopes unsuccessfully – to find their signs in the flesh.[36] Freud's argument, flying as it does in the face of three centuries of anatomical knowledge, is a testament to the freedom with which the authority of nature can be rhetorically appropriated to legitimize the creations of culture.

## Did Columbus Discover the Clitoris?

Even if he was not the first anatomist to do so, there seems little question that in 1559 Columbus saw and described the clitoris. But then the other Columbus is said to have discovered America sixty-seven years earlier and his claim rests upon visiting a continent which he took to be Japan, which had been visited by other Europeans centuries before and which was populated by the descendants of much earlier explorers from Asia. Renaldus Columbus's claim is just as complicated.

"This, most gentle reader, is that: preeminently the seat of women's delight," he announced. Is what? His initial mapping is unfamiliar: "These protuberances, emerging from the uterus near that opening which is called the mouth of the womb [*Processus igitur ab utero exorti id foramen, quod os matricis vocatur*]...." But the clitoris we know today does not emerge from the mouth of the *matrix*, whatever that might be. What follows – I quote it in full including passages I have already mentioned – is even more curious:

> ...[that] preeminently [is] the seat of women's delight; while they engage in sexual activity [*venerem*], not only if you rub it vigorously with a penis, but touch it even with a little finger, semen swifter than air flows this way and that on account of the pleasure even with them unwilling. If you touch that part of the uterus while women are eager for sex and very excited as if in a frenzy and aroused to lust [and] they are eager for a man, you will find it a little harder and oblong to such a degree that it shows itself a sort of male member. Therefore, since no one else has discerned these projections and their working, if it is permissible to give names to things discovered by me, it should be called the love or sweetness of Venus [... *illa praecipue sedes est delectionis mulierum, dum venerem exercent, quam non modo si mentula confricabis, vel minimo digito attrectabis, ocyus aura semen hac atque illac pre voluptate vel illis invitis profluet. Hanc eadem uteri partem dum venerem appetunt mulieres, [et] tanquam oestro percitae virum appetunt, ad libidinem concitatae: si attingues, duriusculam et oblongam redditam esse comperies: adeo ut nescio quam virilis mentulae speciem prae se ferat. Hos igitur, processus atque eorundum usum cum nemo*

*hactenus animadverterit, si nomina rebus a me inventis imponere licet, amor Veneris, vel dulcedo appelletur].* [37]

He again calls the organ he is describing here "that part of the uterus" and a third time refers to "those projections" or "processes" which he had earlier described as "coming out of the mouth of the uterus." The reference seems indeed to be specifically the vagina's "prepuce," the outer skin of the female penis long recognized and erotically linked to pudendal pleasure. Columbus does not seem to be describing a newly discovered female penis. In any case, his nomenclature is decidedly odd and imprecise. His organ may be the clitoris but it is not the clitoris of modern anatomy.

Because Columbus claims to be discovering the female penis, his account is also unabashedly homoerotic. If the male penis or even the male finger is rubbed against the female, penis semen – presumably hers – flies this way, even though one would think that his would, under the circumstances, also fly. In any case, the ancient homologies are maintained. In the classical one-sex model some other parts of the female anatomy – parts that we would call the cervix, vagina and vulva – are the female penis against which the male's rubs. In Columbus's version a new external female penis is the partner object of the male.

Woman is submerged in the next sentence as well. In one of the few instances in which *mulieres* (women) are the grammatical subject, in the temporal clause they are literally surrounded by desire. *Appetent* (from *appetere*, to be eager for) is repeated to flank *mulieres* (women); the redundant predicate adjectives, *percitae* (from *percire*, to arouse) and *concitae* (from *concitare*, to stir up or excite), attest further to her sexual arousal. But then the sentence takes an unexpected turn and the scientifically objective, presumably male, reader is told that the part of the female anatomy in question will become hard and oblong if touched. (A finger or a penis will do to make her "semen [flow] swifter than air.")[38]

Columbus is clearly not briefing a case for clitoral as opposed to vaginal sexuality. The interest in this disjuncture is entirely Freud's. Rather, he and his contemporaries imagine a cascade of pleasure from the inside out. The cervix, he says, has circular folds so that during intercourse it "may embrace and suck out the virile member"; these folds cause the friction "from which lovers experience wonderful pleasure." Further along, "at the end of the cervix, approaching the vulva," there are several little pieces of flesh and by these as well "pleasure or delight in intercourse is not a little increased." Then finally comes the clitoris.[39]

The simultaneous presence of both an interior and an exterior female penis, both subject to erection, pleasure and ejaculation did not disturb Columbus or other sixteenth- and seventeenth-century writers. To the contrary, it provided a second register on which to play the old tune of hierarchical ordering of two genders in the one flesh. Columbus himself and his contemporaries remained committed to the old notions that women had the same organs as men, and that these organs functioned roughly in the same way.

A more popular literature echoes these views. Jane Sharp's self-consciously commonsensical midwifery guide asserts on one page that the vagina, "which is the passage for the yard, resembleth it turned inward," while two pages later, with no apparent embarrassment, she reports that the clitoris is the female penis. "It will stand and fall as the yard doth and makes women lustful and take delight in copulation." And, with the usual credit given pleasure: "were it not for this they would have no desire nor delight, nor would they conceive."[40] Perhaps Sharp would resolve the dilemma of the two female penises by saying that the vagina only *resembles* a penis while the clitoris actually is one. But she is unworried by the problem.

Sharp was, moreover, as undisturbed by ambiguity as by contradiction. Thus, the fact that the labia fit nicely into both systems of homologies and functioned as the foreskin for both the vagina and the clitoris unasked the question of which one was the true female penis. Indeed, both could be regarded as erectile organs. The reader of another midwifery manual was told that "the action of the clitoris is like that of the yard, which is erection" and that "the action of the neck of the womb [the vagina and cervix] is the same with that of the yard; that is to say, erection."[41]

There seemed to be no difficulty in holding that women had a topological inversion of the male penis within them, which embraced and sucked on the male member, and a morphological homologue without, which worked throughout reproductive adulthood in precisely the same way as the man's. The tip of the clitoris, argues Thomas Gibson, is called the *amoris dulcedo* or *oestrum veneris* because, like the glans of the penis, it is where the sweetness of love, the venereal frenzy, is most intensely felt.[42] Sixteenth- and seventeenth-century writers would have found very curious Helene Deutsch's notion that "the competition of the clitoris which intercepts the excitations unable to reach the vagina...create[s] the dispositional basis of permanent sexual inhibition," or Marie Bonaparte's contention that "clitoroidal women" suffer from one of the stages of frigidity or protohomosexuality.[43] Rather, as Nicholas Culpepper put it in 1675, "it is agreeable both to reason and authority, that the bigger the clitoris in a woman, the more lustful they are."[44] And lust, of course, was thought to be immediately relevant to the ultimate purpose of sexual intercourse: reproduction. It is "by stirring the clitoris [that] the imagination causeth the vessels to cast out that seed that lyeth deep in the body," explained Jane Sharp.[45] The erection of both penis and vagina, said another authority, is "for motion, and attraction of the seed."[46] Presumably the "spermatical vessels," the "handmaidens to the stones," as Philip Moore called them a century earlier, "carried the excitement from the external organs to the testes [what we would call ovaries] within."[47]

Columbus claims to have made a very precise discovery in the female reproductive anatomy while at the same time he remained rooted in a conceptual universe that contained no women, only a colder version of man. The controversy over precedence must be understood in this context. It was fraught with language inadequate to genital specificity, a language of the one-sex body in which corporeal difference threatened always to collapse into sameness. Barriers of gender, precariously imposed on one flesh, were consequently all the more important.

The absence of a standard anatomical nomenclature for the female genitals, and reproductive system generally, testifies, however, not to the haplessness of Renaissance anatomists but to the absence of an imperative to create incommensurable categories of male and female through words. The issue here is not the vast elaboration in most languages of terms for organs and functions that are risqué or shameful. The point is rather that until the late seventeenth century it is often impossible to determine, in medical texts, to which part of the female reproductive anatomy a particular term applies.[48] Language constrains the seeing of differences and sustains the male body as the canonical human form. And, conversely, in the one-sex model even the words for female parts ultimately refer to male organs. The post-eighteenth-century words – vagina, uterus, vulva, labia, clitoris – do not have their Renaissance equivalents.[49]

"It does not matter," says Columbus with more insight than he was perhaps aware, "whether you call [the womb] matrix, uterus or vulva."[50] And it does not seem to matter where one part stops and the other starts. He does not want to distinguish the true cervix — the "mouth of the womb" (*os matricis*) which from the outside "offers to your eyes...the image of a tenchfish or a dog newly brought to light," which in intercourse is "dilated with extreme pleasure," and which is "open during that time in which the woman emits seed" — from what we would call the vagina, "that part into which the penis [*mentula*] is inserted, *as it were*, into a sheath [*vagina*]."[51] (Note the metaphoric use of "vagina," the standard Latin word for scabbard, which was otherwise never used in the medical literature for the part to which it applies today.) But Columbus offers no other term for "our" vagina: he describes the labia minora as "protuberances [*processus*], emerging from the uterus near that opening which is called the mouth of the womb..." (the same location as the clitoris).[52] The precision Columbus sought to introduce by naming the true "mouth of the womb" *cervix* vanishes as the vaginal opening becomes the mouth of the womb and the clitoris one of its parts. The language simply does not exist, nor need exist, for distinguishing male from female organs clearly. The haze of one sex still hangs over genital differentiation.

This same sort of tension is evident in other anatomists. Fallopius is anxious to differentiate the cervix proper from the vagina but has no more specific name for it other than "female pudenda," a part of a general "hollow" (*sinus*). The Fallopian tubes, as he describes them, are not patent tubes that convey eggs from the ovaries to the womb but rather hollow twin protuberances of sinews (*neruei*) that penetrate the peritoneum, without seeming to have an opening into the uterus. Fallopius remains committed to a male-centered system and, despite his revolutionary rhetoric, assumes the commonplace that "all parts that are in men are present in women."[53]

Caspar Bauhin (1560-1624), professor of anatomy and botany in Basel, sought to clear up the nomenclature but with an equal lack of success because one sex was too deeply embedded in language. He begins, from a modern perspective, promisingly, "Everything pertaining to the female genitalia is comprehended in the term 'of nature' [*phuseos*], and the obscene term cunt [*cunnus*]." Clear enough. But then Bauhin informs his readers that some ancient writers called the male genitalia *phuseos* as well. Among the terms he offers for the labia is the Greek *mutocheila*, meaning snout, with its obvious phallic connection, or more explicitly translated, "penile lips." (The latter is the more likely sense in an age whose greatest anatomist could regard the cervix as an erectile organ.)[54]

The conflation of labia into foreskin, of female into male, is however much older. A tenth-century Arabic writer, for example, points out that the interior of the vagina "possesses prolongations of skin called the lips" which are "the analogue of the prepuce in men and has as its function to protect the matrix against cold air."[55] For Mondinus, author of the major medieval anatomy text, the labia become a bifurcated foreskin:

> They [the labia] hinder entrance of air and external matter into the neck of the womb or bladder as the skin of the prepuce guardeth the penis. Therefore...Haly Abbas calleth them *praputia matricis* [prepuce of the uterus, of the vagina?].[56]

Likewise in Barengario's text, a major Renaissance illustrated expansion of Mondino, *nymphae* refers to both the foreskin of the penis *and* the foreskin of the vagina, i.e., the labia minora.[57] John Pechy, a popular English writer during the Restoration, revises this trope to accommodate the new female penis so that the "wrinkeled membranous production cloath the clitoris [not the vagina] like a foreskin."[58]

Much of the controversy around who "discovered" the clitoris arose out of precisely this sort of blurring of metaphorical and linguistic boundaries that, in turn, were the consequence of a model of sexual difference in which unambiguous names for the female genitals did not matter. A web of words, already pregnant with a theory of sexual difference or sameness, thus limited how genital organs would be seen and discussed. There were no terms in the Renaissance for what, since the eighteenth century, have been construed as essential signs in the body of incommensurable difference. The boundaries of organs themselves and what could be known about them constrained and were constrained by the openness of the language in which they could be thought.

Who then discovered the "clitoris"? Fallopius says he was the first to see the organ and makes much of it. After trying to straighten out the terminological confusion between vagina and cervix he announces "but these are trivial matters; weightier things to follow":

> This genital [clitoris], because it is concealed among the fatter parts of the pubis, it therefore is hidden even from the anatomists and thus I was the first who detected that same thing in previous years and any others who speak or write about this, *be assured that they*

*learned of the thing itself either from me or from my followers.* You will find the outermost gland of this penis ["*penis*," not the more common word "*mentula*"] straightaway in the upper part of the outer genitals itself where the "wings" [i.e., the labia minora] are joined or where they begin.[59] (Emphasis added.)

This seems straightforward enough: Fallopius says he saw it first. But even though Fallopius advertises his skills and his precedence, he elsewhere shifts to the rhetoric of a Renaissance humanist tracing a word or idea back to classical Antiquity. Like Copernicus he wants to proclaim both his originality *and* his rootedness in tradition:

> ...in book 3, section 21 [of the *Canon*], Avicenna mentions something situated in a certain part of the female genitals that he calls a penis [*virga*] or *albathara*. Albucasis in book 2, section 1, terms this part the penis [*tentigenem*, literally tenseness] which is accustomed sometimes to come to such an increase that women having this can copulate with others as if they were men.[60]

Fallopius then goes on to say that the Greeks called the structure in question *kleitoris*, from which the "lewd verb, 'to touch the clitoris'," is derived. "Our anatomists," he laments, have neglected it. Such neglect might justify the detailed description which I quoted earlier but scarcely the aggressive claim of priority. Two professional imperatives seem to be at war here: the anatomist's desire for personal glory through besting his contemporaries, immediate predecessors and the ancients, and the humanist's concern for recovering the classical past. In any case, it is difficult to say whether Fallopius discovered the clitoris because by his own account he both did and did not.

Bartholinus, a major anatomist of the early seventeenth century, is similarly puzzled. How is it possible, he seems to be asking, that "Fallopius arrogates to himself the Invention or first Observation of this Part; and Columbus gloriously, as in other things he is wont, attributes it to himself," while the organ in question has been known to everyone from the second-century physicians Rufus of Ephesus and Julius Pollux to the Arabic anatomists Albucasis and Avicenna.[61]

A half century later Regnier De Graaf argues that Columbus had no right to name something that had been sighted, named and renamed by generations of anatomists stretching back to the Greeks. Hippocrates, he says, had called it *columnella*, little column, from the Greek *kios*; Avicenna named it *albatra* or *virga*, the rod; to Albucasis it was the *amoris dulcedo*, the sweetness of love; and to others still it was the *sedes libidinis*, seat of lust, the *irritamentum libidinis*, the goad to lust, the *oestrus Veneris*, the frenzy of Venus. It was known to still other ancient anatomists, he reports, as *nympha*, the water goddess.[62]

De Graaf missed some names. Julius Pollux, the second-century compiler of medical word lists, says that in the cleft of the female pudenda, "the throbbing bit of flesh in the middle is the *nymphē* or *myrton* [because it resembled a myrtle berry?] or *epidermis* or *kleitoris*."[63] Other terms in the literature include *tentigo*, tension; *cauda muliebris*, *coles muliebris*, or *mentula muliebris*, all versions of "woman's penis" since *cauda* means literally "tail" as did penis in its earliest usage, while *mentula* was the standard classical obscene term for the male organ. *Crista* [as in cockscomb] and *landica* occurred in nonmedical texts.[64]

But perhaps Columbus was not being quite as self-aggrandizing and wrongly dismissive of his predecessors as Bartholinus and De Graaf suggest. Since Antiquity there had obviously been a metaphorical association between the penis and what we would call the clitoris. But the latter's erotogenic power, which Columbus regards as its essence, had been far less explicitly recognized. And because of this, the various words listed above did not quite mean what "clitoris" meant after the sixteenth century.

I will at least try to brief a case for Columbus. In the first place, De Graaf was mistaken in attributing to classical or Arabic writers those terms — "sweetness of love," "venereal frenzy," "seat of lust," "spur of lust" — which referred, not to the structure, but to the function of the clitoris. With the possible exception of "spur of lust," all these terms were either first used by Columbus or derived from his description. Furthermore, although all modern translators and some ancient authorities tell us that terms like *nympha* and *tentigo* mean "clitoris," they were used in such a way as to obscure precisely *what* they meant.[65]

To be sure, some early uses seem wholly transparent. "Kleitoris" first appears in the verb form *kleitorizein* in Rufus of Ephesus (second century A.D.), who tells us that it means "to touch [the *nymphē*] lasciviously." Moreover, Hyrtl, philologist and professor of anatomy at the University of Vienna while Freud was there, explicitly notes that Rufus was not confusing the singular form of the noun with the plural *nymphae*, i.e., the labia minora: *nymphē* =the muscular piece of flesh in the midst, which some call the "hypodermis" and others the "kleitoris," Hyrtl says, citing Rufus.[66]

But when we consider how, for example, Galen uses the word *nymphē* it is apparent that he is not interested in the specificity of anatomical and erotic signification that would be commonplace after Columbus. The part called *nympha* (or *nymphē*), he writes, "gives the same sort of protection to the uteri that the uvula gives to the pharynx; for it covers the orifice of their neck by coming down into the female pudendum and keeps it from being chilled."[67] Perhaps the clitoris does resemble the uvula with which it is also linguistically related (see n.57). In addition, one can certainly make a case for the metaphorical connection in ancient texts between the vagina=*valvē*, i.e., an organ that breathes in and out, and the throat. But Galen's anatomy remains difficult to interpret. The clitoris does not come down into the pudendum to cover the mouth of the vagina. Moreover, Galen assigns the same function to the "outgrowths of skin at the ends of the two pudenda," that is, to the labia minora that also act as covers to keep the uterus warm.

Soranus, the great second-century gynecologist, has no more interest in the clitoris as an erectile, erotogenic organ: it, the *nymphē*, "is the origin of the two labia and by its nature it is a small piece of flesh almost like a muscle; and it has been called 'nymphē' because this piece of flesh hides like a bride."[68] But then so do the labia minora, which he does not distinguish by name and which are associated with nymphs because of their alleged function of directing the urine.

The same sort of muddle arises regarding the word *tentigo* as a putative synonym for clitoris in the translations of the Arab physician Albucasis. It comes from the verb *tendere*, meaning "to stretch"; as a noun it means "tenseness" or "lust" and was used in Antiquity to refer to an erect penis and even to an erect *landica*, in other words, clitoris.[69] Therefore, when Thomas Vicary, surgeon to Henry VIII, wrote in 1548 (before Columbus published his work) that the vulva "hath in the middest a Lazartus pannicle, which is called in Latin *tentigo*," the reference would seem to be unambiguous. *Tentigo* in early seventeenth-century English still bore the word's Latin meaning: "a tenseness or lust; an attack of priapism; an erection." The structure's location as Vicary describes it allows even less doubt that it is the clitoris. But when he reports on the functions of this part, its "two utilities," he seems to be discussing an entirely different organ. There is no mention of pleasure or sexual arousal: "The first [utility] is that by it goeth forth the urin, or else it should be shed throughout all the Vulva: The seconde is, that when a woman does set hir thies abrode, it altereth the ayre that commeth to the Matrix for to temper the heate." What the name led us to expect, a female penis, turns out to be a pair of workaday flaps, a dual purpose female foreskin.[70] But whatever Vicary means, it is impossible to translate across the chasm that divides his world from ours.

The nomenclature is finally straightened out in the generation after Columbus when *nymphae*, i.e., the plural of *nympha*, was first used by Adrianus Spigelius (1578-1625; the last of the great Vesalian line in the chair of anatomy at Padua) to mean what *nymphae* means today, the labia minora. Thus, right after a precise new erotic center is defined in women's bodies, language comes to articulate that definition. *Nymphae* and *clitoris*, "wings" and "rods," went their separate linguistic ways. By the early seventeenth century the term "clitoris" came to have its modern meaning: a female homologue of the penis which is the primary locus of sexual pleasure.[71]

Ironically, the first use of "clitoris" in English denies this. In 1615 Helkiah Crooke, an English anatomist of some note, argued against all sorts of male/female homologies — the Galenic assignment of the vagina as the female penis as well as the novel description of the clitoris in that role. The clitoris, he says, is not a penis because it does not have "a passage for the seede." It may seem that Crooke is here striking a blow against the epistemological basis of the entire one-sex model until one looks more carefully at his argument against the vagina being a penis. "Howsoever the necke of the wombe shall be inverted, yet it will never make the virile member." Why? Because "the yard consisteth of three hollow bodies," the "two hollow nerves" and a "common passage for seed and urine," while "the necke of the womb hath but one cavity." Clearly, "three hollow bodies cannot be made of one." Moreover "neither is the cavity of a man's yard so large and ample as that of the necke of the wombe." In short, the penis is not a vagina because it is thrice hollow or because it is not hollow enough![72]

Claude Duval in 1612 used the difference between the clitoris and the penis to establish the sex of a man mistaken for a woman and the great seventeenth-century specialist in legal medicine Paulo Zachias likewise distinguishes between the penis and the enlarged clitoris of some women on the basis of the latter's lack of a duct.[73] In 1779 the English surgeon John Hunter summed up the wisdom of two centuries by pointing out that precisely "the part common to both" was the sign of a person's true condition.[74]

But these sorts of arguments do not take away from Columbus's claim. Perhaps he did discover for medical science the organic source of the "sweetness of Venus." Or perhaps he did not. It does not matter — or it is difficult to say — because the dominant medical paradigm of his day held that there was only one sex anyway, differing only in the arrangement of a common set of organs. The problem in Colombus's day and well into the seventeenth century was not finding the organic signs of sexual opposition but understanding heterosexual desire in the world of one sex. Being sure that "jackdaw did not seek jackdaw," that "like did not seek like" as Aristotle had put it, took tremendous cultural resources. It was by no means certain that each time nature would "be to her bias drawn," that, as in the end of *Twelfth Night*, nature would swerve from a straight path and make sure that male and female would couple. The Renaissance shared this concern with Freud. But the clitoris was only a very small part of the problem, if a problem at all, when the entire female genitalia were construed as a version of the male's.

In much Renaissance writing about what might be called the social problem of the clitoris, the issue is making sure that women engage in sexual intercourse as befits their station and not as befits men. By the eighteenth century when the notion of two opposite sexes made heterosexual coupling natural — opposites attract — the problem of the clitoris became the same as that of the solitary penis: masturbation. The threat to society was solitude, not collapse into homoeroticism, which was, by now, more safely "against nature" in a reductionistic sort of way.

### The Clitoris as Social Problem

In Western Europe the most dramatic attack on the clitoris — clitorectomy or excision — was for practical purposes never undertaken until the notorious and quickly condemned antimasturbatory operations of the 1870s. The procedure was widely known, but only in the context of what *other* people did.

From Antiquity to at least the late nineteenth century it was thought that the clitoris of Egyptian women, and more generally of women in hot climates, grew preternaturally large. These unfortunate creatures suffered from what seems to have been conceived of as a racially and geographically specific clitoral hypertrophy that required surgical treatment.[75]

Not all classical reports of clitorectomy concern anatomical deformation. The

Greek geographer Strabo observes in his account of travels through North Africa and the eastern Mediterranean that Creophagi males "have their sexual glands mutilated and the women are excised in the Jewish fashion." He elsewhere noted that the Jews circumcised males and excised females, though he does not offer clitoral enlargement as the reason for these practices. Presumably, cultural factors instead were at work.[76]

The sixth-century Byzantine physician Aetius of Amida and Paulus Aegineta were more straightforwardly clinical in their allusions. Aetius discusses the *nymphae* in their pathological condition:

> This organ in some women attains such a size that it may eventually constitute a deformity and lead to a feeling of shame. And further, it is greatly irritated by constant contact with the clothing and stimulates venery and coitus. On that account it appeared feasible to the Egyptians to amputate the nympha before it became too large, especially before the marriageable virgins were to be assigned. The amputation is done in the following manner....

He then describes how the woman is to be seated, presumably leaning backward on a stool or small table. A young man supports her from behind with his arms under her knees thereby keeping her legs raised and apart. The surgeon takes hold of the offending flesh — which is presumably the covering of the clitoris and the labia minora — and excises them, being careful not to cut too deeply.[77]

Paulus, in describing the same operation, suggests that perhaps clitorectomy is not quite so routine nor so much an attack on excess female sexuality generally but, rather, that it is a measure to be used against women who cross gender boundaries in the sexual act. "In some women," he reports,

> the nympha is excessively large...insomuch that, as has been related, some women have had erections of this part like men, and also venereal desires of a like kind. Wherefore, having placed the women in a supine position, and seizing the redundant portion of the nympha in a forceps....[78]

He describes essentially the same procedure as does Aetius. However we interpret Paulus's clinical rationale, it is clear that clitorectomy was rejected in the West until the nineteenth century. Robert James, the compiler of a standard eighteenth-century medical encyclopedia, quotes the accounts I have cited, reports that the operation is practiced among Arabians and Egyptians to remove "from newborn girls whatever was indecently prominent in that part" and assures his readers that "such an

operation is indeed rarely practiced among Europeans."[79] In a remarkable seventeenth-century compilation of the anthropological lore of bodily transformations,
John Bulwer similarly associates clitorectomy with the barbarity of "the other." In
Arabia, he notes, a people called Creophagi circumcise ("Judaically") not only the
men, but women also; "the women of the Cape of Good Hope also excise themselves,
not from a notion of Religion, but as an ornament." And most worthy of scorn,

> [in] Ethiopia, especially in the Dominions of Prester John, they Circumcise women.
> These Abassines have added errour upon errour, and sin upon sin, for they cause their
> Females to be circumcised.... A thing which was never practiced in Moses Law, nei-
> ther was there ever found any expresse Commandment to do it; I know not where the
> Noselesse Moores learned it....[80]

The only account of clitorectomy in Western Europe that I have encountered
arises not from the victim's excessive sexual lust, nor even from her erotic encounters with another woman, but from her having pretended to be what she was not.
Like those men and women accused of having lain with their own sex under the
pretense of being the opposite, Henrica Shuria stands accused of having violated
some supposedly self-evident sumptuary law of the body; she was charged as a woman
who duplicitously played the part of a man, as if a peasant had dressed up as a lord
with intent to deceive.

Her accusers claimed that Shuria was "a woman of masculine demeanor who had
grown weary of her sex." She dressed as a man, enlisted in the army and served as a
soldier at the siege of Sylva Ducis under Frederick Henry, stadholder (1625-47). She
seems to have kept out of trouble until after the war when, as a civilian, it was presumably more difficult for her to sustain a male persona. It was then that she was
accused of "immoral lust,"

> for sometimes even exposing her clitoris outside the vulva and trying not only licen-
> tious sport with other women...but even stroking and rubbing them...so that a cer-
> tain widow, who burned with immoderate lusts, found her depraved longings so well
> satisfied that she would gladly – except for the legal prohibition – have married her.[81]

Her clitoris, it was said, "equalled the length of half a finger and in its stiffness was
not unlike a boy's member." Shuria was convicted and sentenced to death, though
it is not clear whether her primary offense was "sodomy" – essentially placing some
body part in the wrong orifice – or very nearly getting away with being a female

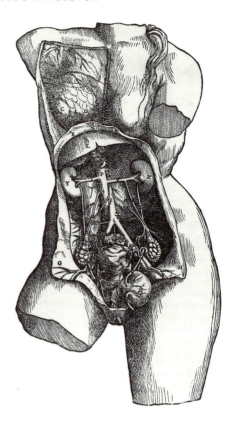

From Vesalius, *De humani corporis fabrica*,
Bâle, 1543 (Paris, Bibliothèque nationale).

bridegroom. But, in any case, instead of being put to death as various great jurists had recommended, "this 'tribas' finding a merciful judge, was, as it were, nipped in the bud, and sent into exile." The widow, though punished in an unspecified manner, was allowed to remain in the city.[82]

The great French surgeon Ambroise Paré gives a complex account of the same sort that discusses female genital mutilation in the context of exorcism and the exotic East. But it also speaks to a more general cultural concern about the "naturalness" of heterosexual union, of the mating of opposites. The "nimphes" of women, he informs his lay audience, "two excrescences of muscular flesh" which cover the urinary meatus and "which hang and, even in some women, fall outside the neck of the womb; lengthen and shorten as does the comb of a turkey, principally when they desire coitus; and when their husbands want to approach them, they grow erect like the male rod...."[83]

So far this seems to be much like the other accounts of clitoral excitation that arises from the rubbing of penis on "penis," or from the focusing of diffuse lust. But Paré then unexpectedly turns to a discussion of what he takes to be a more serious problem, i.e., the performance by females alone of what would otherwise occur

116

between men and women. In the course of heterosexual loveplay, the "nimphes" swell "so much so that [women] can disport themselves with them, with other women." This externally visible erection renders them "very shameful and deformed being seen naked" and a surgeon must be called to cut out what is superfluous and subject to abuse. By this time it is not clear whether Paré is warning men about women who during marital sex might prefer to engage in masturbation or homo-erotic practices, or whether he is alluding to the "problem" of clitoral hypertrophy among Eastern women, i.e., only to that class of women in whom the "nimphes" "fall outside the neck of the womb," and who shamefully act like men. The question of who sees their "shameful" condition when naked is also left unspoken.[84]

Moreover, the case that Paré gives to assure his readers that his account is "as true as it is monstrous and difficult to believe" is so fraught with crosscurrents of meaning that its specific illustrative power is greatly confused. The venue is North Africa. In Fez, we are told, there lives a group of female "prophets," exorcists, who give people "to understand that they have familiarity with demons." These women change their voices so that one thinks that the spirits are speaking through them; they live from gifts people leave for the demons *and* they "rub one another for pleasure, and in truth they are afflicted of that wicked vice of using one another carnally." More sinister still than speaking in the voices of men and having sex like men, they use the spirit's voice to ask beautiful women who consult them to pay by "carnal copulation." And to further complicate matters their patients apparently come to enjoy this form of remuneration, feign sickness and send their husbands to fetch the healers. The poor dupe, whose permission is required for his wife to visit the prophetesses, is thereby made the instrument of his own cuckolding. Indeed, the benighted husband might even prepare a feast for the whole lecherous band. Some husbands, however, get wise to the ruse and drive the putative spirits out of their wives' bodies with a good clubbing, or "deceive them by the same means as the prophetesses have done" (presumably by having sex with themselves?). There are in Africa — so the story ominously ends — "castrators" who "make a trade of cutting off such caruncles, as we have shown elsewhere under *Surgical Operations*."[85]

Once again the offense — in addition to trafficking with demons — is deception and inversion, not perversion. The lowly would be high, women would play the part of men. The narrative slipperiness of Paré's account belies its diffuse anxiety about a sexual world turned upside down. This story is also a curious turn on the quite common trope of exorcism and sexual exploitation. Men who cast out demons, charges Samuel Harsnett in his condemnation of exorcists and exorcism in sixteenth-century England, seem to prefer young women to old because they writhe more actively when the spirits are wrenched from their bodies. These charlatans further exploit their position by touching the cross to the genitals of their patients. Harsnett's condemnation is Protestant propaganda but it was a commonplace of the anticlerical literature of the Middle Ages and the Renaissance that priests and monks hid their sexual exploits behind priestly or monastic garb. The Fez prophetesses seem therefore in good male company.[86]

And finally, Paré's account might be regarded as a kind of medical pornography that plays on the erotic power of the one-sex model. He was asked by the medical faculty of Paris, and he agreed, to cut the passages I have quoted from his popular book on monsters in which they first appeared. (They ended up in his *On Anatomy*, a book less appealing to, and presumably less read by, the laity.) It is difficult to believe that in either context the passages in question could have been written primarily for their prurient interest since the vast bulk of the surrounding material is decidedly unerotic. But by the late seventeenth century similar accounts in popular medical books have an unambiguously naughty quality. "The Lesbian Sappho would never have acquired so wicked a reputation [*une si méchante réputation*] if this part [the clitoris] had been smaller," Nicholas Venette writes in his best-selling sex guide regarding the organ which "is often abused by lascivious women." Clitoral sexuality — masturbation, stimulation by men, or "rubbing" with another woman — finds its way into eighteenth-century pornography and is a commonplace by the nineteenth century.[87]

This, however, is not the occasion to analyze male erotic interests in particular practices. Paré's tale and Venette's coy aside are very much part of that genre of titillating literature that purports to allow men a view into the secret lives of women.[88] When among themselves, they seem to be saying, women rub *their* penises together. But since sex between men and women is metaphorically construed in a wide range of contexts as the friction of two like parts — whether these be the male penis with the vagina or the clitoris — tribadism, women "rubbing" one another, would become merely another variation on an old theme. Indeed, all sex becomes homoerotic. Clitoral arousal — and male homoerotic acts — as signs of their practitioners' intrinsic sexual deviance, of their being "in-between sexes," would have to await the eighteenth century's redefinition of man and woman as being essentially different sorts of creatures. Lesbianism and homosexuality as categories were not possible before the creation of men and women as opposites, thereby leaving room in-between for those whose bodies (and/or psyches) made a choice impossible. Thus, the elaboration in medical literature, as well as in pornography of a "new" female penis and specifically clitoral eroticism, was a re-presentation of the older homology of the vagina and the penis, not its antithesis.

By the nineteenth century the problem of the clitoris was like that of the penis: the solitary vice. "Clitorisme," according to the *Dictionnaire encyclopédique des sciences médicales*, is not found in ordinary dictionaries but finds a place here. It is the act in which women substitute by "a kind of artifice" the pleasures reserved for love between the two sexes. "It is, for women, the same thing that masturbation is for men." These two definitions are, of course, not versions of one another. The first refers primarily to love between women, to what the "dames de Lesbos" do. But this concerns the author less than young women who learn, from bad company or bad literature, to touch their clitorides and who then become addicted to the practice. Eventually, however, the two definitions merge. Women who masturbate do not do so alone; they make converts, and by exciting their clitorides enough develop a sort of penis themselves (perhaps through some unspoken Lamarckian mechanism). They even act as men, and sink further and further into drink and debauchery. "See further 'Masturbation,' " the entry concludes.[89]

Clitorisme leads to the collapse of the social order, the *Dictionnaire* argues. But abuse is not quite like male masturbation in that it leads not just to self-destruction but to homosexuality as well. The solitary vice has a social outcome even if it is a perverted one. Clearly the Renaissance male's fear of being left out is still alive but is secondary to the massive new concern with masturbation as an offence not so much against chastity as against society.

By the late nineteenth century the clitoris takes on still another signification. No longer an encouragement to lesbian practices, it becomes in the work of forensic anthropologists like Lombroso a mark of excessive heterosexuality, the mark of the prostitute. (Parent du Chatellet, the major early nineteenth-century expert on the subject, had declared on the basis of considerable observation that prostitutes did not have unusually large or in any way remarkable clitorides.)

But Freud is not part of this history. His concern is much more that of the Renaissance, of getting bodies whose anatomies do not guarantee the dominance of heterosexual procreative sex to dedicate themselves to their assigned roles. However, he is at the same time a product of nineteenth-century biologism that postulates two sexes, each with their distinctive organs and physiologies, and of an evolutionism which guarantees that even if the genital parts are not born to make heterosexual intercourse natural, they will somehow adapt. In the end, the cultural myth of the vaginal orgasm is told in the language of science. And thus, not because of but despite neurology, a girl becomes the Viennese bourgeoise ideal of a woman.

### Postscript

When I finished the foregoing essay I remained uneasy that I had not offered a coherent version of Freud's argument once it could no longer be regarded as grounded in neurology. In other words, if Freud knew – as I show – that the migration of erotic sensibility from the clitoris to the vagina could not be interpreted as the result of prior anatomy or of anatomical development (for example, the supposed accession of pain receptors in neonates) then how did he think it might be interpreted? I offer the following reconstruction.

In the first place Freud remained a Lamarckian all his life. He believed in the inheritance of acquired characteristics which he generalized to include traits of the psyche – aggressions and needs, for example. "Need" in a Lamarckian sense, he wrote to his colleague Karl Abraham, is nothing other than the "power of unconscious ideas over one's own body, of which we see remnants in hysteria, in short, 'the omnipotence of thought.'"[90]

Hysteria is the model for mind over matter. The hysteric, like the patient who feels pains or itches in a missing limb, has physical symptoms that defy neurology. The hysteric's seizures, twitches, coughs and squints are not the result of lesions but of neurotic cathexes, of the pathological attachment of libidinal energies to body parts. In other words, parts of the body in hysterics become occupied, taken possession of, filled with energies that manifest themselves organically. (The German noun *Bezetsung* is translated by the English neologism "cathexis." The verb *besetzen* also has the sense of "charged as is a furnace, or tamped down, as is a blasting charge, or put in place as is a paving stone or a jewel.")

Freud knew that the natural locus of woman's erotic pleasure was the clitoris and that it remained competitive with the necessary cultural locus of her pleasure, the vagina. Marie Bonaparte reports that her mentor gave her Felix Bryk's *Neger Eros* to read in which the author argues that the Nandi engage in clitoral excision on nubile seventeen and eighteen year old girls so as to encourage the transfer of orgiastic sensitivity from its "infantile" zone to the vagina, where it must necessarily come to rest. The Nandi were purportedly not interested in suppressing female pleasure but merely in facilitating its redirection to social ends. Freud drew Bonaparte's attention to the fact that Bryk must have been familiar with his views and that the hypothesis regarding Nandi orgasmic transfer was worth investigating.

Bonaparte's efforts to discover the fortunes of "clitoroidal" versus "vaginal" sexuality in women whose clitorides had been excised proved inconclusive but she did offer a theoretical formulation of the transfer of erotic sensibility which fits my understanding of Freud's theory not only in the *Three Essays* but also in *Civilization and Its Discontents* and in his 1931 papers on female sexuality. "I believe," writes Bonaparte,

> that the ritual sexual mutilations imposed on African women since time immemorial...
> constitute the exact physical counterpart of the psychical intimidations imposed in child-
> hood on the sexuality of European little girls.[91]

Society takes the bisexual body of a little girl and forces its erotic energies out of their infantile phallic place where nerves ensure pleasure and into the vagina where they do not. "Civilized" people no longer seek to destroy the old home of sensibility — an ironic observation for Bonaparte, since she collected cases of European excision and herself underwent painful and unsuccessful surgery to move her clitoris nearer her vaginal opening so that she might be "normally orgasmic" — but enforce the occupation, i.e. cathexis, of a new organ by less violent means.

If we put all of this together, Freud's argument might work as follows. Whatever polymorphous perverse practices might have obtained in the distant past, or today among children and among animals, the continuity of the species and the development of civilization depend upon the adoption by women of their correct, that is nonphallic, vaginal, sexuality. For a woman to make the switch from clitoris to vagina is to accept the feminine social role that only she can fill. Each woman must adapt anew to a redistribution of sensibility which furthers this end, must reinscribe on her body the racial history of bisexuality. But neurology is no help. On the contrary. Thus, the move is hysterical, a recathexis that works against the organic structures of the body. Like the missing limb phenomenon, it involves feeling what is not there. Becoming a sexually mature woman is therefore living an oxymoron, becoming a lifelong "normal hysteric," for whom a conversion neurosis is termed "acceptive."

NOTES

1. Renaldus Columbus, *De re anatomica* (Venice, 1559), bk. 11, ch. 16, pp. 447-48. The sentences from which my excerpts are taken read: "Therefore, since no one has discerned these projections and their working, if it is permissible to name things one has discovered [discovered by me], it should be called the love, or sweetness of Venus [*Hos igitur processus, atque eorundum usum cum nemo hactenus animadverterit, si nomina rebus a me inventis imponere licet, amor Veneris, vel dulcedo appelletur*]." Having described the exact location of the clitoris he says, "And this, most gentle reader, is that: preeminently the seat of women's delight [*et haec lector candidissime illa, illa praecipue sedes est delectionis mulierum*]...."

2. For a review of this literature up to 1968, see the *Journal of the American Psychoanalytic Association* 16.3 (July 1968), pp. 405-612, which is made up of a series of articles discussing Mary Jane Sherfey's "The Evolution and Nature of Female Sexuality in Relation to Psychoanalytic Theory," in vol. 14 of the journal. Sherfey's article subsequently came out as a book, *The Nature and Evolution of Female Sexuality* (New York: Vintage, 1973). The view that female orgasm is essentially vaginal, i.e., the view that "equates the occurrence of intercourse with the occurrence of female orgasm," and then proceeds to give an adaptationist account of its evolution is brilliantly criticized in a forthcoming book by Elizabeth A. Lloyd of the Department of Philosophy, University of California, Berkeley. Her views are summarized in Stephen J. Gould, "Freudian Slip," *Natural History* 2 (1987), pp. 14-21.

3. Robert Scholes, "Uncoding Mama: The Female Body as Text," in *Semiotics and Interpretation* (New Haven: Yale University Press, 1982), pp. 130-31 and *passim*.

4. Sigmund Freud, *Three Essays on the Theory of Sexuality* (1905), trans. and edited by James Strachey (Avon: New York, 1962), p. 123.

5. *Ibid.*

6. *Ibid.*, p. 124.

7. *Ibid.*, p. 123.

8. Denis Diderot, *L'Encyclopédie*, "La jouissance" (Neuchâtel, 1765), vol. 5, p. 889.

9. On the one-sex model see my *Bodies, Pleasures, Sexual Differences* (Cambridge, Mass.: Harvard University Press, forthcoming), especially chs. 2 and 3; and "Orgasm, Generation, and the Politics of Reproductive Biology," *Representations* 14 (Spring 1986).

10. Richard von Krafft-Ebing, *Psychopathia Sexualis* (London: Staples Press, 1965), p. 31.

11. *Reference Handbook of the Medical Sciences* (1901), vol. 7, p.171. For Hyrtl, who taught anatomy at the University of Vienna while Freud was studying there, see below n.64. The Grimms define "kitzler" as clitoris or female rod, i.e., "weibliche rute," and trace these associations back through a number of earlier forms. "Kitzlerin" is defined as "titillans femina," but the usage given is "the emperor Maximilian called one of his blunderbusses the 'kitzlerin.' "

12. *Ibid.*, p. 172. These "end bulbs" take their name from Wilhelm J.F. Krause (1833-1910), and are found not only in the penis and the clitoris but also in the conjunctiva of the eye and in the mucous membranes of the lips and tongue.

13. *Ibid.*, p. 168, emphasis added.

14. E.H. Kisch, *The Sexual Life of Women* (English trans., 1910), p. 180. Kisch was professor at the German University in Prague; his *Sterilität des Weibes* (Wien and Leipzig, 1886) is a major summary of the literature on female sexuality and reproductive biology.

15. *Dictionnaire encyclopédique des sciences médicales* (Paris, 1813), vol. 18, p. 138.

16. *Ibid.*, vol. 99, pp. 230-88. The vagina, this article reports, is longer in blacks than in whites, corresponding, presumably, to the supposedly larger penis of the black male.

17. George Ludwig Kobelt (1804-57) was a German physician and the eponymous discoverer of Kobelt's network — the junction of the veins of the vestibular bulbs below the clitoris — and several other structures of the genito-urinary system. His *Die Männlichen und Weiblichen Wollusts-Organe des Menschen und verschiedene Saugetiere* (1844, Frieburg in Brisgau) is the basis for the English text which I have generally followed with slight emendations. For the English, see *The Classic Clitoris: Historic Contributions to Scientific Sexuality*, ed. Thomas Power Lowry (Chicago: Nelson Hall, 1978).

18. *Ibid.*, p. 23.

19. *Ibid.*, p. 38.

20. *Ibid.*, p. 43.

21. *Dictionnaire encyclopédique des sciences médicales*, vol. 5, pp. 373-75; for "Clitorisme" see pp. 376-79.

22. *Ibid.* (Paris, 1821), vol. 56, pp. 446-49. "Vagine" began to refer to the organ to which it refers

today in the late seventeenth century. Prior to then the nomenclature of the female anatomy was enormously imprecise because, in my view, anatomists had no great interest in defining a stable *female* interior sexual organ. See Laqueur, *Bodies, Pleasures, Sexual Differences*, ch. 3. As late as 1821 a reference work still found it necessary to note that serious mistakes arose from such lexical imprecision.

23. *Description anatomique des parties de la femme, qui servent à la génération* (1708), p. 8.

24. *Ibid.*, p. 13.

25. *Ibid.*, pp. 9, 13-14. Mariceau points out that the clitoris does not emit semen because it has no urethra.

26. *Ibid.*, pp. 20-22.

27. Jacques Duval, *Traité des hermaphrodites* (Rouen, 1612; repr. Paris, 1880), p. 68. The clitoris because it is so like the penis is also the organ that can be used to distinguish the sexes. Duval saves a man who had been mistaken for a woman from being burned at the stake for having sex with another women by finding "her" clitoris, rubbing it and producing an ejaculation which proved the organ in question to be a penis and its owner a man. See Stephen Greenblatt's rich discussion of this case, "Fiction and Friction," *Shakespearean Negotiations* (Berkeley and Los Angeles: University of California Press, 1988), pp. 66-94.

28. Anonymous, *My Secret Life*, ed. G. Legman (New York: Grove Press, 1966), p. 357.

29. *Tableau de l'amour conjugal* (London: "Nouvelle édition," 1779), pp. 20-21; there were twelve eighteenth-century editions of the English version *Conjugal Love; or the Pleasures of the Marriage Bed Considered*. I owe this information to Roy Porter who is writing an introduction to a modern reprint of Venette.

30. "Infantile Sexuality," in *Three Essays*, p. 93.

31. I am indebted in my account of the "aporia of anatomy" in Freud's essay on feminity in the *New Introductory Lectures* to Sarah Kofman, *The Enigma of Woman* (Ithaca and London: Cornell University Press, 1985), esp. pp. 109-14.

32. I argue more generally against the tenability of the sex/gender distinction in ch. 1 of *Bodies, Pleasures, Sexual Differences*.

33. Gayle Rubin, "The Traffic in Women: Notes on the 'Political Economy' of Sex," in *Toward an Anthropology of Women*, ed. Rayna R. Reiter (New York and London: Monthly Review Press, 1975), pp. 179-80 and 187.

34. Claude Lévi-Strauss, *The Savage Mind* (Chicago: University of Chicago Press, 1962), pp. 46ff. and ch. 2 generally.

35. *Civilization and Its Discontents*, trans. James Strachey (New York: W.W. Norton, 1962).

36. Rosalind Coward, *Patriarchal Precedents: Sexuality and Social Relations* (London: Routledge and Kegan Paul, 1983), p. 286.

37. *De re anatomica* 11.16.447-48.

38. *Ibid.* 11.16.446-47. I owe this novel and important grammatical analysis of Columbus entirely to my research assistant, Mary McCary of the Comparative Literature Department, Berkeley.

39. Columbus, *De re anatomica*, "Concerning the womb or uterus," 119.16.445.

40. Jane Sharp, *The Midwives Book, or the Whole Art of Midwifery Discovered, Directing Childbearing Women How to Behave Themselves in Their Conception, Breeding, Bearing and Nursing Children* (London, 1671), pp. 40, 42.

41. *Ibid.*, pp. 45-46; Mayern et al., *Complete Midwives Practice*, 4th ed. (1680), p. 67.

42. Thomas Gibson, *The Anatomy of Humane Bodies Epitomized*, 4th ed. (London, 1694), p. 199; *oestrus* in Latin means a gadfly or horsefly and figuratively a frenzy.

43. Helene Deutsch, *The Psychology of Women: A Psychoanalytic Interpretation* (New York: Grune and Stratton, 1944), pp. 229-38, 319-24 *passim*; Marie Bonaparte, *Female Sexuality* (New York: International Universities Press, 1956), pp. 3, 113-15; on Bonaparte's resorting to surgery to cure her own frigidity by having her clitoris repositioned at the vaginal orifice, and more generally, for what is at stake in the debate about the locus of female sexuality, see Naomi Schor, "Female Paranoia: The Case for Psychoanalytic Criticism," in *Breaking the Chain: Women, Theory, and French Realist Fiction* (New York: Columbia University Press, 1985), p. 183, n.20 and *passim*. Nicholas Culpepper, *A Directory for Midwives: or, A Guide for Women* (London, 1675), p. 22.

44. *Ibid.*, p. 22.

45. Sharp, *The Midwives Book*, p. 45.

46. John Pechey, *The Compleat Midwives Practice Enlarged*, 5th ed. (London, 1698), p. 49.

47. Philip Moore, *The Hope of Health* (London, 1565), p. 6.

48. I have not studied the nomenclature for the male reproductive anatomy thoroughly and I know of no general study of the subject. There are to be sure many different words for penis, testicle or scrotum but in my reading the referents of these terms are unambiguous. Perhaps this is the linguistic correlative of the corporeal telos generally: the male body is stable, the female body more open and labile.

49. Ovary, or its modern equivalents in other languages, was simply not used, in any form, until the late seventeenth century. The standard terms for the organ that we now understand to be an ovary were "female testicle" and its variants, like "woman's stones."

50. Columbus, *De re anatomica* 11.16.443.

51. *Ibid*. 11.16.445, emphasis added. *Mentula* was an obscene word for penis in Antiquity but became the standard term in the Renaissance; see Robert Adams, *The Latin Sexual Vocabulary* (London: Duckworth, 1982), p. 9. "Vagina" was not used in Latin in its modern sense but referred to a tube or sheath where something, usually a sword, is stuck. It seems to have been used humorously as "anus." See James N. Adams, *The Latin Sexual Vocabulary* (Baltimore: Johns Hopkins University Press, 1983), p. 115.

52. *Ibid*., pp. 447-48. Columbus, like all other Renaissance anatomists, refers to the ovaries as testes that are slightly larger and firmer than the males and that are contained within rather than pendant.

53. Fallopius, *Observationes*, pp. 193, 195-96.

54. Caspar Bauhin, *Anatomes* 1. 12. 101-02. "Porcus" (pig) was apparently a Roman nursery word for the external pudenda of girls; Adams, *The Latin Sexual Vocabulary*, p. 82. Perhaps the allusion is to a perceived resemblance between the part in question and the end of a pig's snout?

55. Jacquart and Thomasset, *Sexualité et savoir médical au Moyen Age* (Paris, 1985), p. 34, quoting Al-Kunna al-maliki. I am translating from their French text. I do not know what Arabic word they translated as clitoris. They do however give "*lèvres*" as an alternative translation and in the context it is clear that the labia minora are the referent.

56. *The Anatomy of Mondinus*, in *Fasciculo de medicine*, ed. Charles Singer, 2 vols. (Florence, 1925), vol. 1, p. 76 and n.64.

57. Jacopo Berengario da Carpi, *Isagogae Brevis*, ed. and trans. by L.R. Lind as *A Short Introduction to Anatomy* (Chicago, 1959), p. 78: "at the end of the cervix little skins are added at the sides; these are called prepuces." In referring to the penis: p.72, "a certain soft skin surrounds this glans; it is called the prepuce...." Hyrtl, *Onomatologia anatomica: Geschichte und Kritik der Anatomischen Sprache der Gegenwart* (Vienna, 1880) gives "nymphae" as meaning both labia and prepuce. See entry 248, "nymphae und myrtiformis."

58. Pechy, *The Complete Midwives Practice Enlarged*, p. 49 generally, and the actual quote is from *A General Treatise of the Diseases of Maids, Bigbellied Women* (1696), p. 60.

59. Gabrielis Fallopius, *Observationes anatomicae* (Venice, 1561), p. 194; for an excellent survey of what is said about the female external genitalia during the Middle Ages see Jacquart and Thomasset, *Sexualité et savoir médical*, pp. 62-66, and 66 for a French translation of this passage.

60. *Observationes anatomicae*, p. 193. Albertus Magnus uses the term "virga" for both the penis and what must be the clitoris and says that manipulating the latter will cause a woman to have the delight of intercourse and have an orgasm. See James Rochester Shaw, "Scientific Empiricism in the Middle

Ages: Albertus Magnus on Sexual Anatomy and Physiology," *Clio Medica* 10.1 (April 1975), pp. 60-61.

61. [Caspar] Bartholinus, *Anatomy Made from the Precepts of His Father, and from Observations of All Modern Anatomists, Together with His Own* (1668), p. 75. This book is a translation of Thomas's (1616-80, the discoverer of the lymphatic system) 1641 revision of Caspar I's (1585-1629) famous text, the *Institutiones anatomicae*. It was Caspar II (1655-1738) who gave his name to the greater vestibular, i.e., the Bartholinus glands, which lubricate the lower end of the vagina during coitus.

62. Regnier De Graaf, *New Treatise Concerning the Generative Organs of Women*, trans. and ed. H.D. Jocelyn and B.P. Setchell, *Journal of Reproduction and Fertility*, supp. 17 (Dec. 1972), p. 89 (p. 17 in the original) and nn.35-39; De Graaf is the eponymous discoverer of the ovarian follicles, though he mistook the follicle that bears his name for the egg.

63. Julius Pollux, *Onomasticon* (Leipzig: Teubner, 1900), p. 174. I owe the translations from the Greek to Mary McCary.

64. Joseph Hyrtl, *Onomatologia anatomica*; "Clitoris-Kitzler"; and Adams, *The Latin Sexual Vocabulary*, pp. 7-98; this whole semantic field needs exploration. For example, Jocelyn and Setchell argue, n.36, that De Graaf is mistaken in claiming that *kios* was an ancient term for clitoris. In fact, they say, the word applied to the uvula and to a kind of cancerous growth that may appear on the genitals. But Galen compared the *nymphē* (clitoris in modern translations) to the uvula which is probably why De Graaf made the connection. Liddell and Scott give as a meaning of "kios=column," "cartilage of the nose," in addition to "uvula" and "wart." Adams, p.35 and n.2, points out that a similarity was observed in Latin authors between the penis and the nose. In the Middle Ages, and I think in much subsequent folklore as well, the size of the nose reflects the size of the male genitals. *Nasus*=nose is also used in *Priapus* 12.14 to refer to the clitoris. Thus penis comes to be the structural homologue of clitoris via a common resemblance to the nose!

65. Jocelyn and Setchell, the editors of De Graaf's *New Treatise*, point out these errors without drawing attention to their significance; Albucasis in fact used the term *tentigo*. Although Hyrtl, *Onomatologia anatomica*, gives *irritamentum libidinis* as a common Arabic term I have found it in no source; Jocelyn and Setchell cannot track it down either but think that it may be an allusion to a lascivious dance called *irritamentum veneris languentis* in Juvenal 11.167.

66. Rufus of Ephesus, *Du nom des parties des corps*, in *Oeuvres de Rufus d'Ephèse*, ed. Charles Daremberg (Paris, 1879, 1963), p. 147, i.e., lines 110-12 of the accompanying Greek; Hyrtl, *Onomatologia*, entry 248, "nymphae und myrtiformis."

67. Galen, *On the Usefulness of the Parts of the Body* (Ithaca: Cornell University Press, 1968), vol. 2, p. 661.

68. Soranus, *Gynaecology*, ed. and trans. Owsei Temkin (Baltimore: Johns Hopkins University Press, 1956), p. 16.

69. Albucasis uses the term in his *Chirurgia* 2.71: regarding *tentigo* see Hyrtl, "clitoris"; Adams, *The Latin Sexual Vocabulary*, 103-04 and the *Oxford English Dictionary*.

70. Thomas Vicary, *The Anatomy of the Bodie of Man*, ed. F.J. and P. Furnivall (Oxford: Early English Text Society, 1888), p. 77. By the late seventeenth century *tentigo* seems to have meant quite precisely "clitoris," as in the title of Andre Homberg's Jena dissertation, *De tentigine, seu excrescentia clitoridis* (1671), listed as a reference in the entry "clitoris" of the *Dictionnaire encyclopédique des sciences médicales* (Paris, 1813).

71. The claim for Spigelius's primacy is made in Hyrtl, *Onomatologia anatomica*, "nympha"; his *De humani corporis fabrica* (Venice, 1627) was published posthumously; see Charles Singer, *A Short History of Anatomy and Physiology from the Greeks to Harvey* (New York: Dover, 1957), p. 163.

72. Crooke, *Microcosmographia: A Description of the Body of Man* (London, 1615), p. 250. The distinction Crooke notes between the penis and the clitoris may not have been apparent to Columbus. He knew of the usual course of the male and female urethra but when asked by a "female hermaphrodite" to cut off her "penis" and widen the opening of the vagina he refused. "I, who frequently longed to perceive the distinctions between these implements, put her off with words." He thought the operation was life-threatening. *De re anatomica* 15, 494-95, in the section "Concerning Things Which Rarely Happen in Anatomy."

73. Zachias, *Quaestionem medico-legalium* (1661), vol. 2, p. 502, par. 16.

74. John Hunter, "Account of the Free Martin," in *Philosophical Transactions of the Royal Society of London* 69 (1779), p. 281. A "free martin" is the cow calf of a litter of two in which the other is a bull calf; the cow calf in such instances is hermaphroditic and sterile.

75. It is not clear from ancient accounts whether the clitoris or labia minora are at issue. The famous Hottentot Venus was displayed as a grotesque example of genital hypertrophy in early nineteenth-century Europe. See Stephen Jay Gould, *The Mismeasure of Man* (New York: Norton, 1981). In 1879 Theodore Bischoff, a major figure in German physiology, studied the genitals of women from various countries and of certain primates. He concluded that the women of some races, some Africans and the Japanese, had especially small labia majora, that certain Africans had large labia minora and that the clitoris in no race was so large as to generally protrude from their covering. He argued against an evolutionary interpretation of the relationship between human and primate genitals. Th. L.W. Bischoff, *Vergleichend anatomische Undersuchugen über die äussern weiblichen Geschechts-Organe des Mensche under der Affen* (Munich, 1879), esp. pp. 27-28, 64.

76. Strabo, *Geography*, ed. H.L. Jones (London: Loeb Classical Library, 1966-70), 16.2.37 and 16.4.9.

77. Aetius of Amida, *Tetrabiblion*, translated from the Latin edition of 1542 by James Ricci (Philadelphia, 1950), bk. 16, ch. 103, p. 107, and n.1, p. 163.

78. *The Seven Books of Paulus Aegineta*, translated from the Greek in 3 volumes by Francis Adams, (London: Sydenham Society, 1856), vol. 2, p. 381, sec. 70. I am uncertain as to whether Paulus regarded the "extirpation of the nympha" as a more or less routine practice or as the surgical cure for a pathological condition. The passage quoted precedes a discussion of the removal of uterine tumors; the section itself is sandwiched between accounts of hermaphrodites and of various bloody excrescences.

79. Robert James, *Medicinal Dictionary* (London, 1745), vol. 3, "Clitoris"; Dr. Johnson helped James plan this work and wrote the biographical entry for Paulus Aegenita.

80. J.B. (John Bulwer), *Anthropometamorphoses: Man Transformed: or, the Artificial Changeling* (London, 1653) p. 380. This remarkable book is a sustained attack on "artificiality" and a vindication of what he calls the "regular beauty and honesty of nature." The book, which deserves careful study, must be regarded in connection with Bulwer's pioneering work on sign language for the deaf and on the development of theatrical and oratorical gestures which precisely mirrored states of mind. See B.L. Joseph, *Elizabethan Acting* (London, 1951), ch. 1. On the pages prior to the one cited he condemns male circumcision, which was regarded by others as diminishing male pleasure and hence procreative potency. Someone writing in Fallopius's name speculates that the Jews practice circumcision so that they will be less distracted by the pleasures of the flesh and better able to serve God. Gabriellis Fallopius, *De decoratione* (1560), "Concerning Correcting a Short Foreskin," p. 49.

81. I have taken this account from Nicolaas Tulp (1593-1674), *Observationum medicarum libri tres* (Amsterdam, 1641), pp. 3, 35, 54, 244 as quoted in Latin by L.S.A. von Romer, "*Der Uranismus in den Niederlanden bis zum 19. Jahrhundert, mit besonderer Berucksichtigung der grosen Uranierverfolgung in Jahre 1730*," *Jahrbuch für Sexuelle Zwischenstufen*, vol. 8, pp. 378-79; I am grateful for this reference to Kent Girard. The context is a discussion of the *Codex Batavus*'s prescription of death by drowning for buggery (Poena in paederatus est capitalis.... Apud nos merguntur dolio aqua pleno) and death by unspecified means for "Tribadic women, whether clitoratrices or fricatrices [*Tribades feminae, clitorizontes seu fricatrices, morte puniuntur*]...." This passage makes clear how different seventeenth-century categories are from our own and how difficult it is to understand precisely what action, state of mind or condition in Shuria's case was thought offensive. Note that there is no reference here either to "lesbian" or "homosexual," both nineteenth-century coinages. *Tribades* is the Latin form of the Greek verb *tribien* meaning "to rub." *Fricatrice* is from the Latin *fricare* meaning "to rub." Indeed, Tulp

notes parenthetically that *fricare* is what the Greeks called *tribien*. *Clitorizontes* must be a variant of the Greek *kleitorebeis*, which meant to "rub lasciviously." Tulp defines it as "trying lascivious sport with other women" which Shuria presumably did; but when he goes on to say that she "*even* stroked and rubbed them" viz. *tribien*, which by implication is worse, the import of "lascivious sports" becomes less clear again. "Fricatrice" in early seventeenth-century English seems to have meant a lewd woman, as in Johnson's *Volpone* 4.2: "To a lewd harlot, a base fricatrice." Perhaps the distinction is one that Ludovico Maria Sinistrari (1622-1701), professor of philosophy and then theology at Pavia, makes in his account of sodomy between merely rubbing genitals and actually putting the clitoris or penis in the inappropriate "vase," i.e., into the anus in the case of men; into the anus of male "sucubi," or the vagina or anus of women in the case of female sodomites. Only the latter is true sodomy, the more horrible crime punishable by death. Ludovico Maria Sinistrari, *De sodomia* (Latin-French edition), par. 22, which summarizes pars. 9-21. Sinistrari's lengthy account of other people's views on this subject, on what being a *fricatrice* or a *tribade* might be, emphasizes my point that there was no language for what we would take to be homosexuality and that, while words existed to describe more or less precisely male "unnatural acts," they failed in specifying female practices.

82. Tulp, *ibid*. It has been argued that Chief Justice Edward Coke (1552-1634) warned, in the context of a case regarding the Marshalsea Court's jurisdiction in a particular matter, that clitorectomy might be used to punish whores who, after three previous warnings and lesser punishments (e.g., being brought before the steward and having her name recorded, being detained in prison, and having her hair cut and shorn), persisted in plying their trade within the court's precincts. This is based on a misreading of the Latin. In fact, the court is imposing for the fourth offense a more permanent and inescapably public disfigurement: "if a fourth time they be found, then let their upper lips [*superlabia*] be cut lest they yearn for desire from someone else [i.e., solicit further; *Quae quidem si quarto invenient, tunc aputentur eis superlabia, ne de caetero concupiscant ad libidem*]"; see *The English Reports*, 77, pp. 1041-42 (Edinburgh and London, 1907); Sinistrari, *ibid.*, par. 22, provides further evidence for the foreignness of clitorectomy in the West. The clitoris of a most respectable nun in a convent near Pavia burst out in 1671, he reports. She was upset by this strange accident and was troubled by "temptations of the flesh." She called a doctor who tried various softening medicines. When he found that the organ remained erect, he cut it off, thereby, Sinistrari remarks, much endangering his patient's life and health. The surgeon later confessed that he resorted to this maiming because he did not know the "doctrine of the clitoris" which he subsequently learned from Bartholinus's *Tabulae anatomicae*. I do not quite see how knowing Bartholinus's views on the subject would have changed his approach to the case.

83. I have taken this account from Ambroise Paré, *On Monsters and Marvels*, trans. with an introduction by Janis L. Pallister (Chicago: University of Chicago Press, 1982), p. 188, n.35. See n.60 above for an account of its provenance.

84. *Ibid.*

85. *Ibid.*; Paré gives as his source the early sixteenth-century Arab geographer Leo Africanus's *History of Africa.*

86. On Harsnett, see Stephen J. Greenblatt, "Shakespeare and the Exorcists," in *Shakespeare and the Question of Theory*, ed. Pat Parker and Geoffrey Hartman (New York and London: Methuen, 1985). Anti-clerical literature not only played on the heterosexual exploits of priests and monks but also made much of the propensity of men and women in orders to engage in homosexual activities. Perhaps the point is that men and women outside the constraint of society will revert to like loving like, jackdaw seeking jackdaw.

87. Paré's paragraph on the so-called *nymphae* was shortened or lengthened again in the various 1573, 1575 and 1579 editions of the book on monsters before being relegated to the section on the womb in *De l'anatomie de tout le corps humain* (1585). The section from Leo Africanus was apparently the only case in which Paré gave in completely to his would-be censors. It was cut from the *Oeuvres* by 1579. See Paula Findlen's paper, "French Popular Medical Literature and the Issue of Sexuality in the Sixteenth and Seventeenth Centuries" (National Endowment for the Humanities Summer Project, 1984), pp. 13-15; I am grateful to Findlen for allowing me to use her work. Nicholas Venette, *Tableau de l'amour conjugal* (Parme, 1687), 1.1.18, or see the English edition *Conjugal Love, or the Pleasures of the Marriage Bed*, 20th ed. (London, 1750), p. 19.

88. See, for example, the seventeenth-century pornographic tale *The School for Venus*, ed. with introduction by Donald Thomas (London, 1972); and more generally Roger Thompson, *Unfit for Human Ears* (Totowa, N.J.: Rowman and Littlefield, 1979), pp. 30, 90, 158-175, and *passim*.

89. *Dictionnaire* (1813), vol. 5, pp. 376-78.

90. Freud to Abraham, Nov. 11, 1917, cited in Peter Gay, *Freud: A Life for Our Times* (New York: W.W. Norton, 1988), p. 368.

91. Marie Bonaparte, *Female Sexuality*, p. 203.

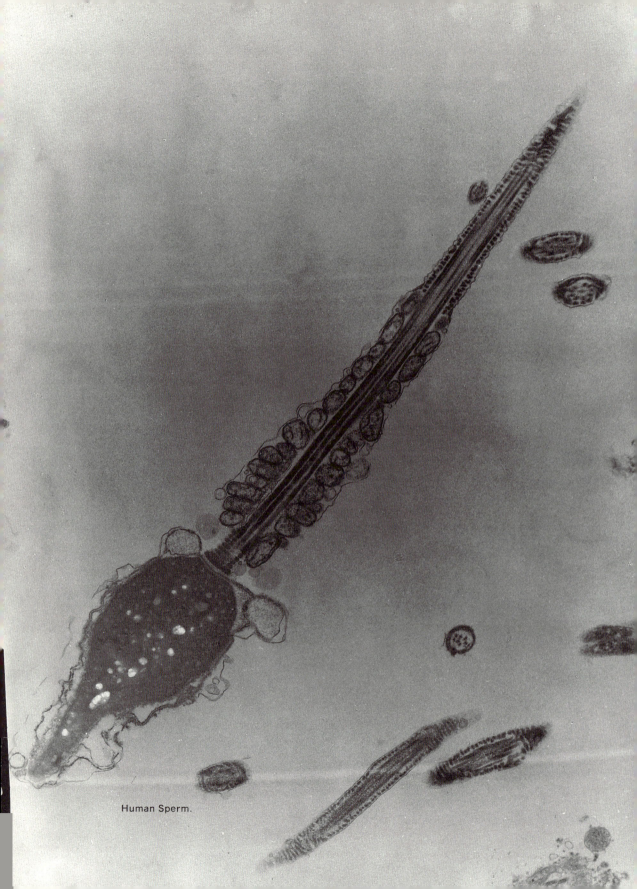

Human Sperm.

# Subtle Bodies

*Giulia Sissa*

## The Body of Semen

The authors of a recent article noted that the asymmetry between the fact that the semen is donated, the uterus only loaned, relates to a fundamental division at the heart of our current theories of filiation.[1] We are used to assuming that between a mother and the fruit of her womb, there is a bond of blood and body. In contrast, a father is linked to his legitimate offspring essentially on the basis of an assumption. In Roman law, the link of paternity was always defined as a matter of opinion, although that did not necessarily imply distrust as to who had in truth fathered the child. Rather, the definition referred to a particular dogma accepted on the position of a father, as such, in relation to the mother and her children.[2] That definition and the fact that it was the social institution of marriage that guaranteed the relationship between a man and his wife's children suggest that in our imaginary representations it is more natural for us to dissociate semen from paternity than childbirth from genetic maternity. That hypothesis is supported by the fact that AID (artificial insemination by donor) is considered a perfectly acceptable social practice, whereas the notion of a surrogate mother is often found distressing and shocking, for it introduces the possibility of drawing distinctions between the uterine mother, the ovulating mother and the social mother, and that is something that upsets our image of a single, true maternal body, certain beyond doubt. We can tolerate the duplication of a father by a semen donor — a nameless actor who is a purely somatic presence — but we resist the idea that childbearing no longer constitutes maternity. It is all right to efface the father's body, but not the mother's.

In the case of a child born by AID, the child's physical genitor is not the same person as his social father. There can be no doubt that this situation in principle simply represents an extreme manifestation of an institutional concept of patrilineality in which, until very recently – in French law, at least – the biological facts remained completely irrelevant. Historians and anthropologists would have no difficulty in supplying plenty of examples to demonstrate the symbolic nature of a child's link with his father. In Greek law, to cite an ancient society both close to yet very different from Roman society, women had the power to pass on material possessions but not to disown or adopt children. It was, a fortiori, not considered necessary for them to recognize the infants to whom they gave birth. The link between a mother and her child went without saying: it was self-evident, incontravertible and irreplaceable. Thus, a child adopted by a third party was no longer considered as the child of his natural father and he relinquished all connections with the latter's family upon being fully recognized as the direct descendant of his adoptive father. On the other hand, he always remained his own mother's child, from every point of view. Women bear children, but men make them. The links of filiation are made and undone by men since it is they who are empowered to recognize, disown and adopt. They are the masters of whatever the women produce. But their power as masters is the reverse side to the essentially fluid nature of the father–child relationship.[3] Françoise Héritier-Augé has studied the Samo of Burkina Faso and, as an ethnologist, has reflected much upon artificial procreation. Among the Samo, duplication of the paternal role is the rule rather than the exception. Before a betrothed girl enters upon legitimate marriage, she lives for a while with a lover with whom she has sexual relations: as soon as she produces a child she goes to live with her husband, who regards the child as the firstborn of his own marriage.[4] In the Trobriand kinship system, recently reconsidered by C.H. Pradelles de Latour,

> every adolescent girl is paired with one of her real or classificatory brothers, who later becomes the legal father of her children.... As for the father (the husband), even if he is not recognized as the biological father, he is nevertheless believed to mold the children in his image within the womb, thanks to his continuous sexual relations with the mother.[5]

Every individual thus has two fathers: a symbolic one who defines the lineage to which he belongs and with which he is identified (that of his maternal uncle), and a second one whose semen molded his somatic identity.

In short, if we consider these matters dispassionately from a comparative ethnological or historical standpoint, AID hardly seems a novelty except, of course, for the quite exceptional character of the technique used. However, still within the domain of anthropological representations, it is worth considering the gift of semen from a second, and complementary, angle that is no less relevant: namely, that of the semen itself. It is legitimate to consider the consequences of the technical treatment to which the seminal fluid is submitted when it is treated simply as a physical substance. Once collected, stored, frozen and banked, the semen is regarded purely and simply as a substance with particular biological, physical and chemical properties. Furthermore, in AID, it functions as an anonymous secretion whose donor's identity is deliberately effaced. The means of tracing biological paternity are obscured at the outset. No trace of the donor's identity is retained apart from a list of physical characteristics — the color of his eyes and hair, his size and so on — on the basis of which an attempt is made to obtain a child who will look as much like his legal father as possible, for the donor whose physical type most closely resembles that of the legal father is the one who will be selected. The role of the donated semen is simply that of an agent of fecundity. The identity of the genitor is not sought; all that matters is that he should be as much like the father as possible so that even the memory of that other body should not be detectable on the body of the child. It is perhaps by expunging the memory of the real link between the semen in the test tube and the child which it produces that the process of AID is made acceptable.

But the consequence of treating semen quite simply as an effective physical substance, in complete detachment from preoccupations on the score of filiation, is — so to speak — to demythologize its potency. In the Western world, a tenacious tradition surrounds the representation of the male body. One legacy of ancient Greek biology was the notion that semen is itself a humor whose material density, physical weight and body might as well be forgotten. By associating it with lightness, airiness and impalpability, it became possible to explain and glorify its power to transmit the paternal identity.

### The Art of Engendering

Ancient Greek society, like any other, worked out a juridical way of differentiating between a natural father and a legal one, as the institution of adoption shows. But the idea that patrilineal transmission involves more than just a transfer of matter was also elaborated in the domain of the natural sciences. It was thanks to its physical qualities that semen tended toward the immaterial. It was through its role as an engendering agent that it provided the biological basis for a certain model of filiation.[6]

For Aristotle, the semen is the vehicle through which form is transmitted, the form of the father that is reproduced in his offspring. The female body, on the other hand, provides matter. Aristotle understands the relation of form and matter as an opposition of contraries for which there is an empirical paradigm. The matter is the equivalent of the material from which a craftsman fashions an object. In generation, the matter is the blood, that superfluous blood that overflows from the uterus once a month. The form contributed by the semen provides the identity of the being about to be born, for it determines that being's specific characteristics. It acts upon the female matter, triggering the process of coagulation and anatomical differentiation that, when completed, results in the formation of a child who is like, if not identical to, his father. The birth of a female indicates some weakness in the father – excessive youth or age, or sickness – and constitutes a degeneration, as it were, a minimal degree of monstrosity. As the maternal contribution is passive and corporeal, so conversely the role of the father is active and imparts form. The female blood contains the body of the child potentially, for the blood nourishes each part of that body as it is the potential substance of all its tissues. However, the female blood on its own cannot realize the somatic potentialities that it contains. It needs the action of the male to set the development of the embryo in motion.[7]

Now, if Aristotle's theory is to be coherent, it is not enough for him simply to declare the female blood to be a mass of raw, undeveloped, inert and amorphous liquid. It is essential that the male contribute no matter at all. The male simply passes on an identity by virtue of the principle of movement; through his power to impart form, he transmits a soul. Soul, form and movement: the semen is the vehicle for three principles that biologists are likely to consider somewhat abstract and surprising. Movement (*kinēsis*) here is understood as a phenomenon that is in no way physical. When Aristotle declares that "the semen has within itself the movement that the genitor set going," he explains that this *kinēsis* is analogous to the architecture of a house.[8] It is a matter of implementing a project, copying the model that is constituted by the genitor's own form. The only physical aspect of conception is heat but, as we shall see, Aristotle turns even this into a metaphysical quality.

First, let us pause to consider the comparison that Aristotle draws between the act of fashioning an object and the process of conception, for it is far more than just a set of sporadic similes: it constitutes a means of conceptualizing the origin of living creatures.[9] By saying, as Aristotle does, that the semen is a tool (*organon*) that possesses "movement in actuality"[10] and that "it is the shape and form that pass from the carpenter, and they come into being by means of the movement in the material,"[11] it is possible to conclude that "this semen is not a part of the fetus as it develops."[12] Just as no particle of any concrete substance passes from the carpenter to his artifact by being added to the wood on which he is working, similarly not the smallest particle of semen can enter into the composition of the embryo. The father's semen is like the carpenter's instrument: nothing passes from the craftsman's body or from the matter of his tools into the product of his labor. So nothing passes from the father's body or from the matter of the semen to the product of generation. The syllogism has all the force of a consecutive chain of reasoning and all the weakness of an argument that rests upon an unproven analogy. But what is important here is that the assimilation of procreation to a technical craft forces the philosopher to deduce that the semen, as such, is not necessary to the process of conception. The seminal fluid is the accidental vector of a completely different kind of heredity. To make a living creature, there has to be a father, that is to say soul, movement and form, but it was not inevitable that these should be conveyed by a spermatic substance.

> The female always provides the material, the male provides that which fashions the material into shape; this, in our view, is the specific characteristic of each of the sexes: that is what it means to be male or female. Hence, necessity requires that the female should provide the physical part, a quantity of material, but not that the male should do so, since necessity does not require that the tools should reside in the product that is being made, nor that the agent that uses them should do so.[13]

This genetic theory, totally biased toward a father who reproduces his specific identity, leads to a paradox: the denial that it is necessary for semen to exist. Yet semen itself, as a physical reality, undeniably does exist. This raises a delicate question: what happens to this "body" of semen in the process of generation? As a result of confusing procreation and paternity, Aristotle is now forced to give some account of this spermatic residue. He must explain its use and be rid of it.

## Semen Does Not Freeze

There are some animals, namely male insects, that do not emit semen in the course of copulation. Instead, the female introduces her "uterus" into the place where the generative power of the male is lodged.[14] In Aristotle's view, this constitutes clinching empirical proof that semen is not necessary in the exercise of biological paternity. Is one to conclude from this that male insects, insofar as they possess no seminal matter, are exemplary beings? It is a disquieting notion for, on the contrary, the model for all living beings and the most perfect creature of all is man, a large viviparous animal who produces semen. What Aristotle says is: "they [the larger animals] are the ones that emit semen, on account of their heat and their size."[15] Sexual differentiation exists so that, among the superior animals, the better (that is to say the male) should be separated from what is inferior (matter, that is, the female): semen is a further sign that indicates the superiority of animals that are hot-blooded, complex and self-sufficient. It is a residue of food that has been elaborated and turned into blood by the vital heat that produces a gradual concoction. In short, it exists for what might be called reasons of metabolism and also as evidence of the zoological hierarchy.

As for its nature, its material composition, the phenomenon of cooling provides Aristotle with the starting point for his theory on this subject. Why, he asks, does semen, which is white and thick as it emerges from the warm body, then become transparent and liquid like water when it remains in contact with the cold air? It does not behave like water, for water is solidified by cold and made liquid by heat. So, despite the appearance that it adopts in the open air, the seminal fluid is not water. Nor can it be a compound of water and earth, like milk, which is always white and dense, for if it were it would not change when it cools. Semen is milky and watery, yet neither water nor earth-and-water. This is very strange. What can its short-lived thickness consist of? Aristotle's answer is that semen is really a compound of water and hot air, or breath (*pneuma*). When it is hot it is of thick consistency because of air, which forms tiny, invisible bubbles in it: what might be supposed to indicate a solid, earthy nature should instead be understood as a sign of super-refinement. Semen is not heavy; it has the extreme lightness of froth, snow or foam.

The philosopher's first step is thus to classify male seed among the most refined of substances, those in which the texture of the matter is rarefied almost to the point of vanishing. The transformation that is brought about by cold can be explained by the evaporation of the *pneuma*:

> These reasons explain the behavior of semen.... It is coherent and white when it comes forth from within because it contains a good deal of hot *pneuma*, owing to the internal heat of the animal. Later, when it has lost its heat by evaporation and the air has cooled, it becomes fluid and dark because the water and whatever tiny quantity of earthy matter it may contain stay behind in the semen as it solidifies, just as happens with *phlegma*.[16]

Semen contains a few traces of earth but this constitutes no more than the tiniest suggestion of solid matter and gives no justification to the historian and doctor Ctesias of Cnidus, in his belief about the semen of elephants: "He says that it gets so hard when it solidifies that it turns into amber. It does not."[17] A mixture of water and air cannot enter a solid state. Nor can it freeze, for air never freezes.[18]

## A Vanishing Body

It is by observing the reactions of semen to the open air that Aristotle manages to establish its nature. However, that still does not help him to understand what happens inside, in the woman's body, when the newly ejaculated foam meets the mass of maternal blood. It is heat that makes semen fertile: not the dry, desiccating heat of fire but the warmth of breath — the vital heat — which is to be found in all animate beings and in the sun, the heat-giving "father" of organisms that are born by spontaneous generation. So it is breath that acts upon the blood. But to say that semen is fertile because it contains this quintessence analogous to the element from which the stars are constituted[19] is not enough to prove the absolute immateriality of paternity. The *pneuma*, though impalpable, is still a concrete substance. So it is consequently necessary to discover what becomes of the corporeal part of the semen.

"The next puzzle to be stated and solved is this. Take the case of those groups of animals in which semen is emitted into the female by the male. Supposing it is true that the semen that is so introduced is not an ingredient in the fetus that is formed, but performs its function simply by means of the *dunamis* [force] that it contains. Very well; if so, what becomes of the corporeal part of it [*sōmatōdes*]?"[20] The question is as explicit as it is crucial, for therein hangs the legitimacy of Aristotle's genetic theory: to be certain that the father transmits nothing but an identity and a soul, Aristotle must dispel all lingering doubts as to the role that the "body" or corporeal part of the semen might covertly be playing. It is tempting to suppose that it mingles with the blood just as other fluids intermingle with the fluids that they meet. And according to Hippocratic theories of generation, the embryo is indeed formed by the intermingling of the male and female spermatic humors. But Aristotle builds his entire biology in opposition to such a symmetry between the two sexes. And the "body" of the semen, a residue of the body of the father, is in danger of undermining his whole edifice of patrilineality.

The most simple solution is to get rid of it. And that is precisely what Aristotle proceeds to do, in a few sentences:

> Consider now the corporeal part of the semen [*tēs gonēs sōma*]. (That which, when it is emitted by the male, is accompanied by the portion of soul-principle and acts as its vehicle….) This corporeal part of the semen, being fluid and watery, dissolves and evaporates; and on that account we should not always be trying to detect it leaving the female externally, or to find it as an ingredient of the fetus when that has set and taken shape, any more than we should expect to trace the fig juice that sets and curdles milk. The fig juice undergoes a change; it does not remain as a part of the bulk that is set and curdles.[21]

## Aura Seminalis

This "body," already so unobtrusive, dissolves and evaporates: it vanishes. Aristotle does not explain how that can be possible inside a womb. However, Galen was later to pay much attention to this important detail. The doctor challenged the deductions of the philosopher by appealing to plain fact: women do produce a kind of seed; menstrual blood is not the matter that Aristotle's theory of embryogenesis claims it to be. Male semen itself is composed of two parts: the *pneuma*, which is its moving force, and the fluid substance that is destined to become established in the uterus, there to form the initial concrete kernel of the embryo. When the semen falls into the cavity of the uterus, the material humor adheres to its tissues and enfolds the *pneuma*. By so doing, it prevents it from evaporating, which it might otherwise do even in the matrix, as breath is so very volatile. For Galen, it would seem, what matters above all is to prevent the slightest effluvia and the smallest drop of semen from escaping from the female body. Semen *is* a material agent in conception.[22]

Aristotle carries through his representation of semen to its ultimate conclusions: this non-matter is aerial and liquid, so it can fly away and dissolve, making way for a paternity that is biologically pure. But even leaving the whole question of the coherence of Aristotle's theory aside, ancient Western thought is pervaded by the conviction that the male humor is animated by a hot breath. Long before Aristotle, Pythagoras believed that semen was a drop of the brain containing a hot vapor that was the source of the embryo's soul and sensitivity. Plato, for whom the seminal fluid also emanated from the brain, flowing to the penis by way of the spinal column, also believed it to be foam. The pre-Socratic philosopher Diogenes of Apollonia was convinced that when the blood reached the area of the abdomen it became light and grew hot: the seminal liquid was simply its froth, *spuma sanguinis*.[23] As for the gynecologists of the Hippocratic Corpus,[24] they recognized that the female body too was able to secrete a seed analogous to that emitted by males, and they believed it to have the same frothy consistency.[25] In short, despite differing views on the genesis of semen, two ideas about it seem to have become established: it was an extremely refined substance and it was derived from whatever was most precious and vital in the body, either the blood or cerebral matter. Within this weightless foam, the quintessence of the male was concentrated.

Of course, that is an outmoded, prescientific Greek idea. But it was a strong image that endured for a long time, during which it was adapted to a series of models of conception within the European tradition. After Aristotle, the tendency to see the frothy appearance of semen both as its essential quality and as the manifestation of a supreme power was to have a long history stretching from Galen right down to Lamarck. Far from rejecting the idea, the naturalists and doctors who made the greatest contributions to the progress of biology continued to adapt it to the most disparate theories. Even animalculism and ovism had a place for the *aura seminalis*: biologists had no compunction about referring to it, using expressions with a whole variety of nuances: the seminal spirit, fetid particles, an alcalescent vapor, an ethereal fire, a pungent atmosphere....[26] This theory, upheld by the conviction that "semen cannot freeze because air cannot freeze," was originally both serious and sensuous; but it has at last received its ultimate coup de grace in the test tubes of the semen banks used in the AID process.

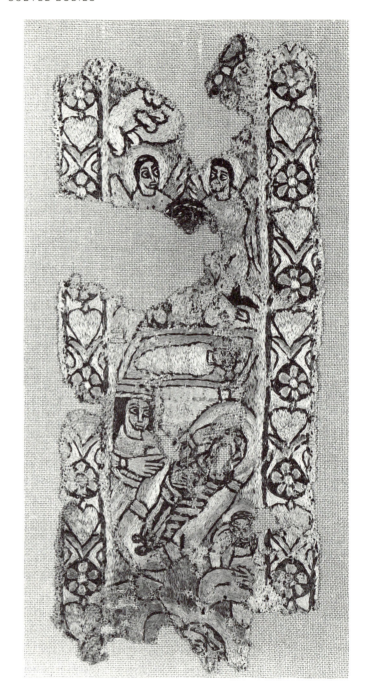

Coptic fabric depicting Mary and Child, Joseph, Solomon and angels (Paris, Louvre).

# The Seal of Virginity

It is the fate of certain phenomena to become signs. They recur in all our lives as part of what is generally accepted and unexceptional, and yet — or perhaps for that very reason — they are facts that speak. What they tell, emphasize and reiterate are things that need to be declared and registered as accepted values. I refer to ritual acts, and I believe that the body is one of their favorite means of expression. To take an example to which the present discussion is to be devoted, marriage is more than just a contractual exchange. In ancient Greece, the marriage ceremonial constituted a public announcement of the sexual contact for which it was...a cover. We shall be returning to this point.

Furthermore, some places in the body or some parts of it, as well as fulfilling their recognized useful functions, also have a role to play as signifiers. Even before we notice how an individual deploys his body, we are conscious that anatomy in itself signifies, whether through physiognomy or in divination through dreams, not to mention medical semiotics or forensic medicine. To return to our particular example, consider how the state of the female sexual organs is supposed to indicate whether or not defloration has taken place. In short, the body is made to operate as a signifier both by rituals that speak of it and by knowledge that makes it speak. The body is a reality of which ritual speaks and is, at the same time, the most telling of objects.

Let us pause to consider the body of a girl in ancient Greece on her wedding day. The *gamos*, or marriage ceremonial, is set up as a theatrical representation of the defloration, or even rape, to which the sexual organs of the *parthenos* (maiden and by extension virgin) are subjected. A scholiast provides confirmation on this point, informing us that the din of the *epithalamium* loudly chanted by the bride's friends gathered outside the nuptial chamber had a very precise function, namely *to cover* the cries of the young bride undergoing the violence of penetration.[1] The chanting covers the cries. But, to judge by the *epithalamia* preserved by tradition, it does so in a remarkable fashion, covering them with more noise in the form of words that allude to what is taking place. We might have expected a ritual that would make it impossible to hear the bride's cries by removing the couple to a distant place or by shutting them away, a ceremony that would offer them seclusion, so that the sexual violence could be consummated far from indiscreet ears. Such was certainly the pattern of events in some circumstances, but only in cases of "secret marriages," or rather, clandestine seductions, furtive meetings that took place — and this is the point — without marriage. A *kruptos gamos* (secret marriage) was the exact opposite of a true marriage. The true *gamos* was altogether given over to din and festivity that surrounded it with light, noise and words in order to conceal sexuality.[2] The event that the body was undergoing was literally enfolded in a poem that, while neither declaring nor concealing it, was nevertheless a sign of it. We shall not dwell upon this strange denial, by means of words, of the sexual relations as they actually took place. Rather, let us note that the defloration was an event that marked the female body, and that the marriage ritual prevented it from passing unnoticed.

The ritual tells of the body. But, as we have already noted, the body itself tells its own story. In this case, there is a natural symptom of the defloration, for the female body bears witness to what has happened to it. In ancient Greece, the totally physical sign of that sexual contact was pregnancy. A swelling abdomen revealed the seduction or violation after the event. This semiotic of consequences was crude in the extreme: there are accounts of fathers who, to make sure of their daughters' virginity, disemboweled them in their quest for a fetus.

Of course, you will say, pregnancy was one sign. But ancient Greece, which gave us the very name of the virginal membrane, surely knew the art of analyzing the hymen. This delicate membrane, so appositely known as the *signaculum* in Latin (a word that loses its etymological derivation from *signum* when translated as "*seal*" in English) seems to exist for one sole purpose: to mark the virgin body with a seal that, once broken, signals the loss of virginity. Is that not what defloration is? A breaching of a seal, a breaking-through, a *ruina* that is both borne by the hymen and indicated by it.

## A Model of Irreversibility

We should not pass too quickly over the Latin language and the whole tradition into which it introduces us, for we ought to have a clear idea of the points of comparison and contrast with Greek ideas on the subject. Let us reread Peter Damian, the eminent expert on canonical law who played such an important part in a series of disputes crucial in restoring probity to Christian thought. His *Letter on Divine Omnipotence*

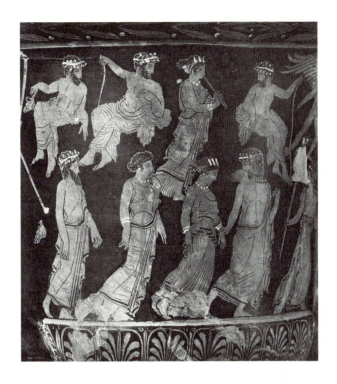

Thanagra crater: bridal procession, 4th century B.C.
(Athens, National Museum).

was probably written in 1067, to Didier, rector of the Abbey of Monte Cassino, and to its community of monks. In the course of a dinner conversation during a visit to the monastery, Didier had cited a remark that Jerome had once made on the subject of divine omnipotence. Jerome was supposed to have said: "I shall speak boldly: although God can do anything, He cannot make a virgin of a girl who no longer is one. He certainly has the power to free her from her distress, but not to restore the crown of her lost virginity to her."[3] Despite God's omnipotence, it is not possible, even for Him, *coronare corruptam*. Defloration is a fact, the ideal model, even, of what is known as a fait accompli, since it constitutes the issue over which divine omnipotence is being called into question. Can God annul what has already happened? Can God reverse the order of events, turn back the flow of time, make what is over and done with come about again? Questions such as these raise many serious problems: in the first place, they affect the very concept of God's experience of duration. Peter Damian's reply is that, for God, duration is all in the present; it is the simultaneous presence of the whole of time, time that is in flow only for mortal beings: in the sight of God there is no yesterday, no tomorrow, only an eternal today, *sempiternum hodie*. It is consequently not in terms of a turning back, reversing the order of what came first and what came later, that the problem should be posed.

Next, the expert on canonical law rejects a hypothesis that he regards as pernicious but that Didier has advanced in support of Jerome's view. This is the idea that, if God cannot accomplish a particular act, it is because he does not wish to. Damian writes as follows:

> But as for you, you maintain that what has been said was certain and well established: God cannot make a virgin of one who is no longer a virgin. Then, with long and prolix arguments, encompassing many questions, you will eventually conclude your explanations with the following formula: God cannot do it for the sole reason that he does not wish to.[4]

Didier was introducing a relationship of cause and effect between wishing to and being able to, and no doubt doing so for laudable motives: namely, to place divine omnipotence beyond reach of doubt by replacing the problem with that of His will, the free will of the Omnipotent. But Peter Damian regarded such a shift as objectively perverse. He argues as follows:

> If God can do nothing apart from what He wishes to do, and if, furthermore, He does

nothing except what He wishes to do, then He can do absolutely none of the things that He does not do.... It follows that whatever God does not do, He is absolutely unable to do.[5]

It is a paradoxical and perhaps surprising conclusion. However, that is the line of argument by which Damian reaches the crucial point. What he does is shift the whole debate to the only domain that seems relevant to him, namely that of ethics. Here, God's power is in no danger of being called into question: the only yardstick by which it is possible to measure the limits of God's actions is the *bonum*, the good. So, yes, God *can* restore a deflowered woman's virginity, just as He can perform countless other miracles. If He abstains from doing so, it must be because he reckons that, though a good thing in itself, the restitution of virginity is not justifiable.

It is unfortunate that after her dishonor (*stuprum*), a virgin must remain deflowered, and it would be good if God restored the seal of virginity in her [*si virginitatis in ea Deus signaculum reformaret*]; but although God never does it — either to keep a woman in a state of fear; or so that she is fearful of losing what she can never recover; or, as is fair and just, so that what she has relinquished as a thing of little value in the midst of carnal blandishments, she shall never recover even through tears and penitence; or, no doubt, so that, reflecting on the lasting marks of her fall within herself [*dum in se ruinae suae signa superesse considerat*], she should persist ceaselessly in seeking more severe remedies for her affliction — if then, for these or other reasons of heavenly providence, a virgin who has been deflowered can never recover her initial virginity, that is absolutely no reason for saying that all-powerful God cannot do it; say rather that He does not wish to, in accordance with His supremely just will, His free choice.[6]

We should therefore attribute to divine wisdom the fact that women are never restored to a state of virginity once they have lost it. God in His wisdom imposes penalties for undervaluing a precious treasure, penalties effected through lasting signs that constantly recall to the mind, conscience and contrition of the guilty woman the memory of what did indeed take place. For the Being capable of curing all illnesses and rectifying all infirmities, it would be child's play to expunge those telltale signs. Repairing the "conclusion" of virginity (*clausola virginea*) would be no trouble to God. "He who from a tiny quantity of semen made the body itself, He who changed it into all the shapes of the body's various members in such a way as to give it human form, who, in a word, made a creature that had not hitherto existed —

could not such a one make that creature intact once more, once it existed and had been spoiled?"[7] The trouble is that this simple action, which would mean nothing to its author, would entail grave consequences for the deflowered woman, for it might make her forget her *lapsus*.

Thus, for Peter Damian, defloration is a happening that marks the body, leaving a *signum* upon it: a broken *signaculum*. But the only interest of his letter would lie in its presentation of one of many examples of divine omnipotence, were it not for the fact that it also constitutes a model expression of the eleventh-century attitude to physical virginity. To be sure, there is more to virginity than *just* the hymen, for, as Damian tells us, moral integrity on its own is enough to turn a prostitute into a virgin. All the same, only *integritas carnis* could truly perfect a refound virginity for, without it, a woman is forever forced to remember what she will henceforth forever lack.

## A Sign That Is Hard To Believe In

The position of the Church Fathers is a very strange one. In the mid-fourth century A.D., Saint Ambrose fired off an indignant letter to the bishop of Verona,[8] guilty of having permitted a midwife to carry out a manual examination on a Christian virgin. He set out two reasons for his protest: in the first place, it was not appropriate for a man of the Church to sanction midwives affronting the intimacy of virgins with their profanatory inspections and probings. Suspicion in itself is offensive and, as for the contact of a hand, this could lead a girl into temptation or even – perish the thought – bring about the very catastrophe that it purported to be investigating. Second, with the backing of medical expertise, Ambrose questioned the infallibility of such a method of verification. He pointed out that doctors themselves declared such an inspection to be of doubtful credibility: that was, after all, the view held by doctors of the greatest antiquity and it was a vexed question even among midwives. What was the point of looking for signs that were dubious and suspect when others that were much more unequivocal could be found, without jeopardizing a woman's modesty? What could be more public than a case of outraged virtue and lost virginity? Chastity transgressed makes itself plain for all to see: the belly swells and the weight of the fetus makes walking awkward, quite apart from the fact that the woman's embarrassment and shame betrays her guilty conscience. Such a deep distrust of anatomy might surprise us, coming as it does from one of the most fervent apologists of Christian virginity. For the writings of Ambrose wax eloquent on the subject of sexual abstinence and, in particular, on the mystery of the birth of Christ. The whole of his treatise entitled *De institutione virginis* is devoted to a commentary on a verse from Ezekiel 44.2, "this gate shall be shut, it shall not be opened [*porta haec clausa erit et non aperietur*]." What can this gate be if not the Virgin Mary, a gate that is closed because of its virginity? Mary is the gate through which Christ entered this world, in a virginal birth, without undoing the genital locks. The hedge of modesty remained intact and the seals of virginity were preserved unbroached.[9] *Porta clausa, claustra, septum, signaculum*: the metaphors follow one upon another, evoking a preserve defended by locks, walls and seals. *Et hortus clausus virginitas et fons signatus virginitas*: virginity is a secret garden, a sealed fountain. Ambrose's advice to girls is to open up their minds, but always to preserve the seal that God has bestowed upon them at birth: *aperi mentem, serva signaculum*.

Physical probes of virginity are coarse since they are used as a pretext for disturbing manipulations, without even providing certain proof. Ambrose sets no store by them. However, according to his discourse on the Virgin Mary, the sexual organs of the Virgin, and hence of every virgin, are sealed. He casts no doubt upon the existence of the hymen. On the contrary, it is a necessary presupposition for the interpretation of the Scriptures: it is the physical detail that makes the coming of the son of a virgin, who must be Unique, something miraculous and truly mysterious. Because of this barrier that is crossed but not pierced, the birth of Christ is a far more marvellous miracle than the birth of Perseus. And the incredulous Salome, who is represented by the Apocryphal Gospels as placing her finger between the Virginal Labia on Christmas night itself, thus touched the truth of a unique happening.[10]

Like Ambrose, both Augustine and Cyprian display utter scorn for such vaginal inspections, regarding them as midwives' practices lacking in respect for the sacredness of virgins.[11] But over and above all this indignation and mistrust, their writings testify to a real belief: namely, that the sexual organs of women carry the mark of virginity, a sign that cannot be reduced to the narrowness of the vagina that Soranus described. Augustine furthermore vouchsafes another precious piece of information that he claims to have found in Varro and that consequently relates to pagan Rome. He tells us, with considerable irony, that the Romans revered a plethora of deities who presided over various moments, each deity being responsible for a particular event. In particular, the various phases of marriage fell under their protection:

> When a male and a female are united, the god Jugatinus presides. Well, let this be borne with. But the married woman must be brought home: the god Domiducus also is invoked. That she may be in the house, the god Domitius is introduced. That she may remain with her husband, the goddess Manturnae is used. What more is required? Let human modesty be spared. Let the lust of flesh and blood go on with the rest, the secret of shame being respected. Why is the bedchamber filled with a crowd of deities, when even the groomsmen have departed? And, moreover, it is so filled, not that in consideration of their presence more regard may be paid to chastity, but that by their help the woman, naturally of the weaker sex, and trembling with the novelty of her situation, may the more readily yield her virginity. For there are the goddess Virginiensis, and the god-father Subigus, and the goddess-mother Prema, and the goddess Pertunda, and Venus, and Priapus. What is this?... Was Venus not sufficient alone, who is even said to be named from this, that without her power a woman does not cease to be a virgin? And certainly, if the goddess Virginiensis is present to loose the virgin's zone, if the god Subigus is present that the virgin may be got under the man, if the goddess Prema is present that, having been got under him, she may be kept down, and may not move herself, what has the goddess Pertunda to do there? Let her blush; let her go forth. Let the husband himself do something. It is disgraceful that any one but himself should do that from which she gets her name.[12]

So Pertunda is the divine personification of a particular task or operation: *pertundere* means to perforate, pierce, penetrate. "After lunch, I lie stretched out and pierce my tunic and mantle," laments a frustrated lover whose lady has left him to languish.[13] This eloquent text implies that, to Romans, virginity suggested the presence of a veil, a taut tissue, which would explain why Soranus, a Greek doctor teaching in Rome, launched his polemic denying the existence of the hymen. It would also explain why it is that the "anatomical" etymology of the name of the Greek marriage song, the *humenaios*, is mentioned by Servius, the author of a commentary on Virgil, but not by Proclus.

However, even if the Church Fathers spoke out against the physical verification of virginity, they stopped short of positively denying the legitimacy and bases of the underlying semiotics. It was left to educated doctors and natural philosophers to deny the existence of the *signaculum* that God was supposed to have given women;

and they did so by appealing to the plain facts: dissection denies the existence of the hymen and observation dissipates the entire fantasy. On the other hand, practicing doctors then turned themselves into ethnographers and psychologists to discover the reasons behind an idea so dear to both men and women, the world over.

> Midwives will certainly affirm that they know a virgin from one that is defloured, by the breach or foundraes of that membrane. But by their report too credulous Judges are soon brought to commit an error. For that midwives can speak nothing certainly of this membrane, may bee proved by this, becaus that one faith that the situation thereof is in the verie entrance of the privie parts, others saie it is in the midst of the neck of the womb, and others saie it is within at the inner orifice thereof, and som are an opinion that they saie or suppose that it cannot be seen or perceived before the first birth. But truly of a thing so rare, and which is contrarie to nature, there cannot be anie thing spoken for certaintie. Therefore the blood that commeth out at the first time of copulation comes not alwaies by the breaking of that membrane, but by the breaking and violating or renting of the little veins which are woven and bespread all over the superficial and inward parts of the womb and neck thereof, descending into the wrinkles, which in those that have not yet used the act of generation, are closed as if they were glewed together.[14]

Those are the words of Ambroise Paré, a Parisian doctor of the late sixteenth century. He was an experienced dissector of dead girls, an attentive reader of Galen, Avicenna and Almensor, and he was intrigued by sexual mores. He took a resolute stand against what he considered to be a common error:

> In som virgins or maidens in the orifice of the neck of the womb there is found a certain tunicle or membrane called of antient writers *Hymen*, which prohibiteth the copulation of a man, and causseth a woman to be barren; this tunicle is supposed by manie, and they not of the common sort onely, but also learned Physicians, to bee, as it were, the enclosure of the virginitie or maiden-head. But I could never finde it in anie, seeking of all ages from three to twelv, of all that I had under my hands in the Hospital of Paris.[15]

According to Paré, the ill-educated included a few misguided "colleagues" (such as "the great and excellent anatomist," Renaldus Columbus), the Africans of Mauritania (where the soiled bed linen is displayed when a nuptial defloration has taken place) and, above all, the midwives and the judges who call upon their evidence. The misunderstanding is widespread, the prejudice hard to correct. And this preconception that lurks and circulates among matrons threatens to obscure medical enlightenment. Paré, the surgeon, is himself no atheist, but he has no hesitation in rejecting as false a "certainty" that is based upon an unfortunate confusion between virtue and *atresia* (the state of being unperforated).

## A Real Being or a Deity of Fable?

Ambroise Paré was no blasphemous and isolated rebel, even if he did engage in this polemic. He was supported by a long tradition of the greatest of the ancient biologists and doctors, Hippocrates and Aristotle, Soranus and Galen. Some of these — Aristotle and Galen — made no mention at all of the virginal hymen, despite their great skill and the attention that they paid to all parts of the body, even the most negligible. Others did speak openly of a membrane that in some cases obstructed girl's vaginas, but always confidently pronounced it to be *pathological*. The Hippocratic Corpus recommends treating the membrane sometimes found in girls with the surgeon's knife.[16] As for Soranus, he is the very epitome of a doctor engaged in controversy over the existence of the hymen. He, for his part, resolutely denied it.[17] Unfortunately, it is very difficult to discover the identities of those whom this doctor practicing in Rome in the second century A.D. was attacking. However, it is easy enough to follow the exchanges in the extension of this same debate that took place between the anatomists of the European classical age. While Paré rallied to the banner of the Greeks, the equally famous Gabrielis Fallopius chose the opposite camp: "There is something worth observing in the female sinus. For there are some anatomists who scorn those who situate the hymen there. But to my mind, the latter do not deserve such derision, for it is true: you can see a fibrous [*nervea*], nonfleshy membrane that comes immediately after the urethra."[18]

Two centuries later, Diderot and D'Alembert's *Encyclopédie* in its turn joined battle against what it considered to be a pseudoscientific, imaginary and imposed notion, worthy only of the most uncultivated and barbarian peoples. So, in conclusion, let us turn to Buffon, that "physician so full of wit and enlightenment." The chevalier de Jaucourt reports his words in the *Encyclopédie*'s article on "Virginité":

Monsieur Buffon tells us that men, being jealous of their liberties of all kinds, have always set great store by anything whose exclusive and first possessors they have believed themselves to be. And that is the kind of madness that made the virginity of girls into something with a "real existence." *Virginity*, which is something moral, a virtue consisting entirely in a purity of heart, became a physical object that was the concern of all and sundry. They have surrounded the subject with opinions, customs, ceremonies, superstitions and even judgments and penalties. The most illicit abuses and the most unjustifiable customs have been sanctioned. They have subjected the most secret of natural parts to inspection by ignorant matrons and exposed them to the eyes of doctors, without realizing that such indecency is an assault against *virginity*. To seek to know it is a violation; and if a girl is put in an indecent position that must shame her internally, that is a veritable defloration.... Anatomy itself casts total doubt on the existence of this membrane known as the *hymen* and also on that of the myrtiform caruncles whose presence or absence were for a long time supposed to indicate defloration or *virginity*, as the case might be. I insist that anatomy justifies us in rejecting these two signs as not only dubious but pure figments of the imagination.

Virginity, then, was not a "physical object," nor did it have a "real existence." Its association with the body was totally metaphorical: it was a "purity of heart." The sexual organs of women were marked by no sign. As for the blood shed when sexual relations took place for the first time, that did not constitute any "real proof" of virginity either. On the contrary, "this would-be sign does not exist in circumstances where the entrance to the vagina has been naturally stretched or dilated." Buffon, like Paré, believed that the quantity of blood that flowed depended upon the relative dimensions of the sexual organs of the two partners. He was less categorical than Paré for, together with a number of other anatomists, he recognized a whole series of possibilities: there are sometimes four protuberances or caruncles, sometimes three or two; sometimes a kind of circular or semicircular ring may be observed, sometimes a wrinkle or a series of small folds. From a strictly anatomical point of view, he thus goes so far as to accept the idea of a half-moon of skin growing around the vagina; and this certainly comes very close to the definition of the hymen given by twentieth-century gynecologists. But what he rejects is the word "hymen" and the image of a taut membrane stretched across the opening of the vagina. It is his belief that, at the age of puberty, a girl's vagina narrows, as a consequence of her growth. The sexual parts, particularly the labia, "are swollen by the abundance of blood and, being thus increased in size, they become tumefied, pressing against each other and sticking together at all the points where they come into immediate contact. The orifice of the vagina in this way becomes narrower than it used to be." This narrowing may take various forms. But whatever its appearance, it is a phenomenon that is connected with a particular age and uncertain and variable circumstances. It should therefore be credited with no semiotic significance.

We began this study by questioning the signs said to indicate virginity and defloration. The answer provided by European medicine is extremely skeptical. In ancient Greece, there was no notion of the hymen. In Rome, Soranus plunged into a debate that was to continue to rage until the end of the eighteenth century. And since then? Modern doctors have resolved the matter once and for all: the hymen does exist. But what they call the hymen is quite different from the sealing membrane that the *Encyclopédie* rejected as no more than a "deity of fable." That kind of hymen no longer has any existence except in the anguished minds of misinformed women. The hymen of medical knowledge today is something akin to the "narrowing" with which many scientists of the past confidently replaced the notion of a gate of virginity.

Notes to The Body of Semen

1. F. Laborie, J. Marcus-Steiff and J. Moutot, "Procréations et filiations: Logiques des conceptions et des nominations," *L'Homme* 95 (July-Sept. 1985); pp. 5-38, esp. pp. 23-24.

2. On this point, see the studies of Y. Thomas, "Pères citoyens et cité des pères," in *Histoire de la famille* (Paris: Armand Colin, 1988); also, "Le ventre: Corps maternel, droit paternel," *Le genre humain* 14 ("La valeur") (Spring-Summer 1986), pp. 211-36.

3. On the juridical aspects of partrilineal and matrilineal transmission in ancient Greece, see A.R.W. Harrison, *The Law of Athens: The Family and Property* (Oxford, 1968), pp. 122-62; also G. Sissa, "La famille dans la cité," *Histoire de la famille*.

4. F. Héritier-Augé, "L'individu, le biologique et le social," *Le débat* 36 (Sept. 1985), pp. 27-32; also, "La cuisse de Jupiter: Réflexions sur les nouveaux modes de procréation," *L'Homme* 94 (April-June 1985), pp. 5-22, esp. p. 14.

5. C.-H. Pradelles de Latour, "Le Discours de la psychanalyse et la parenté," *L'Homme* 97-98 (Jan.-June 1986), pp. 93-106; pp. 97-98 cited.

6. I should like to make it clear that by this I do not mean to suggest that biological facts determine the mode of filiation, but that certain *models* of procreation that purport to convey biological knowledge and truth are already in themselves models of filiation.

7. Aristotle expounded his genetic theory in *Generation of Animals*, trans. A.L. Peck (London and Cambridge, Mass.: Loeb Classical Library, 1953). For a study of the problems raised by this text, see S. Byl, *Recherches sur les grands traités biologiques d'Aristote: Sources écrites et préjugés* (Brussels, 1980), and also S. Campese, P. Manuli and G. Sissa, *Madre materia* (Turin, 1983).

8. *Generation of Animals* (hereafter cited as *GA*) 734b7-17.

9. Aristotle, *Metaphysics*, trans. Hugh Tredennick (London and Cambridge, Mass.: Loeb Classical Library, 1968), 7.9.1034b: "And it is the same with natural formations as it is with the products of art. For the seed produces, just as do those things that function by art. It contains the form potentially."

10. "His hands move his tools and his tools move the material. In a similar way to this, Nature, acting in the male of semen-emitting animals, uses the semen as a tool, as something that has movement in actuality; just as when objects are being produced by any art, the tools are in movement, because the movement that belongs to the art is, in a way, situated in them" (*GA* 730b18-23).

11. *Ibid.* 730b14-15.

12. *Ibid.* 730b11.

13. *Ibid.* 738b20-25.

14. *Ibid.* 739a17-20.

15. *Ibid.* 732a22-23.

16. *Ibid.* 735b32-37.

17. *Ibid.* 736a4-5.

18. Aristotle implies that searching experiments had been carried out in this connection: "Watery substances freeze, but semen does not freeze when exposed to frost in the open air" (*GA* 735a34-36). The reason for this phenomenon is to be found in a general property of air, namely that it does not freeze (*GA* 736a22-23).

19. "In all cases, the semen contains within itself that which causes it to be fertile — what is known as the 'hot' substance, which is not fire or any similar substance but the *pneuma* which is enclosed within the semen or foam-like stuff, and the natural substance which is in the *pneuma*; and this substance is analogous to the element which belongs to the stars. That is why fire does not generate any animal, and we find no animal taking shape either in fluid or solid substances while they are under the influence of fire; whereas the heat of the sun does effect generation, and so does the heat of animals" (*GA* 736b33-737a3).

20. *Ibid.* 736a24-27.

21. *Ibid.* 737a7-16.

22. Galen, *On the Use of Parts* 14.3 and 10; *On Seed*, 2.2. Cf. P. Manuli, *Madre materia*, p. 172.

23. Diogenes Laertius, *Life of Pythagoras*, trans. R.D. Hicks (London and Cambridge, Mass.: Loeb Classical Library, 1979), p. 28: "The semen is a drop of brain containing hot vapor within it; and this, when brought to the womb, throws out from the brain lymph, fluid and blood whence are formed flesh, sinews, bones, hairs and the whole of the body, while soul and sense come from the vapor within."

24. Cf. S. Byl, *Recherches*, pp. 144-45.

25. Hippocratic Corpus, *On Generation*.

26. On the whole of this tradition, see. P. Darmon, *Le mythe de la procréation à l'age baroque*, 2d ed. (Paris, 1981), pp. 75-77.

NOTES TO THE SEAL OF VIRGINITY

1. J.A. Harburg, "Hymenaios (Brautlied)," *Philologus* 3 (1948), pp. 238-46; p. 238 cited.

2. See G. Sissa, *Le corps virginal* (Paris: Vrin, 1987), pp. 110-26.

3. Peter Damian, *Letter on Divine Omnipotence* 2.4.8.

4. *Ibid*. 596c-597a.

5. *Ibid*. 597a.

6. *Ibid*. 599d-600a.

7. *Ibid*. 601b.

8. St. Ambrose, in Epistula 5, *Patrologia Latina*, vol. 16, cols. 891-98.

9. St. Ambrose, *De institutione virginis*, in *Patrologia Latina*, vol. 16, col. 319.

10. *Protevangelium of James* 19.1-20.2; Pseudo-Matthew 13.3-5.

11. St. Augustine, *City of God* (New York: The Modern Library, 1950), 1.18; Cyprian, *Epistula ad Pomponium de virginibus*, in *Patrologia Latina*, vol. 4, col. 364.

12. Augustine, *City of God* 7.9.

13. Catullus 32.11.

14. Ambroise Paré, *Concerning the Generation of Man*, trans. T. Johnson (London, 1649), ch. 42.

15. *Ibid*.

16. Hippocratic Corpus 1.20.

17. Soranus, *Gunaikeia* 1.16-17.

18. Gabrielis Fallopius, *Observationes anatomicae* (Venice, 1561), vol. 2, col. 194.

**Translated by Janet Lloyd.**

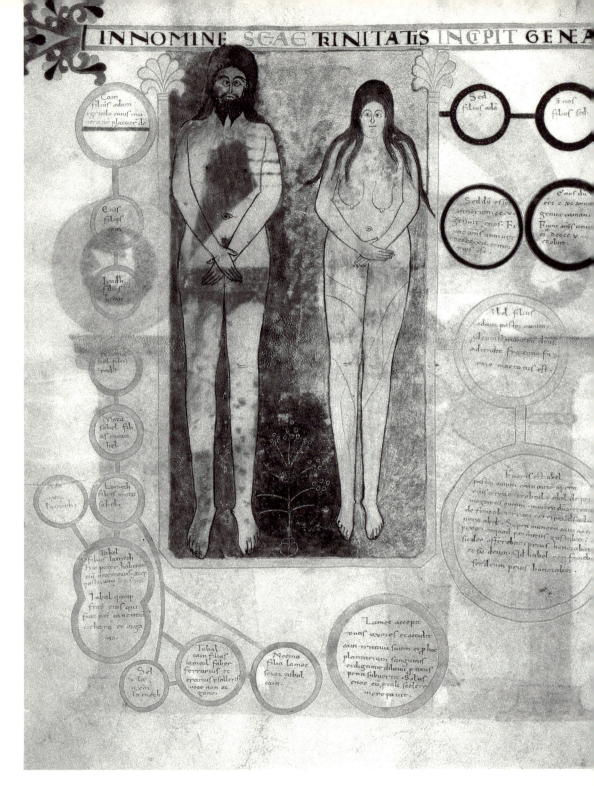

*L'Apocalypse*, Abbey of Saint Sever, 11th century
(Paris, Bibliothèque nationale).

# Semen and Blood:
# Some Ancient Theories Concerning Their
# Genesis and Relationship

*Françoise Héritier-Augé*

Fee-fi-fo-fum
I smell the blood of an Englishman
Be he alive, or be he dead
I'll have his bones to grind my bread
> —English children's song

Adam, Adam, where art thou?
Dese bones gwine to rise again
Heah, Marse Lord, Ise a-comin' now
Dese bones gwine rise again
> —American gospel song

When a child is born, its veins carry a certain amount of blood, but those of the adult carry much more. If blood is lost in the course of life, through accident or according to the laws of nature in the case of women, it is also constantly recreated in the body. Blood is essential to life, life's mainstay. Its presence inside the body denotes life; a living body that is bled white becomes cold, a corpse. Blood and life embody heat. A child, born living and warm, carrying within it that small quantity of blood its body can contain, is the result of a conjunction without which reproduction is impossible; through this conjunction a substance is conveyed from the male body to the female one, a substance that appears necessary to the creation of this new, living human being. However, this substance is not blood, but "seed," or semen. What is more, only nubile girls and women who have not reached menopause — that is, women who lose blood — are able to conceive.

This simple combination of facts, built on commonplace human experience, has been the cause of speculation in all societies. Where do blood and semen come from? How are they constituted inside the body? In what relationship do they stand to each other? What happens when conception takes place? And further still: How does the biological link relate to the social link? What determines descent? How is the continuity between the living and the dead ascertained along the interwoven lines of progeny? What goes into the making of a person? What does he or she transmit in turn? In what way does a child combine what it receives from each of its parents? How can we account for likenesses? And so on.

To these questions and to many others — for the above catalogue is far from exhaustive — complex answers have been provided. Such answers take the form of more or less elaborate theories of the person, aimed characteristically at presenting a coherent, well-ordered world image, fraught with meaning and able to account for its existence and reproduction. Each human group, through the collective and interrelated thinking of its members, produces its own theory. The anthropological outlook takes account of these diverse and original versions and of their inner logical structure. Clearly, these theories have no scientific basis, though they exemplify a mode of thinking that arises, if not from experimentation, at least from observation and experience, and may well be thought of as belonging to a rational order. They are not true for that reason. Instead, they are regarded as true simply because they account satisfactorily for the facts that meet the eye.

Still and all, however diverse and unscientific these theories may be, it appears that only a small number of explanatory models can be built that are capable of answering certain central questions. The thinking involved in the building of such models has to account for the same directly observable empirical data, which leave scant possibilities of choice. The answer, if shaped in the mind that formulates it, is also already shaped by things themselves. Hence, the main point of reflection concerning the genesis of blood and semen — the subject with which I am concerned here — deep-rooted as it is in the anatomy and the physiology of both the human and animal body, comes up against an initial constraint of a purely physical order. I believe that this constraint explains why people living in very different epochs and in very different parts of the world have arrived at remarkably similar theories, as well as why those theories, in their explanatory acuteness and sophistication, sometimes tally with the most modern knowledge on the subject.

Thus, my Samo informants in Burkina Faso make use of their anatomical observations to construct a model that encompasses and qualifies these observations. According to them, both sexes dispose of "sex-water" (the literal translation of *do mu*), which is discharged during sexual intercourse; but only men's sex-water is thick and laden with generative potency. Its encounter with a thickened mass of blood, a kind of blood clot, spinning inside the womb, brings about the conception of a child, provided the clot is in the right position when ejaculation occurs. Sex-water is produced by the male's bones, his joints and his spinal column, which serves as a collector. Impregnation does not take place every time people make love. A particular orientation of the clot is a necessary precondition. When it does occur, an extremely strong suction is believed to be exerted upon the male seed, which is thought to be literally sucked inward. I have often heard that a man who complains at daybreak of aching all over, of back pains and sore knees is teased by the others because his pains are the result of having "made a child" that very night. The pain is ascribed to a brutal, near-total draining of the substance present in the man's bones. This reddish substance, thick and mucilaginous, is called *mu zunare* ("gluey water," or "ropy water") and ordinarily circulates quietly through the human body. It is set into motion by walking or any other physical activity, and turns into blood and semen, a transformation about which I have little information. When impregnation takes place, this gentle alchemy is quickened by a powerful discharge of that particular form of energy and heat which belongs only to man, and is required for impregnation.

Later on, semen turns into blood inside the woman's body, either by reverting to a prior state, if semen is the ultimate stage of a transformational process, or by achieving completion in the form of blood, if semen is only an intermediate stage. In spite of this residual ambiguity, semen and blood would appear to have a common origin: marrow, that of the bones and that of the spinal cord, merged together as a unique entity.

In ordinary times – that is, when a woman is neither pregnant nor nursing – sexual intercourse between spouses provides the wife with a surplus of blood, the largest part of which she loses through her menses, a fact that accounts for the abundance of menstrual blood shed by adult women as compared to nubile girls. When a child is conceived, the husband's seed, transmuted into blood, is vested in the child to which it brings the blood endowment necessary to the support of breath, heat and life. With that end in view, sexual relations must be sustained and assiduous, and the parents must conform to that requirement repeatedly throughout the first seven months of pregnancy (a requirement that, incidentally, is thought to account for the distinctive features that typify a posthumous child). As for the mother, she makes use of her own blood, which she no longer loses, as the raw material for her child's body, including its skeleton.

When the dangerous moment of her lying-in is passed — a time when considerable heat is lost through the expulsion of the child's body in a copious flow of blood — the mother, who is kept warm beside a continuously burning fire and through washing with very hot water, will realize, step by step, the transmutations that pertain exclusively to woman: the gluey substance contained in her bones will turn into milk. Essentially cold by nature, women never manage to make semen, the only body fluid with fecund power. Out of their substance, they obtain a less perfect product, but one that nevertheless taxes all of their capacity for heat. This explains the disappearance of menses, at least during the first months of nursing. All of the heat and all of the substance available goes into milk-making. And though they continue to produce enough blood to cover their own needs, women have none to spare. Man alone has enough heat and potency to produce two distinct body fluids, simultaneously and plentifully.

During the nursing period, sexual relations are normally interrupted. This is a well-known prohibition. The Samo explain it by the fact that semen and milk are similar in nature, though unequal in quality, hence their incompatibility. The intense heat that pervades semen risks burning up the milk. Even through occasional sexual intercourse, the sperm is thought to adulterate the taste of milk, causing the child to turn away crying from the breast, a symptom that makes people suspect that the parents have transgressed the prohibition.

That the mother fashions her infant's skeleton with her own blood may startle us, insofar as the substance contained in the bones later provides fresh supplies of blood for the individual and sperm for the male child. But we are dealing here with a society that is patrilineal (descent through the male line) and patrivirilocal (a son lives with his wives at his father's residence). These facts can be diversely construed; but first of all, let us be rid of an illusion. What we have seen so far should not be taken as meaning that the women transmit something of their own; this always remains a man's affair. A woman inherits blood from her own father who, having received an initial endowment of blood from his father, has also produced blood, day after day in his own bone marrow, constituted by the blood of his mother, and beyond her, by that of his male ancestors in the maternal line.

If, once accepting these premises (the differential contributions of the father and the mother, and the marrow's capacity to produce body fluids), we take them to their logical conclusion, we find the hazy outlines of a sophisticated theory: the infinite regression of those endowments in blood received from male ancestors through the agency of women, even though the endowments that come from the paternal ancestors remain ever-present in the foreground. With every fruitful union new endowments are made, which become obliterated in the course of time, as one passes from one generation to the next. For each grown child, the fraction of blood coming from his or her mother — that is, the fraction constantly generated from the mucilaginous substance within her bones and, behind the mother, from the mother's father — this fraction is thought to accompany that coming from the father at birth, and to precede the fractions coming respectively from the father's mother's father and the mother's mother's father. Those portions coming from more distant ancestors disappear, or remain only as infinitesimal strains.

We are even provided with a threshold of conscious recognition. Indeed, a parallel can be drawn between this theory of the making of a child and Samo marriage rules. Thus, to choose a very precise example, a marriage with a cognate in a collateral line, descended from a female ancestor related to Ego's line through men only, is allowed only at four generations' remove from the common ancestor of the two lines. From this rule we may infer that three intervening generations are necessary to expunge in a child all traces of the physical imprint left in him/her by any ancestor to whom he/she is related through a woman. The prohibitions concerning marriage between such blood relations up to the third generation, and also between cousins who happen to be cognates in a still more complex way, together with other such prohibitions, result in — if they are not aimed at — preventing reinforcement by "agglutination" of those blood lines which we shall call recessive. That is, lines of identical blood or a dominant line and a recessive line of the same blood are not permitted to be rejoined, once they are separate, without a three-generation interval.

Yet another illusion must also be set aside. The dominant strain originating in the paternal line is also a compound, subject to the same regressive pattern as those endowments that come from the maternal ancestors. A man's blood is also renewed during his lifetime through the marrow of his bones, which derives from his mother's blood, and so on. Thus, what this theory expresses, in a social context where descent traced in the agnatic line takes precedence, is that this phenomenon relies more on "speech" and less on blood relationships, insofar as it is based on the common will and public acknowledgment of the social link. As the Samo are wont to say: "Words make descent, and words can take it back." This quite explicit maxim, whose bearing is strongly implemented by the genetic theory of blood, allows us to single out the salient points for this particular society: the individual exists as such only in the diversity of blood lines; and social descent is traced less through transmission by blood than through speech, as the common will voiced and affirmed by the social group. Obviously, each one of these important points would be of a radically different nature in a society that, for example, gave preference to consanguineous unions between close cousins.

If descent is thus construed as one particular path among the several that concur in the advent of an individual composed of flesh, bones and blood, it is also explicitly defined through the communal partaking of food inside the lineage. Group eating is marked out in silhouette by prohibitions peculiar to each group; food generates and renews not only the flesh of the individual, but also his bones and their precious content, which in turn generate blood and semen. Life — which, according to the Samo conceptual scheme, is one of the nine ingredients of man or woman — pervades the world. Every living creature retains a particle of it. Life is conveyed by the blood throughout the body. But if flesh is liable to death and decay, life still endures in a subdued, dormant form inside the bones and disappears totally only when these are burned — a fact that corroborates the idea of a life-conveying blood originating in the bones (Héritier 1977).

I have presented this African example in a brief and necessarily incomplete form. My description purports to show how a coherent, all-embracing scheme is built which encompasses in a single proposition a definition of the individual and a conception of man in society that embraces both the social links among human beings and the natural world. More could be said here about certain key notions,

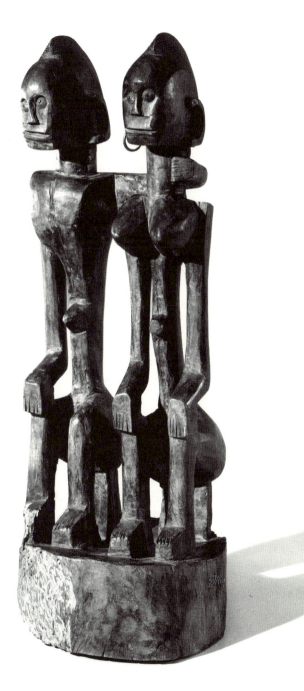

Depiction of a pair of Dogon grandparents, Mali (Zurich, Rietbergmuseum).

165

certain archaic themes, which underlie all these theories, such as the contrasting pair identical/different, which acts as an essential classifier in Samo thinking. The notional system constructed by the observer out of parts of speech and elements of behavior is necessarily imperfect, in that it can never be an entirely closed system. Indeed, for the social actors themselves, it is rarely if ever given as a coherent discourse connecting and integrating in a meaningful context all the salient points we have mentioned: the genetic theory of body fluids and that of the person, the theory of alliance and descent, that of imputed powers and forces. But it is a system that functions only when required, justifying as necessary daily rites, prohibitions and practices. To be sure, from a dialectical perspective, as a system it is not devoid of contradictions.

What has just been said should not be taken to mean that the analysis of any conceptual scheme always rests upon the local theory concerning body fluids, or that the rationale for each act, which functions when required, always derives logically from this same conception of things. The structured ideational scheme, which makes sense and is evolved differently in each society, is made up of mutually definable elements. These add the constraint of their inevitable interaction and reciprocal development to the basic constraint, which derives from the observation of those natural phenomena that must be understood and thus explained – rather in the way stacked weapons assume their characteristic shape only because each weapon leans upon all the others.

In the light of the preceding, the grounds for my assumption – that the explanatory acuteness of such theories sometimes leads them to converge with scientific knowledge because they are deeply rooted in careful observations of human anatomy and physiology – may seem clearer. Thus, for instance, the bone marrow's hematopoietic function is recognized, even if the actual process remains unknown and undescribed, and even if no distinction is drawn between bone marrow and spinal marrow. Likewise, the idea of a progressive obliteration of some ancestors' contributions, calculated in terms of their increasing genealogical remoteness through women, tallies in one sense with the scientific notion of recessivity. The marriage prohibitions obtaining among the Samo between individuals carrying particles of the same blood are not based on eugenics – that is, on the necessity of preventing the possible transmission of consanguineous taints. We are dealing here instead with a fundamental ideological privilege, active in every domain, accorded to the principle of difference rather than that of identity. These prohibitions neatly concur with the idea of a genetic reshuffling of homozygotic factors. What is more, a fecundating principle is understood to be transmitted from one body to another.

I have made a second assumption. The fact that the initial physical constraint consists in the same observable data — the functioning of the human body — means that explanatory theories elaborated quite independently, in different places and at different epochs, coincide in a remarkable fashion on certain precise points, even if the linkage of the diverse elements included in each such cultural scheme shows significant variation. This perspective, if it does not absolutely exclude the existence of mutual borrowing, and the far-reaching diffusion of ideas under peaceable conditions, nevertheless strongly implies that such borrowing is never as successful as when it is cast in a mold to some degree foreordained by certain physiological features built into the structure of the species.

That the Samo theory is not a unique instance — a "hapax" — I should now like to show briefly. I will take as a central point the sequence bone/seed/blood, or more comprehensively, food/marrow/seed and blood,* and examine it on the basis of a few cases, some of which, while civilizationally near to Western cultures, are remote from them in time, while others are part of contemporary ethnographic knowledge. There probably are many other such examples, but the comparative outlook must use the data available, and pertinent cases may be missing. We know that an ethnographic report is simply what the author was able or allowed to see. Moreover, the most fundamental ideas are those people live and breathe by, so naturally that they function, as it were, by preterition, without the need being felt to formulate them. Since every ideational scheme functions that way, traces must be isolated, extrapolated and illuminated, as we shall see in the case of ancient Egypt.

There do exist, however, in the great written traditions, notably in Greek and Hindu thought, texts in which the combination of observable facts have been ordered along rational lines. In the treatise entitled *Generation of Animals*, Aristotle

---

*The theories of the origin of sperm and blood can be classified according to two main themes: they derive from substances already present inside the body or ingested by man; or they are gifts bestowed by supernatural beings. We shall consider here only the first of these explanatory schemes.

expounds admirably upon a series of processes of a biochemical nature, without requiring that substances pass through the bones. Here, blood, milk and sperm are residues (sperm being the only perfect residue) of the transformation of food inside the body. The proof is in "the feeling of weakness which follows upon the slightest emission of sperm, as if the body were deprived of the end product of nutrition" (1.18, 725a5; author's trans.). The process involves the transformation of food into blood, and thereafter — as a result of diverse processing procedures according to sex — into seed by males and milk by females. Man produces sperm because his is a warm nature, such that he possesses a capacity for bringing about an intense concoction of the blood, which transforms it into its purest and thickest residue: sperm, or male seed. Women cannot perform this operation. They lose blood, and at their warmest, they can only succeed in turning it into milk. "Because menses occur, there can be no sperm" (1.19. 727a30). Thus, the ultimate difference between the sexes lies in the fact that one is warm and dry, the other cold and wet, qualities that reveal themselves in their aptitude or inaptitude for achieving concoction." We now have a double transformational sequence: food/blood/sperm, food/blood/milk, which offers a rationalization of the production of fluids as a whole, and above all, orders them hierarchically in terms of a distinction established between the sexes that produce them — a distinction presented as the ultimate rationale and justification of the social order. This same distinction, formulated in hierarchically ordered contrasting terms, necessary to the understanding of the inner workings of fluid production as propounded by Aristotle, is also to be found in conceptual systems in which the male seed is not necessarily thought of as the ultimate stage of blood heating or concoction. We have noted it already among the Samo.

In the Hindu world, as well, semen is considered to originate from food, but the sequence is completed without passage through the blood. But here we are dealing less with an analysis of processes of a somewhat biochemical nature (as in the case of Aristotle) than with what is, strictly speaking, a cosmic vision which integrates all the elements of the universe into a never-ending cycle. Some upaniṣad-s written before 1200 B.C. describe a perfect circle: "From water earth, from earth herbs, from grass food, from food semen, from semen man. Man thus consists of the essence of food" (Taittirīya Upaniṣad 2.1; in Keswani 1962:210-11). Cremation is then conceived of as a necessity: the body consumed by fire rises up in smoke,

desire is the Real — He should be searched out, Him one should desire to understand. He obtains all worlds and all desires who has found out and who understands
that Self."[82] The *Kaṭha-Upaniṣad* (6.14-15) says:

> When are liberated all
> The desires that lodge in one's heart,
> Then a mortal becomes immortal!
> Therein he reaches Brahman!
>
> When are cut all
> The knots of heart here on earth,
> Then a mortal becomes immortal!
> — Thus far is the instruction.

The *Muṇḍaka-Upaniṣad* (2.2.8) provides a similar message:

> The knot of the heart is loosened,
> All doubts are cut off,
> And one's deeds (*karman*) cease
> When He is seen — both the higher and the lower.

## II. The *Garbha-Upaniṣad*

The *Garbha-Upaniṣad* is related to the Atharvanic tradition, as the name of its author,
Pippalāda, illustrates. A short treatise on embryology, it is situated at the crossroads
of several different influences: the *Sāṃkhya-Yoga*, medical texts such as the *Caraka-
Saṃhitā* and *Suśruta-Saṃhitā*, and the *Vedānta*.

Several editions of this *Upaniṣad* are in existence and two of them, found in the
collection *Upaniṣad-Samuccaya* in *Ānandāśramasaṃskṛtagranthāvalī* (1925), include
commentaries by Nārāyaṇa and Śaṅkarānanda. The text that we are publishing here
is from 108 Upaniṣad-s (Bombay: Nirṇaya-sāgara Press, 1925).

In order to better understand the movement of the text, the following parts
should be distinguished: the body's constitution and psychophysiology; the stages
of embryonic and fetal development up until the eighth month; an aetiology of malformations; embryology and soteriology, the ninth month and birth; the correlations between parts of the body and elements of sacrifice; and a brief anatomical

recapitulation. It concludes with the abrupt: "Such is the treatise on deliverance by Pippalāda."

The first part should be understood in light of the *Āyur-Veda*'s classical doctrine. The sections concerning the body, *Śārīra-sthāna*, found in the treatises by Caraka and Suśruta, are especially important. Beginning with a theory of man and spirit based on *Sāṃkhya* ideas, it is followed by an embryology. Our Upaniṣad corresponds quite well with these medical findings. The human body, just like the universe, is made up of the five elements: space (*ākāśa*), wind (*vāyu*, *vāta*), fire (*tejas*, *agni*), water (*āpas*, *jala*) and earth (*pṛthivī*, *bhūmi*). More precisely, while the body is the seat of the psyche (*cetanā*), its material is the result of a modification in these elements (*CS* 4.4.6). It should be pointed out that these elements do not intervene with the body in their pure state, but are combined into complex and various proportions, according to the three main properties (*tri-guṇa*: *sattva*, *rajas* and *tamas*) of "Evolving Nature" (*prakṛti*).

Moreover, the father's semen (*śukra*), which produces the embryo when united with the mother's blood (*śonita*), already contains, from the very start, four of the elements. The *ākāśa* is added during a period of fertility (*ārtava*) when the semen comes into contact with the blood in the uterus (*garbhāśaya*). Yet, in order for an embryo to form, the body's substances (*dhātu*) are not enough, nor is this union between semen and blood. A more subtle element, *manas*, *karman* or *ātman*, is needed (cf. *vijñāna* for the Buddhists). (On this subject see *CS* 4.2-3, *SS* 3.1.16, Vāgbbhaṭṭa, *Āṣṭāṅga-Saṃgraha* 2.2, Cakrapāṇi, *Āyur-Veda-Dīpikā* 4.2.23-27, *Sāṃkhya-Kārikā* 39.)

Now let us turn to embryonic development. According to the doctors, the formation of the heart, the seat of the psyche (*cetanādhiṣṭhāna*), occurs during the fourth and fifth months. During the fifth and sixth months the embryo is endowed with *manas*, spirit, and with *buddhi*, consciousness. During the seventh month the limbs are completed and fortified. In the eighth month vital fluids (*ojo-dhātu*) are passed from the mother to her future child, and a birth during this period is considered dangerous to both of them. In general, the gestation period lasts nine months, but can continue for as long as twelve.

On the determination of sex, as well as on the subject of eunuchs (and hermaphrodites), the Upaniṣad is in agreement with the medical texts. These documents often link malformations and infirmities to a lack or insufficiency of a certain *dhātu* or organic element, such as *tejo-dhātu*, the fire element, in the case of blindness. To what degree do these anomalies come from the parents? The doctors answer: Only when serious faults affect their semen. The Upaniṣad, on the other hand, attributes malformations to a troubled *manas*, which amounts to saying that a child's life and destiny are determined by his parents' mental state. One would think that the Upaniṣad would appeal to the karmic potential already accumulated by the future being. In fact a little later on it does, but to account for the process of individuation, not birth defects. Doctors, however, considered very bad *karman* to be one of the important factors in explaining deformities.

Whatever the case may be, the problem of knowing where this new individual is situated within the complex network of influence is posed. What are the determining factors of his future destiny? They fall into two different categories: on the one hand, the biological material provided by the parents, and on the other, the karmic potential accumulated by the individual from his past lives, passed on continually from himself to himself. Consisting of a certain "psychological continuum,"[83] he is nothing but a subtle body, the holder of residue from past actions. While it never pronounces these words, our Upaniṣad certainly appeals to the karmic chain's continuity in order to explain the process of individuation.

Are these two causal series, the one physical, provided by the parents, the other psychological, provided by the individual himself, entirely distinct — or do they in some way intersect? In effect, by stating that one is born a boy or a girl according to the proportion of the two semens and that a cripple results from the parent's mental troubles, the Upaniṣad makes the individual's entire destiny, in particular his social and religious destiny, depend on the physical series and all the psychophysiological material it provides. A cripple does not have access to the fullness of ritual life, and it matters a great deal whether one is born a boy or a girl in Indian society. The field of merit (*puṇyakṣetra*) is not the same, with all the consequences that this implies. Where does the strict law of *karman* fit in? In order to resolve this problem it would be necessary to reconcile the two causal series into a single schema, which in turn would need to put forward the hypothesis that the subtle body chooses its own womb, according to his latent desires (*vāsanā*) and motivations (*saṃskāra*) already accumulated from past lives.

Let us now consider the fetus's curious monologue, in which we can see the embryology–soteriology relation formed.[84] Completed during the ninth month, the fetus is entirely equipped from a physical, sensory and even intellectual point of view. Due to the *buddhi* he can distinguish good deeds from evil ones and contemplate the Imperishable. Remarkably, he has memories from past lives, a knowledge that is extraordinarily difficult for the adult *yogin* to recapture later on. However, once the child enters the world, he no longer possesses any of these faculties. What has happened in the meantime? The trauma of birth: the child, tightly squeezed in the process, is stunned by the *vaisnava vāya* (defined as *māyā-rūpa* or "form of illusion" in Nārāyana's commentary) and "loses the memory of his births and deaths and no longer knows a good deed from an evil one. To be born is to cross the threshold from memory into oblivion."[85]

Before his birth, finding himself alone and unhappy, locked inside the womb, unable to find a remedy, the fetus makes resolutions: "If one day I am freed from the womb...." A brief eclectic review of the means of deliverance follows: *bhakti*, *śivaïte* or *visnuïte*, *Sāmkhya-yoga* and meditation on the eternal *brahman*. By following certain paths of devotion, a mere touch from the chosen deity is enough to suddenly cancel the law of *karman*. Whatever the case may be, what makes this text so interesting is the close tie it establishes between embryology and soteriology, thanks to the law of *karman*, grasped at the heart of the matter, that is, inside the mother's womb. How does the fetus get out? The linguistic root MUC (*yadi yonyāh pramucye...*) provides the answer, on two different levels: to be born is to be freed from the womb, but deliverance is to be freed from all wombs (cf. *Ch.-Up.* 8.14).

With a play on words, the text returns to its definition of the body as the setting of three psychophysiological fires. It then attempts to relate the three sacrificial fires to three different parts of the body. Other elements and instruments of sacrifice enter in also, corresponding to diverse aspects of the psychophysical organism. All in all, the body is treated as the setting of a transposed sacrifice.[86]

The short list that closes the Upanisad reinforces the idea of the body as nothing but a composed entity ready to decompose, made up of many impurities. He who understands the corporeal mass as such aspires to free himself from it and qualifies for deliverance.

ABBREVIATIONS

Upaniṣad = Up.

Aitareya = Ait.-Up.

Bṛhadāraṇyaka-Up. = BĀU

Caraka-Saṃhitā = CS

Chāndogya = Ch.-Up.

Kauṣitaki = Kauṣ.-Up.

Māṇḍūkya = Māṇḍ.-Up.

Muṇḍaka = Muṇḍ.-Up.

Suśruta-Saṃhitā = SS

Śvetāśvatara = Śvet.-Up.

Taittirīya = Tait.-Up.

NOTES

1. Space (ākāśa), wind (vāyu, vāta), fire (tejas, agni), water (āpas, jala), earth (pṛthivī, bhūmi).

2. The five sense organs and the manas.

3. Qualities perceived by the five senses and the manas. Elements, organs and qualities are arranged according to the following diagram:

| earth | water | fire | wind | space |
|-------|-------|------|------|-------|
| nose | tongue | eyes | skin | ears |
| odors | flavors | forms and colors | touch | sound |

As for the manas, its role is to organize, by sorting through and forming objects out of the raw material taken in by the sense organs. It also develops internal information that it transmits to the ātman.

4. The organism's seven constituents (dhātu) are: organic juices or sap (rasa), blood (rakta), flesh (māṃsa), fat (medas), bones (asthi), marrow (majja) and sperm (śukra). They are made from the organism's three main active principles (tri-dhātu): wind (vāta) in the form of different vital breaths, fire in the form of bile (pitta) and water in the form of serous fluids and secretions (kapha, śleṣman). Together these dhātu furnish [the body with] vital juices (ojas).

5. Fingernails (nakha), hair (keśa), body hair (loma). A more complete list of twelve exists (see Mānava-Dharma-Śāstra 5. 135) which includes nasal mucus, ear wax, eye secretions, phlegmatic secretions, sweat, urine and feces as well. Nails, hair and body hair are cited more often because they are subject to growth and death. Once detached from the body they become impure. These physical impurities are a natural result of the three constituents' (tri-dhātu) functioning.

6. This double origin is blood (śonita) from the mother and sperm (śukra) from the father.

7. What is drunk, eaten, licked and sucked.

8. tejas: "force, flame, burst." It is used here to designate fire's double nature as light and heat.

9. Indians see ākāśa as a hollow (suṣira) in which the wind – rightfully called "the one who makes

the hole" (*suṣirakāra*) – blows. In the human body, *ākāśa* occupies such cavities as the heart, the stomach, the bladder, etc. While the skin's pores ventilate the body, they also serve as a means of entry for *ākāśa*.

10. *piṇḍi-karaṇa*: the action of rolling material (clay, boiled rice, etc.) into a ball with the help of a liquid, such as saliva, with food.

11. The wind functions to circulate and redistribute objects in space.

12. *ākāśa* is omnipresent. Because of this it can offer the space it thoroughly occupies as a gift. Since it is emptiness, it gives the possibility of taking up room, of occupying a place. It thus opposes the idea of closure or narrowness (*aṃhas*) and therefore of anguish.

13. *apāna*: vital breath located at the base of the body that makes its way from top to bottom. This word also means anus, which is how it is used here. The *apāna* breath expels excrement as well as the fetus from the womb.

14. Literally, awake and awakening, thus consciousness and becoming conscious. This word refers to intelligence inasmuch as it means power to obtain a clear and distinct vision of a situation and to arrive at full knowledge of the facts. As the faculty of discrimination and decision making, the *buddhi* (as opposed to the *manas*, which is continually being shaken by solicitations from the outside) brings together the intellectual and intentional aspects of our power of determination.

15. From the root MAN, to think; mental organ, *sensorium commune*. It centralizes the various sensations and perceptions, and holds on to their traces or memories. In return, it projects our intentionality – desires and ideas (*saṃkalpa*) – onto the world.

16. *rasa*: Its most common usage is sap or juice. It can also mean flavor or taste. The theory of the *rasa* involves several different aspects.

As a taste on the tongue, the *rasa*'s counterpart in the real world is water, which produces different flavors by mixing with the other elements, such as earth, fire or air. A predominance of water in the mixture produces a sweet taste (*madhura*); a predominance of earth and fire produces a sour taste (*amla*); of water and fire, a salty taste (*lavaṇa*); of air and *ākāśa*, a bitter taste (*tikta*); of air and fire, a pungent taste (*kaṭu*); and of air and earth, a sharp taste (*kaṣāya*). *Rasa* also refers to the gastric juices produced when the elements are assimilated. Furthermore, this same word is used to designate aesthetic tastes or fundamental emotional tones. The artist must extricate these from their empirical gangue in order to savor them in their pure state.

17. Notes of the musical scale, usually referred to by their first syllables: *sa, ri, ga, ma, pa, dha, ni*. They are listed here as an auditory example. These "sounds," from which melodic themes or *rāga* are composed, are able to provoke a variety of tastes or sentiments whose characters will be accord-

ingly sweet, bitter, awful, soothing, etc.

18. Here we have a list of colors for the eye. They can be related to the "sounds" in the previous sentence that, when composed in melody, are described as each having a specific color.

We are more concerned, however, with the seven *dhātu* found in the following sentence. A specific color is attributed to the diverse liquids circulating in the body's "canals" (*dhamani*, *nāḍi*). Their point of departure is the heart (see *BĀU* 2.1.19, 4.2.3; *Ch.-Up.* 8.6.6; *Kaṭha-Up.* 6.16; etc.). These canals are at the same time nerve circuits that transmit sensory impressions (sounds, colors, odors) as well as information furnished by the *manas* and the *buddhi*. All this put together constitutes the individual's psychophysiological make up. The functions of the *dhātu* thus account for the body's composition.

19. Here it is a question of *kapha* or *sleṣman* (phlegm, lymph). This liquid is related to the *soma*, which is itself related to the moon ("the cold star"), while bile (*pitta*) is identified with the sun's igneous element (*agneya*). See *SS* 3.3.2.

20. This inner fire is a product of the igneous element that circulates throughout the body and gathers in the form of bile. It is fanned by the wind, the motor force that circulates throughout the respiratory system and digestive tract. The heart is not only the seat of organic breath, but also the point of origin for canals conveying blood.

21. According to the commentaries, this word should appear in the following sentence. Just as Prajāpati is born at the end of one year and identifies with this duration, nine to ten months (some say twelve) are needed for the human being to form.

22. The end of menstruation is thought to be an auspicious period for conception. According to *SS* 3.5, the twelve nights following menstruation are favorable to fertilization. *Mānava-Dharma-Śāstra*, 3.46, says: "Each month, after the moment the blood appears, with four distinct days forbidden by decent people, there are sixteen days and sixteen nights that form what we call the natural season of women."

23. The embryo in jelly form, just after conception (*SS* 2.50-51).

24. "Bubble" or "blister," the embryo from the fifth to the seventh day.

25. Lump or spherical mass, the embryo up until the fifteenth day (*SS* 3.14).

26. The word *na-puṃsaka*, translated here as "eunuch," literally means "without virile character." It is also often translated as "hermaphrodite" or one who possesses certain characteristics of both sexes.

27. The "Nonmanifested" (*avyakta*) plus the following seven: the *buddhi* or *mahant*, the "I" or ego (*ahaṃkāra*), and the subtle elements (*tan-mātra*).

28. The sixteen "evolved but no longer evolving" are the five faculty organs of knowledge (*jñāna-*

or *buddhi-indriyāṇi*), the five faculty organs of action (*karmendriyāṇi*), the inner meanings (*manas*) and the five principal raw elements.

29. Making the most of VID's two meanings – (1) to know how to, to know of, to understand; (2) to find, to obtain, to prove – the commentaries annotate *vindati* with *sukha duḥkha sākṣātkāraṃ prapnoti* and *labhate jānīta....* On the whole, the former meaning seems to prevail. This will be made especially clear a little later on when *smarati* and *vindati* are taken up again in a negative form, at the moment of birth.

30. Like those who desert the battlefield, the commentaries tell us, the people who have shared his life (father, mother, children, friends) are no longer there to help him. He must confront the situation alone. The law of *karman* is understood here as being strictly individual.

31. "Great Lord," one of Śiva's names.

32. One of Viṣṇu's names, especially used in reference to his cosmological and yogic aspects.

33. *yantra*: from YAM, meaning to hold back, to curb, to restrain; it signifies any mechanical instrument that clasps and confines. Here it is used for the neck of the womb.

34. "The wind of birth," *sūti-vāyu* or *prasūti-māruta*, referred to here as *vaiṣṇava*, *vāyu*, the wind belonging to Viṣṇu. A particular function of the *apāna*, the wind located at the base of the body, this wind is a violent current of air that expels the child from the womb. "Just as the wind stirs up a wide expanse of water from everywhere, the fetus is stirred up, and in the tenth month he leaves the womb" (*Ṛg-Veda* 5.78. 7-9).

Vedic mythology already associates Viṣṇu with Marut. In his role as the fetus's protector, he is called upon to to consult with them, *Ṛg-Veda* 7.36.9. These invocations, as well as the offerings made to Viṣṇu are found again later, in the *visnubali*, one of the prenatal *saṃskāra* which takes place during the eighth month.

35. The "etymological" meaning of *śárīra* is explained here. The body is where the fires are located (*śriyante*). This is a play on words, something one frequently encounters in the Brāhamaṇa and the Upaniṣad.

The explanation operates on two different levels: physiological and ritual. First of all, the igneous element exists in the organism as bile (*pitta*) which is itself divided into five "fires." Our text cites two of them: *koṣṭhāgni* and *darśanāgni*. The first, the digestive fire (*pācaka*), transforms incoming food in the stomach (*amāśaya*) into cooked food (*pakva*) in the intestines (*pakvāśaya*). The second fire (*ālocaka*) is supposed to light up objects to allow for vision (*darśana*). The three others are: the "coloring" (*rañjaka*), the director (*sādhaka*), and the illuminator (*bhrājaka*). On this subject see J. Filliozat, *L'Inde classique* (Paris: Payot, 1947), vol. 2, p. 153.

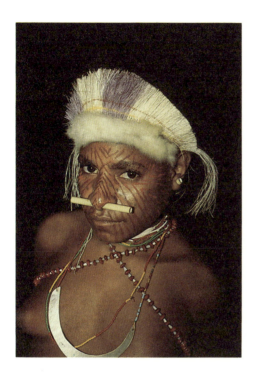
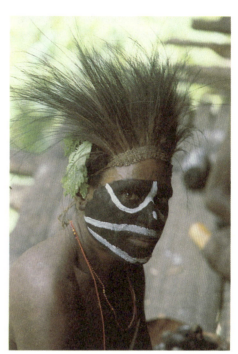

zone

were believed to be at reduced risk of impairing their reproductive future since they had typically fathered several children already. In Awan belief, the purpose of serial copulation was, "to ready the young women for procreative activities by 'opening' the vagina and forcing out any bloody fluids that would harm their husbands and thereby impair successful reproduction" (*ibid.*).

Serial copulation was also mandated in several south New Guinea cultures, but here fears of female sexual pollution were minimal or absent; the emphasis was on fertility in a more positive and general sense. Such was the case, for instance, for the *moguru*, or "life-giving ceremony," which was "the most secret, sacred and awe-inspiring ceremony of the Kiwai people" who lived at the mouth of the Fly River (Landtman 1927:350). The central part of the ceremony entailed the preparation of mingled sexual fluids as life-giving "medicine" for gardens and people:

> In groups, one after another, the men betake themselves to the women's compartments, where soon a promiscuous intercourse is in progress. All jealousy, all marriage rules, otherwise so strongly emphasized, are laid aside, men exchange their wives, and any one may choose any partner he likes, avoiding only his closest blood relations. After the act the men empty the semen into the *baru* [a palm-spathe bowl], and the women add in a similar way to the production of the potent medicine.... Everybody seems to be intent upon contributing as much as possible to the medicine, so that the *baru* should be filled up, and a great number of men, summoned from other villages, render assistance, their wives being among the other women.... The debauchery lasts till early morning, when everybody goes and swims, afterwards drying themselves at a fire and putting on their usual covering. The people then sleep most of the day. This part of the *moguru* goes on several nights, in Waboda, so it is said, till some of the women show signs of pregnancy (*Ibid.*:352).

The sexual "medicine" obtained from this general fertility rite could be used especially to promote the fertility of sago palms (a primary food source) by smearing it on the trunk or tree shoots, and also could be mixed with food and eaten to promote human growth and well-being.

In some Melanesian societies, conception was facilitated by a combination of sexual and nonsexual practices. The following description of the Mekeo of southern Papua delineates "the details of newlywed ritual where the expressed desire for conception of a child is most urgent" (Mosko 1983:25).

The bride each day is fed enormous quantities of boiled plant food along with the broth to increase the amount of womb blood in her abdomen. This sustained engorging results in a few short weeks with the bride becoming quite visibly fat. In indigenous terms, her body is also wet with plenty of skin and blood. During this time she does no work which would divert her blood away from her abdomen. Instead she sits each day inside a mosquito net at the virtual disposal of the groom. He visits her in seclusion as frequently as possible for the purpose of sexual intercourse, and with each act deposits a quantity of male procreative blood or semen in her abdomen. Since considerable quantities of both womb blood and semen are thought necessary to assure conception and avert menstruation, the bride's engorging and her regular intercourse with the groom are sustained for three months minimally.... (*Ibid.*)

All this is not to suggest that beliefs about conception or procreative substance are highly elaborate throughout all of Melanesia. In some if not many Melanesian societies these notions are vague or apparently unimportant, with informants offering little clarity or consistency about how conception or bodily formation takes place. In some societies, like the Telefol, men and women may have views of conception which differ significantly from each other (Jorgensen 1983b). Such discrepancy reinforces Wagner's (1972, 1981) suggestion that "beliefs" do not have uniform normative status within a culture but are forever being shaped and reinvented through creative use (cf. Barth 1975, 1987).

Predominantly, basic notions of procreative conception – whatever their content or clarity – tend in Melanesia to link with a culture's more general notions of gender, growth, nurturance and productive labor. Correspondingly, the complement of conception or growth processes is frequently found in beliefs concerning substance depletion, senescence and death.

## Growth and Nurturance

In the dietary self-consciousness of contemporary America, "You are what you eat" is a popular concept, and one well-reflected in refrigerator posters of the human face or body collaged from food. The literalness and validity of this idea is not wasted on Melanesians, whose daily tie to food production and subsistence labor is very strong. But for them, once again, material substance cannot be divorced from social and spiritual life – food is irrevocably tied to personal relationships and to unseen effects which may enhance or alter its potency. Social and spiritual relations are the preconditions of nourishment and constitution, and the body is conceptualized in terms of them.

## The Mother

The preeminent social relationship of the newborn is to its mother, epitomized through the process of nursing. This pattern is prevalent if not universal in human societies (West and Konner 1976; Konner 1981:30-32), and has a strong influence on images of bodily substance and development in Melanesia. The mother in many Melanesian cultures is symbolized and sometimes explicitly defined as "the woman who gave me breast milk," with the strong sense that "she grew me as a child," or "she gave herself bodily to make my own body." Nursing on demand is common in Melanesia until the child is three or four years old, and in some cultures, such as the Murik of the north New Guinea coast, nursing may persist for last-born children until they are six or seven (Meeker, Barlow and Lipset 1986:39). Correspondent with prolonged nursing, there is an important cultural association in Melanesia between freely given sustenance and healthful bodily constitution. The larger implications are well developed among the Murik:

> [T]he most important qualities expressed by the nursing scene are the generosity, abundance and security provided by the mother and the peace, pleasure and almost intoxicated satiation of the infant. Besides the ideal of the nursing mother–infant, the good mother is also seen as a giver and feeder. A good mother feeds her children whenever they are hungry and indulges their requests for certain kinds of food. Closely related to feeding is the general association of mothers with giving. Each mother hopes that her children will remember her as a generous and abundant source of food. (Meeker, Barlow and Lipset 1986:39)

This orientation is pervasive with many local variants in Melanesia.

## The Mother's Brother

The indulgence and sustenance given the child by its mother is extended in many if not most Melanesian societies with a diffuse sense of bodily support and contribution from the mother's closest blood relatives, particularly her brother or her father. The contribution of such persons is substantial – they have supported the mother herself and then given her to her husband in a connubial relationship. In this sense, maternal relatives have themselves underwritten the development of the woman's offspring.

In terms of bodily and social influence, the mother's brother in Melanesia often has special affinity for the child, and this is commonly reflected in special duties and ritual obligations between them. Very commonly, the mother's brother has a special role to play in the initiation, marriage or funeral of his sister's son. Reciprocally, obligation and tangible repayment are often given by the child's father to the mother's brother (or mother's father). In some societies, as among the Iatmul of the Sepik (Bateson 1936), these social and ritual relationships are very elaborate and complex.

The child's tie with maternal kin, such as the mother's brother, stands in potential opposition to its countervailing affiliation with its father and his kin – particularly in those majority of mainland New Guinea societies where preeminent rights of kin – group identity and/or spiritual essence are transmitted through the male line. This often leads to complementarity or divergence between paternal and maternal kin over their different "substantial" claims on the child – a tension that can have far-reaching implications. For instance, Forge (1972:537) notes that "He [the mother's brother] and his clan sometimes literally own the blood or have a lien on the spirit of their sister's son and do not release him to his patriline [paternal kin] until they receive an often very substantial, final payment of valuables...." Thus, the effective recruitment of a child to its father's clan commonly requires compensatory payment to the child's maternal relatives to reciprocate, abrogate or "pay off" their "blood" contribution to the child (cf. J. Weiner 1982:9-10). In some societies, this sense of blood payment is such that the mother's brother and his kin must be tangibly compensated whenever the blood of their sister's sons is accidentally or violently shed.

The substantial concern with the maternal uncle is intriguingly illustrated among the Daribi of the southeastern New Guinea highlands. Here the mother's brother is considered "just the same as mother," since both of them were formed in the same womb and composed of the same maternal blood (Wagner 1967:64). Given that the child's tie to its mother's brother is irrevocable, the recruitment of a child to its father's group in this nominally patrilineal society is particularly problematic. Payments must be continually made by patrikin to the child's mother's brother to keep the uncle's "ownership" of the child's body at bay.[3] These payments, which are largely comprised of pigs, are intriguingly linked to Daribi notions of conception, since the juices and fat from animals such as pigs are believed to replenish the supply of semen within the human male body (Wagner 1983). At one level, then, Daribi male procreative substance is given as pork to the mother's kin group in reciprocity for the female procreative substance of blood which the mother contributed to the formation of the child. In this respect, Daribi food and sexual transactions reciprocate and complement each other as idioms of bodily formation.

A pattern somewhat complementary to that of the Daribi is found among the Sabarl of the northern Massim (Battaglia 1985). The Sabarl are matrilineal, and here it is the "bone" contributed by the father rather than the "blood" contributed by the mother and mother's brother that must be compensated by the child's natal (matrilineal) clan. Among the Sabarl, this is especially evident at death, when axes that metaphorically represent the corpse of the deceased are given as valuables to the dead person's classificatory "father." Through such means, the bones of the dead person are "harvested" by his or her patrilineal kin. This gift is but one part of elaborate exchanges of "male" and "female" valuables and foods — exchanges through which kinship and gender are established and transacted.

## Male Initiation and Transition to Adulthood

The relationship between bodily substance, social nurturance and growth is particularly pronounced in Melanesian male initiations. Girls in Melanesia are often (though not always) believed to mature "naturally" with less cultural manipulation or interference, while the transition of the boy to adult male is usually considered more difficult and is more ritually marked.[4] In developmental terms, this reflects the tendency for early maternal influence to provide a continuing basis for female gender socialization, whereas boys tend to be pulled outside the sphere of maternal identification to establish a distinct masculine identity. In Melanesia, where gender role dichotomies and oppositions are particularly strong, the resocialization of boys into men is often deeply rooted in notions of bodily transformation. In several regions of New Guinea, it is believed that boys must be ritually resocialized or even cosmologically "reconceived" through male initiations to become men. In some of the more extreme cases, this occurs, inter alia, through a traumatic purging of the boyish feminized self, accompanied by an arduous bodily reconstitution of him in the image of a maturing man.

Common components of male initiation in New Guinea have included prohibition of heterosexual contact and the avoidance of "female" foods.[5] Often, male initiate novices are temporarily secluded bodily from women, and some of the taboos against female contact may last for years. During the period of their seclusion, boys may learn or practice skills of manhood — such as hunting and warfare techniques — and they may learn sacred lore or have cult secrets revealed to them. Frequently, they undergo ordeals of pain, obedience or endurance designed to inculcate masculine strength and forbearance. In some parts of New Guinea, such as the Sepik, Ok and eastern highlands regions, this process is linked with the ritual inducement of bodily changes by purging "female" substances such as blood from the novice, e.g., by bleeding his nose or penis.

Among the most traumatic initiation rites are those of the Bimin-Kuskusmin (Mountain Ok area), who indoctrinate boys nine to twelve years of age into the first of a lifelong series of initiation grades (Poole 1982a). The young novices are, among other things, (a) stripped naked, (b) forcibly washed, (c) deprived of sleep, food and water, (d) harshly rubbed with nettles, (e) forced to eat and then vomit "female" foods, (f) beaten, (g) shaved and bled about the head, (h) pierced with bone daggers through their nasal septa, (i) told they are dying, (j) burned about their forearms with hot fat, (k) force-fed pus from bodily wounds, (l) forced to live in their own bodily filth and (m) repeatedly deceived by initiators concerning the ostensible termination of the ordeals. The general context in which these ordeals are administered is one of antagonism and ridicule (Poole 1982a:122-23).

As Poole summarizes:

[B]oys endure severe privation, extensive degradation, extreme fatigue, constant hunger and thirst, psychological shock, enormous pain, acute illness (including nausea, diarrhea and infection) and other trauma.... In no instances are the boys given any warning of what is to happen. Deceptive, veiled threats often do not lead to what the boys fearfully expect. And ritual violence erupts unexpectedly.... I have witnessed numbers of

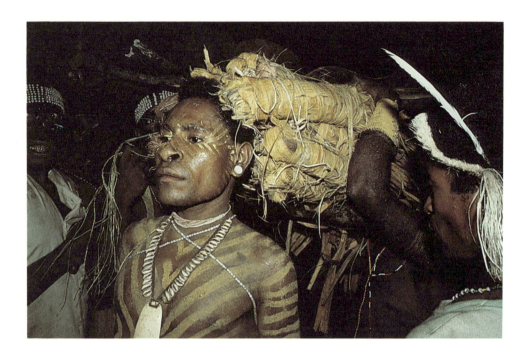

*Gebusi initiate with a heavy bark wig tied to his hair.*

boys lapse into states of uncontrolled, pronounced physical and psychological shock, becoming unconscious or hysterical.... The ritual elders still maintain, nevertheless, that such stress, as long as it is accompanied by knowledgeable control, is completely necessary to the desired efficacy of the *ais am* [first-stage initiation]. (*Ibid.*:138)

Obviously here, the body itself is a key focus of gender resocialization – as feminine substances and associations are purged and masculine ones strongly infused. Poole (1982a) found from interviews and projective tests that novices did indeed change significantly in bodily self-perception and associated gender identification as a result of the rites.

Bodily trauma in male (and female) initiation varies greatly in New Guinea, both in type, severity and/or relative absence. While first stage initiation was typically traumatic in Ok, Sepik and eastern highlands societies, accession to manhood was relatively benign in the intervening Strickland-Bosavi and western highlands areas, where initiate novices were older, usually in their late teens or even early twenties. Among the Gebusi, the main ordeal for these young men was the wearing of a bark wig. While the wig was heavy and pulled tightly on the scalp, it was worn for only a few hours and was discarded by the initiate novice at his own discretion. Among the nearby Kaluli, there was little if any bodily trauma at the ceremonial male seclusion lodge, from which the novices forayed to hunt (Schieffelin 1982). Kaluli novices both accumulated and consumed large quantities of game, and their main proscription was to maintain an attitude of "ritual sobriety" with regard to heterosexuality. Among the Koriki (Purari Delta) peoples of the New Guinea south coast, the *pairama* rites of initiation entailed virtually no trauma at all, despite the pronounced existence of warfare and cannibalism in Koriki society; the boys simply enjoyed themselves in the company of men while they learned aspects of mask-making and other male activities (Williams 1923, 1924). Initiation into a number of the other south New Guinea cults also appears to have been benign, with some exceptions among the Marind-anim (see Williams 1940; Landtman 1927; Zegwaard 1959; cf. van Baal 1966). In the central and western New Guinea highlands, several bachelor and other male cults emphasized symbolic male purification, beautification and masculinization prior to marriage – with a relative absence of prolonged and traumatic ordeals (A. Strathern 1970, 1979a; Meggitt 1964; Reay 1959; Biersack 1982; cf. J. Weiner 1987).

In many cases, transformation of the male body through initiation was as much cognitive as corporeal, with emphasis on learning obligations, prohibitions and ritual knowledge requisite for manhood. This is especially true in the more advanced stages of initiation cults – in societies where initiation was a multileveled process persisting well into adulthood. Particularly in the Ok area, the Sepik and regions of insular and eastern Melanesia, indoctrination into a series of male cults became a lifelong process of acquiring spiritual knowledge and authority, with the cults serving as a preeminent focus of political or economic as well as spiritual life. First stage initiation into such elaborate hierarchies, however, tended in New Guinea to entail prolonged seclusion from women, ritual bleeding of "female" blood and the traumatic enforcement of obedience to male elders. At the end of the ordeals, novices were frequently dressed in elaborate body decoration which indicated their new status and their general beauty, vitality and fertility. Decoration of initiates at higher cult stages has also been quite pronounced in some Sepik and insular sections of Melanesia. Such patterns of costuming and decoration will be considered further below.

## Homosexuality and Bisexuality

In some sections of Melanesia, particularly the southern lowlands of New Guinea and parts of the southern highlands fringe, masculine development was abetted by homosexual insemination – the direct transmission of semen as a life force from men to initiate novices (Herdt, ed. 1984).[6] In different cultures this insemination took place through fellatio, anal intercourse or, less commonly, the rubbing of masturbated semen on the boy's body. Among the Gebusi of the Strickland-Bosavi area, insemination rites were practiced even for male toddlers, who ingested small amounts of their fathers' masturbated semen (Cantrell n.d.). In most regions where homosexuality was practiced, however, it was limited to adolescence and early adulthood, culminating ultimately in bisexuality or in exclusive heterosexuality for full adult men. The male homosexual relationship was in many societies one of social as well as sexual domination of junior boys by their elders, though in other cases the relationship has been more voluntary and/or mutually erotic.

In regional terms, it would be tempting to contrast the south New Guinea emphasis on homosexual growth with the highland New Guinea emphasis on heterosexual depletion – asserting a lowland "semen belt" of homophilia in contrast to a highland "blood belt" of heterophobia. Such a highlands/lowlands contrast, however, is too crude to fit the facts (contrast Lindenbaum 1984, 1987a-b; Whitehead 1986a-b). Important areas of south New Guinea do not practice homosexuality and do not fall into either of these categories, while various parts of northern New Guinea show fascinating permutations of homoerotic and/or heteroerotic custom (e.g., Bateson 1936; Thurnwald 1916; Meeker, Barlow and Lipset 1986). In addition, there are several areas on the southern "fringe" of the New Guinea highlands (Anga and Strickland-Bosavi regions) that combine homoerotic and heterophobic beliefs, e.g., with masculinity enhanced both by homosexual insemination and by heterosexual avoidance, including, in some cases, initiatory bloodletting.

The combination of these complexes is particularly elaborate among the Sambia of the Anga-speaking region, who considered semen a crucial life force which was supplied by homosexual insemination and augmented through the eating of special foods. As Herdt (1984) documents, the acquisition, retention, spending and then replenishment of seminal fluid has been a continuing preoccupation of Sambian men, both in homosexual and in heterosexual relations. These concerns are crosscut by high male anxiety over pollution and debilitation from female womb/menstrual blood and by a rigid and in some ways antagonistic gender polarity. Sambian male initiation rites reflect both these concerns, enjoining, among other things, radical separation from women, copious homosexual insemination, traumatic thrashings, harangues, fasting, food taboos and severe nose-bleeding to purge, strengthen and masculinize the boys (Herdt 1981, 1982a-b, 1987; cf. Godelier 1986).

Among the Etoro of the Strickland-Bosavi area, homosexuality likewise found a complement in gender antinomy, but one that was focused more exclusively on male fears of contamination and depletion in the heterosexual act itself (Kelly 1976). The Etoro apparently did not have harsh initiation procedures, had little domestic gender antagonism, and had little belief in female menstrual pollution. Concern over heterosexual congress, however, led the Etoro to prohibit coitus for between 205 and 260 days per year (*ibid.*:43). The nearby Gebusi, in contrast, present a somewhat different permutation; their strictures about the contaminating influence of female sexuality are more a source of hilarity than anxiety, and indeed Gebusi men seem particularly prone to break their own "rules" of heterosexual and even homosexual propriety (Knauft 1985a-b, 1986, 1987a).

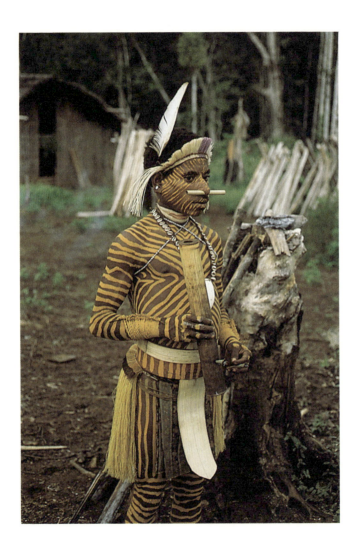

*Young Gebusi man in pre-initiate's costume: elongated phallic covering signals imminent change to bisexual status.*

A much more elaborate pattern of bisexuality is found among the Marind-anim of south coastal New Guinea, among whom both homosexual and heterosexual contact were ritually and socially prescribed (van Baal 1966, 1984). Here, as among several south coastal cultures, semen was considered more an unlimited source of potency than a limited bodily resource. Semen was used to "grow" young boys through regular anal intercourse initiated by their maternal uncles – their *binahor*-fathers – and more promiscuous homosexual intercourse occurred among males at some rites. Nevertheless, semen was considered by the Marind to be an especially potent life force when it was mixed with, rather than separated from, women's sexual fluids. Mingled semen and vaginal fluid were obtained by Marind through rites of serial heterosexual intercourse and were used for numerous life-enhancing purposes; indeed, their usage of mixed sexual fluids was much more elaborate and pronounced than among the Kiwai, described further above.[7] Among the Marind, these rites were particularly traumatic for the female participants, since numerous men of the resident clan copulated serially with only one or two of the younger women present. The very frequent practice of these rites and their attendant female trauma appear to have rendered a significant percentage of Marind women permanently sterile – from infections caused by the chronic vaginal irritation of excessive coitus (South Pacific Commission 1955). Hence the irony that fervent Marind fertility rites actually reduced the demographic viability of their society. Despite their sexual ordeals, however, Marind women were subject to few female pollution restrictions and participated in many activities which were under the exclusive control of men in many other Melanesian societies. Thus, for instance, Marind women exercised significant influence in choosing their spouses, were initiated into a series of initiation grades parallel to those of the men (including ritual insignia), took an active part in almost all in the major cult rituals, and even accompanied men on long-distance head-hunting raids.

These patterns are in some respects the antithesis of the highland patterns described above, in which women were socially and sexually inimical to men. Men from these areas who failed to take adequate purification and precautionary measures against female influence were liable to jeopardize male activities and to themselves become sick or debilitated, or to die. However, as mentioned above, the myriad of specific local patterns preclude any simple dichotomies concerning types of male sociosexual domination or insecurity.[8] In both sexual complexes, for instance, men who are truly strong and energetic are believed potent enough to engage in increased heterosexual activity without suffering adverse effects. While such a belief in highland areas only moderately increased the amount of heterosexual activity (e.g., for politically vigorous polygynists), such a belief along much of the south coast was extended much more broadly and confidently to men generally. A more evenly balanced tension between these poles is evident in several societies of the fringe highlands in north and south New Guinea, in which male pursuit of heterosexuality could be quite active and yet strongly hedged with ambivalence concerning debilitation (e.g., Kelly 1976:41-44; Meigs 1984:16; Buchbinder and Rappaport 1976:20-22).

\* \* \*

In many of the above cases, bodily substances are active metaphors which both engender and reflect wide ranges of social action. Sometimes, a very concrete "economy" of bodily substances is envisaged, with specific practices mandated to mediate the transmission, depletion, replenishment and/or complementarity of these fluids. Such a pattern can be illustrated as well among some matrilineal societies, for example, the Wamira of Milne Bay, among whom blood passed through females creates clan identity and essence, but also causes women to gradually wither and die – as they lose this vital substance through menstruation and childbirth (Kahn 1986:100). At the same time, however, Melanesian beliefs about bodily substance are highly variable in their degree of elaboration and their salience for concrete social action. Often, they are themselves defined or instantiated through ethereal spiritual components or, alternatively, through concrete processes of social organization, labor and production.

## The Adult Body as Active Social Force: Production and Reproduction

Melanesian body-substance beliefs are seldom independent of wider notions of how human action can influence the body. Particularly important here is the relationship between food production, social exchange and bodily welfare. If the "natural" process of reproduction is culturally constituted, bodily nurturance through social and material production is equally subject to sociocultural construction. Productive and reproductive processes are by this means linked in a holistic ecology of bodily constitution.

## Food

The linkage between food and exchange in Melanesia informs images of the body in a number of different contexts. Perhaps most basically, those whose food you consume are those whose labor, land and essence constitute your own being. Most Melanesians concretely appreciate the physical energy used in subsistence cultivation, and the way this is converted into bodily substance to maintain health and well-being. Sometimes the spiritual essence of a clan ancestor or cult spirit additionally infuses or otherwise influences the food that grows on "its" land – and correspondingly infuses or reproduces itself in the bodies of those who eat it.

In the sharing or giving of food, its force or influence is transferred to another person. This makes a gift of food, in a fundamental way, a gift of oneself. Since food in Melanesia is in fact very frequently shared, notions of physical and spiritual force articulate the growth and development of the individual body almost as if intrinsic to the growth and development of the wider social group. James Weiner (1982:27) suggests that for highland New Guinea the frequent sharing of food is indeed culturally equated with the sharing of biogenetic substance. This is in one sense a societal complement to the transmission of biogenetic substance directly, for instance, through homosexual insemination, which occurs in some lowland parts of Melanesia (*ibid.*). As we have seen above, conceptualization of food and of procreative substance crosscut each other in important ways, for example, the consumption of sexual substances may be a special form of nourishment, while, conversely, the eating of particular foods can augment the supply of particular sexual substances.

As might be expected, Melanesian food gifts symbolize in myriad ways the social relationship between the giver and the receiver – both in the type of food given and in its quantity and quality. Food-giving in Melanesia is thus often subject to elaborate culturally-specific conventions concerning who may share food with whom, what kinds of foods may be given, and under what conditions certain foods may or may not be eaten. In short, food is a central link between the body and wider social and cosmological relationships.

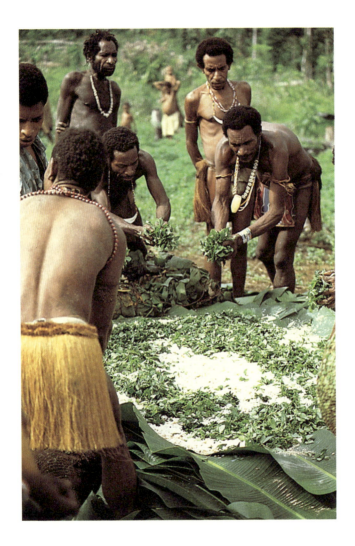

*Feast food: Gebusi men spread edible greens over sago*
*(palm starch).*

Even in its internal characteristics, food is subject to wide ranges of Melanesian symbolism and belief. Often, selected foods are "genderized," with different edible species considered "masculine" or "feminine" based on metaphoric associations of the food's hardness, color, texture, shape or pattern of growth. For instance, milky or greasy foods may be considered to be "like semen," while red pandanus may be considered "like women's blood"; hard or dried foods may be considered relatively "male," while soft, fleshy or watery foods may be considered "female" — in short, mirroring the archetypal body characteristics attributed to males and females themselves. According to their culture-specific associations, specific foods may be proscribed or prescribed for consumption depending on sex, age, initiation grade, marital status or totemic/ritual affiliation of the person intending to eat them. For instance, some species of plants or animals may be proscribed during initiatory seclusion, others during periods of bereavement or mourning. Such dietary strictures explicitly or implicitly bring one's body into physical or mental alignment with the social role being adopted.

In addition to its "intrinsic" properties, eating food also implies trust — that the food given is healthful and untainted. This is particularly important given beliefs in many Melanesian societies that food may be bespelled or poisoned by polluting substances (such as menstrual blood) that can sicken or kill the person who eats it. Even healthy food may pose a danger in the presence of a deceitful guest, since it is frequently believed that food scraps or bodily exuviae may be surreptitiously gathered and bespelled or burned in order to harm the body of the person from whom they have been collected.[9] Food thus articulates the body and its substance in relation to the outside world of social relationships, through which it is maintained or, alternately, maligned.

## Competitive Exchange

In its competitive mode, Melanesian food-giving can become an aspect of aggressive or ostentatious self-presentation. Here we encounter the famous exchange systems of highland and insular Melanesia in which wealth valuables and/or enormous quantities of food — often live pigs or piles of tubers — are given to an individual or group as a show of force and challenge.[10] The receiving group must reciprocate at a later time with an equal or hopefully larger gift if they are to save face and maintain or increase their reputation. In some societies, status competition through food exchange has taken the place of exchanging casualties bodily in warfare; for example, peoples such as the Kalauna who have come to "fight with food" (Young 1971).

In cases of aggressive food exchange, the link between social presentation and internal bodily processes is sometimes quite explicit. To produce a surplus of food for others typically requires personal privation – minimizing one's own food consumption – as well as hard work. The cultural ideal in several insular societies of the Melanesian Massim is thus to have an empty belly but a full storehouse of food – saved for competitive exchange. The corresponding corporeal ideal here is of a body which is very lean, hard, "dry" and light, in other words, highly self-disciplined and unindulgent (Young 1971, 1986; cf. Munn 1986; A. Weiner 1976; Kahn 1986). This notion is often partially tied to gender attributes of male strength and corporeal fortitude, and it is often men who publicly govern the politics of food exchange and who publicly enforce the domestic value of personal privation and hard work.

In several areas of Melanesia, the controlled discipline and authority of adult men is concretely channeled into the growing of special male crops used in prestigious exchanges. Perhaps archetypal here is the growing of long yams by men in parts of the Sepik in northern New Guinea and the growing of yams or taro in parts of the insular Massim and eastern Papua (Tuzin 1972; Harrison 1982; Kaberry 1971; Young 1971, 1986; Fortune 1932:ch. 2; Malinowski 1935; A. Weiner 1976; Kahn 1986; Schwimmer 1973). Sepik yams frequently contain important aspects of the group's patrilineal substance; in some areas each clan has its own distinct "seed line" of yams which must be kept distinct and perpetuated over generations – analogous to the way that yam tubers are themselves thought to proliferate in subterranean genealogies (Tuzin 1972; Harrison 1982). The energies of older men in particular are infused in these long yams, which may grow up to twelve feet in length. In addition to hard work, the yams require elaborate magic and isolation of both grower and crop from female sexual contamination in order to effectively proliferate. The longest yams are given in the most prestigious of competitive food exchanges; their production is a central focus of adult men's lives. In some cases, the huge tubers may themselves be ritually festooned and painted with human costuming appropriate to their owners, whom they literally embody. The ostentatious presentation of these yams puts the receivers in the vulnerable and tenuous position of having to self-present themselves later through counter-gifts of food equal to or larger than those obtained.

Perhaps the best-known examples of competitive gift-giving in Melanesia come from the New Guinea highlands (e.g., A. Strathern 1971; Meggitt 1974; cf. Feil 1984; Lederman 1986). Here the idea of bodily self-presentation is bound up in the items of food insofar as these are a concrete manifestation of one's productive and political prowess. Perhaps more important for the present discussion, highlands exchanges are also accompanied by elaborate body decorations indicating self-enhancement (Strathern and Strathern 1971; M. Strathern 1979). The issue of bodily decoration as an index of the self and the competitive group is one to which we shall return later. In the present context, however, it may be noted that food and wealth items are in many areas of Melanesia ceremonially exchanged for bodies themselves, notably, in marriage or homicide compensation.

## Bodily Exchanges — Marriage

In several areas of Melanesia, including some societies of north and south New Guinea, marriage ideally entails the reciprocal exchange of bodies between different groups — a woman is given in marriage from one kin group in direct reciprocity for one received in return. This true or classificatory "sister exchange" links bodily economy to social relations in a very direct way. In many other parts of Melanesia, however, including the New Guinea highlands, the productive and reproductive powers of the wife — her sexual, child-rearing and labor capacities — are largely transferred along with the woman herself to her husband's group when the latter make a sufficient material payment to the woman's natal kin. This payment or series of payments, termed bridewealth, was in precolonial times comprised largely of pigs, stone axes or shell valuables (e.g., Glasse and Meggitt 1969).

In bridewealth, the wealth and productive embodiments of the husband's group are exchanged for the productive and reproductive powers of the wife. These exchanges are mutually informing aspects of a larger bodily ecology, since in-married wives work to augment the production of pigs — tending, providing and even suckling them for the husband's group. At the same time, the natal kin of the out-married women receive as bridewealth pigs and valuables which they themselves may use in the service of further marital and other exchange transactions, for example, to obtain new wives for themselves. In others words, food, wealth and women are transacted in an encompassing cycle.

This is not to say that women themselves are passive objects in marital or competitive exchange (there has been much debate in the literature about this issue);[11] rather, the dominant ideology is that women and goods are exchanged as complements of one another. For some Melanesian societies, it has been effectively argued that the male exchange of valuables is cosmologically complemented and socially balanced by the reproductive and regenerative value of women (A. Weiner 1976, 1980). In other cases, it has been strongly suggested that, in fact, large elements of spiritual belief and gender ideology promulgate male domination over women (e.g., Godelier 1986; Josephides 1985; Read 1952; Meggitt 1964; Langness 1974; cf. Lindenbaum 1987; M. Strathern 1987).

## Bodily Exchanges — Death

In precolonial Melanesia, the norm of bodily exchange between many groups was that of violent revenge or predation; tribal warfare was endemic in most of pre-pacification Melanesia (see Meggitt 1977; Koch 1974; Langness 1972; Hallpike 1977; Berndt 1962, 1964; Fortune 1939; Schwartz 1963). In many cases an explicit person-for-person model of exchange existed, with killings revenged in a continuing cycle of death-for-death reciprocity (Heider 1979; Larson 1987). Relations of chronic raiding or warfare between groups resulted in substantial homicide rates, especially for men, in many if not most areas of precolonial Melanesia. Among the Mae Enga, for instance, about thirty-five percent of all men ultimately died in warfare (Meggitt 1977:110).[12]

This cycle of killing could often be attenuated, however, by the payment of homicide compensation; in many parts of New Guinea, the giving of pigs or wealth could serve to recompense the close kin of those persons killed in battle or warfare. As such, material payments could be used to end — at least temporarily — blood feuding and revenge between enemy groups.[13]

In most cases, including that of the Mae Enga, various forms of killing, compensation and exchange were ultimately linked. For instance, a truce could be arranged through the payment of homicide compensation, with this compensation itself providing the opening round of material exchanges between the two sides. These continuing exchanges could eventually lead to bridewealth payments and marriage

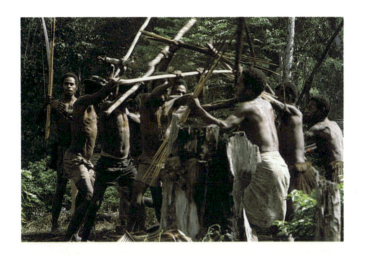

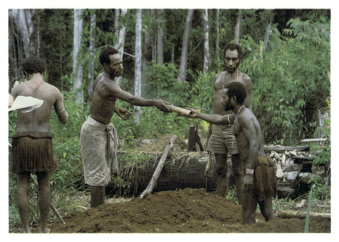

*Death of a Gebusi woman leads to accusation and
violence by kinsmen at funeral.*

*Tobacco pipe passed over grave, signalling an end to hostility.*

between the erstwhile enemy groups. Eventually, however, relations between the intermarried groups could deteriorate, and a pattern of enmity and reciprocal killing reemerge. A long-term cycle could thus develop in which bodily exchanges between groups went through phases of "positive" and "negative" reciprocity: the exchanging of wealth, of wives, of killings and of wealth once again (D. Brown 1977; Schwimmer 1973; Whitehead 1986a-b; cf., Sahlins 1972; Modjeska 1982).

## Cycles of Killing and Regeneration

Cycles linking reciprocity in killing with other forms of exchange were often themselves bound up with larger social and cosmological relationships in Melanesia. During the "negative" exchange of tit-for-tat killing, for instance, the belief was common that the group of the slain victim suffered spiritual as well as social loss. Correspondingly, the ancestral spirits or ghosts of the victimized group commonly demanded revenge. This ghostly anger and malice against the victim's own kin group was typically believed to persist until appropriate retaliation had been completed. Conversely, the killers gloated over or celebrated the victim's death. In some cases, the corpse of the victim might be defiled or mutilated as a sign of ignominy for the deceased's relatives to discover — for instance, left with its genitals stuffed in its mouth (e.g., Meggitt 1977:76), the head of a rival leader displayed on a pike (Reay 1987:90), or the intestines of the victim tied together and strung up (Zegwaard 1959:1037). In other cases, persons killed in warfare were simply butchered, brought home and eaten by the victors (e.g., Knauft 1985b on the Bedamini; Powdermaker 1931:28, on the Lesu in New Britain). Commonly, the attackers celebrated the death with a festive dance, such as the Dani *edai* (Heider 1970, 1979), the Daribi "mock funeral" festival (Wagner 1972:150ff.), or the Purari rite of cannibal celebration (Williams 1924:ch. 14).

An adult man's personal status in precolonial Melanesia was often importantly linked to his killing of others in warfare or raiding — and it was commonly reflected in bodily insignia. In some groups it was believed that the killers gained or incorporated a potent spiritual force from the slain victim. A group's gain or loss in battle casualties was thus articulated directly with beliefs about the spiritual or cosmological welfare of the group as a whole. Such beliefs were especially pronounced in those societies where head-hunting and/or ceremonial killing of captives was practiced (see McKinley 1976). Among the Kwoma of the Sepik, for instance, the killer was believed to supplement his own spirit or *mai*, located in the head, with those spirits of as many persons as he had killed – to the pleasure of his group's own spirits (Williamson 1983:16; Bowden 1983:99,105,110,cf.165). This same head-spirit was embodied in insignia decorations worn by the killer and could be transferred to fertility cult statues, who as masked "heads" were likewise festooned with homicidal insignia.[14]

Among many peoples of the New Guinea south coast, head-hunting and cannibalism were associated quite dramatically with spiritual regeneration. Among the Purari delta peoples, enemies were on occasion ambushed and slain so that their bodies or heads could be ritually fed into the mouths of large wicker spirit-monsters, kept in the sacred rear section of the men's cult house. These wicker monsters, termed *kaiemunu*, embodied the spiritual force of the victorious group, and the "feeding" of them with a human head was a crucial part of Purari male initiation and group rejuvenation rites (Williams 1923, 1924). Among the Asmat of the southwest New Guinea coast, the carefully prepared heads of enemy headhunt victims were highly potent ritual sacrae (Zegwaard 1959; cf. Konrad et al. 1981; contrast Schneebaum 1988). The heads figured prominently in elaborate male initiation rites; through complex rituals enacting death, rebirth and developmental growth, the Asmat novice was imbued with the spiritual identity of the headhunt victim. During one ritual stage, for instance, the novice initiate held the victim's head against his genitals for a prolonged period as part of his symbolic rebirth, and at the end of the rites he indeed received the headhunt victim's name as his own adult appellation. The general recognition of this identity-transformation was so great that the initiated man was immune to attack from the headhunt victim's own relatives; indeed, he could be greeted and even feasted by them as their lost kinsman!

Among the Bimin-Kuskusmin of the Mountain Ok area, the ritual torture and elaborate cannibalism of a captured enemy were the focus of the major public ritual of societal rejuvenation – the Great Pandanus Rite. "In the great pandanus rite...the ritual strength that was transferred to the victim through ritual adornment, sacrifice and endurance of a slow and painful death is said to have been incorporated in all...ritual elders" (Poole 1983:21). Consuming the potent spiritual essence of a corpse's genital tissue appears to have been particularly important in

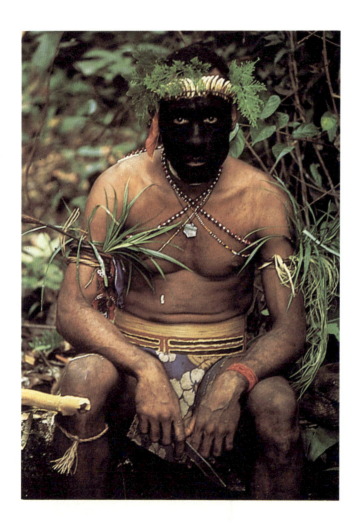

*Face blackened in anger, a young man waits to avenge the death of an uncle.*

the process of Bimin-Kuskusmin spiritual regeneration. Mortuary rites articulated richly with complex Bimin-Kuskusmin beliefs concerning gender and bodily substance were alluded to further above.

A somewhat different permutation is found among the Kiwai of the New Guinea south coast. Among them, "the penis of a slain foe [was] sometimes cut off, threaded on a stick and dried. Before a fight a small piece of it mixed with banana [was] given to the young warriors to swallow, and this [made] them successful in catching and killing male enemies" (Landtman 1927:151).

In some societies, the incorporation of or accession to others' spiritual force was accompanied by serial copulation, as a further aspect of societal regeneration. Among the Purari, mentioned above, the wife of a successful headhunter was placed at the coital disposal of men in the village, who paid material compensation to her husband in return for their sexual access to her (Williams 1923).[15]

In a few cases, the slaying of outsiders had important practical as well as symbolic and cosmological dimensions. The Marind-anim, to the east of the Asmat, were reputed to be among the most inveterate and wide-ranging headhunters in Melanesia (van Baal 1966). Head-hunting raids were undertaken, as among the Asmat, to obtain "head names" for Marind children, but they also occasioned the systematic capture and adoption of victims' orphaned children, who were brought back to Marind territory and raised as full Marind adults.[16] This traffic in children was of such great magnitude that perhaps one-sixth of all adult Marind had in fact been the children of foreign headhunt victims. This large-scale incorporation of outsiders was of particular demographic importance since, as mentioned further above, it appears many Marind women were rendered permanently sterile by the excessive heterosexual coitus enjoined in Marind rituals (South Pacific Commission 1955). The influx of captive children thus countered what was widely recognized to be a very low Marind birth rate. Indeed, the inflow of children was great enough to make the Marind-anim a culturally and territorially expanding group despite a negative internal growth rate. Ultimately, of course, it was Marind spirit beliefs themselves which motivated and intensified this extraordinary cycle — of hypersexuality, infertility, violence and demographic replenishment. These connections are strikingly evident in the elaborate Marind myth and ritual cycle, which emphasizes linkage among impaired copulation, head-hunting and rebirth (van Baal 1966, 1984; cf. Ernst 1979).

## Mortuary Rites

As the essence of slain outsiders is often deemed a potent force, so too, the spiritual force of those who die from natural causes within the community is often potent and subject to social manipulation. While, as discussed below, the primary mortuary emphasis in many Melanesian societies is on how to keep ghostly wrath at bay, the positive power of the deceased is also sometimes harnessed. In a number of societies, mortuary rituals facilitate the amalgamation of the deceased's spirit to the more undifferentiated realm of ancestral spirits, who tend to be the ultimate protectors and overseers of the group's sacred knowledge and success. Some societies in virtually all areas of Melanesia kept parts of the skeleton, particularly the skull of deceased adult men, as relics.[17] In many societies skeletal relics were carefully preserved as important sacrae in cult houses or at sacred sites, sometimes as part of elaborate ritual proceedings or displays.

In the southeast highlands fringe of New Guinea, the emphasis on reincorporating deceased group members was particularly pronounced. In some of these groups, members of the community who died were eaten by their female kin and coresidents to prevent, inter alia, the escape and dispersal of their spiritual force. Among the Gimi this endocannibalism was extensive; the entire body of the deceased was eaten by women, with each woman later receiving a portion of a pig corresponding to the part of the corpse she had eaten (Gillison 1983). This logic was apparently emphatic: "Come to me so you shall not rot on the ground. Let your body dissolve inside me!" (*ibid.*:43; cf. Gillison 1980, 1987). Gimi endocannibalism initiated a process of mortuary regeneration. During the year after death and consumption of the corpse, the skull and jaw of a deceased man were commonly worn by the deceased's mother; thereafter, the bones were placed in rock and tree crevices said to be "like vaginas" in clan hunting grounds and at the borders of the deceased's garden. Eventually, the spirit was reincarnated as a bird of paradise, which continued to reside within Gimi territory. Gimi endocannibalism was thus "the first stage in a process to regenerate the dead, part of the means to maintain the continuity of existence by transferring human vitality to other living things" (Gillison 1983:39).

## Bereavement

In addition to various forms of cannibalism, there is wide variation in Melanesian funerary and mortuary procedures. Commonly the corpse is the focus of grief-stricken mourning among close kin, and of attempts to mollify the spirit of the deceased and/or facilitate its passage to the world of the unseen. Violence to the bodies of the living was often part of this process. Meggitt summarizes for the Mae Enga of the Highlands:

> Relatives attending the initial mourning are expected to demonstrate the extent of their sorrow. Male affines and distant kinsmen tear their hair and beards. A few slice their earlobes so that blood flows over their shoulders. Some of the closest kin of both sexes cut off the tops of fingers. This action also placates the ghost of the deceased, which comes into being at the moment of death when the agnatic spirit leaves the corpse. (Meggitt 1965a:182)

Finger-lopping of young girls appears to have been particularly pronounced among the Dani of the Irian Jaya highlands. Many Dani women by adulthood had by this means lost many or most of the finger joints on both hands (Heider 1979:124ff.). Among the Kaulong of New Britain, the widow of a deceased was strangled to death shortly following her husband's own demise – a practice which was apparently consistently adhered to in precolonial times (Goodale 1980, 1985). Much more commonly in Melanesia, men and particularly women were enjoined to long wailing and keening, and were subjected to mourning taboos of various duration, including food and sexual taboos, restriction of bodily adornment, and circumscribed social activity or seclusion. The severity of mourning procedures typically varied according to the age and sex of the deceased, often being greatest for important adult men and less arduous following the death of women or children.

## Treatment of the Corpse

The status of the deceased was also commonly reflected in the treatment of the corpse. Often, the corpse of an important man was dressed in his full complement of ritual finery and the insignia of his status. Among the Iatmul of the Sepik, an elaborate mortuary display was arranged for important men, portraying iconically their various accomplishments in warfare, ritual, knowledge and exchange (Bateson 1936). Processes of corpse divination also varied depending on the characteristics of the person who died. In parts of the New Guinea interior, corpses of important or unexpectedly deceased persons were inspected before or during decomposition to ascertain if the state of internal parts indicated to the viewers the existence or identity of a sorcerer in causing the person's death.

Among the Gebusi of the Strickland-Bosavi area, corpses of virtually all adults who died from sickness were subject to divinatory procedures (Knauft 1985a:chs. 2, 4). In these the primary sorcery suspects – the person(s) believed to have caused the death – were enjoined to shake the decomposing corpse in a display of their grief. If the eyes of the corpse burst (due to intracranial pressure) or if cadaveric fluid suddenly flowed out of the body cavity, it was taken as a tangible sign that the suspect was indeed guilty of lethal sorcery. The suspect in such cases could be legitimately killed on the spot by the aggrieved without retaliation by the suspect's own kin. The person so executed was then steam-cooked with sago and distributed in a cannibalistic feast, in a procedure similar to that used in the consumption of game animals such as pigs or cassowaries. This act was considered appropriate reciprocity for the sorcerer's prior consumptive killing of the sickness-victim. Killing of sorcery suspects within the community lead to an extremely high Gebusi homicide rate (Knauft 1985a, 1987b; cf. 1987c).

A rather different permutation of corpse divination was emphasized among the nearby Etoro and Kaluli peoples (Kelly 1976, 1977; Schieffelin 1976). Here it was the person who had been killed for practicing witchcraft whose corpse was examined for divination; his or her heart was cut out and exhibited on a stake – a "bright" or "yellowish" heart being thought to indicate that the slain person had indeed been a witch. (The body itself might be consumed thereafter.)

For the Wola, further to the east, the spiritual essence of the sickness-victim's body was transferred to pork, the eating of which was accompanied by omen-taking in which the consumers proclaimed their innocence with respect to the deceased's death (Sillitoe 1987). Among the Marind-anim of the New Guinea south coast, it was the cadaveric fluid of the corpse that facilitated divination; this fluid was apparently drunk by a close relative of the deceased as he or she lay next to the corpse in the grave. During the mourner's ensuing "sleep," his or her dreams were believed capable of disclosing the identity of the sorcerer responsible for the death (van Baal 1966:772). The Marind also believed that shamanic power was transmitted through cadaveric fluid. Novice shamans were enjoined to ingest cadaveric fluid in substantial quantities — the liquid being administrated orally, nasally, and into their eyes until they became quite delirious. Through this ordeal and its accompanying indoctrination, the novice shaman risked death itself to attain the "vision" necessary to see accurately into the world of the spirits and into the world of death (van Baal 1966:888).

Specific mortuary practices and taboos often had as one objective the departure of the deceased's spirit for the world of the dead, this process being facilitated by entreaties or demonstrations of grief by the living. In the absence of such entreaties — and even sometimes when they were carefully followed — the spirit of the deceased was frequently believed to be angry over its worldly death, hence to harbor ghostly malice against living relatives, possibly resulting in sickness or misfortune. The various means by which corpses were disposed reflected, in part, different beliefs concerning the proper departure of the deceased's spirit. In some societies, such as the Dani (Heider 1970, 1979), the corpse was cremated on a funeral pyre. In others, such as the Mae Enga (Meggitt 1965a-b), it was quickly buried, while in many other cases it was mourned for several days before burial. In many Melanesian societies, ranging from at least the Marind-anim in Irian Jaya (van Baal 1966) to the Kwaio in the Solomons (Keesing 1982), the corpse was buried and later exhumed, the bones decorated and reburied again. In many other societies, the corpse was left to decompose partially or totally aboveground, in part so its spirit could disperse.

A more detailed case study illustrates how several of these aspects of funerary custom can combine. Our attention here is on the Daribi of the fringe southern highlands New Guinea; "[t]he mourning of the dead constitutes the most powerful ideological expression in Daribi culture" (Wagner 1972:145). Among Daribi, the corpse was keened by patrikin, spouses and coresidents. Uterine kin of the dead person then arrived and reproached the deceased's clanspeople, accusing them of negligence in allowing the person to die. In precolonial times, the visitors might vent their anger by cutting down food-bearing trees, chopping at houseposts or attacking their opponents by beating them with sticks or slashing at them with axes. The corpse was then left in the residential house for six to ten days, during which time body parts were taken as relics by close descent group and family members:

While the body is still in the house, parts of it, such as the hands, feet or scalp, are occasionally cut off as relics. These are dried over the fire and then pressed beneath a sleeping mat, after which they are worn around the neck as an expression of sorrow. Horobame, of Kurube, wore the dried skin of her son's footsole in this way "because she couldn't see him anymore, he couldn't walk around anymore." (*Ibid.*:147)

After relics were obtained, the closest kin were persuaded to relinquish the remainder of the body, which was placed at midday in an open exposure coffin which also served as a dripping pit for decomposition. The body was removed at sundown, however, when remaining portions of its flesh were to be eaten. The decomposing corpse flesh could be steam-cooked and eaten by the deceased's own clansmen, i.e., the same people whom the deceased "shared meat with" in life, though not by his or her closest family members. Thereafter, the final remains of the corpse were returned to the burial rack, securely covered and tied down with bark. After the corpse had totally decomposed, the bones were recovered and kept in a special "bone house" of pandanus leaves. When this bone house began to disintegrate, the clansmen of the deceased hunted ten to twenty marsupials, the bones of which they burned under the structure in order that the wafting smoke provide a last "sharing of food" with their deceased relative. This act was also believed to reduce ghostly malice. After the ceremony, the bones were taken from the tiny house, put in a new string bag and hung in the central corridor of the longhouse. When, much later, the string bag itself began to disintegrate, the bones were removed and deposited, permanently, in a burial cave or rock shelter. The importance of this process is illustrated in the Daribi belief that ghosts, particularly of those who die unmourned in the bush, may come back and cause sickness. To alleviate this, the Daribi stage *habu* ceremonies which "bring the ghost back to the house." This results in a competitive confrontation between a group of men impersonating the ghost and other men and women acting as longhouse residents. The ghost is ultimately appeased and a communal feast held.

## Mortuary Feasts

Particularly in insular eastern Melanesia, the staging of mortuary rituals to commemorate the dead was an important occasion of wealth distribution and political competition. In economic terms, the death of a powerful political leader ruptured the extensive ties of wealth exchange he had established as the economic and political dimension of his leadership. The reformulation or extension of these relations, undertaken symbolically in commemorative mortuary rituals, allowed new and old leaders to vie in amassing and distributing wealth. By this means, the politico-economic continuance of the society was linked to its spiritual perpetuation and rejuvenation following death, particularly the death of leaders. In some matrilateral groups, such as the Trobriand Islanders, much of this process was under the economic and spiritual control of women (A. Weiner 1976), while in others it was under the more general control of men (Keesing 1982; Wagner 1986; Clay 1986; Errington 1974; Salisbury 1966; Goodenough 1971).

Among the most artistically elaborate mortuary commemorations were the Malanggan of northwestern New Ireland. Closely associated with these ceremonies were elaborate fretted wood masks and other carvings of clan emblem designs (Kramer 1925; Wingert 1962:46ff.,234-39; cf. Meyer and Parkinson 1895; Nevermann 1933; Groves 1935:353-60, 1936). These masks and sculptures, also termed Malanggan, were a genre of commissioned artistic rivalry in which prestige depended upon the Malanggan of a clan's mortuary ceremony being more inventive, elaborate and spectacular than those of others. The intricate meanings of the designs were owned and most fully understood by the clan elders, who commissioned and directed the carvers as well as sponsoring the mortuary feasts at which they were prominently displayed. The Malanggan artwork was itself left to decay when the ceremonies were over.

Developed mortuary feasts also appear to be relatively prominent in some traditional societies of Irian Jaya (e.g., Heider 1979; Serpenti 1965) and include elaborate ancestral statues or fretwork in both north and south parts of the island, for example, among the Asmat in the south and the Geelvinck Bay area in the north (e.g., Konrad et al. 1981; Schneebaum 1985; Gerbands 1967; Wingert 1962:193ff.; cf. Chauvet 1930). Spirit house and totemic art have been particularly developed in the Sepik area in northern New Guinea (Greub 1985; cf. Forge 1965).

In general, the diversity of New Guinea mourning practices reflects the tension between three themes: the cultural constitution of grief, the appropriation or retention of the deceased's spiritual force or essence, and the opposed assertion of difference and antipathy between the world of the living and that of the dead.

# The Body in Its Prime:
# Spiritual Embodiment and Rejuvenation

Because the life of the body in Melanesia is so deeply defined by its web of social
and spiritual relationships, the most spectacular displays of bodily beauty tend also
to be those which reaffirm the social and cosmic rejuvenation of the local group as
a whole. Customs and beliefs of bodily conception, nurturance, productive growth
and death articulate closely with ceremonies that in some way promulgate or promote the strength, vitality, maturation and regeneration of both individuals and their
community (cf. Whitehead 1986a-b).

Even in nonceremonial contexts, Melanesian bodies have exhibited a wide range
of clothing and ornamentation styles. Noseplugs and earplugs, tatoos, scarification,
teeth-blackening, penis gourds and casual ornamentation of leaves, fur or feathers
may in different cultures complement the scant traditional coverings of loincloths,
"ass-grass," fiber skirts or even total nakedness (traditional in parts of the Sepik).
Hairstyles ranged from a shaved head — sometimes at mourning — to intricate long
braids or elaborate wigs. Often different daily clothing styles or insignia carried clear
indices of the sex, age, marital status and political achievements of the individual:
what initiation grade they had attained, how many people they had killed, how many
large exchanges they had transacted, whether they were in mourning and if they
belonged to a special ritual or leadership cult.

In ceremonial contexts, however, the normal body was more greatly transformed,
often in a highly symbolic and richly artistic fashion. In most of Melanesia, the decorated body itself was the preeminent form of art. Ritual costuming took forms as
diverse and creative as Melanesian cultures themselves, being typically a celebra-
tory icon of both the vital self and wider sociocultural and spiritual vitality.

## Costuming and Spirit Impersonation —
## South Coastal New Guinea

In many south coast New Guinea cultures, spectacular body costumes and masks
were associated with mythical beings or ancestral spirits — spirits whose form and
force the wearer of the costume bodily represented or artistically evoked. The
Marind-anim of the south coast used a particularly elaborate array of decorative cos-

tumes which presented various aspects of mythical *dema*-spirits (van Baal 1966). These costumes were employed in an exceedingly complex ritual cycle – on which Marind cosmology depended – through which the travels and activities of the *dema* were enacted, elaborated on and/or revealed to initiates. One of the more spectacular costumes was the *garia* sky-image, a bright semicircular body ornament extending like a huge fan up to six feet over the head and to each side of the wearer. "The ornament is fan-shaped, made of the very light kernel of sago-leaf ribs. The thin, long strips, radially arranged, are lashed together and then painted in various colors, among which white dominates" (*ibid.*:356).

The use and meaning of Marind *dema* costumes was predictably elaborate. The following passage describes the appearance of *Sosom*, one of the principal *dema*:

> The neophytes are brought to the festive grounds and made to sit under the [high] platform, with their backs to the entrance. Some sort of removable fence encloses the place. *Sosom* has donned an enormous headgear made of thin reeds covered with white down. His face is hidden behind the *batend* mask [of scarlet bowerbird feathers], his breast is covered with fiber and a heavy red-brown skirt folds around his limbs. A garland of bright croton-leaves is draped over his shoulders and down his back hang the long strands of his hairdo. Surrounded by men dancing and swinging their bullroarers, *Sosom* proceeds to the festive grounds.... Suddenly the structure moves to and fro, as if a gigantic monster had leapt upon it. A hideous black something descends upon the neophytes: the tail of a monster. The thundering noise has stopped. An eerie silence prevails when the fence is taken away and the uncles and fathers of the boys grasp their arms and drag them out of the enclosure to meet the *dema*. At the same time a hardwood pole [*Sosom's* phallus] is set up and as soon as it stands upright the ordeal starts anew.... At last the *dema* kneels down and in front of the boys his decorations are taken off him. The *dema* is revealed to the boys as an ordinary man. (van Baal 1966:481)

The use of body costumes to represent diffuse spiritual or ancestral forms – revealed to initiates as real men – was pronounced across much of lowland south as well as north New Guinea. Among the Elema of the central south coast, initiation into the wearing of spectacular totemic and spirit-associated masks was both benign and a major social event (Williams 1940). The largest body masks, the *hevehe*, combined in their meaning and symbolism aspects of sea spirits, ancestral spirits, totemic and clan affiliations and considerable artistic elaboration. The masks were made of a light cane and palm-wood frame across which bark cloth was stretched and sewn, painted with intricate inherited designs and fitted at the bottom with a face and gaping sculptured mouth. The masks when worn could stretch twenty-five feet in the air, and yet each was mobile enough to be paraded extensively by a single wearer around the village and on adjoining beaches. Huge vaulted longhouses were built to house the masks, and the elaborate twenty-year cycle of preparing them was a pre-eminent dimension of Elema sociopolitical as well as religious life. In the ultimate display, well over 100 different *hevehe* emerged from their single house for over a month of celebration and feasting — the event constituting the epitome of Elema spiritual and politico-economic effervescence.

## Costuming and Spirit Impersonation — The Sepik

In the Sepik area of north New Guinea, the embodiment of spirits as men in elaborate effigies, masks or noise-making instruments was a crucial aspect of initiatory ordeals and revelations — the Tambaran cult. Women and children were told that the embodiments were truly those of spirits, while the initiation ordeals ultimately revealed to male novices exactly how they were in fact produced and worn or used by men. (These spirit images were linked to elaborate mythical lore and ritual enactment in the process of traumatic masculinization rites occurring in stages throughout the male life cycle.)

The intricacies of this process cannot be detailed here; just one example must suffice. In the ritual climax of the Ilahita Arapesh Tambaran *Nggwal Benafunei*, the initiator elders dress in spectacular costumes and parade themselves in public prior to bestowing their ritual knowledge and its accompanying social status to the next class of initiates – themselves already adult men. Tuzin (1980:221-22) describes the initiators' costumes:

> Except for his eyelashes, all the dancer's facial hair has been removed, and his hairline has been shaved back to expose the front half of his scalp. A yellow oil (*akwalif*) applied to his face gives his skin a much-admired golden glow and uniform texture.... At the center of the artificial hairline a spot of magical red paint (*noa'w*) is applied. Concealed under layers of cosmetic trapping, the *noa'w* is the final, mystic agent of ritual beauty. Its existence is known only to cult members, but its effects are reputedly felt by all.... [T]he decorators exploit virtually every type of pleasing material known to them – feath-

ers, natural fabrics, colorful and/or aromatic leaves, berries, blossoms, shells and sundry other items – to create a costume so striking that the audience will be spellbound by its transcendent beauty. The pièce de résistance is a tall, pointed headdress rising from its point of attachment at the back of the man's head.... The dancer is transformed into a being akin to the Tambaran itself; and, indeed, numerous myths tell of this event permanently changing the mortal protagonist into a spirit entity. The rites of this and the following two days must be judged, then, the climax of Arapesh religious culture.

In the rites themselves, the elder initiators – having previously displayed their transcendent beauty – berate and beat the adult novices. These "initiates" are shoved down a human tunnel into the longhouse. "As each novice disappeared into the dark doorway a sickening thud was heard from within – the wretch's head being crushed under the heel of the Tambaran. By now many of the women [observing from the outside] were sobbing uncontrollably" and the awaiting men were "visibly fear-stricken" (ibid.:236). The "killing" however, was a typical Tambaran ruse:

> As his fear abated and his eyes adjusted to the darkness, the novice beheld the lavishly decked interior: on the right, the gallery wall of spirit paintings running the entire length of the house and festooned with decorated cassowary daggers, mounted birds of paradise and a multitude of shell arrangements; on the left, filling the larger portion of the outer sanctum, a towering line of impassive spirit effigies, and at their feet another line of sculptures in dignified repose. All the remaining floor area was crammed with shells, feathers and daggers." (ibid.:238)

In essence, these adult novices were "seeing for the first time the master works of an artistic tradition whose very existence had been unknown to them" – the artwork associated with the Nggwal Tambaran class into which they were being initiated. (This art was of course extremely secret and was unobserved by women and men uninitiated to this Tambaran stage.) Subsequent phases of the ritual involved the revelation of varieties of sacred flutes and drums, and a two to three month seclusion in which much good food was consumed. At the conclusion, a huge coming-out ceremony was staged in which the new initiates paraded in public the same spectacular costume previously worn by their initiators. A major transfer of ritual knowledge and status was thus enacted.[18]

In some cases, the social and cultural dominance of senior cult members was concretely enacted and reinforced by donning masks of spirits who were angry and vengeful. Through their impersonators, these spirits could wreak poignant social control within their community. In its more extreme forms, this spiritual antagonism could be extremely violent, including several variants of ritual murder. The Tambaran Nggwal, alluded to so artistically above, was on different occasions one such Tambaran; another was termed *hangamu'w*, the human dimension of which was revealed to novices during first-stage initiation:

> Of the 214 *hangahiwa* recorded in Ihahita village, about ten percent have a reputation for murder. Their trappings include crimped cordyline leaves as homicide badges and...the skulls of their victims hung in grisly display around their necks. By donning one of the *hangamu'w* masks, it is said, the wearer becomes possessed of the indwelling spirits of its victims; wild with their passion of revenge, he is likely to kill any living thing that crosses his path. Upon doing so, he supposedly recovers his senses, returns the mask to its place among the others in the spirit house, and, concealing his guilt, joins in the general distress that is agitated when the victim's body is discovered. Moral responsibility is deflected onto the Tambaran itself, which is credited with another killing as evidence of its insatiable appetite. (Tuzin 1982:339)[19]

In general, the violent power of Tambaran and totemic spirits was seen as enjoining public adherence to ritual traditions, taboos and exchange prestation requirements. Tambarans also promoted successful male development and facilitated eminence and success in politico-economic relations and warfare. One of the deepest secrets of the Tambaran initiations was that the spirits were in fact impersonated and controlled by men (cf. Tuzin 1974, 1976, 1980, 1982). Correspondingly, Tambarans expressed diverse desires and personalities, ranging from the beautiful or the extremely violent to the hilarious and ludic.

In many parts of the Sepik and south New Guinea, as well as insular Melanesia, some costumed cult figures were by design outrageously disheveled or clumsy — bogeymen or buffoons who could "terrorize" residents but who were also potent sources of humor and entertainment. In many cases there was a variable or ambiguous boundary between the humor and the danger that such spiritual embodiments could provoke. The extremes of this tension are evident in the traditional initiation to the *tansa* society on Nissan Island in the Solomons (Nachman 1982). Here the grand initiator decorated his penis with yellow, red and white stripes, and — as a central aspect of initiatory revelation — dramatically exposed his penis to the novices. Such behavior was thought to be both outrageous and very funny. In the initiation itself, however, any of the boys who smiled or laughed were said in fact to have been killed, cooked and eaten by the initiators.

### Costuming and Political Achievement — Insular Melanesia

In diverse Melanesian societies, the right to wear or possess powerful spirit masks or insignia was, as in the Sepik, gained through a progressively restrictive process of initiation or political accession; these bodily markers were both symbols of eminent status and the embodiment of spiritual power and authority.[20] In the Tami-Huon area of northeast New Guinea, for instance, distinctive wooden and bark-cloth masks were, like the Tambaran, symbols of "precarious ancestor-spirit beneficence," the beings of which were in control of the secret society and of social propriety generally (Wingert 1962:212; cf. Meyer et al. 1895; Nevermann 1933).

In many insular areas east of New Guinea, however, political hierarchy was even more closely tied to rights over elaborate masks or bodily decorations. Rights to make and/or wear masks or insignia were purchased and these were ceremonially exhibited at elaborate feasts, the staging of which was the hallmark of the aspirant's political success. In Northeast New Britain and the Duke of York Islands, the aspirant's spiritual and political life revolved around the purchase and control of *tubuan* or *dukduk* body masks at mortuary feasts. At these feasts, the deaths of important ancestors or relatives were commemorated (Errington 1974; cf. Danks 1887, 1892; Parkinson 1907; Salisbury 1966, 1970). At such occasions, the society as well as the key individuals at its apex were in a sense symbolically regenerated and reconstituted in political and spiritual well-being — concretely symbolized in the elaborate masks themselves. In many societies of insular and northern Melanesia, as in the Sepik above, the owners of the masks or their henchmen could exercise considerable power and social control when wearing the masks or acting in their name, for instance, attacking followers or extorting their compliance in matters of political support or exchange prestation. In New Caledonia, control of elaborate body masks and an associated mythology of ancestral descendance were significanty tied to chiefly rivalry and authority (Guiart 1966).

The combination of political and spiritual authority established through the control of bodily insignia and decoration was particularly developed in the restrictive secret or public graded cults of New Britain and Vanuatu in eastern Melanesia (Allen 1984; Meyer and Parkinson 1895; Rivers 1914; Deacon 1934; Layard 1942; Allen, ed. 1981; cf. Chowning and Goodenough 1971). Allen (1984:33) summarizes the general characteristics of the graded cult society:

> Wherever the graded society occurs, it consists of a number of ranked grades, entry into which is gained by the performance of ritual based on the sacrifice of pigs with artificially developed tusks, the transfer of payments for insignia and services, and the performance of elaborate dances. Members of the various grades are marked off from one another by their exclusive right to certain insignia, titles and ritual privileges. For the lower grades the complications are minimal and take no heavy toll on the resources or ability of the aspirant. For the higher grades the requirements become progressively more complex and more expensive.... Men who attain the highest rank are believed to acquire or gain access to supernatural powers which they can then utilize in their attempts to control the political aspirations of those beneath them.

The sociopolitical and body-decoration ramifications of public and more secret ritual societies are effectively recounted in Allen's description of a small North Vanuatu island:

> On the tiny island of Mota, with a diameter of less than three kilometers and a population of about 500 persons, Rivers (1914:2:87-129) recorded the existence of no less than seventy-seven secret societies when he visited the community in 1912. Many of these societies had permanent cult buildings in the bush where the members kept their regalia and elaborate headdresses and where they frequently slept and ate.... Each society took great pride in its own unique insignia, masks, dances, and taboos, and each strove to gain members at the expense of the others. Any male of consequence found it imperative to belong to numerous societies — imperative both to advance in the public graded society, and hence aspire to influence and leadership, and as a necessary means of property protection.... The societies displayed numerous Tammany-Hall-style characteristics, including political assassination and general terror tactics. A leader who held high rank in the public graded society and was also a member of powerful secret societies was provided with a degree of institutional support and legitimation not commonly available to Melanesian Big Men. (Allen 1984:32)

It is obvious here that political, economic and religious aspects of Melanesian culture come together through a panoply of powerful and diverse bodily markers.

## Costuming and Societal Rejuvenation — Fringe New Guinea

The political import of bodily insignia and spiritual enactment does not negate the public embrace and enjoyment of the spectacular costume; in important respects it symbolizes the vitality, power and beauty of the society or group of followers as a whole. This dimension of ritual enhancement is present throughout Melanesia but is perhaps particularly pronounced in those regions where status differentials among men are less competitive or invidious. In many of these regions — for example, in fringe areas of the New Guinea highlands — elaborate ritual enactment promulgates health, rejuvenation and/or the overcoming of death for the collectivity at large. For instance, the *habu* ritual described above for the Daribi publicly dispels ghostly influence; it both combats the specter of death and promotes life.

A similar theme is found among the cult and ritual practices of the Lake Kutubu/ Foi peoples to the west of the Daribi (Williams 1977; Weiner 1984, 1986, 1987). Rather than traumatic male initiation, the Foi practiced a myriad of curing cults and organized ritual feasts during mortuary rites as a way of promulgating general fertility. As Weiner (1987:274) suggests in elaboration of Williams (1977): "The prevention of sickness and its implicit converse, the promotion of general fertility is a theme of male definition throughout the southern fringe area of the highlands of New Guinea...." Among the Kaluli, to the west, the spectacular *gisaro* ritual poignantly evoked the memory of the dead and simultaneously asserted the emotional passion of the living (Schieffelin 1976, 1979, 1980; Feld 1982). In the successful *gisaro*, elaborately costumed dancers visiting from other settlements sang songs about the hosts' forest lands and deceased relatives. In response, audience members burned the dancers severely about their shoulders and back — for having aroused such intense grief and sorrow among them. However, the performers continued their dancing and singing unabated. Indeed, they themselves paid compensation to the hosts at the conclusion of the ritual the following morning — in recompense for the emotional anguish that their exquisite performance had evoked in the hosts. Hence, the *gisaro* was a preeminent assertion of Kaluli aesthetic power and reciprocity.

Themes of otherworldly evocation and emotional passion reach a more exuberant and sexual expression further still to the west, among the lowland Gebusi. The Gebusi *gigobra* is a general rite of well-being, typically including a generous feast, an all-night dance, and much singing and joking (Knauft 1985a-b). The dancers

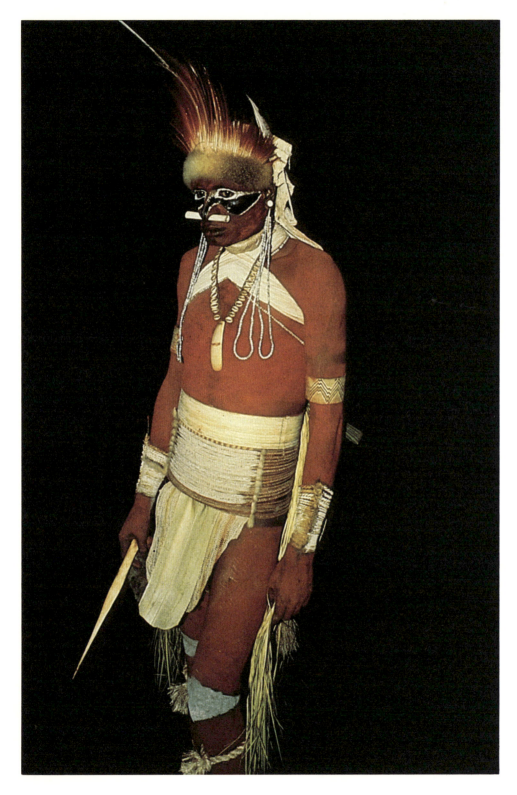

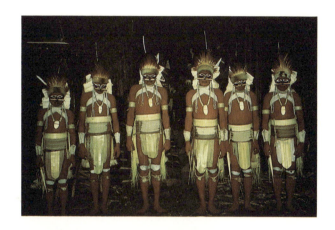

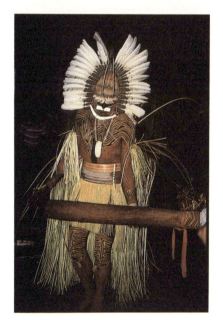

*Gebusi* gigobra *costume.*

*Gebusi initiation costume: a celebration of growth, sexual potency and societal rejuvenation.*

themselves embody on their person the beauty and harmony of the Gebusi spiritual universe. Costume parts worn on the upper half of the body signify spirit-creatures of the upper world, and those on the lower body spirit-forms from the underworld. Thus, for instance, the drum presents a large open-mouth fish or crocodile – the incarnate form of elder male spirits who live in the larger streams and rivers. The top half of the *gigobra* costume, in contrast, presents the above world. The large halo of white headdress feathers comes from the egret, a bird incarnating "male" qualities; the forehead band is fur from the cuscus, a tree-dwelling marsupial spirit-form; and the pearl-shell sliver under the chin is said to present a crescent moon.

The Gebusi dancer as a whole, moving and swaying slowly to the beat of his drum, enacts in his person the beauty, attractiveness and coordinated harmony of Gebusi spirits in their various dimensions. This is an apt metaphor for the social purpose of the dance itself, which promotes healing, conflict resolution and friendly camaraderie. More erotically, the dance is also a context for exuberant public joking and for private attempts to initiate homo- and heterosexual liaisons. This dimension of the ritual is also visually encoded in the symbolism of the dance costume, which is said as a whole to present the red bird of paradise (*Paradisaea raggiana*). This bird is the incarnate form of the beautiful and alluring Gebusi spirit-woman, and is a general symbol of vitality, beneficence and strong erotic attraction. The brilliant red plumage of this bird is portrayed in the red body paint on the dancer, as well as in sprays of red bird of paradise feathers at the back and inside the dancer's white halo headdress. The dark head and gold banding of the bird are reflected in the black eye mask of the dancer, ringed in yellow, and in the black ribbing lined in gold on his trunk and legs.

A further visual semiotic among Gebusi may be illustrated in the costume of the male initiates, also said in general to be an embodiment of the red bird of paradise. In this costume, however, the costume parts are gifts from various men of different settlements who have volunteered to be sponsors of the initiate. The initiate's costume thus displays both the craftsmanship of his allies and his potential ties of political support in various settlements throughout Gebusi territory. When the half dozen or more age-grade initiates process and line up in identical costume, they collectively embody not only the harmony of various spirit forms, but the interconnection of the Gebusi people as a whole. The initiation festivities are in fact the largest collective event in Gebusi society, with the majority of the tribe attending. Once again, however, the elaborate costume also has a pronounced sexual dimension. This is reflected not only in the general red bird of paradise imagery but in the long phallic leaf, said to present the initiate's enlarged penises. This sexual emphasis is particularly appropriate since the young men at the time of their initiation have been liberally inseminated (orally) and have been exhorted to avoid sexual contact with women. As such, they are believed to be at the peak of their physical growth and sexual potency. The term for male initiation is itself "child become big" (*wa kawala*). After initiation, the initiates' much-vaunted virility is released bisexually — first, in homosexual insemination of uninitiated boys, and second, in the active quest for women as sexual and marital partners (Knauft 1987a). These same activities are also pursued at the initiation festivities themselves by the visitors and hosts in attendance.

As Gebusi costuming illustrates, decorative symbolism can be both complex and polysemic. This multivalence is especially apposite for evoking complexly integrated cultural themes of sexual potency, vitality and societal rejuvenation. A similar panoply of themes can be seen in a different cultural context among the Umeda of West Sepik Province, to the north of the highlands (Gell 1975; cf. Juillerat 1986). Among the Umeda, a sequence of elaborately costumed dancers convey rich processes of biological growth, sexuality, reproduction and spiritual regeneration over the course of a nightlong ritual. The first dancers are symbolically associated with cassowaries (large flightless birds) and with elder men, whose active sexuality is indicated by large penis gourds. (These phallic adornments are flapped up and down and clack loudly during the dance.) The ritual proceeds amid many embellishments through a series of painted performers, including sago dancers and sexual buffoons. The rite culminates with the brief dance of red bowmen (*ipele*), who symbolize (among other things) youthful initiates whose penises are bound and who are potent and successful in hunting. Overtly, the ritual is staged to facilitate the growth and fertility of sago (a principal palm-food), but Gell shows its messages to be much richer, including poignant portrayals of gender complementarity, of "natural" reproduction and of spiritual regeneration as it is transferred from one initiation grade to the next. Ultimately, the ritual employs spectacular costuming to enact the rejuvenation and reproduction of Umeda society itself.

## Costuming as Personal Enhancement and Seduction —
## Massim and New Guinea Highlands

The symbolization of beauty, sexuality and vitality are not limited in Melanesia to fringe New Guinea societies. In numerous areas, highly costumed male initiates or dancers are believed capable of attracting women as wives. Frequently, as occurs in much of the New Guinea highlands, young men emerging from initiation-grade or bachelor-cult seclusion are festooned in ritual finery appropriate to their sexual attractiveness or marriageability. In both the New Guinea highlands and the Melanesian Massim, themes of bodily attraction are extended as well to economic or political activities. For the Massim in particular, beauty magic and enhanced appearance increase the individual's ability to attract wealth, as well as lovers (e.g., A. Weiner 1976:ch.5; Munn 1986:101-18). Such beautification is especially important for men in orchestrating successful wealth exchanges and for inducing exchange partners to relinquish their most prized wealth items – such as the famed Kula valuables (ibid.; Malinowski 1922; Leach and Leach, eds. 1983). The kula valuables are in principle themselves forms of body decoration – arm shells and necklaces. However, these valuables are so important that they take on personalities and lives of their own. The history of thier exchange and temporary possession by the inhabitants of the various islands is well-known lore, making the valuables a transcultural repository of renown for the region as a whole. Appropriately, many of the prized valuables are indeed too large and/or important to effectively be worn.

A different permutation of decorative self-actualization is found in the New Guinea highlands. Here costuming is used especially in the context of group status rivalry and display, for example, when large competitive gifts of wealth are given. The stature of participants is justly enhanced by their elaborate decorations – long-plumage headdresses, elaborate face-painting, wigs, shells and other accoutrements too numerous and intricate to describe here (see Strathern and Strathern 1971; Kirk with Strathern 1981; A. Strathern 1975; M. Strathern 1979). While such decoration has been prominent throughout the New Guinea highlands, it has been most thoroughly studied in Mount Hagen (Strathern and Strathern 1971), where the linkage between decoration and deeper aspects of self-enhancement are effectively evident:

> In Hagen thought material success and physical health are alike expressed in a man's bodily condition. A person should be well filled-out, with a gleaming skin, and oiling the

body contributes to it a desired, glossy appearance. Hageners also say that one of the aims of decorating is to make the dancers appear larger: at festivals, where they wear a whole range of ornaments, their enhanced size goes with increased attractiveness; in warfare it makes them impressive and frightens the enemy. (Strathern and Strathern 1971:134)

Not surprisingly, the most impressive and expensive bodily decorations were often worn by or at the direction of the so-called "big-men," those leaders who by dint of personal assertiveness compete effectively at the upper rungs of the shifting status hierarchy. Some bodily insignia specified particular aspects of the big-man's economic or military achievements. Such, for instance, is the *omak*, a set of short bamboo tally sticks laced side by side and hung from the wearer's neck — a bit like a broad but stiff necktie. Among the Melpa, the number of tally sticks — and hence the length of the *omak* — is determined by how many times the man has given away a set of eight or ten major shells in *moka* wealth exchange (Strathern and Strathern 1971).

The term "big-man" is itself frequently a literal gloss of vernacular terms, and big-men *were* sometimes physically big — an association not unrelated to their effectiveness and eminence in warfare (Watson 1967). However, the largess of the big-man, particularly as he reached his prime, was equally if not more evident in economic exchanges, feasting and elaborate oratory; he embodied a special forcefulness, aggression and incisive vitality (e.g., Read 1959; Sahlins 1963; Salisbury 1964; Watson 1967; A. Strathern 1966, 1971, 1979b, 1982 ed.; Meggitt 1971; cf. Keesing 1985b).

While the big-man is in a sense the embodiment of the group, his accomplishments also accrue to his followers and his kin group as a whole; they have contributed their own wealth as part of his gift-giving display. Hence all men — and women — can, on appropriate occasions, decorate themselves elaborately. Commonly, groups of related dancers from a given clan dress in elaborate and near-identical costumes. At the same time, there is, in much highlands costuming, room for a large component of individual creativity. When combined with choice costume parts, this creativity can promote special recognition of the wearer's individuality and power in self-presentation. Individual variation in costuming has had great aesthetic if not also social force in most Melanesian societies.

While subject to personal discretion, the appropriateness of an individual's and a group's choice of costume is — even in the realpolitik of the highlands — also ultimately underwritten by spiritual sanction:

A clan can achieve success only if it has the active support of its ancestral ghosts.... At a festival, a demonstration that an individual or a group is prosperous and healthy itself indicates ghostly blessing. Conversely, failure or disaster is a sign that the ghosts have become angry at some wrong and have withdrawn their help. (Strathern and Strathern 1971:130) This spiritual sanction enforces in broad terms the conformity of costuming with the degree of self-enhancement that the individual or group can legitimately claim. It is in this sense that "the whole act of self-decoration is a kind of omen-taking" (*ibid*.:134).

These themes reflect the more general highlands linkage between spiritual force, bodily vitality, attractiveness and cultural well-being (M. Strathern 1979).

*  *  *

In the most general terms, it may be said that presentation of the decorated body in Melanesia is a celebration of social and cultural vitality in its myriad local dimensions. That this decoration focuses on or about the skin is particularly appropriate, as the skin is the boundary, mediator and index of relationship between the internal self and the collective other (Turner 1980; cf. A. Strathern 1975; M. Strathern 1979). Through its decorations, the body both establishes and indicates self–other relations, particularly in spheres of production and reproduction, substance and spirit. The body in Melanesia is the self-reflecting icon of a particularly rich and varied nature – a performative that sends and absorbs signals of depth and complexity, binding the actor and the audience in intricate webs of experience and meaning.

## Conclusion

The body in Melanesia is intricately tied to cycles of fertility, depletion and regeneration. These include the "natural" cycles of change in the physical environment, the biological patterns of development within the individual body, and the social and spiritual cycles through which interpersonal relationships grow, mature and dissolve. We in the industrialized West tend to divorce these cycles from one another, assuming that our bodily, social and spiritual worlds are largely separate – that they operate according to separate orders of causation. In Melanesia, by contrast, these

254

processes tend to be linked as complementary parts of a single cosmological universe and to be instantiated through a holistic bodily ecology.

This is not to suggest that Melanesian cultural systems form integrated wholes; Melanesian cultural systems have always grown and changed in a dialectical and inconsistent fashion. Certainly, too, bodily ecology is much more developed and/or systematic in some Melanesian societies than in others. It can be argued, however, that the natural world, the anatomical self and the world of social and spiritual relationships are recognized by Melanesians to be integrated in ways that we Westerners largely deny.

This reflects more general differences. While Melanesian cultural systems are full of dialectical tensions and contradictions (particularly in the realms of gender and male status competition), they do not harbor the anxieties of ontological doubt that gnaw the West in matters of mind, symbol and belief. There is little of the radical epistemological schism that we in the West harbor so uneasily — the scientific versus the humanistic versus the pragmatic. This deepest fractionalization of understandings has been foreign to Melanesia. As was so clearly recognized by the great anthropologist Gregory Bateson (1936, 1972, 1979), the symbolic, social and environmental dimensions of life are in fact equally real and intrinsically interconnected. As Bateson also suggested, we neglect an awareness of this holistic ecology only at our own peril and impoverishment. In this respect, Melanesian cosmologies present a major advance over our own.

From this perspective, the relationship between the present account and other forms of inquiry comes into closer view. Certainly it would have been possible to analyze Melanesian bodily beliefs and practices as art — or as artifacts — in and of themselves. This, however, leaves out the indigenous meanings of art and aesthetics — it leaves behind their significance as well as their integration with other aspects of Melanesian life and cosmology.

It would certainly also be possible to generate causal–functional arguments as to why certain trends of Melanesian bodily custom and belief exist in the form they do. Living closer to their biotic environment than we, it is perhaps "natural" that Melanesians have taken basic processes of growth, maturation and death as more poignant and pervasive cultural metaphors than we do. More specifically, it could perhaps be argued that cultural concern with food, disease or bodily privation is foregrounded in those areas of Melanesia where the environment is harsher or morbidity higher; that cannibalism is common where people are plentiful but other sources of protein are not; that male socialization is most arduous where resource competition, social organization or warfare place a premium on collective male toughness and aggression. Correspondingly, competition or restrictiveness over bodily insignia may be greater where material resources, population densities and/or political hierarchies heighten conflict. Perhaps as well, the tendency for adolescent girls to mature more quickly than boys could provide some explanation of male anxiety over impeded physiological development vis-à-vis women.

These arguments cannot be dismissed out of hand. Indeed, our understanding of bodily meanings and practices in Melanesia remains sadly divorced from the sparse comparative information available on subsistence ecology, nutrition and human physiology in this part of the world. However, it is undeniable that Melanesian bodily beliefs and practices have a cultural life of their own. The documented proliferation, spread and especially the incredible diversity of local bodily beliefs and practices in Melanesia are far greater and intricate than any explanation on the basis of genetic, ecological or sociological predicates can reasonably comprehend. A model of the interaction between "natural" ecology and the ecology of cultural belief is perhaps the best that can be hoped for in this respect.

In a different vein, we may consider Melanesian bodily belief against the more recent postmodern emphasis on reflexivity and the relativity of ethnographic perspective (e.g., Marcus and Fischer 1986; Clifford and Marcus 1987; Tyler 1987). Prominent here is the problematic relationship between the viewer and the thing being viewed — between the ostensible objectivity of the subject and the true subjectivity of its object. Certainly self-reflection and relativity of perspective are crucial when considering the body in Melanesia. Our process of ethnographic construction may be subject to deep inquiry, as may the assumption that beliefs or customs are bounded "entities" that can be summarily characterized or generalized about. Certainly as well, our account cannot have been representative of the various sections of Melanesia nor even of the ethnographies available for New Guinea; the personal limitations and biases of the author must be evident here as well.[21] These are important topics that, regretfully, lie beyond our present purview. Likewise, the politics that motivate our own position need to be examined in ways that have only been alluded to above.

In spite of the intrinsic relativity of our perspective, we have tried to make a few substantive characterizations of bodily belief and custom in precolonial Melanesia. In a sense, though, we cannot do otherwise. However filtered or relative our accounts may be, we must at some point rely on our best sources and our best abilities, bracket ontological questions and make the leap of faith which assumes a real world of social and symbolic attributes that we can at least partially capture in our writing. To fail to make this leap of faith, ultimately, would be to keep other cultures in the dark while shining the light of inquiry indulgently on our own personal experience.

It is only the sketchiest of bodily pastiches that we have attempted here for Melanesia. One of the greatest strengths of Melanesian ethnography is the detail and rigor of its published accounts, while to Melanesia itself belongs the rich diversity of indigenous beliefs and customs. Our intent has been more to whet the appetite for appreciating this cultural diversity than to prematurely attempt its grand explanation.

This paper is part of a larger research project funded by the Harry Frank Guggenheim Foundation, whose support is gratefully acknowledged. Support from Emory University for research assistance is also gratefully acknowledged. The author wishes to thank Eileen Cantrell for critical comments on an earlier draft of this paper, though any shortcomings remain his own.

NOTES

1. Given the difficulty of writing consistently in the face of this ambiguity, we have in some instances reluctantly adopted the convention of the "ethnographic present." This present-tense usage does not necessarily mean that the practice or belief in question is today a general practice in the society described.

2. "Patrilineal" indicates that identity in descent groups, such as clans or lineages, is traced through male descent. Matrilineal, in contrast, indicates that kin group identity is traced through females. Melanesian societies exhibit a plethora of descent-group variations, many of them crosscutting or combining aspects of these polar analytic types. It is nowadays generally realized by Melanesianists that simple reference to "matrilineal" or "patrilineal" groups is unduly simplistic; the distinction is made primarily for didactic purposes in the present context.

3. In the absence of sufficient payments by a boy's patrikin, the Daribi maternal uncle may curse the child — believed to cause him sickness or misfortune — or he may even take the child physically as his own.

4. This is not to say that female puberty and initiation rites have been rare in Melanesia, but rather that they have in overall terms been less common and much less elaborate than those for males (see Lutkehaus and Roscoe 1988; contrast Allen 1967; Herdt, ed. 1982).

5. We focus here largely on New Guinea; the subject of male initiation in Melanesia more generally is reviewed in Allen (1967); cf. Herdt, ed. (1982).

6. Reports of female homosexuality in Melanesia have been rare and fragmentary (Herdt, ed. 1984:75 n.10).

7. The fertility of a young Marind-anim woman was thought to be directly tied to her frequency of serial sexual congress with the men of her husband's clan, both upon marriage and whenever she renewed menstruation following childbirth (van Baal 1966). The mingled sexual fluids obtained from the rite were also applied directly to wounds and scarifications to help them heal, mixed with ceremonial food and ingested to enhance growth, placed on plant shoots to promote garden abundance, mixed with sorcery potions to empower them, mixed with other substances to blacken the teeth, and, more generally, used to ensure the potency and success of numerous ritual performances and social activities.

8. This issue is receiving important current attention, though much refinement of it is still needed (cf. Whitehead 1986a-b; Lindenbaum 1984, 1987; Strathern, ed. 1987; Feil 1987:ch.7; see Knauft 1987a).

9. Melanesian sorcery is a vast and intriguing topic; principal sources include Stephen (1986); Zelenietz and Lindenbaum (1981); Fortune (1932); Forge (1970); Young (1983a); Knauft (1985a); Patterson (1974). For a very brief overview see Glick (1973).

10. See, for example, A. Strathern 1971; Feil 1984; Meggitt 1974; Rappaport 1984; Lederman 1986; Young 1971; Oliver 1955; A. Weiner 1976; Malinowski 1922; Leach and Leach 1983; Clay 1986; Errington 1974; cf. P. Brown 1978; Rubel and Rosman 1978.

11. See Feil 1978; M. Strathern 1972, 1980, 1981, 1987; Faithorn 1976; Josephides 1983, 1985; Godelier 1986; Sillitoe 1985; Errington and Gewertz 1987; Keesing 1985a; Young 1983b; cf. Mead 1935.

12. An overview of New Guinea highlands warfare and casualty rates has recently been compiled by Feil (1987:ch.4).

13. In many cases this compensation was paid to kin of slain persons by their allies who had started the war, rather than by the enemy group themselves.

14. The Kwoma statues were closely linked in cult usage with spiritual power in growing yams, fertility, and protection of the group in warfare (Bowden 1983:105ff.,115-17). Indeed, only persons who had killed enemies were believed capable of growing yams, and they alone were automatically permitted to join the most prestigious fertility cult, the *nowkwi* (ibid.:16, 105).

15. Melanesian groups demonstrate diverse linkages between death, copulation and regeneration, on the one hand, and warfare, copulation and depletion, on the other. The former association is seen, for instance, in Trobriand mortuary copulation customs (in association with the death of in-group members):

> During the mortuary wake (*yawali*), which takes place immediately after a man's death, people from all the surrounding communities congregate and take part in the songs and ceremonies which last for the best part of the night. When, far into the night, the visitors return home, it is the custom for some of the girls to remain behind to sleep with certain boys of the bereaved village. Their regular lovers must not, and do not, interfere. (Malinowski 1929:219)

This is perhaps an aspect of female regeneration pronounced in Trobriand mortuary rites and exchange generally (A. Weiner 1976).

The countervailing association between warfare, copulation and depletion is seen among the Murik of north coast New Guinea. Among the Murik, women married to members of the junior moiety grade of the war cult were enjoined to copulate with those of the elder grade to facilitate the transmission of the latter's spiritual authority; when the members of the elder grade had all been successfully seduced, their war-making prowess was symbolically depleted/relinquished, and their authority was officially transferred to the erstwhile junior grade (Meeker, Barlow and Lipset 1986). The belief that copulation is inimical to warfare or long-distance trade (rather than facilitating it) was pronounced in many areas of Melanesia, including much of highland and northern New Guinea. This is somewhat the obverse of the positive linkage between heterosexuality and warfare discussed for the Marind-anim below.

16. Asmat also practiced child- or wife-capture, but to a lesser extent.

17. These areas include parts of the Sepik, south New Guinea, Mountain Ok, insular eastern Melanesia and even the New Guinea highlands.

18. Tuzin (1980: 223) asks, "What does this bestowal entail? Nothing less than renewal of the grand conditions of existence: human and natural fertility, physical security, social harmony, and cultural meaning."

19. Tuzin (1982: 339) describes the *hangumu'w* costume itself as follows: "[T]he *hangamu'w* is a full-body costume consisting of a woven helmet mask, a shoulder area fashioned from coiled strands

of bright orange fruits, and a concealing body curtain of yellow sago fibers. The women are told the half-truth [see below] that these are spirits incarnate, rather than being merely men disguised as such."

20.  While this dimension of masked costuming is most pronounced in insular Melanesia, discussed below, and in the Sepik, it was also nascently present in parts of south New Guinea. Among the Koriki, for instance, men of stature could be initiated into several cults which conveyed on them legitimate knowledge and use of various spirit-masks (Williams 1923, 1924). These rites were paid for by the initiate and culminated in major feasts.

21.  For instance, we have paid relatively more attention to the "flamboyant" cultures of the lowlands, fringe and Ok areas of New Guinea and less to the populous New Guinea highlands than is usually done in regional comparisons. This is perhaps forgivable as a corrective to the lingering tendency to view highland patterns as dominant or archetypal in comparative analysis – with other New Guinea regions conceptualized as negative comparisons. A different problem arises in our relative neglect of Irian Jaya and particularly of insular and eastern Melanesia. Here the problem is my own limited knowledge and the relatively fewer rich ethnographic accounts of traditional practices from these regions (but see Guiart 1956, 1963a-b, 1966; Leenhardt 1947; Layard 1942; Deacon 1934; Harrisson 1937; Allen, ed. 1981; Keesing 1982; Oliver 1955, 1971; Hogbin 1965; Blackwood 1935; Powdermaker 1933; Parkinson 1907; Oosterwal 1963; van Baal 1966; Serpenti 1965; Heider 1970, 1979; Koch 1974; Pospisil 1958, 1963a-b).

Bibliography

Allen, Michael R.

1967    *Male Cults and Secret Initiations in Melanesia*. Melbourne: Melbourne University Press.

1984    "Elders, Chiefs, and Big Men: Authority Legitimation and Political Evolution in Melanesia," *American Ethnologist* 11, pp. 20-40.

Allen, Michael R. (ed.).

1981    *Vanuatu: Politics, Economics and Ritual in Island Melanesia*. New York: Academic Press.

Baal, Jan van.

1966    *Dema: Description and Analysis of Marind-Anim Culture (South New Guinea)*. The Hague: Martinus Nijhoff.

1984    "The Dialectics of Sex in Marind-anim Culture," in *Ritualized Homosexuality in Melanesia*. Edited by Gilbert H. Herdt, pp. 128-67. Berkeley: University of California Press.

Barth, Fredrik.

1975    *Ritual and Knowledge among the Baktaman of New Guinea*. New Haven: Yale University Press.

1987    *Cosmologies in the Making: A Generative Approach to Cultural Variation in Inner New Guinea*. Cambridge: Cambridge University Press.

Bateson, Gregory.

1936    *Naven: A Survey of the Problems Suggested by a Composite Picture of a Culture of a New Guinea Tribe Drawn from Three Points of View*. Cambridge: Cambridge University Press. (2d ed.: Stanford, Cal.: Stanford University Press, 1958.)

1972    *Steps to an Ecology of Mind*. New York: Ballantine.

1979    *Mind and Nature: A Necessary Unity*. New York: Bantam.

Battaglia, Debbora.

1985    " 'We Feed Our Father': Paternal Nurture among the Sabarl of Papua New Guinea," *American Ethnologist* 12, pp. 427-41.

Berndt, Ronald M.

1962    *Excess and Restraint: Social Control among a New Guinea Mountain People*. Chicago: University of Chicago Press.

1964  "Warfare in the New Guinea Highlands," *American Anthropologist* 66.4 (special issue), pp. 183-203.

Biersack, Aletta.
1982  "Ginger Gardens for the Ginger Woman: Rites and Passages in a Melanesian Society," *Man* 17, pp. 239-58.

Blackwood, Beatrice.
1935  *Both Sides of Buka Passage: An Ethnographic Study of Social, Sexual, and Economic Questions in the North-Western Solomon Islands*. Oxford: Clarendon.

Bowden, Ross.
1983  *Yena: Art and Ceremony in a Sepik Society*. Oxford: Pitt Rivers Museum.

Brown, D.J.J.
1979  "The Structuring of Polopa Feasting and Warfare," *Man* 14, pp. 712-32.

Brown, Paula.
1978  *Highland Peoples of New Guinea*. Cambridge: Cambridge University Press.

Buchbinder, Georgeda and Roy A. Rappaport.
1976  "Fertility and Death among the Maring," in *Man and Woman in the New Guinea Highlands*. Edited by Paula Brown and Georgeda Buchbinder, pp. 13-35. Washington, D.C.: American Anthropological Association (Special Publication no. 8).

Cantrell, Eileen M.
n.d.  "Gebusi Gender Relations." Ph.D. Dissertation (in progress) at the Department of Anthropology, University of Michigan, Ann Arbor.

Chauvet, S.
1930  *Les Arts Indigènes en Nouvelle-Guinée*. Paris.

Chowning, Ann, and Ward H. Goodenough.
1971  "Lakalai Political Organization," in *Politics in New Guinea*. Edited by Ronald M. Berndt and Peter Lawrence, pp. 113-75. Nedlands, Australia: University of Western Australia Press.

Clay, Brenda Johnson.
1977  *Pinikindu: Maternal Nurture, Paternal Substance*. Chicago: University of Chicago Press.

1986    *Mandak Realities: Person and Power in Central New Ireland*. New Brunswick, N.J.: Rutgers University Press.

Clifford, James and George E. Marcus (eds.).

1986    *Writing Culture: The Poetics and Politics of Ethnography*. Berkeley: University of California Press.

Comaroff, Jean.

1985    *Body of Power, Spirit of Resistance: The Culture and History of a South African People*. Chicago: University of Chicago Press.

Counts, Dorothy and David Counts.

1983    "Father's Water Equals Mother's Milk: The Conception of Parentage in Kaliai, West New Britain," *Mankind* 14, pp. 46-56.

Danks, B.

1887    "On the Shell Money of New Britain," *Journal of the Royal Anthropological Institute* 17, pp. 305-17.

1892    "On Burial Customs of New Britain," *Journal of the Royal Anthropological Institute* 21, pp. 348-56.

Deacon, A. Bernard.

1934    *Malekula: A Vanishing People in the New Hebrides*. London: George Routledge.

Ernst, Thomas M.

1979    "Myth, Ritual and Population among the Marind-Anim," *Social Analysis* 1, pp. 32-53.

Errington, Frederick K.

1974    *Karavar: Masks and Power in a Melanesian Ritual*. Ithaca, N.Y.: Cornell University Press.

Errington, Frederick K. and Deborah Gewertz.

1987    *Cultural Alternatives and a Feminist Anthropology: An Analysis of Culturally Constructed Gender Interests in Papua New Guinea*. Cambridge: Cambridge University Press.

Faithorn, Elizabeth.

1976    "Women as Persons: Aspects of Female Life and Male-Female Relations among the Kafe," in *Man and Woman in the New Guinea Highlands*. Edited by P. Brown and G. Buchbinder, pp. 86-95. Washington, D.C.: American Anthropological Association (Special Publication no. 8).

Feil, D.K.

1978 "Women and Men in the Enga *Tee*," *American Ethnologist* 5, pp. 263-79.

1984 *Ways of Exchange: The Enga Tee of Papua New Guinea*. Queensland, Australia: University of Queensland Press.

1987 *The Evolution of Highland Papua New Guinea Societies*. Cambridge: Cambridge University Press.

Feld, Steven.

1982 *Sound and Sentiment: Birds, Weeping, Poetics, and Song in Kaluli Expression*. Philadelphia: University of Pennsylvania Press.

Forge, Anthony.

1965 "Art and Environment in the Sepik," *Proceedings of the Royal Anthropological Institute of Great Britain and Ireland* (1965), pp. 23-32.

1970 "Prestige, Influence and Sorcery: A New Guinea Example," in *Witchcraft Confessions and Accusations*. Edited by Mary Douglas, pp. 257-75. London: Tavistock.

1972 "The Golden Fleece," *Man* 7, pp. 527-40.

Fortune, Reo F.

1932 *Sorcerers of Dobu: The Social Anthropology of the Dobu Islanders*. London: E.P. Dutton. (Reprint: New York: Dutton, 1963.)

1939 "Arapesh Warfare," *American Anthropologist* 41, pp. 22-41.

Gell, Alfred.

1975 *Metamorphosis of the Cassowaries: Umeda Society, Language and Ritual*. London: Athlone.

Gerbrands, A.A.

1967 *The Asmat of New Guinea: The Journal of Michael Clark Rockefeller*. New York: Museum of Primitive Art.

Gillison, Gillian.

1980 "Images of Nature in Gimi Thought," in *Nature, Culture and Gender*. Edited by Carol MacCormack and Marilyn Strathern, pp. 143-73. Cambridge: Cambridge University Press.

1983 "Cannibalism among Women in the Eastern Highlands of Papua New Guinea," in *The Ethnography of Cannibalism*. Edited by Paula Brown and Donald Tuzin, pp. 33-51. Washington, D.C.: Special Publication of the Society for Psychological Anthropology.

1987    "Incest and the Atom of Kinship: The Role of the Mother's Brother in a New Guinea Highlands Society," *Ethos* 15, pp. 166-202.

Glasse, Robert M. and Mervyn Meggitt (eds.).
1969    *Pigs, Pearlshells, and Women*. Englewood Cliffs, N.J.: Prentice-Hall.

Glick, Leonard B.
1973    "Sorcery and Witchcraft," in *Anthropology in Papua New Guinea*. Edited by H. Ian Hogbin. Melbourne: Melbourne University Press.

Godelier, Maurice.
1986    *The Making of Great Men: Male Domination and Power among the New Guinea Baruya*. Cambridge: Cambridge University Press.

Goodale, Jane C.
1980    "Gender, Sexuality and Marriage: A Kaulong Model of Nature and Culture," in *Nature, Culture and Gender*. Edited by Carol MacCormack and Marilyn Strathern, pp.119-43. New York: Cambridge University Press.
1985    "Pig's Teeth and Skull Cycles: Both Sides of the Face of Humanity," *American Ethnologist* 12, pp. 228-44.

Goodenough, Ward.
1971    "The Pageant of Death in Nakanai," in *Melanesia: Readings on a Culture Area*. Edited by L.L. Langness and John C. Weschler, pp. 279-92. Scranton, Pa.: Chandler Publishing.

Greub, Suzanne (ed.).
1985    *Authority and Ornament: Art of the Sepik River, Papua New Guinea*. Basel, Switzerland: Tribal Art Centre/Meier+Cie AG Schaffhausen.

Groves, William C.
1935    "Tabar Today: A Study of a Melanesian Community in Contact with Alien Non-Primitive Cultural Influences," *Oceania* 5, pp. 224-40, 346-60.
1936    "Secret Beliefs and Practices in New Ireland," *Oceania* 7, pp. 220-45.

Guiart, Jean.
1956    *Un Siècle et demi de contacts culturels à Tanna, Nouvelles-Hébrides*. Paris: Musée de L'Homme.

1963a "La Structure de la chefferie en Mélanesie du Sud," Paris: Université de Paris (Travaux et Mémoires de l'Institut d'Ethnologie, 66).

1963b *The Arts of the South Pacific*. Translated by Anthony Christie. London: Thames and Hudson.

1966 *Mythologie du masque en Nouvelle-Calédonie*. Paris: Musée de l'Homme.

Hallpike, Christopher R.

1977 *Bloodshed and Vengeance in the Papuan Mountains: The Generation of Conflict in Tuade Society*. Oxford: Clarendon.

Harrison, Simon J.

1982 "Yams and the Symbolic Representation of Time in a Sepik River Village," *Oceania* 53, pp. 141-62.

Harrisson, T.H.

1937 *Savage Civilisation*. London: Gollancz.

Heider, Karl G.

1970 *The Dugam Dani: A Papuan Culture in the Highlands of West New Guinea*. Chicago: Aldine.

1979 *Grand Valley Dani: Peaceful Warriors*. New York: Holt, Rinehart & Winston.

Herdt, Gilbert H.

1981 *Guardians of the Flutes: Idioms of Masculinity*. New York: McGraw-Hill.

1982a "Sambia Nosebleeding Rites and Male Proximity to Women," *Ethos* 10, pp. 189-231.

1982b "Fetish and Fantasy in Sambia Initiation," in *Rituals of Manhood: Male Initiation in Papua New Guinea*. Edited by Gilbert H. Herdt, pp. 44-99. Berkeley: University of California Press.

1984 "Semen Transactions in Sambia Culture," in *Ritualized Homosexuality in Melanesia*. Edited by Gilbert H. Herdt, pp. 167-211. Berkeley: University of California Press.

1987a *The Sambia: Ritual and Gender in New Guinea*. New York: Holt, Rinehart & Winston.

1987b "The Accountability of Sambia Initiates," in *Anthropology in the High Valleys: Essays on the New Guinea Highlands in Honor of Kenneth E. Read*. Edited by L.L. Langness and Terence E. Hays, pp. 237-81. Novato, Cal.: Chandler and Sharp.

Herdt, Gilbert H. (ed.).

1982 *Rituals of Manhood: Male Initiation in Papua New Guinea*. Berkeley: University of California Press.

1984 *Ritualized Homosexuality in Melanesia*. Berkeley: University of California Press.

Hogbin, Herbert Ian.

1965 *A Guadalcanal Society: The Kaoka Speakers*. New York: Holt, Rinehart & Winston.

1970 *The Island of Menstruating Men: Religion in Wogeo, New Guinea*. Scranton, Pa.: Chandler Publishing.

Jorgensen, Dan.

1983a "The Facts of Life, Papua New Guinea Style," *Mankind* 14, pp. 1-12.

1983b "Mirroring Nature? Men's and Women's Models of Conception in Telefolmin," *Mankind* 14, pp. 57-65.

Josephides, Lisette.

1983 "Equal But Different? The Ontology of Gender among Kewa," *Oceania* 53, pp. 291-307.

1985 *The Production of Inequality: Gender and Exchange among the Kewa*. New York: Tavistock.

Juillerat, Bernard.

1986 *Les Enfants du sang: Société, reproduction et imaginaire en Nouvelle-Guinée*. Paris: Éditions de la Maison des Sciences de l'Homme.

Kaberry, Phyllis M.

1971 "Political Organization among the Northern Abelam," in *Politics in New Guinea*. Edited by Ronald M. Berndt and Peter Lawrence, pp. 35-73. Nedlands, Australia: University of Western Australia Press.

Kahn, Miriam.

1986 *Always Hungry, Never Greedy: Food and the Expression of Gender in a Melanesian Society*. Cambridge: Cambridge University Press.

Keesing, Roger M.

1982 *Kwaio Religion: The Living and the Dead in a Solomon Island Society*. New York: Columbia University Press.

1985a "Kwaio Women Speak: The Micropolitics of Autobiography in a Solomon Island Society," *American Anthropologist* 87, pp. 27-39.

1985b "Killers, Big Men, and Priests on Malaita: Reflections on a Melanesian Troika System," *Ethnology* 24, pp. 237-52.

Kelly, Raymond C.

1976 "Witchcraft and Sexual Relations: An Exploration in the Social and Semantic Implications of the Structure of Belief," in *Man and Woman in the New Guinea Highlands*. Edited by Paula Brown and Georgeda Buchbinder, pp. 36-53. Washington, D.C.: American Anthropological Association (Special Publication no. 8).

1977  *Etoro Social Structure: A Study in Structural Contradiction*. Ann Arbor: University of Michigan Press.

Kirk, Malcom with Andrew J. Strathern.

1981  *Man as Art: New Guinea*. New York: Viking.

Knauft, Bruce M.

1985a  *Good Company and Violence: Sorcery and Social Action in a Lowland New Guinea Society*. Berkeley: University of California Press.

1985b  "Ritual Form and Permutation in New Guinea: Implications of Symbolic Process for Sociopolitical Evolution," *American Ethnologist* 12, pp. 321-40.

1986  "Text and Social Practice: Narrative 'Longing' and Bisexuality among the Gebusi of New Guinea," *Ethos* 14, pp. 252-81.

1987a  "Homosexuality In Melanesia," *The Journal of Psychoanalytic Anthropology* 10, pp. 155-91.

1987b  "Reconsidering Violence in Simple Human Societies: Homicide among the Gebusi of New Guinea," *Current Anthropology* 28, pp. 457-500.

1987c  "Managing Sex and Anger: Tobacco and Kava Use among the Gebusi of Papua New Guinea," in *Drugs in Western Pacific Societies: Relations of Substance*. Edited by Lamont Lindstrom, pp. 73-98. Lanham, Md.: University Press of America.

Koch, Klaus-Friedrich.

1974  *War and Peace in Jalemo: The Management of Conflict in Highland New Guinea*. Cambridge, Mass.: Harvard University Press.

Konner, Melvin J.

1981  "Evolution of Human Behavior Development," in *Handbook of Cross-Cultural Human Development*. Edited by Ruth H. Munroe, Robert L. Munroe and Beatrice B. Whiting, pp. 3-52. New York: Garland STPM Press.

Konrad, Gunter, Ursula Konrad and Tobias Schneebaum.

1981  *Asmat: Life with the Ancestors*. Glasshutten, West Germany: Friedhelm Bruckner.

Kramer, A.

1925  *Die Malanggane in Tombara*. Munich.

Landtman, Gunnar.

1927   *The Kiwai Papuans of British New Guinea*. London: Macmillan. (Reprint: New York: Johnson Reprint Co., 1970.)

Langness, L.L.

1967   "Sexual Antagonism in the New Guinea Highlands: A Bena Bena Example," *Oceania* 37, pp. 161-77.

1972   "Violence in the New Guinea Highlands," in *Collective Violence*. Edited by James F. Short and Marvin E. Wolfgang, pp. 171-85. Chicago: Aldine.

1974   "Ritual Power and Male Domination in the New Guinea Highlands," *Ethos* 2, pp. 189-212.

Larson, Gordon F.

1987   "The Structure and Demography of the Cycle of Warfare among the Ilaga Dani of Irian Jaya." Ph.D. Dissertation at the Department of Anthropology, University of Michigan. Ann Arbor.

Layard, John.

1942   *Stone Men of Malekula*. London: Chatto and Windus.

Leach, Jerry and Edmund R. Leach (eds.).

1983   *The Kula: New Perspectives on Massim Exchange*. Cambridge: Cambridge University Press.

Lederman, Rena.

1986   *What Gifts Engender: Social Relations and Politics in Mendi, Highland Papua New Guinea*. Cambridge: Cambridge University Press.

Leenhardt, Maurice.

1979   *Do Kamo: Person and Myth in the Melanesian World* (1947). Translated by Basia Miller Gulati. Chicago: University of Chicago Press.

Lewis, Gilbert.

1980   *Day of Shining Red: An Essay on Understanding Ritual*. New York: Cambridge University Press.

Lindenbaum, Shirley.

1984   "Variations on a Sociosexual Theme in Melanesia," in *Ritualized Homosexuality in Melanesia*. Edited by Gilbert H. Herdt, pp. 337-62. Berkeley: University of California Press.

1987   "The Mystification of Female Labors," in *Gender and Kinship: Essays Toward a Unified Analysis*. Edited by Jane F. Collier and Sylvia J. Yanagisako, pp. 221-43. Stanford, Cal.: Stanford University Press.

Lutkehaus, Nancy and Jim Roscoe (organizers).

1988　"Female Initiation in the Pacific," paper presented at the Symposium of the Annual Meetings of the Association for Social Anthropology in Oceania. Savannah, Ga.

Malinowski, Bronislaw.

1916　"Baloma: The Spirits of the Dead in the Trobriand Islands," *Journal of the Royal Institute*, 45. (Reprint: B. Malinowski, *Magic, Science, and Religion*. Garden City: Doubleday Anchor Books, 1954.)

1922　*Argonauts of the Western Pacific: An Account of the Native Enterprise and Adventure in the Archipelagoes of Melanesian New Guinea*. (Reprint: New York: E.P. Dutton, 1961.)

1927　*The Father in Primitive Psychology*. New York: W.W. Norton.

1929　*The Sexual Lives of Savages in North-Western Melanesia*. London: George Routledge & Sons. (Reprint: Boston: Beacon Press, 1987.)

1935　*Coral Gardens and Their Magic: A Study of the Methods of Tilling the Soil and of Agricultural Rites in the Trobriand Islands*. 2 vols. London: Allen & Unwin.

Marcus, George E. and Michael M. Fisher.

1986　*Anthropology as Cultural Critique: An Experimental Moment in the Human Sciences*. Chicago: University of Chicago Press.

McKinley, Robert.

1976　"Human and Proud of It! A Structural Treatment of Headhunting Rites and the Social Definition of Enemies," in *Studies in Borneo Societies: Social Process and Anthropological Explanation*. Edited by G.N. Appell. Special Report no. 12, Center for Southeast Asian Studies, Northern Illinois University.

Mead, Margaret.

1935　*Sex and Temperament in Three Primitive Societies*. New York: William Morrow. (Reprint: New York: Dell, 1963.)

Meeker, Michael E., Kathleen Barlow and David M. Lipset.

1986　"Culture, Exchange, and Gender: Lessons from the Murik," *Cultural Anthropology* 1, pp. 6-73.

Meggitt, Mervyn J.

1964　"Male–Female Relationships in the Highlands of Australian New Guinea," in *New Guinea: The Central Highlands*. Edited by James B. Watson. *American Anthropologist* 66.4, pp. 204-24.

1965a  *The Lineage System of the Mae-Enga of New Guinea*. Edinburgh: Oliver and Boyd.

1965b  "[Religion of] The Mae-Enga of the Western Highlands," in *Gods, Ghosts and Men in Melanesia: Some Religions of Australian New Guinea and the New Hebrides*. Edited by Peter Lawrence and Mervyn Meggitt. Melbourne: Oxford University Press.

1971  "The Pattern of Leadership among the Mae-Enga of New Guinea," in *Politics in New Guinea*. Edited by Ronald M. Berndt and Peter Lawrence, pp. 191-206. Nedlands, Australia: University of Western Australian Press.

1974  " 'Pigs are our Hearts!': The *Te* Exchange Cycle among the Mae Enga of New Guinea," *Oceania* 44, pp. 165-203.

1977  *Blood Is Their Argument: Warfare among the Mae Enga Tribesmen of the New Guinea Highlands*. Palo Alto, Cal.: Mayfield.

Meigs, Anna S.

1976  "Male Pregnancy and the Reduction of Sexual Opposition in a New Guinea Highlands Society," *Ethnology* 15, pp. 393-407.

1984  *Food, Sex, and Pollution: A New Guinea Religion*. New Brunswick, N.J.: Rutgers University Press.

1987  "Semen, Spittle, Blood, and Sweat: A New Guinea Theory of Nutrition," in *Anthropology in the High Valleys: Essays on the New Guinea Highlands in Honor of Kenneth E. Read*. Edited by L.L. Langness and Terence E. Hays, pp. 27-43. Novato, Cal.: Chandler and Sharp.

Meyer, A.B. and R. Parkinson.

1895  *Schnitzerein und Masken von Bismark Archipelago und Neu Guinea*. Koningliches Ethnographiches Museum in Dresden, pub. 10. Dresden.

Modjeska, Nicholas.

1982  "Production and Inequality: Perspectives from Central New Guinea," in *Inequality in New Guinea Highlands Societies*. Edited by Andrew J. Strathern, pp. 50-108. Cambridge: Cambridge University Press.

Mosko, Mark.

1983  "Conception, De-Conception and Social Structure in Bush Mekeo Culture," *Mankind* 14, pp. 24-32.

Munn, Nancy D.

1986  *The Fame of Gawa: A Symbolic Study of Value Transformation in a Massim (Papua New Guinea) Society*. New York: Cambridge University Press.

Nachman, Steven R.

1982 "Anti-humor: Why the Grand Sorcerer Wags His Penis," *Ethos* 10, pp. 117-35.

Nevermann, H.

1933 *Masken und Geheimbinder in Melanesien*. Berlin.

Newman, Philip L. and David J. Boyd.

1982 "The Making of Men: Ritual and Meaning in Awa Male Initiation," in *Rituals of Manhood: Male Initiation in Papua New Guinea*. Edited by Gilbert H. Herdt, pp. 239-86. Berkeley: University of California Press.

Oliver, Douglas.

1955 *A Solomon Island Society*. Boston: Beacon Press.

1971 "Southern Bougainville," in *Politics in New Guinea*. Edited by Ronald M. Berndt and Peter Lawrence, pp. 276-97. Nedlands, Australia: University of Western Australia Press.

Oosterwal, Gottfried.

1961 *People of the Tor: A Cultural-Anthropological Study on the Tribes of the Tor Territory (Northern Netherlands New-Guinea)*. Assen, the Netherlands: Van Gorcum.

Parkinson, R.

1907 *Dreissig Jahre in der Sudsee*. Stuttgart: Strecker und Schroder.

Patterson, Mary.

1974 "Sorcery and Witchcraft in Melanesia," *Oceania* 45, pp. 132-60, 212-34.

Poole, Fitz John.

1981a "Transforming 'Natural' Woman: Female Ritual Leaders and Gender Ideology among Bimin-Kuskusmin," in *Sexual Meanings*. Edited by Sherry B. Ortner and Harriet Whitehead, pp. 116-65. Cambridge: Cambridge University Press.

1981b "*Tamam*: Ideological and Sociological Configurations of 'Witchcraft' among the Bimin-Kuskusmin," in *Sorcery and Social Change in Melanesia*. Edited by Marty Zelenietz and Shirley Lindenbaum, pp. 58-76. *Social Analysis* (Special Issue no.8). Adelaide, Australia.

1982a "The Ritual Forging of Identity: Aspects of Person and Self in Bimin-Kuskusmin Male Initiation," in *Rituals of Manhood*. Edited by Gilbert H. Herdt, pp. 99-154. Berkeley: University of California Press.

1982b "Couvade and Clinic in a New Guinea Society: Birth among the Bimin-Kuskusmin," in *The Use and Abuse of Medicine*. Edited by Marten W. deVries, Robert L. Berg and Mac Lipkin, Jr., pp. 54-95. New York: Praeger Scientific.

1983 "Cannibals, Tricksters, and Witches: Anthropophagic Images among Bimin-Kuskusmin," in *The Ethnography of Cannibalism*. Edited by Paula Brown and Donald Tuzin, pp. 6-33. Washington, D.C.: Special Publication of the Society for Psychological Anthropology.

1984 "Cultural Images of Women as Mother: Motherhood among the Bimin-Kuskusmin of Papua New Guinea," in *Gender and Social Life*. Edited by Anna Yeatman. *Social Analysis* 5, pp. 73-93.

1985 "Coming into Social Being: Cultural Images of Infants in Bimin-Kuskusmin Folk Psychology," in *Person, Self, and Experience: Exploring Pacific Ethnopsychologies*. Edited by Geoffrey M. White and John Kirkpatrick, pp. 183-242. Berkeley: University of California Press.

1986 "The Erosion of a Sacred Landscape: European Exploration and Cultural Ecology among the Bimin-Kuskusmin of Papua New Guinea," in *Mountain People*. Edited by Michael Tobias, pp. 169-82. Norman, Ok.: University of Oklahoma Press.

1987a "Ritual Rank, the Self, and Ancestral Power: Liturgy and Substance in a Papua New Guinea Society," in *Drugs in Western Pacific Societies: Relations of Substance*. Edited by Lamont Lindstrom, pp. 149-96. Lanham, Md.: University Press of America.

1987b "Morality, Personhood, Tricksters, and Youths: Some Narrative Images of Ethics among Bimin-Kuskusmin," in *Anthropology in the High Valleys: Essays on the New Guinea Highlands in Honor of Kenneth E. Read*. Edited by L.L. Langness and Terence E. Hays, pp. 283-366. Novato, Cal.: Chandler and Sharp.

1987c "Personal Experience and Cultural Representation in Children's "Personal Symbols" among Bimin-Kuskusmin," *Ethos* 15, pp. 104-35.


Poole, Fitz John and Gilbert H. Herdt (eds.).

1982 *Sexual Antagonism, Gender, and Social Change in Papua New Guinea*. *Social Analysis* (Special Issue no.12.) Adelaide, Australia.


Pospisil, Leopold.

1958 *Kapauku Papuans and Their Law*. Yale University Publications in Anthropology, no. 54. New Haven: Yale University Press.

1963a *The Kapauku Papuans of West New Guinea*. New York: Holt, Rinehart & Winston.

1963b *Kapauku Papuan Economy*. Yale University Publications in Anthropology, no. 67. New Haven: Yale University Press.

Powdermaker, Hortense.

1931    "Mortuary Rites in New Ireland," *Oceania* 2, pp. 26-43.

1979    *Life in Lesu: The Study of a Melanesian Society in New Ireland*. London: Williams & Norgate, 1933. (Reprint: New York: AMS Press.)

Rappaport, Roy A.

1984    *Pigs for the Ancestors: Ritual in the Ecology of a New Guinea People*, 2d, enlarged ed. New Haven: Yale University Press.

Read, Kenneth E.

1952    "Nama Cult of the Central Highlands, New Guinea," *Oceania* 23, pp. 1-25.

1954    "Cultures of the Central Highlands, New Guinea," *Southwestern Journal of Anthropology* 10, pp. 1-43.

1959    "Leadership and Consensus in a New Guinea Society," *American Anthropologist* 61, pp. 425-36.

Reay, Marie O.

1959    *The Kuma: Freedom and Conformity in the New Guinea Highlands*. Melbourne: Melbourne University Press.

1987    "The Magico-Religious Foundations of New Guinea Highlands Warfare," in *Sorcerer and Witch in Melanesia*. Edited by Michele Stephen, pp. 83-120. New Brunswick, N.J.: Rutgers University Press.

Rivers, W.H.R.

1914    *The History of Melanesian Society.* 2 vols. Cambridge: Cambridge University Press.

Rubel, Paula G. and Abraham Rosman.

1978    *Your Own Pigs You May Not Eat: A Comparative Study of New Guinea Societies*. Chicago: University of Chicago Press.

Sahlins, Marshall D.

1963    "Poor Man, Rich Man, Big-Man, Chief: Political Types in Melanesia and Polynesia," *Comparative Studies in Society and History* 5, pp. 285-303.

1972    "On the Sociology of Primitive Exchange," in *Stone Age Economics*. Edited by Marshall D. Sahlins, pp. 175-285. Chicago: Aldine.

Salisbury, Richard F.

1964 "Despotism and Australian Administration in the New Guinea Highlands," in *New Guinea: The Central Highlands*. Edited by James B. Watson. *American Anthropologist* 66.4, pp. 225-39.

1966 "Politics and Shell-Money Finance in New Britain," in *Political Anthropology*. Edited by M. Schwartz and A. Tuden. Chicago: Aldine.

1970 *Vunamami: Economic Transformation in a Traditional Society*. Berkeley: University of California Press.

Schieffelin, Edward L.

1976 *The Sorrow of the Lonely and the Burning of the Dancers*. New York: St. Martin's Press.

1979 "Mediators as Metaphors: Moving a Man to Tears in Papua New Guinea," in *The Imagination of Reality: Essays in Southeast Asian Coherence Systems*. Edited by Alton L. Becker and Aram A. Yengoyan, pp. 127-44. Norwood, N.J.: Ablex Publishing.

1980 "Reciprocity and the Construction of Reality," *Man* 15, pp. 502-17.

1982 "The *Bau A* Ceremonial Hunting Lodge: An Alternative to Initiation," in *Rituals of Manhood: Male Initiation in Papua New Guinea*. Edited by Gilbert H. Herdt, pp. 155-201. Berkeley: University of California Press.

Schneebaum, Tobias.

1985 *Asmat Images: From the Collection of the Asmat Museum of Culture and Progress*. Minneapolis: Crosier Mission/Sowada.

1988 *Where the Spirits Dwell: An Odyssey in the New Guinea Jungle*. New York: Grove Press.

Schwartz, Theodore.

1963 "Systems of Areal Integration: Some Considerations Based on the Admiralty Islands of Northern Melanesia," *Anthropological Forum* 1, pp. 56-97.

Schwimmer, Eric.

1973 *Exchange in the Social Structure of the Orokaiva*. New York: St. Martin's Press.

Serpenti, Laurentius.

1965 *Cultivators in the Swamps*. Assen, the Netherlands: Van Gorcum.

Sillitoe, Paul.

1985 "Divide and No One Rules: The Implications of Sexual Divisions of Labour in the New Guinea Highlands," *Man* 20, pp. 494-522.

1987    "Wola Sorcery Divination," in *Sorcerer and Witch in Melanesia*. Edited by Michele Stephen. New Brunswick, N.J.: Rutgers University Press.

South Pacific Commission (Population Study S-18 Project).

1955    Rapport van het Bevolkingsonderzoek onder de Marind-anim van Nederlands Zuid Nieuw Guinea.

Stephen, Michele (ed.).

1987    *Sorcerer and Witch in Melanesia*. New Brunswick, N.J.: Rutgers University Press.

Strathern, Andrew J.

1966    "Despots and Directors in the New Guinea Highlands," *Man* n.s. 1, pp. 356-67.

1970    "The Female and Male Spirit Cults in Mount Hagen," *Man* 5, pp. 571-85.

1971    *The Rope of Moka: Big Men and Ceremonial Exchange in Mount Hagen, New Guinea*. Cambridge: Cambridge University Press.

1972    *One Father, One Blood: Descent and Group Structure among the Melpa People*. London: Tavistock.

1975    "Why Is Shame on the Skin?" *Ethnology* 14, pp. 347-56.

1979a   "Men's House, Women's House: The Efficacy of Opposition, Reversal, and Pairing in the Melpa *Amb Kor* Cult," *Journal of Polynesia* 88, pp. 37-51.

1979b   *Ongka: A Self-Account by a New Guinea Big-Man*. New York: St. Martin's.

Strathern, Andrew J. (ed.).

1982    *Inequality in New Guinea Highland Societies*. Cambridge: Cambridge University Press.

Strathern, Marilyn.

1972    *Women in Between: Female Roles in a Male World, Mount Hagen, New Guinea*. London: Seminar (Academic) Press.

1979    "The Self in Self-Decoration," *Oceania* 59, pp. 241-57.

1980    "No Nature, No Culture: The Hagen Case," in *Nature, Culture and Gender*. Edited by Carol MacCormack and Marilyn Strathern, pp. 174-223. New York: Cambridge University Press.

1981    "Self-interest and the Social Good: Some Implications of Hagen Gender Imagery," in *Sexual Meanings*. Edited by Sherry B. Ortner and Harriet Whitehead, pp. 166-91. Cambridge: Cambridge University Press.

Strathern, Marilyn (ed.).

1987    *Dealing with Inequality: Analysing Gender Relations in Melanesia and Beyond*. Cambridge: Cambridge University Press.

Strathern, Andrew and Marilyn Strathern.

1971    *Self-decoration in Mount Hagen*. Toronto: University of Toronto Press.

Thurnwald, B.R.

1916    *Banaro Society: Social Organization and Kinship System of a Tribe in the Interior of New Guinea*. *American Anthropological Association Memoirs* 3, pp. 253-391.

Turner, Terence S.

1980    "The Social Skin," in *Not Work Alone: A Cross-cultural View of Activities Superfluous to Survival*. Edited by Jeremy Cherfas and Roger Lewin, pp. 112-43. Beverly Hills, Cal.: Sage.

Tuzin, Donald F.

1972    "Yam Symbolism in the Sepik: An Interpretive Account," *Southwestern Journal of Anthropology* 28, pp. 230-54.

1974    "Social Control and the Tambaran in the Sepik," in *Contention and Dispute: Aspects of Law and Social Control in Melanesia*. Edited by A.L. Epstein. Canberra: Australian National University Press.

1976    *The Ilahita Arapesh: Dimensions of Unity*. Berkeley: University of California Press.

1980    *The Voice of the Tambaran: Truth and Illusion in Ilahita Arapesh Religion*. Berkeley: University of California Press.

1982    "Ritual Violence among the Ilahita Arapesh: The Dynamics of Moral and Religious Uncertainty," in *Rituals of Manhood: Male Initiation in Papua New Guinea*. Edited by Gilbert H. Herdt, pp. 321-57. Berkeley: University of California Press.

Tyler, Stephen A.

1987    *The Unspeakable: Discourse, Dialogue and Rhetoric in the Postmodern World*. Madison: University of Wisconsin Press.

Wagner, Roy.

1967    *The Curse of Souw: The Principles of Daribi Clan Definition and Alliance in New Guinea*. Chicago: University of Chicago Press.

1972    *Habu: The Innovation of Meaning in Daribi Religion*. Chicago: University of Chicago Press.

1981    *The Invention of Culture*. 2d ed.: Chicago: University of Chicago Press.

1983    "The Ends of Innocence: Conception and Seduction among the Daribi of Karimui and the Barok of New Ireland," *Mankind* 14, pp. 75-83.

1986    *Asiwinarong: Ethos, Image, and Social Power among the Usen Barok of New Ireland*. Princeton, N.J.: Princeton University Press.

Watson, James B.

1967    "Tairora: The Politics of Despotism in a Small Society," *Anthropological Forum* 2, pp. 53-104.

Weiner, Annette B.

1976    *Women of Value, Men of Renown: New Perspectives in Trobriand Exchange*. Austin: University of Texas Press.

1980    "Reproduction: A Replacement for Reciprocity," *American Ethnologist* 7, pp. 71-85.

Weiner, James F.

1982    "Substance, Siblingship and Exchange: Aspects of Social Structure in New Guinea," *Social Analysis* 11, pp. 3-34.

1984    "Sunset and Flowers: The Sexual Dimension of Foi Spatial Orientation," *Journal of Anthropological Research* 40, pp. 577-88.

1986    "Blood and Skin: The Structural Implications of Sorcery and Procreation Beliefs among the Foi of Papua New Guinea," *Ethnos* 51, pp. 71-87.

1987    "Diseases of the Soul: Sickness, Agency and the Men's Cult among the Foi of New Guinea," in *Dealing with Inequality: Analysing Gender Relations in Melanesia and Beyond*. Edited by Marilyn Strathern, pp. 255-77. Cambridge: Cambridge University Press.

West, M.M. and Konner, M.J.

1976    "The Role of the Father: An Anthropologial Perspective," in *The Role of the Father in Child Development*. Edited by M.E. Lamb. New York: Wiley.

Whitehead, Harriet.

1986a   "The Varieties of Fertility Cultism in New Guinea: Part 1," *American Ethnologist* 13, pp. 80-99.

1986b   "The Varieties of Fertility Cultism in New Guinea: Part 2," *American Ethnologist* 13, pp. 271-89.

Williams, Francis E.

1923    "The Pairama Ceremony in the Purari Delta, Papua," *Journal of the Royal Anthropological Institute of Great Britain and Ireland* 53, pp. 361-87.

1924   *The Natives of the Purari Delta*. Territory of Papua, Anthropology Report, no. 5. Port Moresby: Government Printer.

1940   *Drama of Orokolo: The Social and Ceremonial Life of the Elema*. Oxford: Clarendon Press.

1977   "Natives of Lake Kutubu, Papua," in *"The Vailala Madness" and Other Essays*. Edited by Eric Schwimmer, pp. 161-331. Honolulu: University Press of Hawaii.

Williamson, Margaret Holmes.

1983   "Sex Relations and Gender Relations: Understanding Kwoma Conception," *Mankind* 14, pp. 13-23.

Wingert, Paul S.

1962   *Primitive Art: Its Traditions and Styles*. New York: Oxford University Press.

Young, Michael W.

1971   *Fighting with Food: Leadership, Values and Social Control in a Massim Society*. Cambridge: Cambridge University Press.

1983a  *Magicians of Manumanua: Living Myth in Kalauna*. Berkeley: University of California Press.

1983b  "Our Name Is Women; We Are Bought with Limesticks and Limepots: An Analysis of the Autobiographical Narrative of a Kalauna Woman," *Man* 18, pp. 478-501.

1986   "The Worst Disease: The Cultural Definition of Hunger in Kalauna," in *Shared Wealth and Symbol: Food, Culture, and Society in Oceania and Southeast Asia*. Edited by Lenore Manderson, pp. 111-27. Cambridge: Cambridge University Press.

Zegwaard, Gerard A.

1959   "Headhunting Practices of the Asmat of West New Guinea," *American Anthropologist* 61, pp. 1020-41.

Zelenietz, Marty and Shirley Lindenbaum (eds.).

1981   *Sorcery and Social Change in Melanesia*. *Social Analysis* (Special Issue, no. 8). Adelaide.

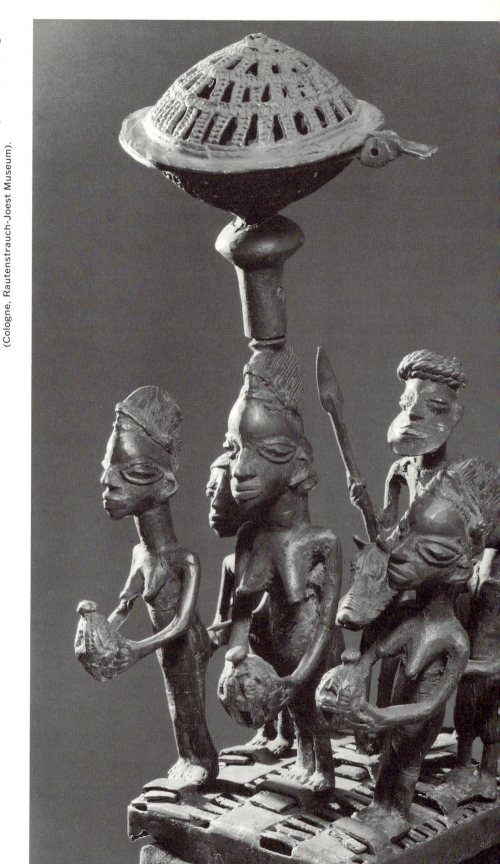

Queen with two servants followed by the King. Yoruba art, Nigeria (Cologne, Rautenstrauch-Joest Museum).

# Older Women, Stout-Hearted Women, Women of Substance

*Françoise Héritier-Augé*

No observer of Western society will deny the emphatic male domination by which it is marked. Subordination of the female is obvious in the political, economic and symbolic realms. Few women represent the people in local or central government (in the executive branch and in administration). Economically, women are generally relegated to the domestic sphere, and they never escape it completely: women who hold salaried positions must, in effect, combine the two kinds of activity. If they engage in nondomestic activities, women rarely reach the top levels of their profession, the positions of responsibility, leadership, prestige. In the symbolic terms transmitted through tradition and childhood education, the recognized and valued activities are those that men carry out. In addition, a range of value judgments highlights characteristics deemed natural, and therefore unchangeable and manifest, in the behavior, the accomplishments and the feminine "qualities" or "faults" that are viewed as typical of the sex. A negative discourse presents women as creatures of the irrational and the illogical, devoid of critical intelligence, nosy, indiscreet, gossipy, incapable of keeping a secret, given to routine, unimaginative, uncreative — especially where intellectual or artistic endeavors are concerned — timid and cowardly, slaves to their bodies and their feelings, ill-suited to controlling and judging their passions, inconsequent, hysterical, fickle, untrustworthy or even treacherous, cunning, jealous, envious, incapable of friendship among themselves, undisciplined, disobedient, immodest, perverse — Eve, Delilah, Galatea, Aphrodite.... Then there is another, apparently less negative configuration of terms: delicate homebodies, unsuited to intellectual or physical adventure; sweet, emotional, requiring peace, stability and the comfort of home; inclined to shirk responsibility; incapable of decisive behavior or abstract thinking; gullible, intuitive, impressionable, tender and chaste — women by nature need to be subjugated, guided and supervised by a man. In both cases, and passing over contradictions between the two versions (hot-blooded woman, cold-blooded woman; pure woman, polluting woman), one can see this symbolic discourse refers to a feminine *nature* — morphological, biological, psychological. These lists of characteristics have a negative or unvalorized cast, whereas the lists of corresponding male characteristics are positive or valorized. There is a major sex and a minor sex, a "strong" sex and a "weak" sex, a "strong" spirit and a "weak" spirit. The natural, congenital weakness of women implies and legitimizes the subjection even of their bodies.

We will not ask here whether the unequal relation of the sexes in Western society can and ought to change, and if so, according to what standards. Rather, we will ask two very different questions. Can one say that male domination is *universal*? If so, what is the *origin*, the explanation for this fundamental inequality between the sexes?

\* \* \*

It is not at all certain that we have a complete count of all the human societies that exist or once existed. Certainly all known societies have not been described. And when they have been, it has not necessarily been done in such a way as to reveal, case by case, the nature of the relationship between men and women. With these reservations, which imply the absence of an absolute scientific proof, there is a strong statistical probability, stemming from a study of anthropological literature on the subject, that male supremacy is universal.

One criticism of this affirmation, from a feminist viewpoint, is that most anthropological studies have been conducted by men. To which one might add that when such studies are conducted by women, the latter of necessity share in the dominant ideology of their own society, which valorizes masculinity, and that, as a result, they take a greater interest in the men's world, which is considered more interesting and, in any case, more accessible. This double bias, ethnocentric and androcentric, would mean that one sees other societies through one's own eyes and, more specifically, through the eyes of the man, who dominates in our society. Finally, the world of women being especially secret and closed to an anthropologist — particularly a male — our means of approaching them is men's vision of their own society. The women of societies studied in this way are thus seen with doubly masculine eyes,

282

a fact that would explain the image dominant in anthropological literature of their humbled status.

One cannot completely reject this argument, but it seems appropriate to restrict its import on several counts: first, if one concedes that female anthropologists share in the dominant ideology of their own society, it is a contradiction to suppose that, in other societies, women could have a set of representations that differed radically from those of the men. Second, the natural tendency among anthropologists is to take an interest in the exotic and what is most removed from their own culture; so it is not at all obvious that men would be incapable of seeing and noting the cases where women play an important and active role, at some remove from the canons of our own culture. What is more, one cannot say whether a massive breakthrough effected by anthropologists who are women and feminists would not reveal further, and so far unknown, handicaps in the study of the world of women. Finally, a recent study (Whyte 1978) shows, on the basis of statistical correlations between variables for the position of women and the sex of the observer in the case of ninety-three populations, that the latter given is of negligible importance. The author concludes that studies done by men are not necessarily exhaustive and reliable, but that one finds in them no systematic distortion that would present the status of women as abnormally low. A greater abundance of documents supplied by female observers would produce a more accurate view of the role women play, but would not necessarily indicate that their situation is better than generally believed. For example, it is true that, as early as 1939, Phyllis Kaberry corrected the image Malinowski had provided of Australian aboriginal women – humble, deferential to men, spurned, cast out from the sacred. But for all that, she does not reverse their story's general import.

A second objection to the statistical probability of universal male domination (based on the examination of anthropological documents) is that it does not accord much attention to history. This argument is presented in two different ways. In the great societies of the present day, one can observe a leveling process centered on domination of a patriarchal type, even as women are deprived of the rights or privileged positions they once held, under the influence of several factors: the established religions, both Judeo-Christian and Islamic; the development of commerce and industry that favors new kinds of activity and therefore upsets positions already gained; the incidence of colonialism, which conveyed and aggravated the other two factors in areas where it took hold. One response is that it is difficult to see how established religions favoring the role of men could have sprung up and developed in complete defiance of the dominant ideology. In the same way, it is difficult to see why, if women were dominant in a given area in political, economic and ideological terms, they would have been incapable of adapting to the social transformations brought about by economic change or colonization. In any case, the leveling under discussion probably manifested itself by the aggravation of a condition rather than its gradual inversion.

The second version of the argument from history refers to the well-known evolutionary theory, derived from theses of Bachofen (1861), of a primitive matriarchy. According to this theory, there was an initial stage of humanity characterized by an ignorance of physiological paternity, by a cult of God-mothers and by the domination of men by women in politics, economics and ideology. This is not the place to engage in a critique of evolutionary theories of humanity; let us simply note that the term "matriarchy," which conveys the idea of feminine power, has been and is still frequently used to refer to what are, in actuality, cases of matrilineality – where the principal rights are those of men born into filiation groups defined by women – or to refer to mythic cases like that of the Amazons.

From an anthropological point of view, the human society that seems to have come closest to the definition of matriarchy is that of the Iroquois (Brown 1970). They have been studied by many authors, beginning with the famous work of the Jesuit Father Joseph Lafitau (1724) and the story published by Seaver (1880) concerning the life of Mary Jemison. In the six Iroquois nations, the women were not treated with deference or accorded unusual attentions, and it seems, according to Morgan, that the men considered themselves superior, devoting all their energy to long-range hunting – a hunt could last a year – or to war. But the women, or at least a few of them, seem to have enjoyed rights or powers rarely equaled elsewhere.

Filiation was traced through the women and residence was matrilocal. Women of the same line lived in the same long-house with their husbands and children, under the supervision of "matrons" selected by means of which we unfortunately have no exact knowledge. The matrons, who supervised and organized life in the long-houses, also organized the women's agricultural work, a female prerogative they exercised in common in collective fields belonging to the women of that line. The matrons themselves allotted the cooked food family by family and to guests and members of the Council. The matrons were represented, if not at the Great Council of the Six Iroquois Nations, then at least at the Council of Elders within each nation, by a male representative who spoke in their name and made their voice heard. The voice of the matrons was not, in fact, a negligible voice, since they had the right to veto a war, if the war project did not please them. In any case, they could prevent the execution of a projected war that didn't meet with their approval simply by forbidding the women to give warriors the provisions — dried or concentrated food — they had to take along. Judith Brown believes the Iroquois matrons owe their elevated status to the fact that they control the economic organization of the tribe (they also allot the fruits of the men's hunt), which is plausible given a favorable matrilineal social structure. The major productive activity of the women — that is, hoe-cultivation — is not incompatible with the activity of tending young children. According to the same author, there are, interestingly enough, only three types of economic activity that allow this combination of chores: gathering, hoe-cultivation and traditional commerce (which does not mean that every society in which these activities are practiced accords women privileged positions). Lastly, it is not a matter of indifference that it is the matrons who enjoy significant status among the Iroquois. We will come back to this point later on.

Those in search of an original truth turn for support to the study of societies that we consider the most "primitive" (even though they, too, have a history): the hunter-gatherers, populations that practice neither agriculture nor husbandry and live from direct appropriation of the fruits of nature through hunting, fishing, catching insects and small animals, picking berries, fruit and wild grains.

At the present time, there are an estimated thirty hunter-gatherer peoples. They do not offer a unified picture of male–female relations that one might suppose to be a relic of a single, original model. But it would appear that all of them display the existence of male supremacy, albeit with enormous variations, ranging from a protoequality of the sexes among certain Indian fishing peoples (Anaskapi) to a protoslavery of women among the Ona (Selk'nam) of Tierra del Fuego (cf. Chapman).

It is true that among certain hunter-gatherers — notably in Australia and Africa —

the women enjoy substantial autonomy. Maurice Godelier explains this by noting that, in these cases, there is no difference between domestic and public economy, since there is no private property and the family unit is not strictly conjugal. The men impose no physical constraints: when the group travels, its course is chosen to combine good hunting and good gathering; the women move about freely and make their own decisions.

But these "idyllic" portraits ought not to conceal the existence of other groups belonging to the same economic type, where relations between men and women are marked by violence. Anne Chapman describes a people among whom the women have no rights, where a man can strike, injure or even kill his wife without reproach, where the women, held in contempt, on a daily basis know nothing but brutal subjection and, during periodic male initiation rites that sometimes last several months, terror and violence inflicted by the masked celebrants. It is worth noting here that a myth of origins justifies this dependent state.

In the beginning, Chapman tells us, the men lived in abject submission and were forced to carry out all tasks, including domestic ones, and to wait on their wives. These lived together in the women's big hut, from which emanated the roar attributed to terrifying masks. Moon was a guide to the women. This continued until the day that Sun, a man among men, bringing game to the ritual hut to feed the women, overheard the young women mocking the credulity of the men; then he understood that the masks were not the emanations of supernatural forces directed against men, but a plot concocted and used by women to keep the men in a state of dependency. So the men strangled all the women with the exception of the very young girls, whose memory was untouched, and they reversed roles. Moon went back into Sky, where she still seeks to avenge herself on Sun: the eclipses of the sun show this. This reversal justifies absolute male power. Women are kept ignorant of their original state; the myth is transmitted only to men during their initiation; like the men, the women see Moon and the beings associated with her as enemies of the human race, because they know them to be hostile to their brothers, sons and husbands.

This is a perfect example, if ever there was one, of the mythical — that is, purely ideological — nature of the theme of primitive matriarchy, and one that occurs in a patriarchal society of the most "primitive" sort. It is not an isolated example. Among the Baruya of New Guinea, not hunter-gatherers but farmers who also engage in male initiation, men are taught during such rites that it was women who originally invented the bow and the ceremonial flutes. Men stole them after breaking into the menstrual hut where these objects were hidden. Ever since, men alone have known how to use them – the flute is a means of communicating with the world of the supernatural – and are thus granted a complete supremacy (Godelier). The Dogon of West Africa have a myth that women were similarly dispossessed of their power over the world of the sacred when men stole from them the red-tinted fiber skirts on the ceremonial masks. In all these cases, one is dealing with societies that exhibit a pronounced masculine power, a social organization they justify by reference to a mythical, originary matriarchal condition. But one must not conclude from this that the myth of a primordial matriarchy is universal, and that this universality is proof of its historical character, which would in turn lend support to evolutionary theories. The story of the same founding reversal is occasionally based on very different premises, because it is precisely this theme of the founding reversal – this myth of a world upside-down that needs setting right – that is the structural fact, and not the specific content, of each story. Thus, among the lagoon-dwellers of the Ivory Coast, matrilineal societies that assign power to the male also evoke in their myths an opposite primordial state, based this time on patrilineal institutions. The River demands that the group sacrifice a child before letting it cross over. The chief's wife refuses to give up her son; the chief's sister gives up hers, in order to save her brother and the entire group. The chief then decides that, in the future, the transmission of power and wealth will occur, not through the wife's son, but through the sister's son, the uterine nephew. But here no female violence is committed to take power from the men. The men have it and keep it: two women – a wife, a sister; two female positions conceived as diametrically opposed and in the name of which the chief promulgates a new law governing filiation – the egoism of the wife–stranger, the altruism and devotion of the blood–sister. But the chief is already a man, and the position of chief remains the man's.

The fact is that a myth does not deal in history: it conveys a message. Its purpose is to confer legitimacy on the existing social order. The Ona, Baruya and Dogon examples explain how the social order, incarnate in the preeminence of the male, is based on violence against women. The myth states explicitly that every culture, every society is based on sexual inequality and that this inequality is an act of violence. Does this mean that we have to believe in actual, intentional acts of violence at the outset, acts that established the social order? Do we have to believe in a historical dispossession, or is this simply a self-justifying discourse the society presents to itself in order to explain a situation actually produced by a number of unintended, objective causes? We will return to this point later on.

We have said mythology legitimizes the established social order. Nevertheless, not all societies have elaborated myths, properly speaking, to "justify" male domination, to give it meaning. All of them have an ideological discourse, though, a body of symbolic thought that has the same function of justifying man's supremacy in the eyes of all members of the society, women as well as men, because they all share by definition in the same ideology, inculcated from childhood on.

These symbolic narratives are built on a system of binary oppositions, of dualities, that contrast series like sun and moon, high and low, right and left, clear and opaque, bright and dark, light and heavy, front and back, dry and wet, male and female, upper and lower. One recognizes here the symbolic framework of Greek philosophical and medical thinking as we find it in Aristotle, Anaximander and Hippocrates, where the equilibrium of the world (as well as that of the human body and its humors) is based on the harmonious blending of these opposites, with any excess in an area provoking disorder and/or illness. In Greek thought, the central categories are hot and cold, dry and wet, and these are directly linked to masculinity (hot and dry) and femininity (cold and wet). In an apparently inexplicable fashion, they are assigned values, positive on the one side, negative on the other, though there is a certain ambivalence about the dry and the wet, which do not in themselves have strong positive or negative values, but acquire them by association in different contexts. Thus, in the scheme of the body, the hot and the wet are on the side of life, joy, comfort, and thus positive; the dry and the cold are on the side of death, and thus negative (the dead are thirsty). But in the scheme of the seasons, the dry is positively associated with summer heat, the wet negatively associated with winter cold. In the sexual scheme, women who as living bodies are hot and wet, but who become cool and dry as a result of menstruation, ought to be drier than men. But the male is hot and dry, associated with fire and positively valued; the woman is cold and wet, associated with water and negatively valued (Empedocles, Aristotle, Hippocrates). Aristotle says that, *by nature*, the sexes differ in their aptitude for "cooking" the blood to produce their particular bodily humors: women's menstrual secretions are an incomplete and imperfect form of sperm. Sperm, a rarefication and purging of the blood by intense concoction, is the purest of substances, elaborated to the last possible degree. This relation of perfection to imperfection, purity to impurity, which is the relation of sperm to menstrual flow, thus of male to female, presupposes as a result a fundamental, natural, biological difference in the aptitude for concoction: because man is from the start hot and dry, he accomplishes to perfection what woman, who is naturally cold and wet, can only accomplish imperfectly, in her moments of greatest heat, in the form of milk.

This philosophical–medical discourse, which gives a scholarly form to popular belief, is really an ideological discourse, like myth. The correlations among the binary oppositions bear no relation to a given reality, but rather relate to the positive or negative values attributed from the outset to the terms themselves. Like myth, this discourse performs the function of justifying the order of the world, the social order. Thus, in a perfect union of myth, the taxonomy of vegetables and the ideological relations of the sexes, Marcel Détienne (1977) explains, on the basis of mythological tales about Hera's solitary conception of Ares and his sister Hebe, why only women eat lettuce, a cold, wet soup vegetable: it is excellent for the onset of menstruation and a smooth flow of blood, but a corollary is that it frustrates pleasure. This is why men never eat it, fearing impotence and the loss of desire and pleasure (lettuce made Adonis impotent). Sexual pleasure is by rights a man's pleasure; women must content themselves with conception and must prepare themselves for it by eating the right foods.

Greek thought has certainly molded our own Western culture, as we shall see below. But how — other than on the basis of constants typical of the symbolic use of such material, specifically, the social relation of the sexes — does one explain that this same logic of opposites, of binary oppositions valued positively and negatively, appears in societies where the influence of Greek thought has just as certainly not been felt?

Among the Inuit of the central Arctic (Saladin d'Anglure 1978), Moon is a man and Sun his sister; turning the Greek example around for certain of the terms under consideration, "the cold, the raw and nature are assigned to man, the hot, the cooked and culture are assigned to woman"; and the myth of origins makes of women nothing more than "cloven men." The first woman was born of a man, and procreating woman is nothing more than a sack, a container that temporarily harbors a human life generated by man. Always relegated to the domestic realm, woman can only leave the masculine order in which she is confined by a literal evasion that leads to her death from exhaustion in the snow and cold.

Many other examples – African, Indonesian, American, etc. – could be offered (cf. Héritier 1978; Ingham 1970). In all cases, clustered symbolic concentrations give their meaning to social practices. In other cultures, naturally, binary systems other than those based on the hot and the cold may refer to the same practices or, as with the Inuit, a binary system based on the hot and the cold may invert all or a part of the series of related associations. In effect there is no rationale in these choices based on the objective apprehension of a natural given, even if they appear naturally legitimate. One must view these binary oppositions as cultural signs and not as bearers of a universal significance. The significance inheres in the existence of the oppositions themselves and not in their content; they are the language of social intercourse and of power.

Always and everywhere, ideological discourse bears the trappings of reason. Our own cultural discourse, inherited from Aristotle, also grounds an instituted social relation on biological differences, on a supposedly eternal nature. In this regard, for example, it is interesting to consider the scientific and medical discourse of the nineteenth century, as it is expressed in the writings of Julien Virey (cf. Knibiehler 1976). By successive shifts, he goes from a binary-type characterization of the sexes to a legitimation of the domination of one sex over the other, pretending to the most modern, objective, rational scientific argument drawn from the observation of a biological given. And yet he offers us nothing here other than the discourse of Aristotle, of the Inuit, or of the Baruya of New Guinea (Godelier). For Virey (1823), the ideal couple is "a dark, hairy male, *dry*, *hot* and impetuous, who finds the other sex fragile, *wet*, smooth and pale, timid and modest." It is the energy of sperm that gives married women self-assurance and boldness: "it is certain that the male's sperm permeates the woman's organism, vivifies all of its functions and *heats* them up." Because of her supple, delicate integuments and of a ramification more intensive than in men of the nerves and blood vessels beneath the skin, woman has an "exquisite" sensitivity. This exquisite sensitivity makes her particularly apt for pleasure, with passions that are easily inflamed; and thus, she has a natural tendency to profligacy, depravity and a lack of concentration or reflection, the latter being acts eminently and naturally male. The same sensitivity that suits a woman for the care of children, the sick and the aged also produces dangerous passions in her, which is why a man must watch over her closely. Virey writes: "Because woman is weak by her very constitution, Nature therefore wished to make her submissive and dependent in the act of sexual congress; therefore, she is born for kindness, tenderness and even patience, docility; therefore, she must bear the yoke of restraint without complaint in order, by her submission, to ensure harmony in the family" (*De l'éducation*, 1802).

It seems to me that, in contrast to what Yvonne Knibiehler has written, this is not an individual, "naively" phallocentric view influenced by stereotypes of the era, but, rather, it is the elaborated expression of commonly shared archetypes in scholarly form. The text, in a reasoned manner that would claim to be "scientific," translates popular value judgments of the kind enumerated above. The text continues along Aristotle's line of thinking, which itself was a rational elaboration of much earlier archetypes, and it prefigures the discourse of alienist and hygienist doctors of the nineteenth century in particular on female hysteria, as well as Freud's on penis envy: woman lacks sperm and the natural capacity to produce it.

As we have just seen, the symbolic narrative always legitimizes masculine power, whether because of the initial violence women inflicted on men and, thus, because they misused power when it was in their hands (the myth of the Ona of Tierra del Fuego); or because of their natural, biological incapacity to reach a higher level, that of man. In any case, man is the natural measure of all things: he creates the social order. According to Godelier, the Baruya of New Guinea express this same idea directly: women are disorder; they may be more creative than men, but in a muddleheaded, disorganized, impetuous, unreflecting way. Thus, at the beginning of time, they invented the flutes and the bow that men subsequently stole and that signify their power. But the women strung the bow backward and killed blindly, anarchically, all around them. After stealing the bow, the men shouldered it properly: ever since, they have killed with deliberation. Where creative women bring disorder, man brings order, the reasonable measure of things. Thus speak mythology and symbolic discourse.

★  ★  ★

So how does one explain the very special status of the Iroquois matrons, among other examples? Judith Brown (1970) claims that historical sources don't enable us to know what the matrons, heads of the long-houses, were called. But she herself, following other authors, refers to them as "elderly heads of households." We shall postulate that they were, in all likelihood, women of advanced age and that, if their turn as head of the household did not come automatically, by mere succession, they were elderly women of greater strength than others, in character, in spirit, in authority. Thus, our hypothesis is that the term "matrons," used by earlier authors, refers to elderly women – or to put it differently, speaking the physiological truth, to women who have reached or passed the age of menopause.

Menopause is not a subject on which one finds much information in the anthropological literature: it is a subject one does not think about, an embarrassing subject, a censored – if not a taboo – subject. One speaks of advancing age, of old age as a stage in life, but not of the threshold where everything tips. Nevertheless, generally it seems that, in anthropological reports dealing with women, the status of an individual tends to change in two situations: in old age, which is to say, at menopause; and in the case of sterility – which is to say, in those situations where women are not or are no longer able to conceive.

In a very interesting article, Oscar Lewis (1941) writes about what the Piegan Indians of Canada call "manly-hearted women." In this society, described as completely patriarchal, the ideal of feminine behavior consists in submission, reserve, kindness, modesty and humility. However, the Piegan acknowledge another type – women who do not behave with the modesty and reserve of their sex, but, rather, behave aggressively, arrogantly, boldly. They are modest in neither speech nor deed: some urinate in public, like men; some sing men's songs; some join in men's conversations. This behavior goes hand in hand with a perfect mastery of the tasks they perform, male as well as female. They do everything more quickly and better than anyone else. They tend to their affairs without interference or support from men and they sometimes forbid their husbands to do anything without their approval. They are thought to be sexually active and unconventional in their love habits, but they themselves claim to be more virtuous than other women. They do not have to fear being dragged into the public forum for adultery, because they are known to defend themselves by sorcery. Nor do they fear the mystic consequences of their acts. Finally, they have the right, like men, to organize sun dances and to participate in the ordeals. They have the "power."

What does it take to be recognized as a manly-hearted woman among the Piegan? Oscar Lewis indicates that it takes a combination of two characteristics: first, one must be rich and hold a high social position; second, one must be married. It also helps to have shown prophetic signs in childhood, to have been a father's favorite daughter, given in marriage with a dowry of horses. A poor woman is beaten and mocked if she presumes to behave like a manly-hearted woman. Some women do not become manly-hearted until they have been married and widowed several times, inheriting each time a part of the wealth of their dead husband. Having become manly-hearted, they marry (following a male pattern) men younger than themselves (from five to twenty-six years, according to Oscar Lewis's statistics), whom they dominate in all ways.

So marriage is absolutely necessary if one is to become manly-hearted, and it is marriage that brings wealth and elevated status. It is too bad that no more is known of the Piegan system of thought, but it is very likely that Aristotelian ideas of the kind articulated by Virey ("a married woman is somehow more virile, more masculine, more self-assured, more resilient than a timid, fragile virgin...quite fat women commonly lose their rotundity in marriage, as though the energy of the sperm had impressed on their fibers a greater tension and dryness"; *De la femme*) are very close to their own. Man, the character of a man's sperm, makes woman, the character of the woman.

There is one further condition necessary to becoming a manly-hearted woman. It is not explicitly listed among those which the informants mentioned. This should not surprise us, since it is the condition sine qua non (the strength of representational systems is that they work by elision: the essential, what goes without saying, is never mentioned) — one must be of an advanced age. Among the 109 married women of Oscar Lewis's sample, fourteen are of the manly-hearted type. One is forty-five years old, another forty-nine, the others between fifty-two and eighty. Only a single one is thirty-two. As a result, Oscar Lewis adds to the two preceding criteria the third one of "maturity." But this word is doubtlessly too weak. For the bulk of the sample, the women are beyond the age of fertility and they have been through menopause. No allusion is made to the children any of them may have brought into the world. This is a pity, since it would have been interesting to know whether the thirty-two-year-old listed as a manly-hearted woman had had any pregnancies or not. In any case, Oscar Lewis himself comments that disagreements among informants about the manly-hearted character of this or that woman only arose for the youngest ones.

Menopause and sterility elicit notions, attitudes and institutions that vary sharply from one society to another, but that can nevertheless be explained according to the same symbolic logic. If the Piegan or Iroquois pattern is not unusual in reference to elderly women, other societies, African ones in particular, consider the menopausal woman who is suspected of continued sexual activity to be a dangerous woman. She concentrates heat and she may be accused of witchcraft, especially if she is poor and widowed and thus does not have the "power" to respond to the charge and defend herself. This does not in fact contrast with the Piegan example, though at a quick glance this might seem to be the case: the manly-hearted woman who mocks accusations of all kinds, because she has the "power" to respond to them with impunity through witchcraft, must, by contrast, be wealthy and married.

In the high Middle Ages in the West, according to Michel Rouche (1985), the elderly, widowed woman is "at the turning point of sex toward death." Her libido is dangerous. If she keeps her dowry, she becomes a powerful and dominating personality. But she also stands for the feared and hated model of the witch, the blood-sucking vampire and cannibal.

In most so-called "primitive" populations sterility — in the woman, that is, since male sterility is generally not recognized — is considered an absolute abomination. But this is not always the case. Thus, among the Nuer of east Africa, a woman recognized as sterile, which is to say one who has married and remained childless a certain number of years (until menopause, perhaps?), returns to her own family, where from then on she is considered as a man — "brother" to her brothers, paternal "uncle" to her brothers' children. As an "uncle" she will be in a position to build up a herd, just like a man, from her share of the cattle paid as a bride price on her nieces. With this herd and the fruits of her personal industry, she will in turn be able to pay the bride price for one or several wives. She enters into these institutionalized matrimonial relations as the "husband." Her wives wait on her, work for her, honor her, show her the courtesies due a husband. She hires a servant of another ethnic group, usually a Dinka, of whom she demands services including sexual services for her wife or wives. The children born of these relations are hers, call her "father" and treat her the way one treats a male father. The genitor has no role other than subaltern: he may have affective ties to the products he has engendered, but he remains for all that a servant, treated as such by the woman–husband, as well as the wives and children. He is paid for his services with the gift of a cow, an "engendering fee," each time one of the daughters he has produced gets married.

Whether absolute or relative – that is, caused by age or by menopause – sterility and the social corpus of institutions and behavior it occasions can always be explained according to the patterns of symbolic representation analyzed above. It is evident, in any case, that the sterile woman is not or is no longer a "woman" properly speaking. Whether negatively or positively, failed woman or failed man, she is more of a man than a woman. So *it is not the sex but the capacity for fertility that makes up the real difference between male and female*, and male domination, which we must now attempt to comprehend, is ultimately the control, *the appropriation of a woman's fertility when she is fertile*. What remains – that is, the psychological factors, the special aptitudes that make up a society's images of masculinity and femininity and are assumed to justify the domination of one sex by another – is a product of education, and thus of ideology. Therefore, there is no maternal instinct (in the commonly understood sense) that would have maternity be a purely biological matter and would maintain that woman, determined by her nature and thereby self-evidently, has an avocation for child care and, what is more, for the domestic. Maternity is a social fact just as it is a fact of biology (the same holds true for paternity; see N.C. Mathieu 1974), and there is nothing about the biological fact itself that explains the ineluctable process which, by way of the maternal instinct, assigns woman domestic tasks and a subordinate status.

The bodily appropriation of fertility in the male is doomed to failure: it can never be more than simulated (this does happen). So appropriation takes the form of control: appropriation of women themselves, or of the products of their fertility; distribution of women among the men. Women are fertile, inventive, create life; but man brings order, regimentation, political order. His control is made all the easier by the handicap that comes with fertility: a pregnant or nursing woman is less mobile than a man. Thus, it has been shown that, among the Bushmen, nomadic hunter-gatherers who have no domestic animals for milking and among whom, therefore, the child may nurse to the age of three or more, a man covers 5,000 to 6,000 kilometers a year, a woman 2,500 to 3,000.

This restricted mobility does not in and of itself imply an inferior physical capacity (nor, a fortiori, inferior intellectual capacities); however, it has been used to justify a certain distribution of tasks in prehistoric societies of wild men, hunter-gatherers, who lived completely from their natural surroundings (we know that agriculture and husbandry are relatively recent inventions in the history of humanity). Men hunt large animals and protect the unarmed from predators of every kind; women care for the unweaned young and gather foodstuffs easier to obtain than large game (one cannot hunt easily with a baby on one's hip). This is a division of labor born of objective constraints and not of a psychological predisposition in either sex to the chores assigned them, or of a physical constraint imposed by one sex on the other – this division of labor does not carry any inherent principle of valorization.

The social control of women's fertility and the division of labor between the sexes are, in all probability, the two axes of sexual inequality. But one must still grasp the mechanism that makes this inequality into a valorized relation of domination/submission.

Kinship is the general matrix of social relations. Man is a being who lives in society; all society is divided into groups based on kinship, and it overcomes this initial division through cooperation. The primary institution leading to solidarity among groups is marriage. A group that counted only on its own internal resources to reproduce itself biologically, that practiced incest and incest alone, would vanish if only through a reduction in numbers: a brother and sister conjoined produces one household instead of two. The exchange of women between groups is an exchange of life, since women give children and their fertility to people other than their immediate kin. This is no doubt the crucial element in male domination, embodied in the economic constraints of the distribution of chores: the reciprocal refusal by men to profit from the fertility of their daughters and sisters, of the women in their group, for the profit of foreign groups. The rule of exogamy basic to every society must be understood as the rule of the exchange by men of women and their fertility. What is remarkable is that, through special rules of filiation and alliance, they always initially appropriate the women in their group as well as the women given in exchange for their own. It is only here that violence and force can be invoked as a final explanation.

The appropriation of women's fertility, which is vital for the constitution and survival of any society through the exchange of women, goes hand in hand with the confinement of women in a maternal role. One has the image of the *Mother* and of the nursing mother. This is made all the more easy because the child is kept on the breast for many months. Weaning, in societies unfamiliar with artificial nursing and modern nutritional techniques for babies, occurs at two and one-half or even three years. The child knows only its mother as a food source during these years and will continue to turn to her for food after weaning; and it will do so all the more "naturally" because a restriction to the nursing role, to the role of keeper and care-giver, will have occurred. The mother may be placed on a pedestal, greatly respected, idealized – this still does not contradict the idea of male power itself.

The appropriation and control of women's fertility, a restriction of women to the nursing role that is facilitated by the child's dependence on her for food – this seizing of sorts has been accompanied by the invention of specialized technical skills, that is to say, by the male sex's exclusive use of certain techniques which require an apprenticeship but from which the female's physical makeup does not in any way exclude her. Men have created a preserve, just as there was a private, inaccessible preserve for women, that of biological reproduction. Thus, to take another example from the hunter-gatherer peoples, from the Ona of Tierra del Fuego (Chapman), bow-hunting is the men's responsibility. They learn how to make bow, arrows and in some cases poison. They learn at a very early age how to use a bow, and this apprenticeship is reserved for them. Chapman shows that, without a fitting apprenticeship, women are physically unable to use this object. The preserve of technical skill of a highly specialized nature, a corollary of the distribution by sex of primary tasks and one based on objective constraints, results in another restriction of women to tasks that certainly require knowledge and skill (but are not sex-specific: men can also gather in times of scarcity) but that will never be a part of the male preserve. What matters here is not that a few women manage, from time to time, to enter into this preserve; it is the very justification for the existence of a preserve that is being called into question.

We may add to that the work of the mind, the ideological creativity we saw at work in the symbol systems set forth above: an unequal value is assigned to the tasks performed, having nothing to do with the amount of work performed or the mastery of its execution. Thus, in hunter-gatherer societies, the women's contribution by gathering can occasionally amount to more than seventy percent of the food supplies of the group. But that does not matter: the real prestige accrues to the role of hunter. Here we face the ultimate mystery. Because, it seems to me, the raw material of the symbolic is the body — the prime place for the observation of sensory data — and because for any complex problem there can only be solutions that refer to explanations based on simpler and simpler data until they run up against elementary facts, I would propose that the reason for this is possibly a feature anchored in the female body (and not an incapacity for the concoction of sperm). What man values in man, then, is no doubt his ability to bleed, to risk his life, to take that of others, by his own free will; the woman "sees" her blood flowing from her body (Do we not, in French, usually say "voir," to see, for "avoir ses règles," to have one's period?) and she produces life without necessarily wanting to do so or being able to prevent it. In her body she periodically experiences, for a time that has a beginning and an end, changes of which she is not the mistress, and which she cannot prevent. It is in this relation to blood that we may perhaps find the fundamental impetus for all the symbolic elaboration, at the outset, on the relations between the sexes.

We wish to thank Edizioni Einaudi for authorizing this adaptation of "Maschile/Femminile," which appeared in Italian in vol. 8 of the *Enciclopedia Einaudi* (1983) and in French in *Les Cahiers du Grif* (Éditions Tierce, winter 1984-85).

BIBLIOGRAPHY

Bachofen, J., *Das Mutterecht*. Stuttgart, 1861.

Brown, Judith R., "A Note on the Division of Labor by Sex," *American Anthropologist* 72 (1970), pp. 1073-78.

———, "Economic Organization and the Position of Woman among the Iroquois," *Ethnohistory* 17.3-4 (1970), pp. 151-67.

Chapman, Anne, *Drama and Power in a Hunting Society: The Selk'nam of Tierra del Fuego*. Cambridge,

London and New York: Cambridge University Press, 1982.

Détienne, Marcel, "Potagerie de femmes ou comment engendrer seule," *Culture: Quadrimestrale di studi storico-culturali* 1 (July 1977), pp. 3-8.

Godelier, Maurice, "Le sexe comme fondement ultime de l'ordre social et cosmique chez les Baruya de Nouvelle-Guinée: Mythe et réalité," in *Sexualité et pouvoir*. Edited by Armando Verdiglione. Paris: Payot, 1976.

Héritier, Françoise, "Fécondité et stérilité: La traduction de ces notions dans le champ idéologique au stade pré-scientifique," in *Le fait féminin*. Paris: Fayard, 1978, pp. 383-96.

Ingham, John M., "On Mexican Folk Medicine," *American Anthropologist* 72 (1970), pp. 76-87.

Knibielher, Yvonne, "La nature féminine au temps du code civil," *Annales* 31.4 (1976).

Lewis, Oscar, "Manly-hearted Women among the North Piegan," *American Anthropologist* 43 (1941), 173-87.

Lloyd, G.L.B., "The Hot and the Cold, the Dry and the Wet in Greek Philosophy," *Journal of Hellenic Studies* 84 (1964), pp. 92-106.

Mathieu, Nicole-Claude, "Paternité biologique, maternité sociale," paper presented at the 8th World Conference of Sociology (ISA Research Committee on Sex Roles in Society), Toronto, 1974.

Pécaut, Myriam, "Le pur et l'impur," in *Lettres de l'École Freudienne* 20 (March 1977), pp. 101-11.

Reiter, Rayna B., *Toward an Anthropology of Women*. New York and London: Monthly Review Press, 1975.

Rouche, Michel, "The Early Middle Ages in the West," in *History of Private Life*, vol. 1. Cambridge: Harvard University Press, 1987.

Tillion, Germaine, "L'enfermement des femmes et notre civilisation," in *Le fait féminin*. Paris: Fayard, 1978.

Virey, Julien Joseph, *De la femme, sous ses rapports physiologique, moral et littéraire*. Paris, 1823.

———, *De l'éducation*. Paris, 1802.

———, *Dictionnaire des sciences médicales*. Panckoucke, 1811-22.

Whyte, Martin King, "Cross-cultural Studies of Women and the Male Bias Problem," *Behaviour Science Research* 13.1 (1978), pp. 65-86.

**Translated by Leigh Hafrey.**

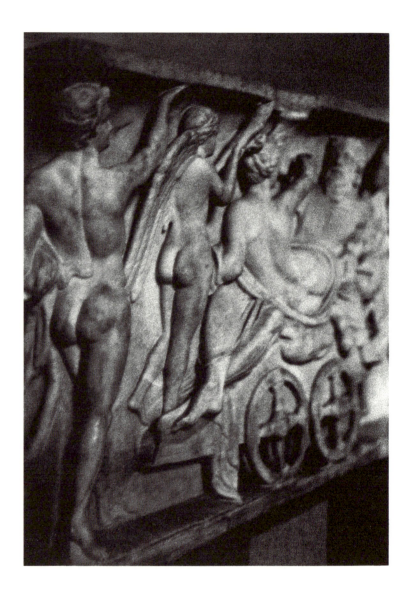

The Marriage of Dionysus and Ariadne. Roman bas-relief, 140-50 A.D.
(Munich, Staatliche Antikensammlung und Glypotethek).

# Personal Status and Sexual Practice in the Roman Empire

*Aline Rousselle*

## Statuses and Feelings

"The household would know how to mourn: the slave enfranchised under the will has one way of showing sorrow, the client mentioned with praise another, another the friend honored with a legacy."[1] In this passage we learn from Fronto that tears were governed by an etiquette determined by social relations; it is worth adding to this that women have their own particular way of shedding them. It was not for his tears themselves that Hadrian was censured, but rather for shedding them in a womanly way (*muliebriter*).[2] All attitudes relating to human feeling were similarly governed and to flaunt the code would be exceptional behavior that would not pass unnoticed. One purpose of education and, according to Plutarch, even of truly philosophical instruction was the promotion of those social norms:

> For through philosophy and in company with philosophy, it is possible to attain knowledge of what is honorable and what is shameful, what is just and what is unjust, what, in brief, is to be chosen and what avoided, how a man must bear himself in relation to the gods, with his parents, with his elders, with the laws, with strangers, with those in authority, with friends, with women, with children, with servants; that one ought to revere the gods, to honor one's parents, to yield to those in authority, to love one's friends, to be chaste with women, to be affectionate with children, and not to be overbearing with slaves.[3]

In this passage, Plutarch mentions seven categories of people in relation to whom a free male citizen of the upper classes was taught from childhood how to behave. In this respect, Plutarch proves himself a good conservative, quite untainted by the extremism of Musonius for whom just the same moral laws applied "to the elderly and to children, to the strong and to the weak,"[4] and even to women.[5] The feelings

301

and behavior that were tolerated and expected from free male citizens (and, even within that category, from men of specific different statuses) were regulated and apportioned according to the statuses of the individuals with whom those citizens happened to be involved. It is from the point of view of this code of distribution that I should like to take up the question of sexuality and the changes which it underwent in the course of classical Antiquity. It is only by studying the customary use that male citizens made of the bodies of others that we can hope to understand the precepts of morality propounded by Musonius, Epictetus, Philo, Flavius Josephus and Clement of Alexandria.

In the second century, philosophy was seen as a means to living a good life. Philosophical training is frequently presented as an individual quest, so we tend to have a picture of young Roman nobles journeying abroad to sit at the feet of the great teachers exiled in Greek lands (not that their exile usually affected the language of their teaching). But if it were simply a matter of individuals, we would not be able to understand why so very many exiles and so very many communal suicides occurred in the course of the first century. Atticus, a Platonist in Plutarch's circle, [6] writes:

> The whole of philosophy is thus divided into three parts: what is called the ethical domain, the physical domain and the logical domain. The first of these makes an honest man of you and guides entire households toward perfection.

In other words, the ethical side of philosophy is a collective domestic exercise.

There were no such things as bodies in general: in this domain, as in every other in the Roman Empire, we must take into account juridical (as well as social) status,[7] freedom, citizenship, family status (whether or not enjoyed with full rights), membership of the orders and, finally, degrees of honor (to which there was a sexual dimension).

## Status and Reproduction:
## A "Demeco-System"[8] or a Social One?

Our study of the question of sexual behavior should also take into account the overall social arrangements affecting reproduction: the reproduction of the civic body and the reproduction of society, involving links between the biological generation of slaves on the one hand, and of citizens, on the other. Angus McLaren's book on reproduction in modern times[9] has prompted me to think in a more general fashion about a number of patterns of behavior that I had already discerned in the world of the Roman Empire. The most significant of these had seemed to me to be the abstinence observed by wives, an abstinence which I attributed to two factors: first, the facilities (offered by concubines or slaves) that were enjoyed by husbands within their own households; second, repulsion that was likely to have been felt by Roman wives themselves, as they may well have been deflowered before the age of twelve.[10] I still subscribe to that opinion, in part at least. Now, however, I think that the attitudes of these aristocrats call for further consideration. Roman wives encouraged their husbands to seek pleasure elsewhere;[11] understanding wives, such as the wife of Scipio Africanus, would qualify for high praise.[12] Plutarch advised wives to be tolerant of their husbands' sleeping with concubines (*hetairae*) or servants (*therapainides*)[13] in a text in which he nevertheless also advised a husband to forswear "the very pleasure from which he tries to dissuade his wife." Given that there was no question of denying him a concubine, presumably what Plutarch was forbidding the husband was indulgence in certain sexual acts. In the same treatise, he writes that a good wife "ought, especially when the light is out, not to be the same as ordinary women." Contrary to Paul Veyne,[14] the point is not that a man ought to extinguish the light before making love to his wife, but that the ancients generally did extinguish the light and make love before they went to sleep — that was the best time to do so, the time recommended by the doctors.[15] We also know, from Epictetus, that sexual temptation was considered to be stronger in the dark: "Yes, but if you put a bit of a wench in his way, what then? Or if it be in the dark, what then?"[16] What Plutarch is saying is that in the dark, some women lose all modesty, whereas a legitimate wife ought never to make love like a courtesan.[17]

The distribution of the citizen's sexual activities may be regarded both as a social means of stabilizing reproduction and also as a way for free women, probably of the upper classes, to space out or limit their pregnancies.[18] I should add that, despite the fact that many effective, if dangerous prescriptions for stimulating menses did exist in Rome — that is to say, abortive potions used when a pregnancy had started — the right of decision in this domain was not legally the woman's.[19] The sexual relations between men and boys in Greece may similarly be regarded as a socio-demographic means first and foremost, as a means of sparing the lives of female citizens who might otherwise be killed by too many pregnancies and also as a means

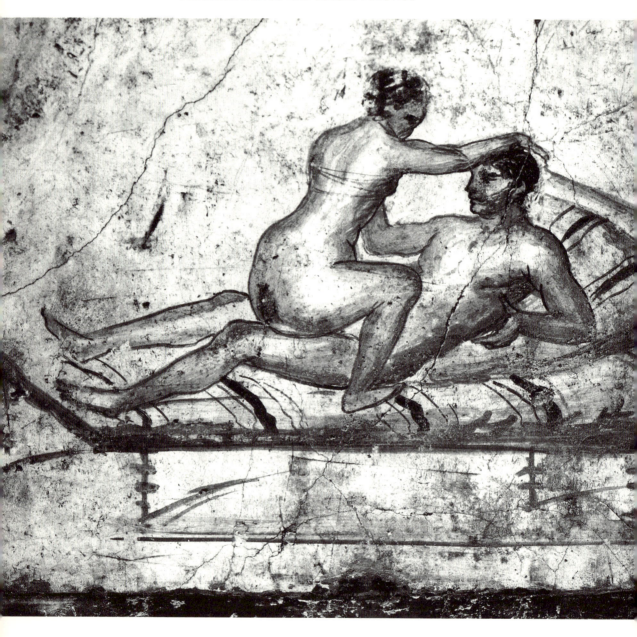

Erotic scene from a Roman fresco (Pompeii, House of the Vettii).

of limiting the number of illegitimate children who, in Athens, could under no circumstances accede to the status of citizens. The feelings of a married citizen father toward his illegitimate children, born from women other than his wife, were probably not the same in Greece as they were in Rome; and the difference was not necessarily the result of a straightforward evolution. All the same, I do not believe that the problem as a whole has hitherto been raised or tackled, much less resolved. Greek texts of the classical period discouraged citizens from fathering bastards. Seven centuries later, Plutarch was doing likewise. Not only was it harmful to the city to fill it with individuals of dubious and uncertain status, even if they were free on account of their fathers being citizens, it was also, in Plutarch's day, a concern that such children would suffer from inferiority their whole lives long.[20]

The Greeks (or, at any rate, the Athenians) seem to have shown some concern for those of their biological descendants who survived; there was a kind of conscience, shared by their civilization in general, regarding biological fact, biological filiation. This conscience manifested itself in the way they felt about whatever bastards they had fathered, and it testifies to an appreciation of the practical aspects of the situation. In Athens, a boy who was made a prostitute against his will was irredeemably defiled; he lost the freedom of speech that defined a full citizen and was thus reduced to the status of a second-class citizen. In Rome, however, if a citizen was violated by an enemy, he retained both his honor and status, just as a wellborn daughter or an honorable wife subjected to rape preserved their rights as matrons.[21] If we bear in mind the crucial importance of the status of citizenship in every field of thought, we shall be in a better position to understand the so-called "populationist" speeches of Augustus as they have come down to us.

Augustus had read out to the Senate a speech first delivered at least a century earlier, in the year 131, by one Metellus Macedonicus[22] and he had also made it known, in the form of an edict, to the people as a whole.[23] It is probably an extract from the speech which Aulus Gellius, in his *Attic Nights*, attributes to another Metellus, one who was censor in 102.[24] Thus, not only had the problem been recognized long before Augustus, but, furthermore, it had been posed in the very same terms. Aulus Gellius tells us that Metellus was a censor when he addressed the people (by which we should understand the *comitia centuriata*) in a speech designed to encourage

Romans to marry, that is, to take legitimate wives. The function of the censor was to preserve the purity of the Senate membership and to divide the citizens into the five census classes. These were still, at this date (before Marius's reform of 117), essential for military conscription to which the lower classes contributed fewer men than the upper classes. The censor was the only person in Rome likely to have some demographic idea of the number of Roman citizens, for he alone dealt with, if not statistics, at least the figures provided by his latest census. This was the period between the two Gracchi, two years after the death of King Attalus of Pergamum who had bequeathed his kingdom to the Roman Republic. The Eastern wars had filled the households of Rome with Greek slaves, both male and female and from every cultural and social level. Not enough emphasis has been laid upon the fact that, during the second century B.C. (the period of the greatest influx of slaves to Rome), those slaves were Greeks. The general tone of the Roman attitude toward slaves consequently stemmed from their attitude toward Greeks and also from the attitude of the Greeks themselves toward their own slaves.[25] A century earlier, Plautus had been writing comedies about characters who bore misleading Greek names though they were ruled by Roman law. The slaves in those plays, with their pseudobarbarian origins (such as "the Cathaginian") were slaves in a town — Rome — where the vast majority of the slave population was already Greek.[26] Now, Plautus's plays are full of the obscene vocabulary of Attic comedy, in which slaves are constantly said to be penentrated by their masters. The problem is far from being whether "the Greeks" taught the Romans about love between men; it lies, rather, in understanding in what ways contact with the Greeks affected Roman homosexual love. It seems to me that the inferior, servile position of defeated Greeks in Roman households must have helped to impart an aspect of power to the sexual relationship obtained in a partnership involving two men, one of whom was master, the other slave.[27]

Let us return to Metellus's speech, repeated by Augustus, as it is recorded by Aulus Gellius:

> If we could get on without a wife, Romans, we would all avoid that annoyance; but since nature has ordained that we can neither live very comfortably with them nor at all without them, we must take thought for our lasting well-being rather than for the pleasure of the moment. It seemed to some of the company that Quintus Metellus, whose purpose as a censor was to encourage the citizen body [*populus*] to take legitimate wives

[*ad uxores ducendas*], ought not to have admitted the annoyance and constant inconveniences of the dowry [*rei uxoriae*] and that to do this was not so much to encourage as to dissuade and deter them.[28]

Aulus Gellius then takes the trouble to name and cite a rhetorician who supported Metellus's speech and then expressed his own opinion on this matter, concluding his remarks as follows: "having admitted the existence of annoyances notorious with all men, and having thus established confidence in his sincerity and truthfulness, he then found it neither difficult nor uphill work to convince them of what was the soundest and truest of principles — that the city cannot be safe without numerous legitimate marriages [*civitatem salvam esse sine matrimoniorum frequentia non posse*]." It is important to understand to what that "we" who cannot "live at all" without marriage refers and also the meaning of this "nature" as a result of which Romans cannot live comfortably with their wives yet cannot live at all without them. If we translate *populus* and *civitas* as "the citizen body," the matter becomes clearer: it is not individuals who suffer from the diminishing number of legitimate marriages, but the citizen body as a collectivity. The text identifies each individual citizen with the city itself, that is to say, with the citizen body as a whole. As for "nature," how, if there were no legitimate marriages, could it occasion a total lack of satisfaction? Certainly, human nature, biology pure and simple, can be satisfied without marriage. Rather, what is being discussed here is a specific kind of nature, one which allows Roman law to speak of a *filius naturalis*, a natural son or grandson, only when the son is the biological descendant of his *pater*, the man who hold paternal power over him. Wherever it is a matter of citizenship and the law, in order to understand "nature" we must refer to the definitions of "natural son" and "natural father" and "natural grandfather" that are given in articles of the *Digest* in the chapter devoted to adoptions, since the rights of natural succession are directly opposed to those of succession through adoption. A natural son is thus set in opposition to an adopted son; any children of an adopted son remain under the power of their "natural grandfather," and the title of "natural father" is given to the man with paternal power who gives his son to be adopted by another.[29] Thus, what is meant by "nature" is a chain of three linked generations of citizens comprising a natural grandfather, a natural father and a natural son/grandson. It is this nature that can in no way be satisfied in the absence of children born from legitimate marriages. It is not real nature, which we should call biology; rather, it is a nature that is at once juridical, controllable and controlled.[30]

In this period, Roman citizens by birth still could not marry freed women. As relayed by Dio Cassius, Augustus's speech similarly encouraged Romans to make new citizens by fathering legitimate natural sons:[31] "You are betraying your country by rendering her barren and childless." (At this point, Dio first uses the term *steriphē*, meaning "victim of female sterility," and then *agonos*, meaning "male sterility.") "How can the State be preserved if we neither marry nor have children?... What you want is to have full liberty for sexual violence [*hubrizein*] and defilement [*aselgainein*]."[32]

The problem is set out fairly and squarely: the reproduction of the citizen body could be controlled by keeping a check on a man's relations with his wife, his relations with his dependents (whether men, women or children), which were relations of force (*hubrizein*),[33] and also those of his relations that defiled a citizen (we shall be defining these presently). And when it came to providing sons for the fatherland, they could only be either natural — in the sense defined above, biological and legitimate — or else adoptive. By reverting to this speech, Augustus certainly made the point that the civic body was in danger of failing to reproduce itself by natural filiation and of doing so, instead, firstly through adoption and secondly through regular programs of manumission conferring citizenship. The adoptions themselves were likely to be of illegitimate children who had been born of a slave woman and subsequently freed. So what Augustus feared was to see the Roman people, the citizen body, turn into a people of freedmen; in other words, that with each generation a citizen would be replaced by a man he had freed, either his own son by a slave woman, the son being subsequently freed, or a freedman whom he had made his heir. It was a solution that made it possible to have sons without taking a wife who would be protected by her status of matron and by her dowry. Augustus was trying to set the situation in order. First, he authorized all citizens (except senators) to enter into legitimate marriages with freedwomen. Next he ruled that citizens must be both married and the fathers of children before they could come into inheritances. He also limited the possibilities of adoption: a man could only adopt if he already had a legitimate wife. That was likely to create obstacles, as his wife and her father might wish first for sons of their own blood. He also introduced regulations of a Malthusian nature regarding manumissions that carried with them the rights of citizenship for the freedman. The most important of these legal measures was that which authorized marriages between freeborn men and freedwomen. It allowed citizens of the middle and lower classes to choose one of their slave women, free her, and marry her so that they could wield paternal power over the children that man and wife produced together.

Plutarch says that Roman citizens had children so as to be able to inherit.[34] They were certainly not the only ones to be calculating when it came to the matter of descendants, and their calculations involved limiting their contact with their wives and reserving most of their sexual energy for external liaisons. Philo of Alexandria knew what he was talking about when it came to the Greco-Roman world and the laws passed by Augustus. We may believe him when he tells us that citizens (the only category to be taken into account) were no longer concerned about fathering children when they took male sexual partners.[35] What they were doing in such cases was limiting their descendants to children who would put them in a position to inherit. Having done so, they could turn elsewhere for pleasure.[36]

In classical Greek society, as in the society of the Roman Empire, citizen wives were shielded from pregnancies, both by their own abstinence and by the opportunities, available to their husbands, to find sexual pleasures elsewhere. The situation is not that of an eco-demography in which the statistics apply to the entire population. Instead, it is truly that of a socio-demecography in which a small section of the population maintained its level of reproduction, or even decreased it, by safeguarding the health and lives of its wives through abstinence. Meanwhile, for the other strata of the population, there were no means of regulation other than those sought by the mothers themselves and those upon whom they were dependent: it would take the form of abortion. Such forms of regulation were not demecological; rather they were a matter of individual decision and they differed depending on the social status of those concerned, in accordance with the various laws (or imperial edicts) that applied. No legal measures were taken to control the birthrate and reproduction of noncitizens, foreigners or slaves.

## The Law, Acts and Statuses

As we pursue our discussion, let us remain within the juridical framework that invariably defined acts of all kinds by making it clear who was acting and upon whom. It

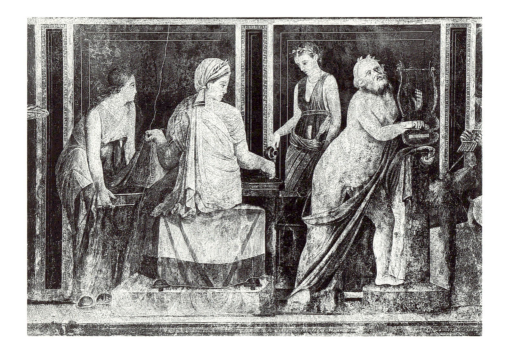

Roman fresco (Pompeii, Villa of the Dionysian Mysteries).

was a matter not just of social but also juridical status, which affected the extent of an individual's participation in the life of the city.

The inhabitants of the Roman world constantly had to be aware of whom they were dealing with. Once again, here is an example: a husband who caught his wife in adulterous *flagrante delicto* had the right to kill her lover. However, it was a limited right, for the only lovers liable to such summary execution were slaves, men who had been freed by the wife, the husband or other members of the family, and individuals who belonged to the category of the infamous (*famosi*), that is to say actors, gladiators, beast-fighters, singers, dancers, prostitutes and procurers – or quite simply, those who happened to be born from an infamous parent, something that was not immediately discernible.[37]

The status of women was easily recognizable since only matrons, that is to say honorable, untouchable women, wore the matron's robe and cloak (the *stola* and the *palla*), while infamous women (*famosae, proborosae*) wore togas when they went out. An honorable woman or girl who went out dressed as a servant forfeited her protection against rape and sexual propositions, and their aggressors were recognized to have extenuating circumstances.[38] A free man could be recognized from his ring. His costume did not mark him out from other men, for the Senate had ruled against distinctive apparel on the grounds that "the slaves would begin to count our number."[39] Generally speaking, distinctions of dress were dictated by work, as it was impossible to work wearing a toga. Nevertheless, jurists did attempt to establish distinctions of dress between "the clothes peculiar to men, to children and to women and those that they all wear, and the clothes of slaves. The latter wear shirts, tunics and cloaks of linen, or some other material."[40] If a man was not to be at risk, he needed to know whether it was safe for him to make advances to a particular woman or man in the street: honorable women and high-born girls and free young boys, who were citizens wearing the *toga praetexta* and a *bulla* round their necks, were all immediately recognizable from their appearance: as far as they were concerned, a man would have no difficulty in avoiding accusations of debauchery. But in many other cases, the matter was not so simple.

## What Citizens Could Demand of Dependents
Beauty, intelligence and strength are oblivious to status, as are the feelings they inspire.

But, into the relations implied by these feelings, status introduces an element that transforms them into a power game — and it is one that operates in both directions.

### What Could Be Demanded of Dependent Girls.

A free man could choose from among his slaves born in the house[41] a little girl whom he decided to free and bring up to be his concubine. As soon as she was twelve, she acquired the legal status of concubine and matron, just as at this same age, a freeborn daughter given away by her father well before the age of twelve, acquired the legal status of legitimate wife (as did a little freed girl who was legitimately married). If the freed girl had children, what was their status? Like most other manumissions, that of a female slave was a private act which took place within the household, in the presence of a few friends. Clearly, if the master wished to make the girl his concubine or wife, he freed her before she reached the age of thirty which, since the *Lex Aelia Sentia*, had been the legal age for manumission with the possibility of Roman citizenship. In Rome, the manumission of a slave younger than thirty years old had to take place in the pesence of five senators and five knights; in the provinces, before twenty citizens named in the special list of *recuperatores*. But these girls, freed in the household to become wives of their masters, did become genuine citizens.[42]

For concubines, the situation was different. A woman freed before the age of twelve to become the concubine of her master and, later, the mother of one of his children — a woman who could be accused of adultery and was thus committed to fidelity — transmitted her freedom to her child but not the right to citizenship.[43] This was one of the reasons why Augustus declared that citizens were not producing enough children for the city. Furthermore, I imagine that abortions often took place in cases where the master was also legally married. As I have already suggested, the methods of birth control used by legitimate wives were probably abstinence, the postpartum taboo and prolonged breast-feeding; concubines, who were of lower status, had abortions. This is confirmed in the *Apostolic Tradition* written by Hippolytus of Rome in the first half of the third century: "If a man's concubine is his slave and she has raised his children, she will hear the word…otherwise she will be turned away." In other words, the Church tried to make sure that a slave concubine did not abort or expose her children.[44] This would explain why, as the inscriptions show, so few children were born to freed women.[45] It should be added that slave women who were freed later in life, being bought by a companion who had also been freed, would probably have had their children before their manumission, in which case they would have given birth to slaves.

Given that certain women were reserved for certain men and that free and honorable young boys (the sons of noninfamous families) were protected against acts of sexual aggression, there were some sexual acts that could not take place between honorable male and female citizens. Those acts would consequently be demanded of a man's dependents, over whom the master enjoyed total power in this domain: I refer to acts of *impudicitia* (debauchery).[46]

***What a Master Could Obtain From Slave Boys.*** Sexual power relations of this kind produced the distinctive systems that the Romans applied to love between men. Masters made use of dependent girls as well as boys, and we know from Christian authors that children exposed to this kind of abuse were brought up to be prostituted at a very early age. When a slave boy struck his master as pretty and charming, the latter would sometimes decide to prolong this graceful period of his life by castrating him. The doctor Heliodorus wrote: "Since some powerful men often oblige us — despite ourselves — to make eunuchs, I must give a short account of how this operation is carried out."[47] Domitian prohibited operations of castration, as did Nerva after him.[48] But eunuchs were then imported to make up for the shortage. Sporus, whom Nero called his wife, had been castrated before puberty: he had a tender, beardless face and no male characteristics at all. The philosopher Favorinus had been castrated at a very early age in order to prevent the changes of puberty, as we learn from Lucian, who relates how Demonax used to tease Favorinus.[49] Some masters wanted to delay the appearance of male characteristics and male sexual activity in their favorite young slaves for as long as possible, but they were not prepared to have them emasculated. Marcellus, the fifth-century doctor from Gaul, lists a number of methods for preventing sexual maturity: *Eunuchis sine ferro faciendis remedia physica et rationibilia diversa de experimentis* (Physical aids for making eunuchs without the knife and various rationales concerning the experiments).[50] Some were magic, pure and simple — a pestle tipped with a wreath and placed under the bed; others involved chemical magic — a drink containing the congealed drips from around the wick of a lamp that had been allowed to burn out; other methods were medical — eating lettuce seeds was recommended.[51] All of this is *Si quem coire noles fierique cupies in usu venerio tardiorem* (If you do not wish someone to copulate and desire a delay in his sexual activity). In the same chapter, Marcellus also mentions some mechanical methods of preventing sexual activity, such as infibulation.

Here we come to an important point. The Roman, like the Greeks, thought that in pederasty — that is, the love of young men — the position of the *erōmenos* (the loved one) should only be adopted during the period beginning with the onset of puberty and should end later at variable age. This applied solely to *erōmenoi* who were citizens. But the Latin documents are concerned chiefly with slave *erōmenoi* and the masters who sought their love.[52] These masters would not give them their freedom, but they would promise it. Hence, inscriptions such as the following: "The freedom that I had been promised was refused me, but my early death has rendered it eternal,"[53] (although this particular inscription does not relate to the kind of situation that we are discussing). One of the most repugnant events in the history of Roman society occurred following the murder of the city prefect, Pedanius Secundus.[54] After a long debate in the Senate, four hundred slaves were put to death, as the law demanded. Tacitus notes that Secundus had promised freedom to a slave, but he had then put off the act of manumission indefinitely. Both men, master and slave alike, were in love with a young *exōletus* slave (that is, a man who made himself available for the role of sexual partner). It seems to have been a classic case: the master seeking the services of one slave by promising to free another with whom the first slave was in love.

We have now seen what a master could demand of a slave, whether young or not so young, and sometimes also of his freedmen. Furthermore, he could abuse the wives of his freedmen with impunity. So, we can also understand how it was that such masters might well have been haunted by a fear of their slaves becoming the lovers of their own wives.[55]

We have briefly examined the acts that represented one alternative to the procreation of citizens, acts for which Augustus, according to Dio Cassius, rebuked the Romans: namely, acts of violence (*hubrizein*) perpetrated, obviously enough, upon inferiors —either slaves or unprotected individuals, such as all those from the categories legally defined as infamous. Such acts could, by and large, neither be restricted nor be prevented. Legal developments aimed at protecting dependents were, however, in the offing.

On the other hand, the law could intervene, both effectively and promptly, in the cases of the other two alternatives mentioned by Dio Cassius: first, temporary liaisons, if they were between individuals who were full Roman citizens; and second, what Dio refers to using the verb *aselgainein*. In both cases, I disagree with historians who think that Augustus's laws on adultery were never applied and that there was no suppression of so-called passive homosexuality. It is, after all, reasonable to suppose that there was a link between Augustus's rebukes and the laws he introduced.[56]

Let us take as our starting point the existence of a particular status that was defined by, among other things, sexual behavior, namely the status of infamy. The infamous were people — men, women and children — who lived in or were born into the world of prostitution, the theater or the games, and it was a status by which one was marked forever. The *Lex Aelia Sentia* even laid down that a slave originally employed in the arena and later freed could never accede to full citizenship.[57] Not until the edict promulgated by Septimius Severus was it ruled that a woman who had been prostituted as a slave should not remain tainted by infamy once she had been freed.[58] Under Augustus's laws, the sanction for adultery was infamy both for the woman, who was deprived of her matron's rights and costume and thereby also of the right to enter into a Roman marriage (*conubium*) with her lover or, indeed, any other Roman, and also for the guilty lover. A compliant husband who had turned a blind eye to his wife's infidelity was considered as a *proxeneta* and he was also reduced to the status of infamy. When, under Severus, a fiancée or a girl given in marriage at a very early age became liable to prosecution for adultery, it was stipulated that her compliant husband should also be reduced to infamy.[59] Infamy was even more closely associated with a man daring to marry such a woman knowing that she no longer had the right to wed for this precise reason.[60] What is important here is the idea of contamination, for by acting in this way a citizen would defile not only himself but also the city to which he belonged. It is necessary to distinguish between the loss of *conubium* and the status of infamy: a freed woman who had been her former master's wife or concubine, and who left him without his consent, lost her status of matron but was nevertheless not reduced to that of infamy. The status of infamy embraced a specific class of individuals who were excluded from the city. That it was truly a matter of defilement is indicated by the term *stuprum* (debauchery) which was applied to the specified acts that brought about such exclusion. A woman's adultery, the fleeting sexual relations entered into willingly by girls of high birth, widows or divorcees, were all acts of debauchery which affected the woman in the same way as her partner.[61] Even the remarriage of widows — including those not subject to mourning (such as the erstwhile wives of traitors) — before the legal period of ten months had elapsed, resulted in reduction to infamy for all those involved — the woman, the man who married her and the bridegroom's *pater* who was responsible for him.[62] The defilement involved was regarded as affecting the city: this can be inferred from a fragment of Seneca on the subject of the modest wife "who was an example to her age, though in those days indecency was held to be a *monstrum* [a religious danger] to the city, not a vice."[63]

Historical and literary works document the application of such laws. Tacitus, in his *Annals*, cites two women who were certainly degraded for bad behavior in contravention to the Julian laws: Lepida, who is described as *infamis*, and Albucilla, who is called *famosa*. Both adjectives have a precise juridical meaning and refer to public convictions.[64] Shortly after the death of Augustus, Lepida was repudiated by her elderly husband, who was himself childless, and accused of carrying the child of her lover. Even before Augustus's reign, one could bring legal actions for marriages concluded in contravention to the regulations. Suetonius tells us that Caesar annulled a marriage concluded before the expiration of the period required for a divorced woman.[65] A few years later, Augustus is said to have reduced to infamy all husbands who had failed to respect the period during which both widows and divorcees were supposed to suffer from a "disturbance of the blood" (*turbatio sanguinis*).[66] He condemned to death a freedman of whom he was very fond for having committed adultery with a matron.[67] A case is also related of a patrician youth accused of adultery, who defended himself before the Senate and was granted mercy because he happened to be the landlord of the house in which Augustus had been born.[68] Under Tiberius, sentences for debauchery were passed upon women who believed themselves to be protected since they had taken the precaution of applying to the *aediles* for a "license for debauchery" — in other words, they had already declared themselves to be prostitutes.[69] Dio Cassius tells us that in the early years of the reign of Septimius Severus, two thousand lawsuits for adultery were pending.[70]

Let us now turn to the sexual relations between men. Here, we find the same pattern of convictions and degradation of civic status. When sexual relations between males are considered, the question that arises more often than not is whether any repressive legislation relating to them existed in Rome; and the discussion which then follows generally concentrates solely on the *lex Scantinia*, whose date and contents remain unknown.

There can be no doubt that boys from good families were protected against sexual aggression by the laws passed by Augustus, just as were wellborn girls and matrons. Their aggressors would be convicted of debauchery in exactly the same way. The question to be resolved is whether any laws existed that forbade Roman citizens, in particular those from the senatorial and knightly orders, from adopting the so-called passive position in sexual relations between men. Historians all agree that the position was universally despised;[71] so much is clear from the texts and from the insults of the time.[72] But few historians can find evidence of any penal sanctions in such cases. In 1956, however, Max Käser established a connection between first, the *Lex Iulia Municipalis*, a law that Caesar introduced, relating to the organization of a number of cities with Latin rights, where epigraphical evidence exists; and second, the rules that barred certain Romans from pleading in the tribunals as postulants, that is to say, acting there on behalf of those — such as women, blind people and children under guardianship — who were not permitted to represent themselves. The prohibition was certainly a mark of civic degradation.[73] What this proves is that civic acts were forbidden not only to those who had sold their bodies, that is to say, prostituted themselves (and in this respect, Roman law tallied with Athenian law)[74] but also to all those suspected of allowing themselves to be treated sexually as women, *muliebria pati*, which is precisely what prostitutes were despised for doing. However, the point here is not the scorn in which they were held, but the possibility of their being legally sentenced to civic degradation.

If we accept that what is known as "Metellus's" speech (as recorded by Aulus Gellius and Dio Cassius, the one in Latin and the other in Greek) does indeed reflect Augustus's legislation, we should establish a parallel between the legal measures listed by Suetonius: "He revised existing laws and enacted some new ones, for example on extravagance, on adultery and chastity [*pudicitia*], on bribery and on the encouragement of marriage among the various classes of citizens [the orders],"[75] and the rebukes that this speech addresses to the Roman people. Bribery here meant the practices to which some citizens resorted in order to acquire posts as magistrates: *pudicitia* had always been one of the requirements for such appointments. If we accept what is suggested by the instances in which the word occurs in most texts, namely, that in the case of a man, the precise meaning of *impudicitia* is acceptance of the so-called feminine position in homosexual relations, we must also recognize that Augustus passed a law sentencing those found guilty of it to civic degradation. This was the last of the solutions that citizens might adopt in order to avoid having legitimate sons born of their own blood: *aselgainein*, as Dio Cassius puts it, using a word which, in the Greek idiom of the Roman period, denoted not only the defilement of adultery in the case of a woman[76] but also the situation of the *pathicus*, the man who was prepared to adopt the position of a woman. The texts of Suetonius and Dio Cassius confirm that men were indeed convicted for this kind of behavior, just as they confirm that women were convicted for adultery.

In the reign of Tiberius, Germinius Rufus, who was suspected of having consented to provide his male partners with all the pleasures that they desired, was accused of *malakia*, softness. The charge was eventually changed to impiety. He was found guilty and committed suicide, his wife deciding to commit suicide with him.[77] Dio Cassius also records that guardians were appointed for a number of Senators because they lived *aselgos*, indecently, in the precise sense of the term.[78] The appointment of a guardian implies that they had lost their legal capacities so, for example, they could no longer plead in a court of law. But the best example is that of the two brothers Rufus and Proclus Scribonius, both of whom were governors of parts of Germania. Dio writes that they both had the same *tropoi*, or tendencies — a term that he always uses to refer to men's preference for sexual relations with other men, and to evoke the dubious acts that such relations implied.[79] They were recalled from Germania by Nero, who was in Illyricum at the time, and it was there that, before coming to trial, they committed suicide. If we associate this double suicide with that of Germinius Rufus, we should also connect the two incidents with the laws on the *capitis deminutio*, which honored the wills of senators whom the Senate had declared to be enemies and who had forestalled their executions by committing suicide.[80] Dio Cassius notes that the Scribonii brothers "committed suicide to avoid being sentenced, in the sight of all, to *atimia*," *atimia* in the penal as well as the moral sense. Greek *atimia* (the forfeiture of civic rights, which initially meant that one might be killed with impunity by any citizen) was a penalty applied under both Greek and Roman law during the Empire. It was one of the possible calamities that could befall one, and one which the ancient authors often mention, as Atticus does in a list that includes "physical infirmities, poverty and *atimia*."[81] *Atimia* is the Greek term that corresponds exactly to the Latin *infamia*, as can be seen in a passage of Dio Cassius, in which Trajan, upon acceding to power, swears that he will not put any honorable man to death or subject him to infamy (*atimasoi*).[82]

An accusation of indecency was so dangerous that one proconsul, teased by a Cynic for having his body-hair removed, would have had that philosopher executed had Demonax not intervened to prevent this.[83]

Accusations of "indecency" could be based on no more than bearing and style of dress, which is borne out by books on physiognomy as well as by literary works.[84] A man's laxity in dress immediately prompted the suspicion that he accommodated the desires of other men, desires specifically defined as those which men would normally satisfy with their male slaves.[85]

One of the most forceful arguments against the existence of any legislation designed to deter citizens, particularly those from the upper orders, from engaging in a passive role in sexual relations between men is the fact that the documentation supporting it is so late, dating from the second century at the earliest. Against this, I would first consider the *Lex Iulia Municipalis* and the evidence conerning similar measures prohibiting certain individuals from pleading in the law courts on behalf of others (postulation) which Max Käser has presented so convincingly. It is, I think, legitimate to add to this the evidence provided by two Jewish writers of the first century, Philo and Flavius Josephus. Both emphasize that sexual relations between men were punishable by death under Jewish law, an assertion for which the Bible provides no corroboration at all. Let us take a closer look at these texts.

Philo associates sexual relations between men with a drop in the birthrate, exactly as did the speech that Dio Cassius attributes to Augustus. Again like Dio Cassius, he uses both the terms that denote "sterility," *agonia* in the case of males, *steirosis* in that of females. And it is essentially the "orders" of the upper classes that are concerned: "the best kind of men become scarce."[86] Elsewhere, he repeats the argument: the pederast "does his best to render cities desolate and uninhabited,"[87] which is exactly what Dio Cassius reports Augustus as declaring "You are betraying your country by rendering her barren and childless; nay more, you are laying her even with the dust by making her destitute of future inhabitants. For it is human beings that constitute a city, we are told, not houses or porticoes or marketplaces empty of men."[88] Philo also refers to cases of defiled men being excluded from civic rights: "Knowing that in assemblies there are not a few worthless persons who steal their way in and remain unobserved in the large numbers which surround them...."[89] And in his treatise *On Abraham*, he evokes that image of empty towns again: in the land of Sodom, "they accustomed those who were by nature men to submit to playing the part of women...they were corrupting the whole of mankind. Certainly, had Greeks and barbarians joined together in affecting such unions, city after city would have become a desert, as though depopulated by a pestilential sickness."[90] As in Augustus's speech, a connection is established between certain forms of sexual behavior, the loss of civic rights and a demographic threat that particularly affects the upper classes. So when elsewhere Philo tells us that androgynous individuals may be killed with impunity, we can guess the point that he is making.

Philo is at pains to explain the Jewish laws, that is, to draw parallels between them and the Greek and Roman laws. When speaking of assemblies, he explains that Judaism excludes from them a number of categories of individuals: first, men defiled by their effeminate behavior; second, eunuchs castrated at a very tender age and still in the full bloom of their beauty; third, female prostitutes; and fourth, the sons of prostitutes.[91] Such measures would be familiar to a Roman from his own institutions. Speaking of "androgynous beings," those who become androgynous through desire, Philo tries to make sure that his Greek and Roman readers understand him: "These persons are rightly judged worthy of death by those who obey the law, which ordains that the man-woman who debases the sterling coin of nature should perish unavenged, suffered not to live for a day or even an hour, as a disgrace to himself, his house, his native land and the whole human race."[92] What he has in mind is not Jewish law, nor the fact that Jewish law condemned homosexuals to death; what all this is really about is the existence of hermaphrodites in Rome and the defilement thereby brought upon the city. By playing on the term "androgynous," which he applies to "men who change themselves into women," Philo is able to assimilate applying the death penalty to Romans convicted of "indecency" to the destruction of "monsters" on religious grounds. Next, he draws a parallel between, on the one hand, pederasts and eunuchs (castrated in order "to heighten still further their youthful beauty," who are "each of them a curse and a pollution of his country") and, on the other, the category of effeminate men affected by the Greek laws against *atimia* and the Roman ones against *infamia*. On the basis of the Greek or Roman reader's understanding both of the defilement produced by a monster and of the degradation of citizens who take the passive role in sexual relations between men, Philo proceeds to try to win his approval for the Jewish death penalty for pederasty and castration. Flavius Josephus's *Against Apion* confirms the fact that Jewish law condemned homosexuals to death.[93] This treatise was written at least half a century after Philo's observations; and during that half-century, the Jewish citizens of the city of Rome itself had had a chance to become even more closely identified with Roman life and institutions. It may well have been at this point that, prompted by Roman law — that is, Augustus's rulings on "indecency" — a more severe interpretation of the Jewish law (Deuteronomy 23, 17) was introduced.

The attitude of Christian authors before Constantine toward sexual relations, of whatever type, between men was more or less that adopted by Philo. That is to say, they extended to all such relations the condemnation that Roman law and public opinion meted out to men who accepted the position reserved for slaves in homosexual acts. In my own view, there can be no doubt that this condemnation was largely prompted by a recognition of the element of power which entered into such relationships. Tertullian calls them criminal. And Suetonius refers to them in the same terms in the following passage: "of these charges or slanders [*crimines*], he [Augustus] easily refuted that for unnatural vice [*impudicitia*]."[94]

When Augustine, writing at the beginning of the fifth century, condemned the ceremonies devoted to the Mother of the Gods, he encapsulated all the remarks noted above:

> In any case, however they interpret her rites as symbols referring to nature, it is not according to nature, but against nature, for men to play the part of women sexually. And yet this malady, this crime, this indecency, of which even men of depraved character can hardly be compelled under torture to make confession, is a part of their sacred rites of which they freely make profession.[95]

Augustine uses the very same terms as those that were earlier applied to the laws on postulation: he speaks of *muliebria pati* and the certainty that this practice is a crime, telling us that in his own day, torture was used to confirm the guilt of the accused.

During the Roman Empire, the various types of sexual demands made by male citizens, particularly those from the upper classes (the orders), were distributed between (their) wives, concubines, infamous women and male and female slaves. Such matters were governed by a social code and they were also codified legally, even though they were considered to reflect emotions and desires. One simply did not feel the same emotions and desires for individuals of different statuses. As soon as Roman society, which included both Jews and Christians, came to realize that it was possible to have just the same feelings for wives as those previously reserved for intellectual friendships between men, and to have exactly the same feelings for slaves and dependents as those previously reserved for legitimate wives, the whole edifice crumbled. Furthermore, the condemnation of the sexual abuse of dependents brought in its wake condemnation of the sexual abuse of all the sexual acts similar to those that used to be demanded of them.

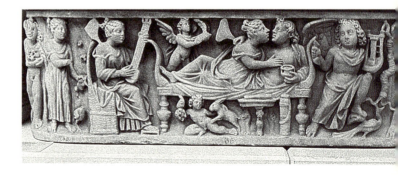

Cupid and Psyche (London, British Museum).

An earlier version of this essay was delivered in 1985, first in Paris, at the seminar organized by Nicole Loraux and Yan Thomas at the Ecole des Hautes Etudes en Sciences Sociales, and subsequently in Princeton at the invitation of Peter Brown and the Committee for Late Antique Studies. I should like to express my thanks to all those whose criticisms and comments were so helpful to me.

NOTES

1. M. Cornelius Fronto, *Correspondence*, ed. C.R. Haines, (London and Cambridge, Mass.: Loeb Classical Library, 1955). Cf. Tacitus, *Annals* trans. John Jackson (London and Cambridge, Mass.: Loeb Classical Library, 1962), 3.1, which describes Agrippina's return with the ashes of Germanicus: "The little flotilla drew to shore, not with the accustomed eager oarsmanship but with an ordered melancholy. When, clasping the fatal urn, she left the ship with her two children, and fixed her eyes on the ground, a single groan arose from the whole multitude; nor could a distinction be traced between the relative and the stranger, the wailings of women or of men." Even men of the upper classes were shedding tears: see Ramsey MacMullen's remarks, "Romans in tears," *Classical Philology* 75 (July 1980), pp. 254-55. On tears in general: Anne Vincent-Buffault, *Histoire des larmes* (Paris and Marseilles: Rivages, 1984).

2. Spartian, *Hadrian SHA* 14.5. To the examples provided by R. MacMullen (see above n.1), it is worth adding that of Vespasian weeping in the Senate when it refused to allow the succession to pass to Titus: Dio Cassius, *Roman History*, trans. Earnest Cary (London and Cambridge, Mass.: Loeb Classical Library, 1968), 66.12.

3. Plutarch, *The Education of Children*, trans. Frank Cole Babbitt (London and Cambridge, Mass.: Loeb Classical Library, 1960), 7E. Compare the attitudes recommended toward clients, wards and relations, Gellius 5.13.1ff. Here, however, I am noting what for us is a matter of feelings but for the Romans was governed by status. See also Plutarch, *On Affection for Offspring, Can Virtue Be Taught?* trans. W.C. Helmhold (London and Cambridge, Mass.: Loeb Classical Library, 1962), 439E, where he defines the relations "of a household, a city, a marriage, a way of life, a magistry."

4. Musonius 54.

5. *Ibid.*, 56-57.

6. Frag. 1 or 2.1, p. 38, Flornit 176.

7. Saara Lilja, in "Homosexuality in Republican and Augustan Rome," *Commentationes humanarum litterarum*, Societas Scientiarum Fennica 74 (1983) stresses the need to take account of "the social status of persons involved in homosexual relations," and is quite right to do so. However, it is primarily a matter of juridical status.

8.  In his inaugural lecture at the Collège de France, "L'histoire immobile," published in *Annales E.S.C.* (1974), pp. 673-91, on pp. 679-80, Emmanuel Le Roy Ladurie used the expression "eco-demography" (éco-démographie) to refer to a society's methods of regulating its reproduction: "It is true that the methods (quite undeliberated) employed by the classical system to stabilize itself in this way have little to recommend them to our own day and age. (I am thinking, for example, of epidemics: these truly were an element in an eco-system that associated human beings with their biological environment – that is to say the attacks of bacillae and other, predatory, species. The model I am briefly evoking here is thus a matter of fact and eco-demography: it is not intended to be either normative or attractive.)" Instead of using the term eco-demography, one could adopt the concept of "demecology" current in paleontology; see J. Roger, *Paléontologie générale*, "Sciences de la Terre" 1 (Paris: Masson, 1974). We could then speak of a demeco-system. But in the case of all human societies, a socio-demeco-system obtains, a social system grafted onto the combined evolutions of a population and its environment. On these ideas current in paleontology, see Lucienne Rousselle, "La Paléodémécologie: une ouverture nouvelle vers la compréhension des phénomènes d'interaction entre les organismes fossiles et leur environnements," *Bulletin de l'institut géologique du bassin d'Aquitaine* 21 (1977), pp. 3-11.

9.  Angus McLaren, *Reproductive Rituals* (London and New York: Methuen, 1984). See Aline Rouselle, review in *Le mouvement social* 137 (1986), pp. 121-24.

10.  See A. Rousselle, *Porneia: On Desire and the Body in Antiquity*, trans. Felicia Pheasant (New York: Basil Blackwell, 1988), ch. 6.

11.  J. Boswell, *Christianity, Social Tolerance and Homosexuality: Gay People in Western Europe from the Beginning of the Christian Era to the Fourteenth Century* (Chicago: University of Chicago Press, 1980), p. 62 n.4.

12.  Valerius Maximus 6.7.1; cf. Jerzy Kolendo, "L'esclavage et la vie sexuelle des hommes libres à Rome," *Index: Quanderni di studi Romanistici, International Survey of Roman Law* 10 (1981), pp. 288-97: knowing of her husband's relations with a slave woman, she freed the latter when Scipio died (p. 289).

13.  Plutarch, *Advice to Bride and Groom*, trans. Frank Cole Babbit (London and Cambridge, Mass.: Loeb Classical Library, 1967), 140B.

14.  Paul Veyne, *L'elégie érotique romaine* (Paris, 1983), p.100.

15.  See Rousselle, *Porneia*, p. 30.

16.  Epictetus, *Discourses*, trans. W. A. Oldfather (London and Cambridge, Mass.: Loeb Classical Library, 1967), 1.18.21-23. On all this, see my chapter "Gestes et signes de la famille dans l'Empire Romain," in *Histoire de la famille*, ed. Christiane Klapisch, André Burguière, Martine Ségalen and

Françoise Zonabend (Paris: Armand Colin, 1986), 1, pp. 231-69 (bibliography, pp. 612-13).

17. See also Plutarch, *On Listening to Lectures*, trans. Frank Cole Babbitt (London and Cambridge, Mass.: Loeb Classical Library, 1969), 37D: "Some of our young men, as soon as they lay aside the garb of childhood, lay aside also their sense of modesty."

18. We should bear in mind that female skeletons discovered in Greece indicate, on the average, five full-term pregnancies: see Mirko Grmek, *Les maladies à l'aube de la civilisation occidentale* (Paris, 1983) p. 148, citing J.L. Angel, "The bases of Paleodemography," *American Journal of Physical Anthropology* 30 (1969), pp. 427-38 for the neolithic period down to the Iron Age. For the classical period, see J.L. Angel, "Paleoecology, Paleodemography, and Health," a paper delivered at the 9th International Congress of Anthropological and Ethnological Sciences, Chicago and Detroit, Aug. 28–Sept. 8, 1973, summarized and discussed by Sarah Pomeroy, *Goddesses, Whores, Wives and Slaves: Women in Classical Antiquity* (New York, 1975), p. 68. See Emmanuel Le Roy Ladurie, "Biographie de la femme sous l'Ancien Régime," in *Panorama des sciences humaines*, ed. Denis Mollier (Paris, 1973), pp. 626-28.

19. A. McLaren's research into the responsibility for this decision is one of the best parts of *Reproductive Rituals*.

20. Plutarch, *The Education of Children* 1B. That is the reason why fathers should abstain from fleeting relationips with free courtesans and concubines.

21. On rape in Rome and Greece, see Aeschines, *Against Timarchus*, trans. Charles Darwin Adams (London and Cambridge, Mass.: 1958), Loeb Classical Library, p. 13: a youth prostituted by his father lost his freedom of speech; cf. K.J. Dover, *Greek Homosexuality* (London: Duckworth, 1978), p. 44. On freedom of speech, the basis of Athenian political rights, M.I. Finley, *Politics in the Ancient World* (Cambridge, 1983). A Roman citizen who was taken prisoner and raped by the enemy preserved his honor intact: Justinian, *Digest* 3, 1, 1, 6: "Si quis tamen vi praedonum vel hostium stupratus est, non debet notari." Cf. Boswell, *Christianity, Social Tolerance and Homosexuality*, p. 75 n.61. On this point Jerôme Bérnay-Vilbert, "La répression de l'homosexualité dans la Rome antique," *Arcadie* 21.250 (October 1974), pp. 443-55, is mistaken on p. 444, where he follows P. Grimal's view. Compare the situation of a wellborn girl who suffered rape: Justinian, *Digest* 49, 5, 14, 7-8 (Ulpian): "Quae vim patitur, non est in ea causa, ut adulterii vel stupri damnetur."

22. Livy, *Periocha* 59. The speaker knew what he was talking about: twenty seven members of his family addressed him as "Pater." Cf. Yan Thomas, "Parricidium, 1: Le père, la famille et la cité," *MEFRA* 93 (1981), p. 659 n.47.

23. Suetonius gives the speech a title: *De prole augenda*. See *Lives of the Twelve Caesars: Augustus*, trans. J.C. Rolfe (London and Cambridge, Mass.: Loeb Classical Library, 1970), 89.

24. Aulus Gellius, *Attic Nights*, trans. J.C. Rolfe (London and Cambridge, Mass.: Loeb Classical Library, 1961), 1.6.1-2.

25. We are here moving back and forth between two different periods, that of one or other Metellus (131 or 102) and that of Augustus. On slaves under the Empire: Mary L. Gordon, "The Nationality of Slaves under the Early Roman Empire," *Journal of Roman Studies* 14 (1924), pp. 93-111, shows that it is extremely difficult to infer the ethnic origin of slaves in Italy from our basic epigraphical sources. On this point, she criticizes Tenney Frank, to whose calculation she draws attention. Of five thousand names of slaves taken from the *CIL* that relate essentially to the period of the Roman Empire, T. Frank found 2,874 to be Greek, 2,126 Latin. He assumed the Greek names to denote a Greek or Eastern origin. Mary Gordon lists a number of ways in which slaves names were chosen, pointing out how they could falsify Frank's conclusions. However, this problem is of little concern to us since we are dealing with a speech delivered in the second century B.C., for which there are no inscriptions that could be used as a basis for any statistical study. For Heikki Solin Greek names in general belong neither to slaves nor to Greeks: see "Noms grecs à Rome," in *Colloques internationaux du CNRS* 564 (Paris, 1977). Both fashion and also literary and other influences ought to be taken into account. On the "nationality" of slaves, see the bibliography in Zvi Yavets's *Le plèbe et le prince* (Paris, 1984), p.23 n.2. Ramsey MacMullen, "Roman attitudes to Greek Love," in *Historia* 31 (1982), pp. 484-502, considers this matter but without taking into account the fact that the Greek attitude toward slaves might affect the attitude of Romans toward the Greeks who had become their own slaves.

26. Louis Pernard, "Le droit romain et le droit grec dans le théâtre de Plaute et de Térence," Thèse de droit de Lyon (Lyons, 1900), pt. 2, p. 49ff. In an article on civic degradation for male prostitution in Athens, Johannes Michael Rainer, "Züm Problem der Atimie als verlust der bürgerlichen Rechte insbesondere bei männlichen homosexuallen Prostituirten," *RIDA*, 3d ser., 33 (1986), pp. 89-114, compares the Greek horror felt for men who undergo anal penetration with African practices upon defeated enemies.

27. I in no way wish to suggest the very controversial idea that it was the Greeks who taught the Romans pederasty. Paul Veyne "L'homosexualité à Rome," *Communications* 35 (1982), pp. 26-33, esp. pp. 27-28: considers the opposite view to be correct: "Should we really believe that Rome learned of this kind of love from the Greeks, who were its masters in so many other domains? If the answer is 'yes,' the inference must be that love between men is a perversion so rare that one people can only have learned of it from another who set a bad example. If on the other hand, it would seem that pederasty was indigenous in Rome, the conclusion must be that it would be astonishing, not for a society to know of love between men, but for it not to. What calls for an explanation is not the tol-

erance of the Romans, but the intolerance of modern societies. The right answer is surely the second one." On the basis of no evidence other than the plays of Plautus, MacMullen ("Roman Attitudes") takes the opposite view.

28. In this translation, the usual interpretation adopted by most English and French versions has been modified. Here is the text in Latin: "Si sine uxore pati possemus, Quirites, omnes ea molestia careremus; sed quoniam ita natura tradidit, ut nec cum illis satis commode, nec sine illis ullo modo vivi possit, saluti perpetuae potius quam brevi voluptati consulendum est." I have retained the reading of *pati* given by J.C. Rolfe, Loeb, 1954, pp. 30-33. Other scholars have preferred *esse* or *vivere*. I have also modified the usual translations of the important points indicated where the relevant Latin words follow the English translation. As will be appreciated, it is important to recognize that Roman law requires that we should render *populus* as "the citizen body" and *res uxoria* as "dowry," and not as "people" and "married life" or the "annoyance and constant inconveniences of the married state." Even Paul Veyne falls into the common error as a result of failing to identify *res uxoria* as the technical expression used to refer to the dowry: see *Histoire de la vie privée* (Paris, 1985), p.49.

29. Justinian, *Digest* 1, 7, 26, 29, 30, 31, 40.

30. On this matter in general, see my contribution, "La nature du citoyen" to the colloquium on the body and the citizen, organized by Nicole Loraux and Yan Thomas, École des Hautes Études en Sciences sociales, Paris, 21-23 January 1988 (forthcoming).

31. Dio Cassius 56.5-7.

32. For a definition of the word *hubrizein*, see K.J. Dover, *Greek Homosexuality* (London: Duckworth, 1978), pp. 51-63.

33. *Ibid.*, p. 51.

34. Plutarch, *On Affection for Offspring* 493E.

35. J. Boswell, *Christianity, Social Tolerance and Homosexuality*, p.55. See Philo, on homosexuality: *De specialibus legibus* 1.325, 3.37-42; *Som.* 1.126; *De vita contemplativa* 59-61; *Rer. div. her.* 274; *Gen.* 4, 38; *De Abrahamo* 135-36. Philo's complete works are available in English translation by F.H. Colson (London and Cambridge, Mass.: Loeb Classical Library, 1958). See also the closing passage of this article.

36. For a discussion of the nonreproduction of men who love men, see Boswell, *Christianity, Social Tolerance*, pp. 9-10.

37. See E. Cantarella, "Adulterio, omicidio legittimo e causa d'onore in Diritto romano," *Studi in onore di Gaetano Scherillo* (Milan, 1972), vol. 1, p. 250. The same applies to the definition of parricide: it is important to define both the murderer and the victim, for the law varies in this respect.

For example, Constantine defined the murder of a son by a father as parricide, which was an innovation in Roman law. See Yan Thomas, "Parricidium, 1: Le père, la famille et la cité," pp. 649-50.

38. Justinian, *Digest*, 47, 10, 15, 15 (Ulpian): "Si quis virgines appellasset, si tamen ancillari veste vestitas, minus peccare videtur."

39. Seneca, *De Clementia*, trans. John W. Basore (London and Cambridge, Mass.: Loeb Classical Library, 1963), 1.24.1.

40. Justinian, *Digest*, 34, 2, 23, 2 (Ulpian). See Marcel Morabito, *Les réalités de l'esclavage d'après le Digeste* (Besançon and Paris, 1981), p. 190.

41. These slaves were relatively numerous and helped to keep the slave population up to strength when warfare was providing fewer slaves. The situation as regards Egypt has been studied by Iza Malowist, "Les esclaves nés dans la maison du maître et le travail des esclaves en Egypte romaine," *Studii classici* 3 (1961), pp. 147-62. These slaves were either produced by a free man, probably the master, and a slave woman, or else by two slaves.

42. There were particular laws governing the status of slaves freed privately: *Lex Aelia Sentia* in 4 A.D., Gaius 1.42-46; *Lex Junia*, Gaius 1.22 and 3.56; a fragment of Dositheus 6, 7, from 18 A.D. tells us that these laws laid down that the slave freed without any of the public procedures acquired his freedom but not citizenship. There was one exception to this rule: Gaius 1.19: a girl freed privately so that her master could marry did become a citizen.

43. A. Rousselle, "Concubinat et adultère," *Opus* 3 (1984), pp. 75-84.

44. Hippolytus of Rome, *Apostolic Tradition* 16.23, ed. G. Dix (London, 1968), p. 27.

45. G. Fabre, *Libertus: Recherches sur les rapports patron affranchi à la fin de la République Romaine* (Lille, 1982), vol. 1, pp. 333-36.

46. On the possible sexual demands made of freedmen: Seneca the Elder, *Controversiae* 5, pref. 10, cited by Paul Veyne, "La famille et l'amour sous le haut Empire Romain," *Annales E.S.C.* (1978), pp. 35-63; see also M.I. Finley, "Slavery and Humanity," in *Ancient Slavery and Modern Ideology* (London, 1980), pp. 93-122; Jerzy Kolendo, "L'esclavage et la vie sexuelle des hommes libres à Rome," *Index: Quaderni di studi Romanistici, International Survey of Roman Law* 10 (1981), pp. 288-97; and on political disqualification for "sexual services" in Rome as a problem in the granting of citizenship, Augusto Fraschetti, "A proposito di ex-schiavi e della la loro integrazione in ambito cittadino a Roma," *Opus* 1 (1982), pp. 97-103. See also J.N. Adams, *The Latin Sexual Vocabulary* (London: Duckworth, 1982), p. 163 on the vocabulary connected with such a sexual *officium*: the occurrences of this word and also of its equivalent *patientia*.

47. Paul of Aegina, *Surgery* (French trans. R. Brian, *Chirurgie*, Paris, 1855) echoes a chapter by

Oribasius, *Medical Collection*, which followed Heliodorus. There were two methods: crushing and excision. On eunuchs, A. Rousselle, "L'eunuque et la poule: La logique de la reproduction," *Mi-Dit: cahiers méridionaux de psychanalyse* 2-3 (June 1984), pp. 57-65. In this article, I showed that it was known how to perform the vasectomy described by Galen in his treatise *On Seed*. It was well known that men who were castrated many years after puberty, as in the case of the Gauls, retained their male characteristics and their sexual activity. Only those castrated as children never came to sexual maturity. A counterproof is provided by the account of Thévenot's travels: "Most part of these officers are Eunuchs... heretofore it was thought enough to geld them, but a Grand Signor having one day, as he was walking, perceived a Gelding covering a Mare, so soon as he was come home, ordered all that the Eunuchs had remaining to be cut clear off, and since that time it hath been the constant custom to cut all clear off to the Belly, which is done when they are but about eight or ten years old": J. de Thévenot, *Travels into the Levant*, trans. A. Lovell (London, 1687). See also, for example, Flavius Josephus, *Against Apion* 2.270. This difference between different kinds of eunuchs is not noted by any of the scholars who have studied the Galli, Graillot, Carcopino and Nock included. On eunuch slaves: Peter Guyot, *Eunuchen als Sklaven und Freigelassene in der griechisch-römischen Antike*, band 14; *Stuttgarter beiträge zur Geschichte und Politik* (Stuttgart: C.-R. Chantraine, 1980) Hist. z. 234, 1982, pp. 141-42.

48. Dio Cassius, *Roman History* 18.7. See Marcel Morabito, *Les réalités de l'esclavage d'après le Digeste* (Besançon and Paris, 1981), p. 187 and n.489, juridical references: *Digest* 48, 8, 6 (Venuleius): 9, 2, 27, 28 (Ulpian, Vivianus); 48, 8, 4, 2, repeats Hadrian; 37, 14, 6, 2 (Paul). Until the time of Justinian, eunuchs could enter into legitimate marriages and adopt children, but could not inherit, see G. Fabre, *Libertus* vol. 1, p. 285; vol. 2, pp. 214-15 n.6. See Yan Thomas's contribution to the Loraux/Thomas colloquium (above, n.30).

49. Lucian, *Demonax* 12, 13. In truth, Lucian's hero is Demonax, and he was not a bit concerned about Favorinus, the beardless philosopher. Polemon, the physiognomist, gives Favorinus as an example of a eunuch: cf. Elizabeth C. Evans, "The Study of Physiognomy in the Second Century A.D.," *Transactions of the American Philological Association* 72 (1941), pp. 96-108.

50. Marcellus, *De medicamentis liber* 33.65, ed. M. Niedermann, *Corpus-medicorum latinorum* 5 (Leipzig and Berlin, 1916).

51. According to the Greek tradition, lettuce was an anti-aphrodisiac for males: see M. Detienne, *Dionysos Slain* (Baltimore, 1979). For the Egyptian tradition, on the other hand, it was an aphrodisiac: see A. Rousselle, *Porneia* (Paris, 1983), p. 221.

52. It would be interesting to make a collection of allusions to masters in love, trying to win the love of a male or female slave. In the main, they occur as rhetorical examples of being enslaved

by the senses, and are to be found particularly in Philo, Epictetus and Libanius, where this is a quite common theme in which there is never any question of giving the loved ones their freedom until they have made some response.

53. Buecheler, CLE 1015. Cf. W. Den Boer, *Private Morality in Greece and Rome*, (Leyden: Brill, 1977), p. 217; G. Fabre, *Libertus*, vol, 1.6, pp. 153-57, suggests that sexual services were a condition of *spes libertatis*. Cicero and Tiro come to mind.

54. Tacitus, *Annals* 14.42.

55. E.g., Lucian, *The Downward Journey or the Tyrant* and *Alexander the False Prophet* (London and Cambridge, Mass., Loeb Classical Library, 1968).

56. I would recommend consulting the bibliography compiled by Eva Cantarella, "Adulterio, omicidio leggitimo e causa d'onore in Diritto romano," pp. 243-44; to which should be added Francisco Grelle, "La 'correctio morum' nella legislazione Flavia," *ANRW* 2, Principat 13 (Berlin and New York, 1980), pp. 340-65 and Leo Ferrero Raditsa, "Augustus's legislation concerning marriage, procreation, love affairs and adultery," *ANRW* 2 Principat (Berlin and New York, 1980), pp. 278-339.

57. Gaius, *Institutes* 1.12.

58. Justinian, *Digest* 3, 2, 24 (Ulpian).

59. *Ibid.*, 48, 5, 14.

60. *Ibid.*, 48, 5, 30: debauchery of oneself, in this case.

61. See A. Rousselle, *Porneia*, ch. 5.

62. Justinian, *Digest* 3, 2, 11.

63. L. Annaei Senecae Fragmenta, *De matrimonio* 70; Teubner, p. 431.

64. Lepida, *Annals* 3.22: "Quirinius, post dictum repudium adhuc infensus, quamvis infami ac nocenti miserationem addiderat"; Albucilla, *Annals* 6.47: "multorum amoribus famosa Albucilla" and 48: "stuprorum eius ministri, Carsidius Sacerdos praetorius ut in insulam deportaretur, Pontius Fregellanus amitteret ordinem senatorium." The terms *infamis* and *famosa* are often wrongly translated as "decriée" in French and "notorious" in English, as for example by Amy Richlin, "Sources on Adultery at Rome," in *Reflexions of Women in Antiquity*, ed. Helen Foley (New York and London, 1981), p. 338. The idea of moral condemnation does not go far enough: it was also a matter of a degraded juridical status. The same applies to other occurrences of *famosus* in Tacitus, *Histories* 5.2.1: Jerusalem, *famosa urbs*; Blaesus, whose death is *famosa*: *ibid.*, 3.38.1; Suetonius, *Tiberius* 25: "feminae famosae...famosi iudicii notam sponte subibant": the "infamous women themselves asked to be recorded as having been judged infamous."

65. Suetonius, *Lives of the Twelve Caesars: Julius* 43: "Although there was no suspicion of adultery":

this is a clear indication that a woman could go and live with a man other than her husband, thereby manifesting that the first marriage was over.

66. Justinian, *Digest* 3, 2, 11.

67. Suetonius, *Lives of the Twelve Caesars*: *Augustus* 67.

68. Suetonius, *Lives of the Twelve Caesars*: *Augustus* 5.

69. Tacitus, *Annals* 2.85. Michèle Ducros, "La crainte de l'infâmie et l'obeissance à la loi (Cicero, *de republica* 5.4, 6)" *REL* 57 (1979), pp. 145-65, p.161 n.1, associates this text with those that prevented male citizens found guilty of infamy from becoming magistrates, but she does not see that a woman judged to be infamous forfeited the very thing that, for her, was essential to her rights as a citizen: namely, her right to marriage.

70. Dio Cassius, *Roman History* 76.16.

71. J. Boswell, *Christianity, Social Tolerance and Homosexuality*, p. 24 reminds us of Plato's discussion of "effeminate men," but makes no attempt to define "effeminate." See also Paul Veyne, "L'homosexualité à Rome," *Communications* 35 (1982), pp. 26-33, for example p. 29: immense scorn fell upon any free male who played the "passive" part in a homosexual relationship or was, as it was called, *impudicus* (for that is an often overlooked meaning of this word) or *diatithemenos*. See, above all, Ramsey MacMullen's observations in "Roman Attitudes to Greek Love," *Historia* 31 (1982), pp. 484-502.

72. See Jean Taillardat, *Suétone: 'Peri blasphemon, Peri Paidion'. Des termes injurieux, Des jeux Grecs* (Paris, 1967); also, G. Vorberg, *Glossarium eroticum* (Reprint: Hanau and Mainz, 1965), e.g., s.v. "mollis," p. 363.

73. Max Käser, "*Infamia* und *ignominia* in dem römische Rechtsquellen," *Zeitschrift der Savigny-Stiftung für Rechtsgeschichte: Römanistische Abteilung* band 73 (1956), pp. 220-78, in particular p. 235. *Lex Iulia Municipalis*: "queive corpore quaestum facit"; to be compared with Digest 3, 1, 1, 6, "removet autem a postulando pro aliis et eum qui corpore suo muliebria passus est [except when the sexual acts are undergone in the course of war]." The verb *pati* is also used to indicate that a girl has arrived at puberty: *viri patiens*: see C. Lécrivain, C. Daremberg and E. Saglio, s.v. "Matrimonium," in *Dictionnaire des antiquités Grecques et Romaines d'après les textes et les monuments*, vol. 3, (1877-1919). Ducros's article, "La crainte de l'infâmie" concentrates too much on the Republic to be useful here. Furthermore, I cannot agree that "infamy in this period was not a juridical concept" (p. 160). Besides, the whole of this article, like Käser's, concerns infamy in general, not infamy for reasons of indecency. Plato's *Laws*, 836C-E shows that what is meant is men playing a passive role, like women, his point being that men should not be used as if they were women.

74. See, as well as Dover, *Greek Homosexuality*, Johannes Michael Rainer, "Zum Problem des

Atimie als Verlust der bürgerlichen Rechte insbesondere bei männlichen homosexuellen Prostituierten"; and Giulia Sissa's contribution to the Loraux/Thomas colloquium.

75. Suetonius, *Lives of the Twelve Caesars*: *Augustus* 34: "leges retractavit et quasdam ex integro sanxit, ut sumptuarium et de adulteriis et de pudicitia, de ambitu, de maritandis ordinibus."

76. Messalina: Dio Cassius, *Roman History* 60.18. Nero and young boys: *ibid.*, 51.9; Vitellius: *ibid.*, 65.2; Domitian: *ibid.*, 67.6.

77. *Ibid.*, 58.3.

78. *Ibid.*, 57.2-3.

79. *Ibid.*, 64.17, 61.11. On *tropos*, see Dover, *Greek Homosexuality*, pp. 69, 82, 83 n.5.

80. Justinian, *Digest* 4, 5 on the *capitis deminutio*; and *Digest* 4, 5, 5, 7. *Atimia* by itself does not translate the Roman prohibition of fire and water, which Dio Cassius translates literally, for example at *Roman History* 56.27.

81. Atticus, frag. 2.15; ed. and trans. into French by E. des Places (Paris: Collection des Universités de France, 1977), p. 44. See also Plutarch, *The Ancient Customs of the Spartans* 237C: loss of civic rights in perpetuity for having kissed a boy.

82. See Dover, *Greek Homosexuality*, p. 131 on the verb *atimazein* and the meaning of *atimoun* in Aristotle, namely, to deprive of the rights of citizenship.

83. Lucian, *Demonax* 50.

84. For example, the anonymous Latin treatise on physiognomy, French trans. and commentary by Jacques André, ed. *Traité de Physiognomonie* (Paris: Collection des Universités de France, 1981); to be compared with Aulus Gellius's descriptions, *Attic Nights* 30.5; Musonius 19.21; and Lucian's descriptions, *Demonax* 50 and *Alexander the False Prophet* 3 and 5. On clothing, Aulus Gellius, *Attic Nights* 6.12, on long-sleeved tunics: a man wearing one of these, who "at banquets...reclines on the inner side of the couch with a lover" was suspected of being fond of men (*virosus*): "Does anyone doubt that he does what wantons [*cinaedi*] do?" Suetonius makes use of all these ingredients in his critical description of Caesar (chs. 45-49). Similarly, Dio Cassius, *Roman History* 43, on Caesar. On effeminate men, Boswell, *Greek Homosexuality* p. 24ff. and p. 50 n.20, on the terms "active" and "passive."

85. See Amy Richlin, "The Meaning of *irrumare* in Catullus and Martial," *Classical Philology* 76 (January 1981), p.40-46; and, more generally, J.N. Adams, *The Latin Sexual Vocabulary*. Clearly, there was never any question of censuring a master for using a slave in this way, as Jérôme Bernay-Vilbert mistakenly supposes, "La répression de l'homosexualité dans la Rome antique," p. 454.

86. Philo, *De vita contemplativa* 60.

87. Philo, *De specialibus legibus* 3.39.

88.  Dio Cassius, *Roman History* 56.5.

89.  Philo, *De specialibus legibus* 1.325.

90.  Philo, *De Abrahamo* 135-36.

91.  Philo, *De specialibus legibus* 1.325.

92.  *Ibid.*, 3.38. The French ed. Mosès (Paris, 1970) *Sources Chrétiennes* 25, p. 83 has "inverti" where the text has "androgynous." I have retained the Latin reading. Philo, *ibid.*, 3.42, favors extermination for passive men whom he describes as "androgynous." In this same period, Musonius, frag. 21, was also assimilating "effeminate" men to androgynous beings. On the condemnation of "androgynous beings," in particular by Plato, see Marie Delcourt, *Hermaphrodites*, Coll. latomus 68 (1966), p. 48. Cf. Aulus Gellius, *Attic Nights* 9.4, 16: " 'hermaphrodites'...were formerly termed *androgyni* and regarded as monsters, but now are instruments of pleasure."

93.  Flavius Josephus, *Against Apion* 2.199.

94.  Suetonius, *Lives of the Twelve Caesars*: *Augustus* 71. See Marie Delcourt, *Stérilités mystérieuses et naissances maléfiques dans l'Antiquité classique* (Liège and Paris, 1938), on the elimination of hermaphrodites in Greece and Rome.

95.  Augustine, *City of God*, trans. William M. Green (London and Cambridge, Mass.: Loeb Classical Library, 1963), 6.8.

**Translated by Janet Lloyd.**

zone

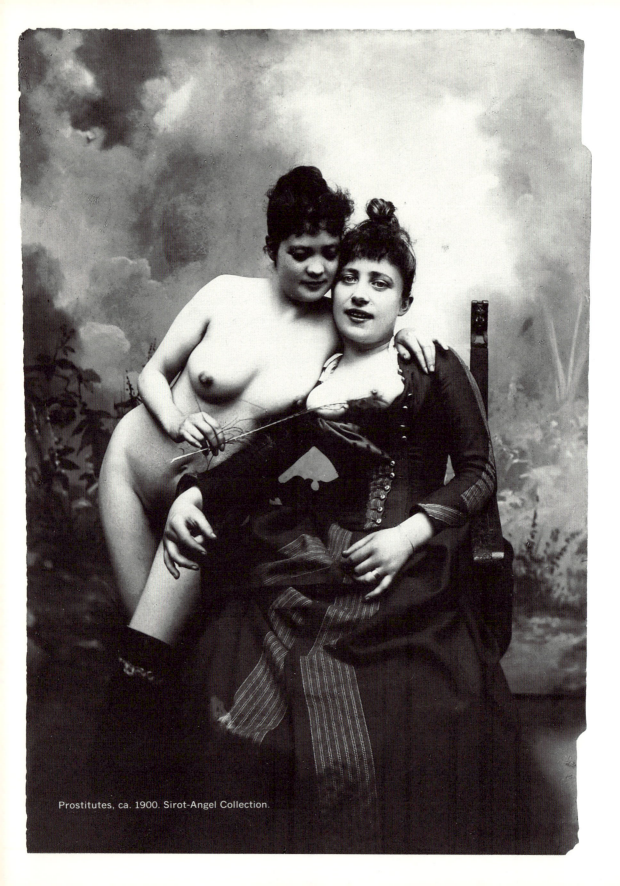

Prostitutes, ca. 1900. Sirot-Angel Collection.

# The Social Evil, the Solitary Vice
# and Pouring Tea

*Thomas W. Laqueur*

I want to sneak up on a cultural interpretation of the purported fact, widely held among nineteenth-century observers, that prostitutes are barren. My general point is that talk about sex is about a great deal else than organs, bodies and pleasures.

It is striking, for example, how little the Greek Church Father Gregory of Nyssa is explicitly concerned with sexual intercourse or desire in his tract *On Virginity*. Instead he returns again and again to the pain of human existence – as long as men, "these mortal creatures, exist and look upon the tombs of those from whom they came into being, they have grief inseparably joined to their lives" – and specifically to the enormous anxieties of social reproduction. "Assume that the moment of childbirth is at hand; it is not the birth of the child, but the presence of death that is thought of, and the death of the mother anticipated." He enumerates the emotional commitment of being a parent: one's efforts on behalf of a child's happiness, success, life itself. Marriage, in short, is a momentous investment in the future of the social order.[1]

And virginity is a very different sort of commitment, a commitment of the soul, and by no means of the body alone, to a new and different community in Christ. As Peter Brown has recently argued, "the debate about virginity [in the early Church] was in large part a debate about the nature of human solidarity. It was a debate about what the individual did and did not need to share with fellow creatures."[2]

I make this detour in order to turn attention away from sexuality as an innate human quality that needs to be, and is, repressed in various ways at various times, or even as a historically contingent construct, following Foucault and Nietzsche, which is woven into the sinews of power. I want instead to dwell on the constitutive connection between the sexual and the social body. "Society haunts the body's sexuality," as Maurice Godelier puts it; but the body's sexuality also haunts society.[3] It proclaims deep and conflicting cultural ambitions and anxieties.

In the nineteenth century, virginity is of course no longer the issue. But the body's sexuality, the specters of prostitution and masturbation this time, still haunts society. Their names bespeak their threat: the social evil; the solitary vice. Both terms are new and both reveal the perceived new dangers of very old practices.

I want to consider briefly the political and sexual radical Richard Carlile's treatment of the latter – the solitary vice – to emphasize how much the concern for masturbation can be construed as a concern about "the nature of human solidarity," and how little it appears to be a worry about excess or wicked sexual desire. Sociability and not repression is at stake. Carlile's *Every Woman's Book* is a sustained attack on conventional sexual morality, a plea for freeing the passions and a practical guide to birth control. Love is natural and only its fruits can and should be controlled, marriage laws constrain excessively a passion that should not be forced or shackled and so on. Carlile advocates Temples of Venus for the controlled, health-preserving, though extramarital satisfaction of female desire – he thought that five-sixths of deaths from consumption among young girls resulted from want of sexual commerce and perhaps as much as nine-tenths of all other illnesses as well.

But on the subject of masturbation Carlile the sexual radical is as shrill as the most evangelically inspired moralist or alarmist physician. Born of the cloister or its modern equivalents where a diseased religion turns love into sin, "the appeasing of lascivious excitement in females by artificial means" or the "accomplishment of seminal excretion in the male" is not only wicked but physically destructive as well. Masturbation leads to disease of mind and body. Indeed the "natural and healthy commerce between the sexes" for which he offers the technology is explicitly linked to the abolition of prostitution, masturbation, pederasty and other unnatural practices.[4]

The contrast could not be clearer between a fundamentally asocial or socially degenerative practice – the pathogenic, solitary sex of the cloister – and the vital, socially constructive act of heterosexual intercourse. But the supposed physical sequelae of masturbation seem almost a secondary reaction to its underlying social pathology. The emphasis in "the solitary vice" should perhaps be less on "vice," understood as the fulfillment of illegitimate desire, than on "solitary," the channeling of perfectly healthy desire back into itself. The debate over masturbation that

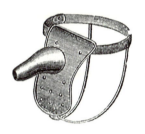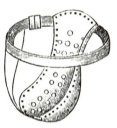

raged from the eighteenth century onward might therefore be understood as part of the more general debate about the unleashing of desire upon which a commercial economy depended and about the possibility of human community under these circumstances — a sexual version of the classic "Adam Smith problem."

Prostitution is the other great arena in which the battle against unsocialized sex and its dangers in a potentially fragmented culture was fought. "Whoring," of course, had long been regarded as wicked and detrimental to the commonweal but so had drunkenness, blasphemy and other disturbances of the peace. Not until the nineteenth century did it rise to being "*the* social evil," a particularly disruptive, singularly threatening vice. How this happened is a long story of which I want to tell only a small part.

Prostitutes were generally regarded as an unproductive commodity. Because they were *public* women; because so much traffic passed over their reproductive organs; because in them the semen of so many men was mixed, pell-mell, together; because the ovaries of prostitutes, through overstimulation, were seldom without morbid lesions; because their fallopian tubes were closed by too frequent intercourse; or, most tellingly, because they did not feel affection for the men with whom they had sex, they were thought to be barren, or in any case very unlikely to have children. One writer went so far as to argue that when prostitutes did become pregnant it was by men they especially preferred, and that prostitutes who had been transported to Van Diemen's Land reformed themselves, set up new domestic situations and suddenly found themselves fertile.[5]

Of course not every expert would agree. Indeed Jean Baptiste Parent-Duchâtelet, one of the most genuinely gifted nineteenth-century specialists in public health, whose study of prostitution is but the most famous of a series of pioneering works, insisted that there was nothing special about prostitutes. They did not have unusually large clitorides and were, therefore, not attracted to prostitution by excessive sexual desire; insofar as they had fewer children it is because they practiced abortion or birth control. Prostitution, he argues, is not inherent in bodies; in its modern form it is instead purely a pathology of commercial urban society. But in disagreeing with the general wisdom Parent is allying himself with what I take to be the main interpretive thrust of the idea of the barren prostitute.

To get at this I want to go back to the high Middle Ages when the "observation" that prostitutes are barren first appears. Aristotle, among others, had pointed out that the womb of a woman who was too hot — and the lascivious nature of prostitutes suggested such an excess of *calor genitalis* — might well be inhospitable to a new "conception." That is, it might burn up the conjoined seeds. But Aristotle did not actually equate prostitution with excess heat. Lucretius points out that prostitutes use lascivious movements which inhibit conception by diverting "the furrow from the straight course of the plowshare and [making] the seed fall wide of the plot." But this observation is in the course of a discussion of why "obviously our wives can have no use" for such wiggles.[6]

The reasons given in late medieval and Renaissance literature for the barrenness of prostitutes are several: excess heat, as mentioned above; a womb too moist and slippery to retain the seed; and the mingling of various seeds — in short, reasons very much like those given by nineteenth-century doctors. But I want to draw attention to another, less explicitly physiological explanation, which links the problem of barrenness with a more general derangement of the body politic. A twelfth-century encyclopedist, William of Conches, explains why prostitutes who engage frequently in the sexual act rarely conceive. Two seeds are necessary for conception, he reminds his readers, and prostitutes "who only perform coition for money and who, because of this fact feel no pleasure, emit nothing and therefore engender nothing." A sixteenth-century German doctor makes a very similar argument. Among the causes of barrenness, Lorenz Phrysen notes "a lack of passion in a woman for a man as, for example, the common women who work only for their sustenance."[7]

There is nothing unexpected here, at least to those who have read any medical literature written before the eighteenth century. This is another version of the old saw that orgasm is necessary for conception. But why do prostitutes not experience pleasure; why are the "common women" chosen to illustrate the point that an absence of passion causes sterility? The friction of intercourse must be as warming in harlots as in other women, yet their bodies respond differently. Why?

In both of the examples I have cited, money — or, more precisely, a somehow illegitimate exchange of money — provides the missing middle term. Prostitution is sterile because the mode of exchange it represents is sterile. Nothing is produced by it because like usury it is pure exchange. As Howard Bloch argues, it was precisely in the twelfth century and in response to a nascent market economy that usury became of urgent concern to the Church. And the particular wickedness of taking interest, it was held, is that nothing *real* is gained by it. Indeed, Aristotle, on whom Thomas Aquinas bases his case, argues that usury is "the most hated sort" of exchange and is to be particularly censured because it represents the antithesis of the natural, the productive, household economy. It is "unnatural and a mode by which men gain from one another." A perverted economic practice, like perverted sex, breeds abominations or nothing at all:

> Interest, which means the birth of money from money, is applied to the breeding of money because the offspring resembles the parent. That is why of all modes of getting wealth this is the most unnatural.

It is as if usury were incestuous intercourse. Or, as Catherine Gallagher puts it, "what multiplies through her [the prostitute] is not a substance but a sign: money." Prostitution, if one follows this web of connections, becomes, like usury, a metaphor for the unnatural multiplication not of things but of signs without referents.[8]

A deep cultural unease about money and the market economy is couched in the metaphors of reproductive biology; this is Aristotle's formulation. But, more to the point here, fear of an asocial market takes on a new avatar in the claim that sex for money, coition with prostitutes, bears no fruit. This sort of sex is set in sharp contradistinction — one senses especially in the German example — with the household economy of sex, which is quintessentially social and productive. Phrysen elsewhere in the text that I cite develops the metaphor of the productive womb protecting the fetus just as the crust of bread protects the crumbs. The image of baking, warmth and kitchen contrasts with the cool barrenness of those who work, have intercourse, *only* for pay, completely outside the bounds of the household and the household economy.

By the nineteenth century the trope of the barren prostitute had, as I have suggested, already a very respectable seven-century-old pedigree. But the boundaries that it guarded — between home and economy, public and private, self and society — were both more sharply drawn and more fraught with conflict in the urban class society of Europe after the industrial and commercial revolutions than ever before. Or at least so thought contemporary observers. Society seemed to be in unprecedented danger from the market place. And the sexual body bore the widespread anxieties about this danger. (One can, and of course in a detailed study must, be more specific and contextual in making this point. Laura Engelstein, for example, is doing research on the synergistic coupling of urban anti-Semitism and sex for money, more specifically, on the fears of the Jewish prostitute, in late imperial industrializing Russia.)

While masturbation threatened to take sexual desire and pleasure inward, away from the family, prostitution took it outward. Perhaps even more than masturbation it broke the barrier between home and market that, in much social thought, was regarded as the safeguard for human solidarities against the disintegrative forces of the market. The sterility of prostitutes and their other biological defects and dangers (as well as the illnesses resulting from self-abuse) are in this context not warnings against undue sexual pleasure or inadequate sublimation but, rather, representations of the dangers of withdrawal from family and other supposed shelters from money.

The problem with masturbation and prostitution is essentially quantitative: doing it alone and doing it with lots of people rather than doing it in pairs. It is thus in the same category as other misdeeds of number, the withdrawal of the protagonist of Florence Nightingale's *Cassandra* for example, who refuses to pour tea for the household and withdraws alone to her couch. The social context, not the act itself, determines acceptability.

The paradoxes of commercial society that had already plagued Adam Smith and his colleagues, the nagging doubts that a free market economy can in fact sustain the social body, haunt the sexual body. Or, the other way around, the perverted sexual body haunts society and reminds it of its fragility.

NOTES

1. Gregory of Nyssa, *On Virginity*, in *Ascetical Works*, trans. V.W. Callahan; see pp. 14-15, 19, 51 on marriage as a microcosm of earthly commitment.

2. Peter Brown, "The Notion of Virginity in the Early Church," in *Christian Spirituality*, eds. Bernard McGinn and John Meyendorff (New York: Crossroads, 1985), p. 436.

3. Maurice Godelier, "The Origins of Male Domination," *New Left Review* 127 (May-June 1981), p. 17.

4. Richard Carlile, *Every Woman's Book or, What is Love Containing Most Important Instructions for the Prudent Regulation of the Principle of Love and the Number of a Family* (London: Richard Carlile, 1828).

I used an 1892 reprint of the 1828 edition published by the Malthusian League. The tract was originally published in Carlile's *Red Republican* in 1828. See esp. pp. 18, 22, 26-27, 37-38.

5. Edward John Tait, *On the Diseases of Menstruation and Ovarian Inflammation* (London, 1850), p. 54; Michael Ryan, *The Philosophy of Marriage ... with the Physiology of Generation in the Vegetable and Animal Kingdoms*, 3rd ed. (1839), p. 168; Frederick Hollick, *The Marriage Guide or Natural History of Generation* (1850), p. 72; Henry Campbell, *Differences in the Nervous Organization of Man and Woman: Physiological and Psychological* (1891), pp. 211-12; Ryan, *Jurisprudence*, p. 225; George Naphys, *The Physical Life of Women* (Walthamstow, 1879), pp. 77-78.

6. Lucretius, *The Nature of the Universe*, trans. Ronald Latham (Harmondsworth, 1951), p. 170; as far as I can tell, no one cited any evidence for this claim between its articulation in the twelfth century and its going out of favor in the late nineteenth.

7. Regarding excessive moisture as a cause of barrenness see, for example, R.B. [R. Buttleworth?], *The Doctresse: A Plain and Easie Method of Curing those Diseases which Are Peculier to Women* (London, 1656), p. 50. A variant on the heat argument is that an ordinary woman experiences two orgasms, one from the alteration in her cold state caused by the inflow of hot sperm from the male and another from her own emission. Harlots, whose wombs are already hot from excessive intercourse, lack the first. On this claim, see Helen R. Lemay, "William of Saliceto on Human Sexuality," *Viator* 12 (1981), p. 172. She attributes it to William of Conches or some twelfth-century interpolator. William of Conches as cited in Danielle Jacquart and Claude Thomasset, *Sexualité et savoir medical au Moyen Age* (Paris: Presses Universitaires de France, 1985), p. 88; Lorenz Fries (Phrysen), *Spiegel der Artzney* (1546), p. 130: "Die unfruchbarkeyt wirt auch dardurch geursacht/ so die fraw kein lust zu dem mann hat/ wie dann die gemeynen frawlin/ welche alleyn umb der narung willen also arbeyten." My colleague, Prof. Elaine Tennent of the German Department at Berkeley, suggests that while the use of "frawlin" (i.e., "fraulein" in modern German), instead of "fraw" as in the previous clause, supports reading "gemeynen frawlin" as prostitutes, one might construe the clause to refer to common women – peasants – who work *only* to earn their keep rather than, as Luther would have preached, for the greater glory of God. This would fit nicely with the analogies made by Calvin and others between sexual heat or passion and the warmth, the ardor, that the heart ought to feel for God, on which point see William Bouwsma, *John Calvin: A Sixteenth-Century Portrait* (New York: Oxford, 1988), pp. 136-37. Phrysen taught at Strasbourg, a strongly Protestant university. Even if one were to accept this later reading, Phrysen's argument still supports my claim that one's relationship to production and exchange is linked to the body's capacity to procreate.

8. R. Howard Bloch, *Etymologies and Genealogies: A Literary Anthropology of the Middle Ages* (Chi-

cago, 1983), pp. 173-74; Aristotle, *Politics*, in *The Complete Works of Aristotle*, ed. Jonathan Barnes (Princeton, 1984) 1.1997 (1258b1-7); this naturalistic expression of a cultural anxiety, in the case of prostitutes and perhaps also of usury, strikes me as an aspect of the new relationship between the sacred and the profane that Peter Brown discusses in his "Society and the Supernatural: A Medieval Change," *Society and the Holy in Late Antiquity* (Berkeley and Los Angeles, 1982), pp. 302-22, esp. pp. 324ff. Indeed the production of authoritative texts like William of Conches might be construed as evidence for Brown's shift from "consensus to authority." Catherine Gallagher, "George Eliot and *Daniel Deronda*: The Prostitute and the Jewish Question," in *Sex, Politics, and Science in the Nineteenth-Century Novel*, ed. Ruth Yeazell (Baltimore, 1986), pp. 40-41.

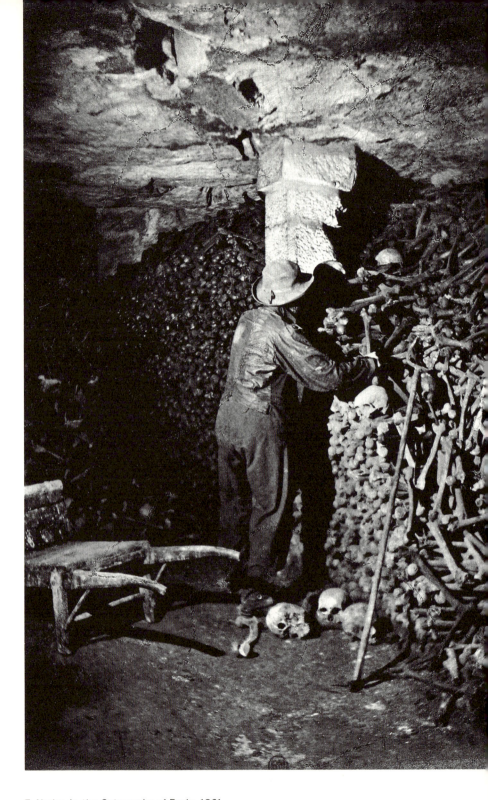

F. Nadar, In the Catacombs of Paris, 1861.

# The Bio-Economics of *Our Mutual Friend*

*Catherine Gallagher*

## Value, Wealth and Illth

Charles Dickens's *Our Mutual Friend* draws on an antithesis that John Ruskin had named in *Unto This Last* (1862) a few years before the novel appeared: that of wealth and "illth." In developing this antithesis, Ruskin began with a question and an anecdote, both of which anticipated in striking detail the opening chapter of Dickens's novel. Ruskin's question was, "[I]f we may conclude generally that a dead body cannot possess property, what degree and period of animation in the body will render possession possible?"[1] In the first chapter of *Our Mutual Friend*, Gaffer Hexam also insists on the absurdity of the idea that a dead man can possess property. He raves,

> Has a dead man any use for money? Is it possible for a dead man to have money? How can money be a corpse's? Can a corpse own it, want it, spend it, claim it, miss it?[2]

Gaffer seems to think that these questions automatically call for a negative reply: "No, a dead body cannot possess property." The novel, however, not only leaves this issue open but also goes on to ask Ruskin's more complicated question, the one that introduces the possibility of "illth": what degree of health, of life, of animation, is necessary before the body can be properly said to possess something? Ruskin's question turns into an anecdote, like the one that opens *Our Mutual Friend*, of drowning and dredging up. Ruskin writes:

> [L]ately in a wreck of a California ship, one of the passengers fastened a belt about him with two hundred pounds of gold in it, with which he was found afterwards at the bottom. Now, as he was sinking — had he the gold? or had the gold him?
>
> And if, instead of sinking him in the sea by its weight, the gold had struck him on the forehead, and thereby caused incurable disease — suppose palsy or insanity — would the gold in that case have been more a "possession" than in the first? Without pressing

the inquiry up through instances of gradually increasing vital power over the gold, . . .
I presume that the reader will see that possession . . . is not an absolute, but a graduated
power; and consists not only in the . . . thing possessed, but also . . . in the possessor's vital
power to use it. (169-70)

Ruskin, then, begins his investigation into the nature of economic value with
death in order, it seems, to root wealth in bodily well-being. Wealth, he concludes,
is the possession of useful things by those who can use them. Useful things are those
that nurture life, and those who can use them are those who are (at the very least)
in a state of bodily animation. To the degree that possessions cause bodily harm, as
in the story of the drowned man, to the degree that they incapacitate or make people ill, they are "illth."

The hero of *Our Mutual Friend*, John Harmon, is closely identified with, indeed,
is identified as, the drowned body dredged up by Gaffer Hexam in chapter one. As a
possessor of gold, he has also been killed by the action of illth because he has been
murdered for the sake of his money. We might say that this story is Ruskin's retold,
although in Dickens's version both the man and the gold have surrogates. George
Radfoot takes Harmon's place and, as Harmon later explains, is "murdered for the
money" by "unknown hands," conceived merely as extensions of what Harmon calls
"the fate that seemed to have fallen on my father's riches – the fate that they should
lead to nothing but evil" (370). Thus, John Harmon is officially drowned and
dredged up at the novel's outset, a victim of illth. After being proclaimed dead, he
staggers dazed through the novel's opening episodes, as if, following the stages of
Ruskin's inquiry, he had reached the state of merely being wounded in the forehead
by his would-be riches. The question that drives the plot is the same as that asked by
Ruskin: What degree of animation in the formerly dead man would be necessary to
render possible his possession of (instead of by) his money? "Should John Harmon
come to life again?" the hero keeps asking. If he were to reanimate himself, gradually working his way from dead to ill to well, could he change illth to wealth?

The point of making these parallels between *Unto This Last* and *Our Mutual Friend*
is not to argue that Dickens got the germ of the novel from Ruskin. It is rather to
direct our attention to a pervasive pattern of mid-Victorian thought, a widespread
insistence that economic value can only be determined in close relationship to bodily
well-being. In several key texts on economics, sanitation, social theory and aesthet-

ics, this "new" way of restructuring economic investigations around the human body took the dead body as a starting place and tried to move toward reanimation. However, as I hope to show through an analysis of *Our Mutual Friend*, this operation often resulted in the reseparation of value (equated with Life) from any of its particular instantiations (or bodies). That is, the attempt to resituate the human body at the center of economic concerns, to rewrite economic discourse so that it constantly referred back to the body's well-being, paradoxically, itself tended to do what it accused unreconstructed political economists of doing: separating value from flesh and blood, conditioning value on a state of suspended animation or apparent death.

Ruskin and Dickens were by no means pioneers in the attempt to pose the question of value in terms of bodily well-being. Indeed, their effort has a history within political economy itself. We normally think of Ruskin and Dickens as part of a specifically literary moral reaction against the Victorian forces of commercialism and social alienation, and political economists are often singled out as the ideological vanguard of heartless laissez-faire capitalism. Certainly, this was often the self-understanding of Ruskin and Dickens. Ruskin quite explicitly wrote *Unto This Last* as a polemic against classical political economy, and Dickens, although far from confronting any system systematically, nevertheless wrote of the "dismal science" as an enterprise devoted to the justification of particular human suffering. Ebenezer Scrooge epitomizes this bland insensitivity to individual pain when he suggests that the indigent ought to die and "reduce the surplus population."

As this quotation suggests, Thomas Malthus's epoch-making *Essay on Population* (1797) was often identified as the most outrageously hard-hearted book in the whole hard-hearted economic canon. Malthus was accused of setting population increase against economic well-being, of viewing a populous nation as one on the brink of disaster. Ignoring the complexities of Malthus's argument as well as its polemical situation inside the debate over the perfectability of man, his humane critics saw in his essay only a devaluation of human life and accused him of trying to found the wealth of nations on the death of babies. The alleged zest with which he described the positive checks to population (death by starvation, infanticide) scandalized many reviewers, who characterized Malthus as a ghoul. He had built death, physical misery and vice (the prevention of conception) into the base of the economic structure. He had inaugurated what was seen as a negative bio-economics in which economic well-being (a balance of resources and consumption) could only be achieved through the devastation or prevention of life.

Like Dickens in his portrayal of Scrooge, Ruskin also implies that Malthusianism is the original sin of political economy, its most blatant act of severing economic value from embodied human life. Hence, Ruskin tries rhetorically to reconnect economic and bodily health through etymology. He derives value from "*valor* from *valere*, to be well, or strong...strong *in* life (if a man), or valiant; strong *for* life (if a thing), or valuable. To be 'valuable,' therefore, is to 'avail towards life'" (168). Ruskin faults the political economists for calculating the values of commodities without regard either to their potential for sustaining and enhancing life or to the ability and willingness of their possessors to activate that potential. Ruskin's economic essays constantly return to this theme: the political economists have abstracted value, severed it from flesh and blood. "The true veins of wealth," he writes, "are purple – and not in Rock but in Flesh...the final outcome and consummation of all wealth is in producing as many as possible full-breathed, bright-eyed and happy-hearted human creatures" (144). That contrast – blood veins in flesh versus metallic veins in rock – is at least as old as the Midas myth, but in the nineteenth century it took on a new urgency and specificity. It was not directed simply against human greed or miserliness but against what many of Ruskin's contemporaries saw as a terribly destructive economic orthodoxy that was determining social reality.

Ruskin's purple veins of wealth statement, like Dickens's characterization of Scrooge, asserts the rights of human bodies against the doctrines of political economy generally and those of Thomas Malthus specifically. In fact, however, on this point Malthus himself fully anticipated these self-proclaimed anti-Malthusians. The relationship between bodily well-being and economic value was not, as Ruskin and Dickens seemed to think, a blind spot of political economy, but was, rather, one of that discipline's most problematic obsessions. And no one had treated the issue in terms closer to Ruskin's own than Malthus himself. I do not have space here to describe the paradoxical complexity of Malthus's *Essay*;[3] suffice it to say that although Malthus undeniably made bodies socially and economically problematic, he did so, paradoxically, by ceding all value to them rather than removing value from them. Hence, Malthus, like Ruskin and Dickens, also polemicized against the abstracting tendencies of other political economists, and although he certainly feared overpopulation, he gave (at least in the first edition of the *Essay*) no definition of value that can distinguish it from flesh. It was Malthus who first deplored Adam Smith's failure to distinguish among commodities on the basis of their *biological* usefulness; indeed, Malthus at times seems an even more fanatical proponent of the idea that value is in flesh than Ruskin, for he goes so far as to suggest that the only productive labor is that which produces working-class food; that is, that the production of more laboring flesh is the sole proper outcome of labor. By this logic, purple veins would indeed be the only true source of the wealth of nations.

When writers like Dickens and Ruskin insisted that health and illness be introduced into the calculation of economic value, they were not adding ideas drawn from some moral discourse distinct from political economy but were, rather, unwittingly emphasizing one element of the logic of political economy itself. The biological aspect of political economy, the emphasis on value derived from flesh, follows from its central premise the labor theory of value. But this very theory simultaneously dislodges considerations of physical well-being from calculations of value. The doubleness of Malthus's attitude toward living flesh, then, was just one instance of the following systematic ambivalence.

Political economists such as Adam Smith took labor to be the source or measure of all exchange value and often calculated the value of labor by the value of the commodities (primarily the food) necessary to replenish the body for the hours of labor expended on another commodity.[4] Thus, the exchange value of any commodity was rooted in biological need; the worker's body was the primary nexus of exchange through which the value of those commodities that reproduce its labor largely determine the value of all other commodities. Adam Smith, for example, argues that all economic exchanges are ultimately rooted in the toiling body. The use of money merely covers over this fact which political economists insisted on revealing: "What is bought with money or with goods is purchased by labour as much as what we acquire by the toil of our own body."[5] However, it is precisely because the "toil of the body" is a universal equivalent determining exchange value that commodities can acquire abstract value independent of their biological usefulness. The very ability to calculate, through the common measure of labor, the relative values of commodities led away from a hierarchy of commodities based on ultimate biological usefulness. The labor theory of value could "equate" a bushel of corn, for example, with

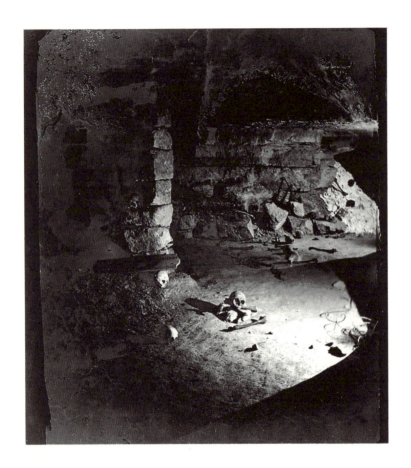

F. Nadar, In the Catacombs of Paris, 1861.

a bit of lace, even though, from another physiological point of view, the corn would seem more intrinsically valuable. The humane critics of political economy resemble Malthus in accepting the premise of the labor theory of value while rejecting its normal implications. The value of a thing, they claim, is at least equivalent to, as Ruskin phrased it, the cost of keeping the artisan for the length of time it takes to make the article "in bread and water, fire and lodging" (25). Biological regeneration is the foundation of all value for the critics as well as the proponents of political economy. But the critics, beginning with Malthus, claim that because the laboring body is the source of all value, commodities that immediately sustain more laboring bodies should be assessed as more valuable than those without direct physiological benefits. Thus, the critics often accord a privileged position to the commodities that are most easily turned back into flesh. Malthus and Ruskin alike, then, wanted economic exchange to proceed from flesh back to flesh by the least circuitous route: life expended immediately converted into life replenished.

Viewed within this context, the emphasis on death in Ruskin and Dickens seems an extension of those very tendencies in political economy that claim to valorize life most fully. For those are the tendencies stressing the commodity's need to have a life-giving potential that makes up for its life-draining origins. In other words, the humane critics of political economy imagine the commodity, the bearer of value, as freighted with mortality, as a sign of spent vitality, in order to demand all the more strenuously that it have a vitality-replenishing potential.

This is the curiously death-centered bio-economics that *Our Mutual Friend* draws out to its most paradoxical lengths. We have already seen that death from illth and the possibility of reanimation are at the core of the novel's main plot. But the book's obsession with the place of human bodies inside systems of economic accumulation and exchange goes far beyond John Harmon's story, and that story can best be illuminated by a view of the novel's overall bio-economics.

To begin once again at the beginning, our introduction to the theme shows us the dead body as a nexus of two kinds of economic exchange. John Harmon is not the only person interested in turning "his" dead body into life. As one of the many kinds of garbage that Gaffer and Lizzie Hexam fish out of the river, the corpse forms a part of their livelihood. It is from this fact that Lizzie is trying to avert her own attention in the opening scene, as she and her father tow the putrefying corpse, which will later be identified as John Harmon's, to shore. In Lizzie's reluctant conversation with her father, the corpse and the river merge in the impersonal pronoun "it": "I — I do not like it, father." "As if it wasn't your living!" replies Hexam. "As if it wasn't meat and drink to you!" (3). The shocking power of this metaphor, which immediately turns Lizzie "deadly faint," is its removal of all mediations between the girl's "living," her sustenance, and the corpse's moldering flesh, which becomes, in this oddly literalizing image, her food. Lizzie's physical reaction is another literalizing metaphor of denial: she would rather turn her own body into the dead white thing than keep it alive on such carrion. This first suggestion of how death might be exchanged for life is the most primitive and horrific of biological economies presented in the novel.

Gratefully, we seem to move immediately on to another. We are relieved to learn, as the passage continues, that although the river has yielded many things that have directly nurtured Lizzie ("the fire that warmed you," "the basket you slept in," "the rockers I put upon it to make the cradle of it"), the dead bodies have been only *indirect* sources of life. They have been sources of money, and hence can be seen by Lizzie and the reader not as food itself but as the wherewithal to purchase food. Gaffer robs the bodies before turning them over to the police and also collects inquest money for having found them. Hence, the bodies are part of a seemingly thoroughly civilized network of economic circulation. Lizzie is also disturbed by this exchange of the body for money; indeed, she claims that the sin of pilfering from the corpses is the root of her shame. However, coming to us as it does in the context of the primitive alternative presented in Gaffer's metaphor, the intervention of money has a double moral impact. On the one hand, it brings the Hexams' living inside the pale of civilization. But, on the other hand, the intervention of money itself seems just a metaphor that would (but can't quite) cover over the reality of vulturism emphasized by Gaffer's and the narrator's insistent metaphorizing. The metaphors of the corpse as a living, of Gaffer as a bird of prey, make the trope of economics — the mediation of money — seem to be a euphemism directing our attention from that which the explicit metaphors reveal: the real exchange *is* life for life.

We are, then, given two ways in which a corpse can be a "living" in this passage, but the distinction between them is collapsible. The more acceptable account (in which the human body is an item of exchange in a money network that fails to distinguish it from other items) is disturbing. But the source of the disturbance, when sought, seems to be the deep secret that money is always ultimately taken out of flesh. That is, the horror is not that human flesh becomes money, but that money is just a metaphor for human flesh. In this respect, the exchange made through the corpse is really not different from any other economic exchange, since all value is produced at the expense of life.

The opening of *Our Mutual Friend*, then, while echoing *Unto This Last*, also carries out its logic to a nightmarish extreme: any commodity qua commodity is expended life. The commodity as dead body merely emphasizes this universal truth, and the further typical humanitarian suggestion that it should immediately become nutrition is then indistinguishable from Swift's "modest proposal." The opening pages of the novel reveal that the humanitarian critique, wishing as it does for the shortest possible circuit between expended and augmented life, conjures up, as a reductio ad absurdum of itself, a fantastic, worse than cannibalistic bio-economy.

As many critics have noticed, Gaffer and Lizzie Hexam are not the only scavengers in the book, the only people making a living out of the dead husks of life. Most of the book's economic enterprises amount to trading in human remains. The Boffin-Harmon dust mounds are only the most elaborate example. They are the assembled debris of a vast number of lives. And they also become, through Mortimer Lightwood's metaphor, the spewed-forth life of old Harmon himself: "On his own small estate the growling old vagabond threw up his own mountain range, like an old volcano, and its geological formation was Dust. Coal dust, vegetable dust, bone dust, crockery dust, rough dust and sifted dust – all manner of Dust" (56).

This is an image of peculiar fixity, seemingly ill-assorted with the characterization of old Harmon as a "vagabond." It de-emphasizes the circulation of debris in the dust trade and transforms the enterprise into Harmon's simultaneous expending and hoarding of his own substance. The expense of his life is a self-burying; dust erupts from him and settles on him, so that accumulation and interment are the same thing. The last we hear of old John Harmon makes his death seem the merest extension of the activity of his life: "He directs himself to be buried with certain eccentric ceremonies and precautions against coming to life" (58).

Old Harmon's whole existence seems to have consisted in "precautions against coming to life." He is the prototypically illthy individual, causing, in Ruskin's phrase, "various devastation and trouble around [him] in all directions" (171). He oppresses and anathematizes his own living flesh and blood, his son and daughter, while he builds up his geological formations of dust. The flesh-and-blood-versus-rock metaphor echoes Ruskin's distinction between the true veins of wealth (purple and in flesh) and the false veins (gold and in rock). The conflation of gold and rock in mountains of dust turns both to death; Mortimer Lightwood, in telling old Harmon's story, makes this explicit. But, at the same time, he calls attention to the clichéd nature of these associations: "[Harmon] chose a husband for [his daughter], entirely to his own satisfaction and not in the least to hers, and proceeded to settle upon her, as her marriage portion, I don't know how much Dust, but something immense. At this stage of the affair the poor girl respectfully intimated that she was secretly engaged to that popular character who the novelists and versifiers call Another, and that such a marriage would make Dust of her heart and Dust of her life — in short, would set her up, on a very extensive scale, in her father's business" (56).

One cannot simply dismiss the associations made here between dust, money and death. Old Harmon was a death-dealer, both in the sense that he traded, like Gaffer Hexam, in the remains of life and in the sense that he converted life into those remains. But the fact that these associations are presented as sentimental commonplaces should make us take a closer look at them, a look that reveals how Harmon's business, like Gaffer's, emphasizes that value *as such* is always life expended and accumulated, stored up, in inorganic form. Hence, Old Harmon's conversion of life into death, his death-dealing, is no different in principle from any other process of realizing value. Moreover, it is certainly preferable to the primitive directness of the carrion economy briefly figured in the opening chapter. Although the passing of life is legible in both Harmon's and Gaffer's commodities, the inorganic garbage already represents the achievement of several steps in the economic process of liberating value from the body.

Hence, despite the dust versus flesh, death versus life metaphors in the passages that introduce us to the dustmen, the transmission of life into inorganic matter and thence into gold is not truly presented as life-destroying in the novel. On the contrary, it is portrayed as a sanitizing process and one in which a pure potential called "Life" is released. This elongated circuit between life expended and life augmented is one of increasing abstraction in which a life-transmitting potential, or power, finds itself outside of human bodies for a long period of time. And the liberation of such a vital power turns out to be the novel's very means of making Life seem valuable.

Little wonder, then, that the revaluation of Old Harmon's legacy is accomplished not by its attachment to a worthy body (as Ruskin would have it), but by its sustained suspension through the apparent death of Young John Harmon. Apparent death is the structural principle of the narrative. Young Harmon, as we have seen, describes himself as being dead but having the potential for reanimation. He is, like riches themselves, the possibility of embodied life in a state of suspended animation. And it is only in this state, when he has not claimed his money but has instead, by sloughing off his supposed body, achieved a kind of ontological oneness with the money as pure vital potential, that he can change illth into wealth. He is dead as its inheritor, and yet he manages the fortune as Mr. Boffin's secretary. "The living-dead man," as the narrator calls him, resolves to remain in this state of suspended animation until he has effaced even his function as manager, until he is a mere "method" by which the money manages itself: "...the method I am establishing through all the affairs...will be, I may hope, a machine in such working order as that [anyone] can keep it going" (372).

Apparent death becomes the only direct access to the essence and value of life. Apparent death is the condition of storytelling and regenerative change. It reveals the value of his own story: "Dead, I have found the true friends of my lifetime still as true, as tender, and as faithful as when I was alive, and making my memory an incentive to good actions done in my name" (372). As John Harmon becomes merely a name, a memory and a fortune, the nugget of value that the story of his life contained is scattered and proliferates. From this vantage point, John Harmon, like an omniscient narrator, can see the complete pattern and know its worth. Even better, like an omnipotent narrator, he can change the story to create more value. He does this by remaining apparently dead as John Harmon to win (disguised as a poor man) the love of the mercenary girl who would otherwise have married him simply for his money. Hence, although the final aim of the dust plot is to prevent Bella's reduction of herself to a commodity, its machinations all depend on Harmon's merger with the fortune, his organic death into it.

John Harmon's plot, then, demonstrates that value, even the value of Life itself, is only discoverable from some vantage point outside of the body. And the novel, moreover, repeatedly relocates value outside the body through processes that resemble the substitution of inorganic wealth for live bodies, even though the origin of wealth in bodies is never effaced. Hence, the fascination of the novel with macabre commodities. If the organic "death" of young John Harmon and his merger with his fortune is one example of the connection between money and the release of vital power, the commodities of Mr. Venus, a preserver of animals and birds and articulator of human skeletons, recapitulates the same point in a grotesquely comic form. While the consciousness of the living-dead John Harmon hovers around the Boffin residence as secretary, the mortal remains of the man whose death has enabled this suspended animation are themselves suspended, it would seem, in Venus's shop. "I took an interest in that discovery in the river," Venus tells Wegg. "I've got up there – never mind, though" (84). Venus buys and sells body parts and also labors to make them dry, stable and hence valuable. Of course, he also has a few fleshy organisms (various preserved babies), but most of his trade is in turning bodies into inorganic representations of themselves. It is this activity that releases value from the body and makes it a "living" for Venus but also bizarrely restores a kind of life to these bodies of representation themselves. As he hands a stuffed canary to a customer, Venus triumphantly remarks, "There's animation!" (81).

The same drawing out of value from the organic body and storing it up, suspending it, in the inorganic characterizes Jenny Wren's doll-making trade. Jenny imagines that the great ladies, whose clothes she copies to make her dolls' dresses, are working for her as models. She imagines that her own effort of "scud[ding] about town at all hours" (435) to see these fashionable clothes is matched by their owners' pains in trying on the dolls' dresses: "I am making a perfect slave of her" (436), she says of one of her "models." And the result of all this sweat is the thing of value, as in Mr. Venus's shop, the inorganic body: "That's Lady Belinda hanging up by the waist, much too near the gaslight for a wax one, with her toes turned in" (436).

All of this metaphoric and imagistic insistence on the bodily origins of the commodity and on its disembodiment, on its transcendence of its organic origins and simultaneous conversion into vital potential, finds its culmination in the explicit vitalism of Rogue Riderhood's revivification. In this episode, Life takes on its pure reality and absolute value only because it has been entirely disembodied. Rogue's body itself is merely a "dank carcase," and no one (besides Rogue's pathetic daughter) has any interest in the fate of the man himself. It is neither body nor spirit that is of concern in this scene, "but the spark of life within him is curiously separable from himself now, and they have a deep interest in it" (443). For the sake of this abstracted entity, "All the best means are at once in action, and every-body present lends a hand, and a heart and soul." But when that potential and hence essential Life begins to instantiate itself in the particular body of Rogue Riderhood, its value dissolves: "As he grows warm, the doctor and the four men cool. As his lineaments soften with life, their faces and their hearts harden to him" (446). "The spark of life," the narrator comments, "was deeply interesting while it was in abeyance" (447).

"Life in abeyance" characterizes not only the temporary condition of Rogue Riderhood but also the condition of John Harmon. As such, as we've seen, it's the condition underlying the narrative itself. Moreover, especially for those who insist most strenuously on the flesh and blood origins of economic value, "life in abeyance" is the definitive condition of commodities and their representation, money. As Rogue Riderhood's suspended animation clearly shows, the curious separation of Life from the body is the refinement and purification of vitality itself. Hence, the humanitarian attempt to place and hold the human body at the center of inquir-ies into the nature of value has a paradoxical result: it leaves the body suspended, apparently dead, while the newly valorized essence, vitality, achieves ever more inor-ganic and even immaterial representations.

This, then, was the destiny of the illth/wealth distinction and of the bio-economy on which it relied: those transfers of vitality that were at the heart of a body-centered economic theory kept proving the dependence of vitality on the suspension of ani-mation in the body, on its apparent death. In Dickens's novel, the illth/wealth dual-ity cannot be said to collapse, but the two terms enter into a dynamic fluctuation that breaks their immediate, one-to-one pairing with their supposed physiological reference points, illness and health. The storytelling, value-creating consciousness, like the consciousness of love, like economic value and the vital force itself are all released from bodies and only exist in their pure form while they remain outside of bodies. In the name of Life itself, the humanitarian critics of political economy repeat the logical trajectory of their antagonists and dislodge the body from the center of their discourse.

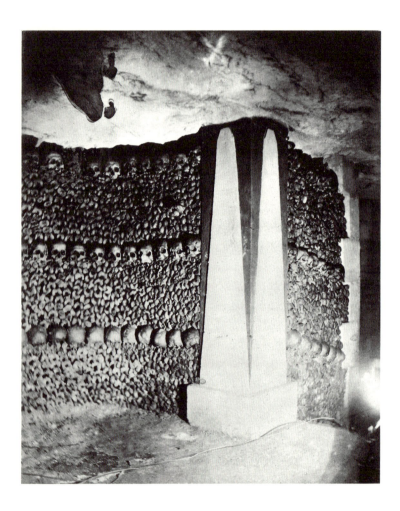

F. Nadar, In the Catacombs of Paris, 1861.

## Value: Wealth and Filth

Or perhaps it would be more accurate to say that the body remains at the center but is deanimated, that what remains at the center are the bodily remains. And this makes it necessary to attend to their disposal. *Our Mutual Friend* is not only interested in getting a living from dead or apparently dead bodies but also interested in getting a living from them as *garbage*, as waste that is being at once disposed of and retrieved, salvaged. We have already seen that in the novel corpse commodities remind us of the life-draining nature of all commodities and hence contain in themselves the illth/wealth duality. But in order to explain why the body should additionally be presented as potential waste and why the novel should be divided between a watery world and a dry, dusty one, I would like to conclude by turning briefly to a slightly different controversy, one that overlaps the concerns of political economy but is not identical to them: the controversy over urban sanitation.

It is difficult for us to recapture the metaphysical weight that sanitary issues bore in mid-Victorian England.[6] The question of how to dispose of decomposing matter was by no means merely technical. It was intermeshed, perhaps even more than political economy, with proofs of God's providence, of nature's beneficence, of human responsibility. There were heated debates over how to dispose of decomposing matter, but there was agreement that such matter had a deep dualism in its nature. It was both illth and wealth. One popular belief held that each nation had a God given capital of fertilizing elements which generated its food as interest. These fertilizing elements included human waste and decomposing human bodies. A way had to be found, sanitary reformers argued, to return this capital to the food-producing earth, for if it were not returned, it would, first, not bear sufficient interest as food to keep the population alive, and second, become itself the seed of death rather than life. For although there was considerable disagreement over how large concentrations of decomposing matter caused disease, everyone agreed that they did. Hence dead and decomposing human matter was organized into the sanitarian's bio-economy as both potential illth and wealth.

For many, the illth/wealth distinction was aligned with a distinction between wetness and dryness: decomposing matter allowed to rot in the river was illth; decomposing matter buried in the ground was wealth. The hero of Charles Kingsley's novel *Yeast* makes this distinction between the wet and the dry; he looks down at the Thames,

> at that huge, black-mouthed sewer, vomiting its pestilential riches across the mud. There it runs...hurrying to the sea vast stores of wealth, elaborated by Nature's chemistry into the ready materials of food; which proclaim, too, by their own foul smell, God's will that they should be buried out of sight in the fruitful, all-regenerating grave of earth; there it runs; turning them all into the seeds of pestilence, filth, and drunkenness. (ch. 15)

Dickens was a vocal supporter of sanitary reform, and he wrote *Our Mutual Friend* during a time when London was undergoing one of its greatest sanitizing projects, the embankment of the Thames. It is not surprising, then, that the book draws on these organizing concepts, imagining the Thames to be a potentially pestilential open sewer full of human refuse. The narrator describes the very waterfront as a place "where the accumulated scum of humanity seemed to be washed from higher grounds, like so much moral sewage, and to be pausing until its own weight forced it over the bank and sunk it in the river" (21). If political economy alone suggests the equation of commodity and life-drained body and suggests that the out-of-body state was the most valuable of all, it is the bio-economics of the sanitarians that lets us see why the novel arranges its inquiry into the nature of wealth around the disposal of human remains. It is within this discourse that the division of the novel's world into wet and dry begins to make sense, that the heroism and horror of dragging bodies out of the river comes into sharper focus. This is the discourse that allows us to understand why Bradley Headstone's internal rot expresses its essential sterility in images of churning water. It lets us understand, too, why the dust world is the place of transformations, why dryness and burial mounds would be the sites of regeneration. Further, it allows us to perceive the association between the river and the potential for tragedy. Characters in the river plot frequently undergo reduction; they have fewer and fewer options as the plot proceeds. On the other hand, the inhabitants of the dust world only apparently reduce themselves. As in the cases of John Harmon, Boffin and Bella, deathliness, insensibility, are only stages in the process of preserving and releasing vital power. That suspended animation on which the release and transfer of vitality depend requires removing the body from the river and entombing it, as Eugene's body is entombed, in a dry place.

Hence, if political economy provides the metaphors that allow value to rest on suspended animation and even to require discardable bodies, the bio-economics of the sanitarians gives us more insight into the novel's obsession with the disposal of the very bodies its own paradoxical logic keeps discarding. The recycling of such garbage–bodies, their conversion from illth to wealth, is the prototypical act of value-creation in this novel. In it, once again, the deanimated body, vitality and value become indistinguishable, causing the terms illth and wealth to lose their physiological reference points.

The whole richly contradictory and fertile mixture is perhaps best summed up in the novel's last conversation between Lizzie and Eugene. Eugene, like John Harmon and Rogue Riderhood, must undergo a period of apparent death, of suspended animation, and for Eugene this period follows Lizzie's retrieval of his garbage-body from the river, where it has been dumped, as John Harmon's was dumped, after a murder attempt. The two love plots work on a complicated series of parallels and inversions centering on images of suspended animation and discardable bodies, but it would take far too much time to trace those complexities here. The salient point for our purposes is that the period of suspended animation or apparent death is the moment when Eugene's life takes on value, and he is able, as John Harmon was able under similar circumstances, to give and receive love. Thus, the familiar pattern is repeated: suspending the body's animation allows the liberation of value.

But furthermore, since Eugene's apparent death is not accomplished with a surrogate body, the equation of the hero's own body first with floating refuse and then with a broken "thing," that is, the emphasis on the body as garbage, is far more pronounced in Eugene's story than it was in John Harmon's. In his speech to Lizzie as his body returns to a state of animation, he stresses this garbage–wealth equation by turning her into both: " 'You have thrown yourself away,' said Eugene, shaking his head. 'But you have followed the treasure of your heart... you had thrown that away first, dear girl!' " (753). Hence Eugene and Lizzie are equally garbage and treasure to one another; indeed, they are treasure because they are garbage. And it is therefore perfectly rational for Eugene to fear the returning health of his body: "in this maimed and broken state, you make so much of me." Lizzie can make much of him, add value to him, only while his body is thus broken. Only while the vitality is somewhere outside his body can he possess this treasure, which is the squandering of Lizzie's life.

And so we seem to be witnessing the regenerative inversion of the horrific life-transfer suggested in the opening scene, for now Lizzie's life becomes the wealth of the cadaver; instead of getting a living off the garbage–body, she spends her life on it. But in *Our Mutual Friend* reversals are never so neat. The expense of Lizzie's life is experienced by Eugene as a heavy debt: "It would require a life, Lizzie, to pay all; more than a life." Instead of inverting the novel's opening scene, Eugene's last words recapitulate it. There really is only one thing he can do to discharge his debt to Lizzie and keep himself in the condition of value he has achieved; we are right back where we started when Eugene concludes, "I ought to die, my dear."

*Our Mutual Friend* incessantly requires the body's suspension as a condition of the valuable life; illness unto death brings wealth. The location of both mortality and vitality, both fatality and regeneration, in decomposition makes us acutely aware that illth and wealth are alike abstractions from the body's particularity. They are alike poised on the vanishing point of those "full-breathed, bright-eyed, and happy-hearted human creatures" the literary humanitarians had set out to vindicate.

### The Apparent Death of the Author

It is remarkable that, despite Eugene's reference to the squandering of Lizzie's life, all of the commodity–corpses, the discarded and suspended bodies in *Our Mutual Friend*, are male. I would like very briefly to sketch an explanation of this fact by linking the apparent death of the male body both to the commodification of women and to this novel's presentation of the author.

The two main plots, as well as several of the subplots, are driven by attempts to save women from becoming commodities. Bella, having escaped the fate of passively "being made the property of others," must then be saved from offering herself on the marriage market. Lizzie is also vehemently opposed to being a passive item of exchange between her brother and Bradley Headstone and must be rescued from the fate of becoming Eugene's mistress, his "doll," and then presumably passing into the world of the common prostitute. The novel reworks this material in tragic, comic, sentimental, satirical and farcical modes in many of the minor plots as well. Even Pleasant Riderhood, who is engaged to Mr. Venus, expresses a fear of being confused with one of her fiancé's skeletal commodities. She breaks off the engage-

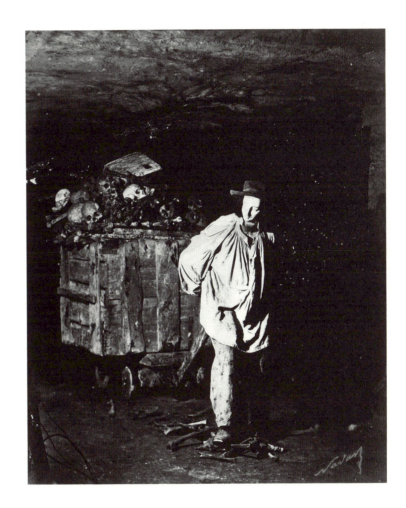

F. Nadar, In the Catacombs of Paris, 1861.

ment because "she does not wish to regard herself, nor yet to be regarded, in that boney light" (129).

Mr. Venus's solution to this problem, his plan for saving Pleasant from an identification with her body as commodity, is a humorous summary of the novel's operations: he promises to confine himself to the articulation of men. In this novel, then, women seem just naturally prone to commodification; but commodification is also the fate from which they must be rescued by men who preemptively enact the condition of suspended animation, the condition, as we have seen, of the commodity itself. Men are knocked out, drowned, dried out, stored up and finally reanimated ("There's animation!") so that women need not undergo any such self-alienation. The state of suspended animation is thus exclusively masculine in *Our Mutual Friend* because it is so naturally feminine.

This masculinity that is achieved through the incorporation of the feminine differs from femininity in its ability to survive its apparent death. Only the men are capable of holding "Life in abeyance"; only they have extra bodies at their disposal. Bella and Lizzie have no such out-of-body possibilities, and hence they are debarred from the process of releasing value and being released as value, as pure vital potential, as *potency* itself.

*Our Mutual Friend*, then, provides an example of how apparent lapses in identity, breaks in the continuity of the self and moments of self-alienation associated with the marketplace finally create the effect of an endlessly resilient, and in this case emphatically male, transcendent subject. Nowhere does this impression of broken, femininized and enhanced male selfhood appear more overwhelmingly than in the novel's postscript, where it is the impression of the author himself. The postscript superimposes a series of authorial impressions, among which the idea of Dickens as a principle of continuity suspended between the apparently discontinuous monthly parts of the novel. The final impression, though, is produced by an anecdote Dickens tells of a train accident that befell him as he was taking a monthly part of *Our Mutual Friend* to the printers. I will close with this last and final paragraph from the works of Charles Dickens:

> On Friday the Ninth of June in the present year, Mr. and Mrs. Boffin (in their manuscript dress of receiving Mr. and Mrs. Lammle at breakfast) were on the South Eastern Railway with me, in a terribly destructive accident. When I had done what I could to

help others, I climbed back into my carriage — nearly turned over a viaduct, and caught aslant upon the turn — to extricate the worthy couple. They were much soiled but otherwise unhurt.... I remember with devout thankfulness that I can never be much nearer parting company with my readers for ever, than I was then, until there shall be written against my life, the two words with which I have this day closed this book: — THE END The author heroically risks his life to deliver his manuscript in this passage and then apparently dies into that commodity, where he remains immortally suspended.

NOTES

1. *"Unto This Last" and Other Essays on Art and Political Economy*, ed. Ernest Rhys (New York, 1932), p. 169. All quotations from Ruskin are from this edition, and subsequent page numbers are given in the text.

2. *Our Mutual Friend* (London, 1974), p. 4. All previous quotations from the novel are from the Oxford University Press edition, and subsequent page numbers are given in the text.

3. The following argument is developed in detail in my article "The Body Versus the Social Body in the Works of Thomas Malthus and Henry Mayhew," *Representations* 14 (Spring 1986): pp. 83-106.

4. This discussion of the labor theory of value is admittedly extremely crude. It ignores the distinctions between Smith's and Ricardo's theories, and between imagining labor to be a common measure of exchange value and imagining it to be the source of that value. It also fails to touch on the issue of the relationship between exchange value and other forms of value as well as the vexed question of how the value of labor itself as a commodity might be either determined or measured. It follows Malthus's analysis of the flaw in Adam Smith's thinking, but I believe it is, nevertheless, accurate in its description of the central role both given to and denied to the laboring body in political economy.

5. Adam Smith, *The Wealth of Nations* (New York, 1970), p. 26.

6. This description of the sanitarian's debate is heavily indebted to Christopher Hamlin's excellent "Providence and Putrefaction: Victorian Sanitarians and the Natural Theology of Health and Disease," *Victorian Studies* 28 (Spring 1985), pp. 381-412.

zone

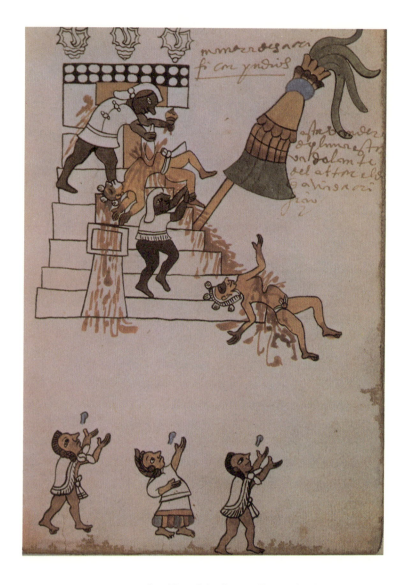

Sacrifice of the Aztecs. From a facsimile of the Tudela Codex, 1553
(Madrid, Museo de America).

# The Meaning of Sacrifice

*Christian Duverger*

***Potential Energy.*** To understand human sacrifice among the Aztecs we must realize that the human organism contains a considerable quantity of potential energy which, technically, can be released.

The Aztecs believed that the energy ration of each individual was determined at the moment of conception, when the *tonalli* descended from the thirteenth sky. At that moment, forces theretofore scattered throughout the universe were concentrated in the embryo; at the moment of birth they would give the newborn his vital autonomy. *Tonalli* means, in fact, "warmth of the sun"; a sunbeam is a *tonalmeyotl*, etc.[1] *Tonalli* partook of the sun and shared some of its qualities. A parcel of global Energy diluted in the cosmos, it also constituted the individual energy supply of each human being, what we might call his "radiance," to retain the solar and thermal connotations of the word.

*Tonalli* was an energy source connected exclusively with life. For example, when an Aztec healer was faced with a prolonged illness showing symptoms of listlessness, his first instinct was to determine whether the patient had lost his *tonalli*, which would portend imminent death. And if his examination confirmed this diagnosis, he would immediately use magical processes to find and recapture the lost *tonalli*. The loss of this energy, serious though it might be, was nonetheless quite frequent, and manifested itself in organic dysfunctions or pathological forms of chronic apathy.[2]

***Religious Organization.*** Every man was thus personally endowed with a charge of teleonomic power that we may refer to as vital energy. However — and this is where intervention became possible — this energy supply seems to have been disproportionate to the needs of life. *Tonalli* was profuse. Though neither unlimited nor infinite, its power far exceeded the necessities of bodily functions, growth and reproduction. This is why the Aztecs believed in a temporary life after death. For them, the dislocation of the human organism was never the result of a breakdown of energy, but, on the contrary, the occasion for the release of surplus energy. In other words, death was always an accident of fate, and no one ever died of old age. Since there was no reason for the excess energy to be consumed suddenly at the moment of death, it was thought to survive for a certain time. The Aztecs symbolically set the period of survival of this individual energy after death at four years. It is known that the Mexica believed that the number four represented stability, whereas five was associated with dissolution, destruction and annihilation.

There are texts that give precise accounts of beliefs concerning the afterlife. After death came the long and arduous journey to Mictlan, the place of the dead.[3] This trek through the underworld was strewn with obstacles: the dead person had to traverse eight jagged mountains and eight parched deserts, face a serpent and brave the glacial "obsidian-bladed wind." At the end of his journey, he reached the nine rivers of hell. "And when four years had passed, the dead arrived at the nine lands of death, where a wide river flows.... It is said that as they strode, they looked at the dogs on the opposite bank. And when a dog had recognized his master, he would jump into the water to fetch him and help him cross....[4] Then, in the nine lands of death, he would perish."[5] The verb *popoloa*, used to describe the end of these wanderings, connotes the ideas of dissipation, destruction, depletion and effacement.[6] Thus, there is no ambiguity: the soul's energy did not outlive the body eternally. The subterranean saga in which the dead were hurled from one ordeal to the next drained them totally. The significance of this hellish adventure becomes clear when one realizes that the Aztecs situated Mictlan in the north, beneath *teotlalli*, that "divine land" from which the Tribe issued. The voyage toward Mictlan was basically a return to the source; the end of the journey was an affirmation of absolute origins. The cycle was complete when all traces of individual existence beyond the river of hell were obliterated.

Viewed from the perspective of life, this postmortem dissipation of energy is clearly wasteful. The trek toward Mictlan was a solitary one, and any consumption of energy for private use was thought to drain potential communal forces. Aztec leaders attempted, therefore, to recycle, for the benefit of the living, the power of the *tonalli* freed by the decomposition of the human organism. Death became a source of energy.

## Energy from Destruction

Putting death to the service of life, sacrifice appears at first glance to be a paradox. It was, however, part of a coherent worldview. Death was thought always to release surplus vital energy, but in cases of natural death, this energy was driven underground, dispersed in the depths of the earth, where it could no longer be used by the living. A way had to be found, then, to stop its escape at the moment of death in order to capture and reuse its life-giving qualities. Since the natural process of death released energy, interrupting the natural course of life would likewise prevent this uncontrolled dissipation of energy. It is thus necessary to influence and even regulate the death rate in order to recuperate life forces. Therefore, ritual murder became a way of storing energy.

Human sacrifice by the Aztecs constitutes, indeed, a practical application of a curious physical phenomenon: if destroying life released energy, then it was only by ritualizing this destruction that the energy could be harnessed. It was the disruption of natural continuity — *rhegma* — that reversed the movement of decomposition. Forestalling the inexorable course of nature transformed the loss of force into a surge of power. Sacrifice, thus, was not so much a question of killing people as it was of killing life. Through the artificial interruption of vital movement, "negentropy" was born.

Thus, sacrifice was not the result of some inhuman, gratuitous barbarism. It was essentially a technology. Of course, for our culture which knows only symbolic sacrifice, such as the Eucharist, the Aztec practices remain puzzling and their efficacy suspect. And yet, it seems that today we use a similar principle for purposes of energy production, in ways that strangely echo the quest of the ancient Mexica. What is the principle behind the splitting of the atom? It aims precisely at the destabilization of certain elements for the purpose of releasing nuclear energy. With the discovery that smashing the nucleus of the atom liberates some of its binding energy, hasn't modern physics penetrated the secret spirit of sacrifice?

The atomic model allows us to carry the analogy further. It confirms in particular the necessity for the artificial disruption of the natural state. It is known that a large number of elements possess naturally radioactive isotopes. Their nuclei, which are unstable, disintegrate spontaneously at periods characteristic of each element. The behavior of this natural radioactivity corresponds to the dissipation of energy in people. Taken to the extreme, it demonstrates the dangerous way that movement slides into immobility, because the endpoint of instability, the stability marked by the cessation of radiation, follows an intense release of energy.

On the other hand, man can split the atom artificially, thereby creating a powerful source of energy. Although the phenomenon of breakdown remains structurally identical, human intent changes its implications. In practice, man must instigate and organize the process in order to exploit its results. But whether he bombards a stable nucleus in order to break it, or he increases the instability of nuclei that are already radioactive in order to induce fission, it is always by causing the breakdown of the atom that man assumes control of the element and can channel the forces released by its disintegration. Does the sacrificial knife not play the same role in Aztec society as the atomic reactor or the particle accelerator in our contemporary society?

What is certain is that just as we feel we are making good use of the atom, the ancient Mexica felt that they were gaining something by the purposeful destruction of life. Their belief in the afterlife of warriors killed in battle testifies to the efficacy they attributed to sacrifice. "Brave warriors, eagles and jaguars that died in war went there, to heaven, to the house of the Sun."[7] The expression "to die in battle" naturally covered sacrificial death, which was the price of combat. Furthermore, the chronicler Sahagún's informants specify clearly: "All those shall go to heaven, to the house of the Sun, who die in war, whether they perish on the battlefield or whether they be captured and killed afterward. They died then, flayed or thrown into fire, or pierced by arrows, or smeared with resin. They all went to the house of the Sun."[8] "And they lived in the east, where the Sun rises. And when the Sun was getting ready to rise, while it was still night, they dressed and armed themselves for war, and marched off to meet the Sun. They pushed it out of the darkness; and they uttered war cries to make it rejoice. They led attacks before it and gladdened it thus. And they carried it to the middle of the sky, to its zenith, to its apogee."[9]

What lies behind these images of popular belief? Is it enough to see in the "paradise" promised to warriors the worthy reward of courage and daring? No, for these dead warriors were not simply honorary figures in the company of the Sun. It is specifically declared that by their death they helped the Sun to rise, and that they carried it and raised it to its apogee. In other words, they brought energy to Energy, they helped supply the reserves of force that were symbolized and embodied by the sun.

The warriors were aided in this task by women who had died in childbirth, the *mociuaquetzque*. Indeed, bringing a child into the world was identified with an act of war, with taking a captive.[10] The woman who died in childbirth thus, by analogy, was promised the afterlife of a warrior. "Women who died in childbirth lived there in the sky, where the Sun sets. . . .[11] And when the Sun was already far along on its path, the women dressed and armed themselves for war; they put on their shields and standards; then they rose toward the zenith to meet the Sun. There, eagles and jaguars held the Sun in their hands. And those warriors, eagles and jaguars, those who had died in war, passed the Sun over to the women. . . . Then it was the women's turn; they brought the Sun down on a palanquin of green feathers, uttering war cries to make it happy. In this way they carried the Sun until it set."[12] This touching depiction of the sun's dependence on people may be compared with other texts, where we see the sun avidly seeking nourishment and guidance. The sun needed an escort to lead the way, for its astral course was a battle that it could not wage alone. It also needed to be carried; the gleaming palanquin allowed it to conserve its energy. And it was the warriors killed in battle — sacrificed on the altar of life — who were chosen to officiate.

This afterlife lasted four years. Then the Sun's acolytes were metamorphosed. Transformed into hummingbirds or butterflies, "here on earth, they sipped nectar from all kinds of flowers."[13]

The consequences of sacrificial death were clearly very different from those of natural death. Underground wanderings are symmetrically contrasted with a march through the heavens alongside the Sun. But whereas the subterranean afterlife was strictly individual, draining away into total disintegration and leading to nothingness, the celestial afterlife of the warriors became a source of vital energy on which the entire community could draw. As they support the sun, the victims' souls service society by supplying energy. And the metamorphosis of those killed in sacrifice into hummingbirds or butterflies, creatures of the sun, completed the process of transforming their afterlife into something tangible. This contrasts with the dissolving function of the *Chiconauhmictlan*, which obliterated forever all traces of existence.

If sacrifice led to the release and recycling of *tonalli* energy, this was undoubtedly, in the Aztec view, because it made use of the principle of destruction. From this point of view, it is instructive to note that in the eyes of the Mexica, *tonalli* became social energy only at the moment of birth. It was the coming into being that released the existential energy, and it did so because this was essentially a process of rupture. This explains why birth was identified with death.[14] There must always be a disturbance in equilibrium, a break in continuity so that life force may be released. The ritual murder of sacrifice, far from being an aberration in the cultural behavior of the Aztecs, fitted perfectly into the logic of their beliefs.

### Games and Death

For the Aztecs, human sacrifice was in no way a hidden act perpetrated in the holy of holies of some distant sanctum by an occult sect of sacrificial priests. The culmination of the Mexica's social life, ritual murder was, on the contrary, surrounded with public rites. A preparatory ritual which was, in one form or another, a sort of game, preceded the sacrifice. Then, finally, the climax of the performance was the ceremonially ritualized killing. These are the two aspects of Aztec sacrifice that we will study closely.

*The Performance.* Sacrificial ceremonies dominated nearly the entire rite. And the ritual established a true "theater of cruelty" complete with that "concrete bite at the heart and the senses" that so intrigued Antonin Artaud.[15] However, Aztec pageantry was characterized by two peculiarities: on the one hand, the prelude to sacrifice was highly ritualized, and on the other, the presacrificial rites were essentially a type of game. Whereas games were prohibited and systematically denounced in official pronouncements, they had an important, institutionalized role in preparations for sacrifice.

*General Proceedings.* Presacrificial games were governed by extremely simple rules: in all cases, they involved intense physical activity; they brought on strenuous exertion and fatigue; and they were mandatory for all victims designated for sacrifice. Within this basic framework there were many variations, but one mandatory element remained constant – the vigil (*tozoztli, tozoliztli*). Even in those exceptional cases where sacrifice was not accompanied by a particularly elaborate ceremony, there was the ritual wake, with its obligatory complement of dances and songs. During the festival of Panquetzaliztli, for example, the slaves' masters took the victims to the temple at Pochtlan. "And there," reports Sahagún, "they were forced to stay up the whole night, singing and dancing."[16] The Nahuatl text specifies that on this occasion the snake dance was performed: "The dancers stood in line, took one another's hand, and formed a large circle.... At top speed they ran, jumped, moved about breathlessly.... And the old men of the area played the drums and sang for them."[17]

During the eighth month of the year, a woman representing the corn goddess Xilonen had to die. "On the eve of the sacrifice, the whole night was spent singing hymns in honor of the goddess: the men and women stayed up all night, not sleeping for an instant; no one closed his eyes, and hymns to Xilonen were sung. At daybreak the dancing began."[18] At other times musicians were brought in to keep the sacrificial victims awake. "At night, the vigil was held at the temple of Tlaloc. Drums beat, flutes played, conch shells were sounded, people sang, the *teponaztli* growled, and sticks were banged together. It was thus that those symbols of the rain gods who were to be sacrificed were kept awake."[19]

No victim was spared this sacred vigil, not even the young children who were sacrificed to the Tlaloques in the first month of the year in order to bring rain. "When the procession had reached the altar of Tozocan, the 'place of the vigil,' those little creatures were kept up the whole night, with priests singing to them to keep them from falling asleep."[20]

The principle of these presacrificial vigils is clear: the prospective victim must first be provoked to fatigue and bodily depletion. Added to sleep deprivation was a four-day fast or a dose of various sedatives or stimulants. The condemned were generally forced to drink *teooctli*, the divine *octli*, until they showed the first signs of intoxication.[21] Or else they were forced to inhale aromatic herbs or mind-clouding perfumes. And in this heavy atmosphere, to the droning rhythms of flutes and drums, without stopping, without a moment's respite, they were forced to dance to the point of exhaustion.

Sometimes the presacrificial dances were not limited to the night before sacrifice, but started several days earlier. Thus, at the "little festival of the lords," the woman chosen to incarnate the salt goddess Uixtociuatl was forced to dance nonstop

for ten days while wearing the ornaments of the goddess. "Covered with these adornments, she danced with women who were also singing and dancing to keep up her
spirits. They all held each other with garlands of flowers and on their heads wore
wreaths made of that fragrant herb called *iztauhyatl* that is like Castille incense. . . .
And the woman who represented Uixtociuatl stayed in the middle. She sang and
danced for ten days with the other women, and after ten days had passed, she began
the vigil; for the whole night, without sleeping, without resting, she danced the
*mitote*, propped up on the arms of the old women. At the same time the male captives who were to be sacrificed before her the next day likewise danced."[22] This
exhausting ludic marathon was a truly hallucinatory spectacle, during which the goddess, staggering with fatigue, overwhelmed by pulsating rhythms and the intoxicat-
ing odors of flowers, had to hang onto the arms of her acolytes to fulfill, beyond
the point of exhaustion, her painful presacrificial dancing duties.

The fact that something as innocuous as dancing could be made into an epic
endurance test in order to fulfill its ritual function is ample evidence of the importance of the presacrificial play activity. And the example of the goddess Uixtociuatl
is far from exceptional. Strenuous exertion, often bordering on overt violence, was
indeed the general rule.

*The Role of Presacrificial Games.* The Aztec attitude toward play seems paradoxical. This was a frugal culture that codified the smallest gesture in terms of efficacy
and proportion. Strenuously opposed to wastefulness, it naturally prohibited any type
of game that depleted energy and concentration. Why then was this forbidden play
activity officially and ostentatiously incorporated into the ritual of human sacrifice?
How could the Mexica reconcile the condemnation of the principle and the insti-
tutionalization of the practice? The answer is simply that the presacrificial games
served a practical purpose that became clear once they were completed.

## From Stimulation to Intoxication

Games are, undeniably, stimulating. They induce a state of excitement in the player,
a specific tension that affects his bodily functions. Games thus mobilize forces that
are usually dormant, drawing upon potential energy that is ordinarily untapped. We
might think, then, that games were purposely used by the Aztecs to concentrate in

the victim the maximum intensity of energy before sacrifice in order to reinforce the effectiveness of the ritual murder.

But we must bear in mind a particular characteristic of the presacrificial rituals. If, from the outside, they seem to have the formal structure of games, they were not played for the sake of play. Beyond the games, there was a trance; beyond the trance, exhaustion. Pushed to the point of no return, the game transcended play, transcended itself in an efficacious and spectacular death by sacrifice.

The presacrificial games seem, then, to have been an application of the logic of total stimulation. Agitating the organism to the extreme was thought to tap the energy reserves of the afterlife, a sizable stock that was ordinarily inviolable, even in the case of natural death. Only the brutality of death by sacrifice could release those forces jarred by the excesses of the presacrificial games. It was thus not the games that drained, destroyed, "emptied" those who were sacrificed; death remained the ultimate instrument of destruction.

Finally, the presacrificial games were not merely a catalyst for the successful outcome of the ritual, but also a precondition for the entire process. Physically, the sacrificial process was facilitated by the agitated state of the victim: the more a system is disturbed, the more easily it breaks down. The organic instability produced by the excitement of the games made the body physiologically more vulnerable, thus facilitating the breakdown of the binding energies.

On a more practical level, the presacrificial games were a way of ensuring the compliance of those who were destined to die. For the treatment inflicted on the victims generally left them dazed, in a sort of secondary state where bodily weakness outweighed panic. It was only at this price that the victims could climb onto the sacrificial altar with apparent resignation. Naturally, there were no policemen guarding the captives, no soldiers forcibly dragging the victims off to execution. Sacrifice was not a punishment[23] and it should never be viewed as a repressive and barbarous act. A ritual in every way, it must be understood as a mystical and magnificent religious act. But to make sure that the system of sacrifice, which was the basis of a particular social order, would not be publicly repudiated by a captive resisting the knife of the sacrificial priest, adequate precautions had to be taken.

Fatalism was an important part of Aztec culture. The principle of predestination was not questioned, and sacrificial destiny could be readily accepted as inevitable.

In addition, Aztec leaders could draw upon a whole range of "ideology" from the classic appeal to courage to the promise of a pleasing and glorious hereafter. These arguments must have appealed to the sensibilities of the warriors who were perpetually conditioned to die with dignity. "O Tezcatlipoca," reads one prayer addressed to the god of war, "grant that all eagle-warriors and jaguar-warriors be worthy. May they all be promised to sacrifice.... May their hearts feel no fear. May they taste the sweetness of obsidian-bladed death. May the double-edged knife bring joy to their hearts...." Further on, referring to warriors killed in combat or in sacrifice: "May their throats and stomachs find repose in the embrace of our mother, our father, the Sun, the lord of the earth.... Everlasting is their abundance, their joy. They sip the nectar of flowers,[24] their chosen flowers, the flowers of joy and happiness...."[25]

If this ideal of virile stoicism in the face of death dictated the behavior of prisoners of war, what was its significance for slaves, women and children? The chroniclers stress that sacrifice was valued as a near godlike honor, and that the victims, therefore, showed no reluctance to undertake this mission.

Nevertheless, the body recoiled instinctively before death. The ecstatic, hallucinatory games that preceded sacrifice seem specifically designed to ensure the composure of the victims. And on careful study of the texts, we realize that, more often than not, the condemned reached the foot of the temple not with head held high and looking straight ahead, but worn and bruised, haggard and drained, like those warriors whose flesh had been flayed in cruel gladiatorial combat, or like the staggering, drugged women who had just danced for ten days without stopping.

Just as the bullfighter's *banderillas* provoke the bull, but also make him bleed, the Aztec's presacrificial games had the effect of both stimulating and weakening the victims.

## The Energy Offering

The value of the presacrificial games derived from their communal character. Individual games, indeed, were officially frowned on because they dissipated energy in ways that were both selfish and gratuitous. But sacrifice and its prelude may be viewed as the archetype of the gift, the offering of an individual or of a restricted group of individuals to society as a whole. Let us consider, for example, the manner in which the captive passed from the hands of his master to those of the priests responsible for the sacred public ceremony. "The day before the prisoners were to die, their captors started dancing at noon. And until midnight, they held a vigil for their captives in their neighborhood temple. And in the middle of the night, they led their prisoners before the fire and cut off a lock of their hair from the crown of the head.... But it was the priests who sacrificed the prisoners. Those who had captured them did not themselves do the killing; they brought them forth as tribute, handed them over as offerings; then the priests seized them, dragging them by the hair to the top of the pyramid."[26]

The rite of cutting off a lock of hair is rich in meanings. It can be interpreted, I believe, as a symbolic death, the death of the captive as possessor of an individual existence. From that point on, he was in a state of stay of execution, deprived of all autonomy, belonging to the indistinct social body, in the realm of his cosmic destiny.

Everything connected with hair in the Aztec world remains mysterious. Nevertheless, much evidence leads us to believe that hair (*tzontli*) was perceived as the seat of the individual's psychic force. It seems to have harbored a certain form of vital power, perhaps even the *tonalli*. For example, sorcerers from whom, unbeknownst to them, a lock of hair had been cut lost their supernatural powers.[27] The flowing hair of courtesans exerted a powerful force of attraction. And the lock of hair shorn from prisoners of war was kept as a talisman and proof of bravery by the captor. Depending on the conditions and circumstances of capture and sacrifice, the trophy-lock was either placed on the inside of the shield used in combat, or suspended from the support beam of the house, or even buried in the ground near the victorious warrior's house.[28] The prisoner, once dispossessed of the warrior's lock of hair, no longer belonged to himself any more than he belonged to his captor; he had become a communal offering and his master kept nothing more than the image of his victory in the form of a lock of hair.

The question remains: Did the presacrificial games draw their value solely from their intimate connection with sacrifice or did they contain their own ultimate justification? All evidence points to the latter. The games were not simply a prelude to the offering: they were in themselves an offering of the most precious matter venerated by the Aztecs — energy. This ritual outflow of energy, far from contradicting the principles of the Mexica economy, was an application of the universal formula

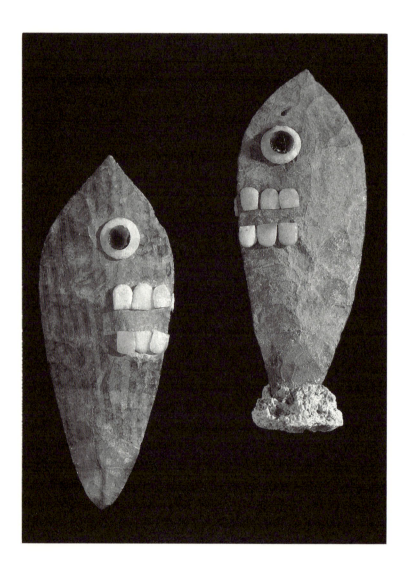

Aztec sacrificial knives (Mexico, Templo Mayor).

for ritual destruction: offer up the part to save the whole, thereby becoming the creditor of the gods.

The presacrificial games were not, then, an anarchic outburst, a conspicuous deviation from Aztec frugality. They played their role in the implacable plan of resistance set up to furnish society with energy resources adequate to its needs and its ambitions.

### The Killing

The killing of the sacrificial victims followed a special rite that was completely distinct from the preparatory games. In the Aztec universe, the quintessential form of human sacrifice was excision of the heart, though naturally, in a society that practiced sacrifice en masse, other forms, such as decapitation and burning, were also known.

*The Archetypal Scenario.* "There were so many diabolical instruments, such as horns, trumpets, cutlasses, and so many burned Indian hearts, with smoke curling around the idols, all congealed with blood, that I would like to send them all to the devil!"[29] Crude and brutal as it is, this exclamation of terrified disgust gives a good summary of the conquistadors' reactions to the bloody practices of the Aztecs. This custom was proof, furthermore, to the conquerors that the religion of Mexico was nothing but idolatry and the work of the devil. As a result, the Spanish chroniclers wrote extensively, if not objectively, on the subject. We can, however, compare their accounts with Nahuatl texts and pre-Hispanic pictographic documents that describe the theme of sacrifice and give us a fairly precise account of this violent, apparently barbaric, rite.[30]

Ordinary sacrifice, the type most commonly practiced, was accomplished by ripping out the heart. For this purpose, the Aztecs used a rounded sacrificial stone, the *techcatl*, which, from the side, looked like a block that was about one meter high and curved at the top.[31] The victim was stretched out over it, back arched and head thrown back nearly touching the ground. Five priests clasped the arms, legs and head of the victim, whose chest pointed toward the sky. The sacrificial priest slashed open the upper abdomen, just below the ribcage, with a flint knife, the *tecpatl*. He then plunged his hand into the chest, grabbed the victim's heart and tore it out, offering it to the sun before placing it in a ceremonial container. Another priest stuck a straw into the open wound and drew out blood, which he splashed generously onto the victim's body. The lifeless cadaver was then thrown from the top of the pyramid down to the bottom of the steps, where his master gathered it up. Meanwhile, at the top of the temple, the chest of another victim had already been carved open.

These are the broad outlines of the sacrificial act as described in many accounts.[32] In some, colorful descriptions are a combination of naiveté and realistic observation, as in these passages by the chronicler Diego Durán: "In the place where the sacrifice was to take place were those butchers and ministers of the devil. They sacrificed the victims by carving open their chests and removing their hearts, and threw them, half-alive, from the top of the temple, whence they rolled all the way to the bottom of the steps, bathed in blood."[33] He continues: "With a knife dropped onto his chest, a man could be sliced open as easily as a pomegranate."[34] Or: "The sacrificer…stretched his hand out in the air to offer the heart to the sun, held it out this way just long enough for an *Ave Maria*, then threw it down to the idols."[35]

Despite the embellishments, the various stages of sacrifice are accurately reported. The most striking thing about this way of administering death is that the knife wound was not intended to kill the victim, but simply to open his chest, allowing the sacrificial priest to plunge his hand into the viscera and rip out the still-beating heart of the sacrificial victim. On this point, all sources agree. Furthermore, several Nahuatl texts provide us with a precise idea of the terminology connected with sacrifice. "The priests laid the captive down on the stone, opened his chest, slit it open: then they cut out the heart, broke the heart strings."[36] To break the vena cava and aorta "as one snaps a thread," the priests used a flint knife: strictly speaking, this was the moment of death. The extraction of the heart was already an offertory gesture.

The description of this cruel and bloody sacrifice makes clear the necessity for a tranquilizing prelude, for other than the drugs sometimes taken during the dances and the introductory games, there was no provision for anesthetization or narcotic substances before the killing. The process must have been all the more painful in that it was done with a firmly mounted, double-edged, spear-shaped flint knife.

Though the main features of killing remained constant in all sacrifices, details varied with the different festivals. Thus, the sacrifices were always conducted by priests (*tlamacazque tlamictizque*), but not always by the same ones. In general, the sacrificer was the high priest of the divinity being honored. In any case, sacrifice seems to have been an exclusively male ministry, apparently a question of custom rather than one of physical strength. Indeed, in medicine bleedings were always done by men.

Variations in the sacrificial ritual involved not only the place of execution but also the time. Sacrifices of solar character took place at noon. This was the case for the festival of Nahui-ollin and the festivals held during the month of Quecholli, celebrated in honor of the god of the hunt. Most often, sacrifices took place at dawn[37] or during the day.[38] But there were also night sacrifices dedicated, for example, to Tlaloc,[39] the planet Venus[40] or the chthonic gods.

A series of details "personalized" the sacrifices proper to each god. When a young man, who had been living for a year like the god Tezcatlipoca, was to die, he climbed to the top of the temple unaccompanied and of his own free will, breaking a flute on each step of the staircase. And his body, instead of being flung haphazardly from the top of the pyramid as custom dictated, was carefully carried down by four of the god's servants. When the women personifying mountains in the festival of Tepeilhuitl were to die, they were carried up on litters to the site of the sacrifice by women. When Uixtociuatl died, the jagged-edged spur of the sawfish was placed on her throat.

It would be pointless to go into detail about all the variants of the fantastic Aztec ritual. Let us simply note that the differences in ceremony in no way affected the fundamental gestures of sacrifice: excision and removal of the victim's heart. The variations concerning the ritual of execution were, however, a response to certain mythological and religious imperatives. Sacrifice was always a performance, and the gestures of the gods represented were governed by an intricate set of details to which the Aztecs reverently adhered.

**The Fundamental Duality.** To say that sacrifice was a form of sun worship is an oversimplification and misinterpretation. Strictly speaking, this formulation is, of course, correct. But we must not lose sight of the dual identity of the Sun, which is at once diurnal and nocturnal. The Aztecs considered this astral body to be not only a creature of light: they attributed to it as well a subterranean, shadowy life that was just as important as its heavenly life. Its nocturnal course was perceived to be a trip through hell, a passage through the bowels of the earth. This is why the sun, in its overall life-bearing quality — what I have referred to elsewhere as the abstract Sun — was always designated by the two-part name Tonatiuh Tlaltecutli, "Sun, Lord of the Earth." Sacrifice made to the Sun thus had a double significance, both solar and earthly, and was the expression of a remarkable complementarity.

In the type of sacrifice by abdominal incision and extraction of the heart, there are two main symbolic components — heart and blood. The solar connotation concerns more precisely the heart element (*yollotl*). They called the sacrificed captives' hearts *quauhnochtli tlazotlil* (the eagle's precious Barbary figs). They seized them and held them up to the sun, the turquoise prince, the flaming eagle. In this way, they nourished it, fed it. And when they had offered the hearts, they placed them in the *quauhxicalli* (the eagle's vase).[41] And they called the captives killed in sacrifice *quauhteca* (men of the eagle).[42] We know that the eagle was the twin of the Sun, one of its figurations in the symbolic world. Everything connected with the eagle thus connoted energy. Numerous paintings, manuscripts and bas-reliefs represent the eagle holding a bloody heart in its claws: this is the familiar image of the Sun feeding on human hearts. In iconography and statuary, the Sun is also represented with the features of the jaguar (*ocelotl*), and thus assumes an image of voracity.

It is perhaps unnecessary to dwell at greater length here on the solar dimension of sacrifice. This is the most obvious and frequently described aspect of all. On the other hand, the earthly side, perhaps because it is less spectacular, is sometimes neglected by analysts. But it complements perfectly the astral dimension of sacrifice.

The earth, indeed, was subject to the law of the cosmos, which is to say, for the Aztecs, an inexorable tendency toward loss and decay. The agricultural rites were therefore not abstract or allegorical fertility rites. Like all Nahua religious acts, they were part of a larger work of revitalization. For example, the characteristic ceremonial tool of the agricultural divinities was the *chicauaztli*, a type of digging stick fitted with a bell, whose purpose was to summon the rain. The word *chicaua* means to revitalize, to strengthen, to bring to life."[43] Beating the *chicauaztli*, rhythmically on the ground, was thus a symbolic sowing of vital forces. The earth had to be nourished in order to be fruitful, in turn. In this perspective, human sacrifice may be viewed, in part as an agricultural rite, with the sacrificial element bearing the earthly value being the blood (*eztli*).

There are countless methods of torture and killing. Sacrifice by tearing out the heart does not seem a priori to be the simplest or the most natural technique. We may therefore infer that it was the result of a deliberate choice made by this society. What is its most striking clinical characteristic? Certainly the amount of bloodshed that results from it. According to experts, excision of the heart by severing the vena cava and the aorta would quickly spill five or six litres of blood.[44] This is the most dramatic hemorrhaging that could be obtained by any means of slaughter. Must we not then infer that the Aztecs instituted this type of sacrifice precisely in order to release the greatest quantity of blood possible? This blood, spurting from the victims, was the precious "jade water," that indispensable *chalchiuatl*, providing energy in the form of agricultural fertility.

If the human hearts destined for sacrifice to the Sun constituted a solid food, the liquid blood was naturally a drink. It was the Lord of the Earth, the chthonic face of the Sun, who drank it; the earth drank this "precious water" in the same way that it absorbed the rains that periodically watered the Mexican fields. This is why Tlaltecutli was always represented as a monster, with a sacrificial knife emerging from his wide-open mouth, ready to gobble up the waves of human blood spilled for him on the altars of Tenochtitlan.

NOTES

1. Fray G. de Molina, *Vocabulario en lengua castellana y mexicana* (1571), ed. Antonio de Spinola (Facsimile: Mexico: Porrúa, 1970).

2. On the loss of *tonalli*, cf. in particular Ruiz de Alarcon, *Tratado de los supersticiones....* (Mexico: Ediciones Fuente cultural, 1953), pp. 136-38.

3. I am speaking here of beliefs that are strictly Aztec. Underground peregrinations are the rule. However, we must note that the Aztecs borrowed from the natives a belief in an eternal earthly paradise, Tlalocan, a place of abundant vegetation located on the coast of the Gulf of Mexico. This particular hereafter was reserved exclusively for those men or women designated by Tlaloc, as, for example, those who had died of dropsy or drowning.

4. A yellow dog was always sacrificed during funerals to allow the dead person to overcome the final obstacle in his journey.

5. "Auh in oncan chiconamictlan oncan ocempopoliooa"; cf. Fray Bernardino de Sahagún, *Historia*

general de las cosas de Nueva España (1582), 4 vols. (Mexico: Porrúa, 1956). Trans. by Charles E. Dibble and Arthur J.O. Anderson as *Florentine Codex: General History of the Things of New Spain*, 13 vols. (Santa Fe: University of Utah and School of American Research, 1950-55), vol. 4, p. 42.

6. Molina, *Vocabularia*, vol. 2, p. 83r.

7. Sahagún, *Florentine Codex*, vol. 7, p. 162.

8. *Ibid.*, vol. 4, p. 47.

9. *Ibid.*, vol. 7, p. 162.

10. The conception of a child seems precisely to have summoned, attracted, focused and concentrated energy flows heretofore dispersed throughout the cosmos. At the moment of birth, the midwife joyously uttered war cries, "for the new mother had just fought a good fight; she had become a brave warrior; she had won a captive, she had captured a baby." *Ibid.*, vol. 7, p. 167.

11. This is why the west was called *ciuatlampa*, "the women's side."

12. *Ibid.*, vol. 7, p. 163.

13. *Ibid.*, vol. 4, p. 48.

14. *Ibid.*, vol. 2, p. 183.

15. Cf. Antonin Artaud, *The Theater and Its Double* (New York: Grove, 1958), p. 131.

16. Sahagún, *Florentine Codex*, vol. 3, p. 52.

17. *Ibid.*, vol. 3, p. 132.

18. *Ibid.*, vol. 3, p. 98.

19. On the Festival of Etzalqualiztli: *ibid.*, vol. 3, p. 83.

20. *Ibid.*, vol. 1, p. 141.

21. Cf., for example, *ibid.*, vol. 3, p. 52.

22. *Ibid.*, vol. 1, pp. 172-73.

23. The death penalty was part of the Aztec penal code, and it was even often applied. But in those cases, the methods of killing were totally different from those used in the rite of sacrificial death. The death penalty could be administered by strangulation, beating, stoning or arrows.

24. Warriors offered in sacrifice were metamorphosed four years later into hummingbirds or butterflies (cf. *supra*, end of "Energy from Destruction").

25. Warrior's prayer at Tezcatlipoca: Sahagún, *Florentine Codex*, vol. 7, pp. 12-13.

26. *Ibid.*, vol. 3, p. 46; see also p. 106.

27. *Ibid.*, vol. 1, pp. 335 and 358.

28. We have little information on the reasons for these variations. The three cases are brought up in the texts with no mention of their particular significance. The knife used for cutting the

hair was called *itztlotli*, "the obsidian falcon."

29. Bernal Díaz del Castillo, *Historia, biografia y geografia de la Nueva España* (1568) (Reprint: Buenos Aires: Espasa-Calpe, 1955), ch. 92, p. 200.

30. In particular: *Codex Laud*, pls. 1 and 8; *Codex Nuttall*, pls. 3, 69, 81; *Codex Selden*, vol. 2, pl. 12; *Codex Borgia*, pls. 19, 21, 33, 40, 42, 45.

31. See, for example, *Codex Nuttall*, pl. 3; *Codex Borgia*, pl. 42.

32. Numerous descriptions in Sahagún, *Florentine Codex*: cf. vol. 3, pp. 46-47, 52, 68, 165, etc.

33. Diego Durán, *Historia de los Indios de Nueva España y Islas de tierra firme*, 2 vols. (Mexico: Ediciones nacional, 1951), vol. 2, p. 86.

34. *Ibid.*, p. 93.

35. *Ibid.*, p. 104.

36. "*quioalteca techcac, coneltequi quioalixtlapana in iielchiquiuh: niman ie concotona, contlatzcotona in yollo*" in Sahagún, *Florentine Codex*, vol. 3, p. 108.

37. E.g., during the seventh, tenth and fifteenth months.

38. E.g., during the first, second, and fifth months.

39. Sixth month.

40. Sahagún, *Florentine Codex*, vol. 3, p. 172.

41. *Quauhxicalli* comes from *quauhtli*, "eagle," and *xicalli*, "gourd," by extension, "container." We therefore do not agree with the translation by Rémi Siméon, who proposes "wooden dish," bringing in the word *quauitl*, "wood." Cf. Siméon, *Dictionnaire de la langue Nahuatl* (Graz, 1963), p. 371. The context suggests a continuing reference to the eagle, and archaeology teaches us that the *quauhxicalli* were usually made of stone.

42. Sahagún, *Florentine Codex*, vol. 3, p. 47.

43. Molina, *Vocabularia* 19: pt. 2.

44. Cf. Dr. Louis Captian, "Les sacrifices humains et l'anthropologie rituelle chez les anciens Mexicains," *Journal de la société des américanistes* 12 (Paris, 1920), p. 212.

From *La fleur létale*, Paris, Editions du Seuil, 1979.
**Translated by Shelley Temchin.**

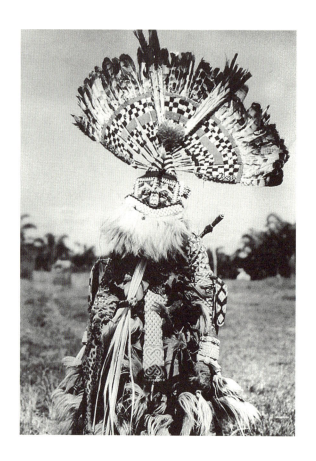

Maashamboy Kuba royal mask, Zaire
(Tervuren, Musée Royal de l'Afrique Centrale).

# The Sacrificial Body of the King

*Luc de Heusch*

In Africa, the body of the king is an illusory production machine. This mysterious body is the site where natural forces mesh with the social order to assure complete fertility, complete fecundity. Often, this precious body must be unblemished and cannot contain any infirmity; further, it cannot age or lose its sexual power.

This unique body is destined to be sacrificed sooner or later. Frazer was the first to discover this, though he did not succeed in discovering the exact meaning of it. He thought that the "divine" kings were put to death before their natural end, or at the close of a reign limited in time, in order to avoid at all costs the danger that the decrepitude of the god-man would lead to the decay of all of nature itself. But the fact is that the sacred king, destined for this sacrificial death, is not a god. It is not as the spirit of vegetation that he is condemned to die, but as a monstrous creature. In central Africa, the Kuba king (*Nyim*) is invested with a dangerous power indispensable to the proper functioning of the universe and society. The *Nyim* derives this exceptional and disquieting mystical power from the enthronement rites, which abolish his ties to the clan. The heir-designate has sexual relations with one of his sisters and marries a great-niece in his own matrilineal family group. He is likened to a fearful sorceror; he is henceforth considered to be filth and the representative of God on earth. Upon his death, he will become a spirit of nature (Vansina 1964: 98-116). He is as fiery as the sun rays that burn the earth, or as the attacking leopard. He is surrounded with a network of prohibitions, and formerly he could not die a natural death.

It is hard to challenge Frazer's central intuition. The "sacred" king, fearful master of natural forces, is condemned to die prematurely, to become a quasi-sacrificial victim at the close of a longer or shorter reign. The ritual execution is written in his destiny, it is the strongest expression of the prohibitions that circumscribe his exorbitant power, his monstrous nature. This symbolic configuration was perfectly elucidated in the case of the Moundang of Chad by Alfred Adler, who rightly reproaches Frazer's successors in Great Britain for having misunderstood the symbolic bases of African royalty (Adler, 1978). "Of course," he writes, "the importance of the religious and mystical values associated with the function of authority were never misunderstood, but the sacred as such was depicted as one means among others for imposing and affirming a power essentially dependent, clearly, on more compelling factors: the ecology, the demography, the social morphology, the economy and lineal and familial structures" (*ibid.*: 25). Thus, Evans-Pritchard, in his famous 1948 *Frazer Lecture*, denied the necessity for ritual regicide as it was practiced most notably by the Shilluk of the Upper Nile. According to Frazer, the king was strangled at the first sign of weakening, since his condition threatened the general fertility. This tradition, Evans-Pritchard declares, is only the fiction of a sociological explanation (Evans-Pritchard 1948). His skepticism seems to me, as it seemed to Adler, unjustified (Adler 1978: 29). Among the Moundang, the specific power attributed to the king of Léré is tied to the possession of magical instruments for acting on fertility and rain. Here, the king reigns over an extra-clanic space in the center of a vast palatial domain which produces the riches necessary for the sacrifices. The monarch is surrounded by a network of prohibitions whose function is "according to Frazer's formulation, as much to protect the king as to protect others from him" (*ibid.*: 39). For this all-powerful being is dangerous. He is situated outside the circuit of exchanges (he acquires numerous wives without matrimonial compensation), he is foreign to the order of the clans and defined by a species of "extra-territoriality" (Adler 1982: 169). Sole beneficiary of war profits, he is "a sort of great predator"; abuse and excess are "the very law of royalty"; they attest to "the vigor of the power and, finally, despite the apparent paradox, guarantee the prosperity of the farmers in the same way as the magic of rain, which he possesses" (*ibid.*: 171).

This very violence gives meaning to the ritual execution of the king. Adler suggests this: the regicide is the supreme prohibition, the ultimate expression of the constraints that circumscribe his exorbitant power and make him unique. He is "at society's limit, somewhat like Archimedes' point, which allows one, if not to lift up the world, at least — which is almost the same thing — to conceive of the union of society and nature" (*ibid.*: 38). The king's cadaver is accursed; it is scalded and its bones thrown into a flooded river, which carries them far away. "If the sovereign's body or even a part of his body were buried in the ground, the latter would become sterile and the population would be threatened by the worst calamities" (*ibid.*: 380).

It is within this perspective that one must interpret the modalities of regicide to which, according to Frazer, the king of the Lunda, the *Matiamvo* (*Mwant-Yav*) was subjected in central Africa. He was condemned to die a violent death when his subjects had had enough of his "insatiable demands." The story, as reported to a Portuguese expedition by a subordinate chief, is worth dwelling on for a moment. When the decision was made to put an end to the sovereign's life, he was forced to engage in war. If he did not die on the battlefield, a new battle was waged during which the king and his people were abandoned. At this point, he decapitated his wives and relatives himself, then awaited his own death seated on his throne, decked out in his most beautiful adornments. A functionary dispatched by a powerful neighboring chief would come and execute him savagely by decapitating him after cutting off his four limbs. The mutilated trunk would be buried, while the head, arms and legs would be bought back for a ransom (Frazer 1890; Veldez 1861: vol. 2, 194ff.).

This story can be compared with the tradition relating to the power of the sacred Lunda chief who rules over the Pende of Zaire, the *Mwata Kombana*. The latter accedes to power at the price of a twofold transgression: incest and murder. He unites ritually with his sister while several of his close relatives are killed in secret. These victims are no doubt used in the construction of a belt made of human nerves and tendons which the chief wears around his loins. What is strange is that, sooner or later, this ritual object is supposed to cause sterility in the *Mwata Kombana*, mystically responsible for fecundity and prosperity (Sousberghe 1963: 62, 69). From this belief we learn that the power of the chief's life is limited in time. It affirms, as it were, the symbolic death of the possessor of power as sacred monster.

These accounts confirm the ambivalence toward the royal body. The somber description I have borrowed from Frazer clearly implies that the people condemn the king to death for his very excesses. Let us explore the problem in greater depth.

Among the Bolia of Central Zaire, all power is related to witchcraft, as though the latter were the formidable, transcendent source of all efficacy. This serene amorality may be rather surprising to Westerners accustomed to the dichotomy of good and evil.

Mbomb'lpoku, the chief of the *elima* nature spirits, only comes into contact with the great chiefs, who associate with him but once in their lives, at the moment of their investiture. They then maintain more familiar relations with the subordinate *elima*, who are their wives. But for most mortals, commerce with the *elima* is dangerous. One must be presented to them by ancestors and the cost of that meeting is always a human life (Van Everbroeck 1961: 77). Contact with the supernatural world is always related to witchcraft, and because of this, the Bolia chiefs may be considered ambivalent creatures. One could say that in this case, power is the exercise of a permissible witchcraft (*iloko*), since it implies the mediation of an ancestor. The latter appears in a dream to one of his descendants and informs him of his desire to initiate him into the *iloki*, at the same time warning him that he will first have to offer up the life of someone close to him – a blood nephew, a sister, his mother, a child, a wife – to the *elima* spirit from whom he derives the mysterious power (*ibid.*: 87). The contract is drawn up by the ancestor himself, assisted by the shadow (*asisa*) of the interested party. This initiation into the clan's witchcraft (*iloki i bokundi*) confers dangerous destructive powers, but its beneficiary will not necessarily practice this formidable art. In any case, it is only after having benefited from this knowledge that one may aspire to political office, a specialized form of witchcraft.

Van Everbroeck distinguishes two particular forms of *iloki*. The first is the *iloki i loboko*, the power over the ground. In order to become chief of the earth (*nkumu i loboko*), it is indispensable to acquire it from an *elima* spirit by means of a human life. This exchange confers the faculty of "knowing everything that happens, in the visible world as well as in the invisible," within the boundaries of that domain of which he is proprietor (*ibid.*: 92). The summoned spirit proves to be kindly: he explains to the new chief of the earth how he should go about securing the general prosperity, how he should combat the criminal action of the sorcerers. The spirit also grants him the power to curse the ground and its inhabitants in order to establish his authority (*ibid.*: 93). Superior political power is designated by the term *ekopo*. In order to define its essence, the term witchcraft is once again joined to it: *iloki y ekopo*. The initiating ancestor transports the candidate chief into the ruins of his former residence. He summons together all the spirits of the village who, in return for the promise of a human life, confer on both of them the strength to go before their chief Mbomb'lpoku. The candidate chief will have to bring Mbomb'lpoku several victims chosen from among his relatives in order to be invested with "power over the men, animals and fish of his future chiefdom" (*ibid.*: 95).

If the Bolia represent an extreme case, they nevertheless shed light on the general problematic of sacred power. For whatever reason, sacred power always implies transgression such that the king appears as a dangerous creature, one who is between nature and culture, in a place where the power of life is also a power of death, a place where he exposes himself to becoming a sacrificial victim.

Every year, this threat weighs on the king of the Swazi, who accumulates in his own person the "defilement" of the year that has just passed. At the time of the summer solstice in the southern hemisphere (December 21), when the sun comes to rest in its "southern house," the Swazi king is the principal actor in a great cosmic game (Kuper 1947: 197-226), during which a black bullock, taken from a common man, is put to death. This animal is the substitute for the sovereign and on this occasion proclaimed "bull of the nation." Various substances are extracted from the victim's body and combined in the composition of a magic potion administered to the sovereign to revitalize him. Later, in an atmosphere of excitement that approaches paroxysm, the king is veritably transformed into a nature spirit. A headdress of black feathers falls over his shoulders, hiding his face; on his forehead he wears a band of lion skin. His body is covered in green leaves. Brandishing a shield in his left hand, he executes a mad dance before the young warriors, who address him by the title of "Thunder." This typically Frazerian king, promoted to a new existence after the substitute sacrifice, truly incarnates the living forces of nature. After having disappeared several times, this triumphant king appears one last time, brandishing a greenish gourd, which he throws in the direction of the warriors. The acts performed by the king throughout this ritual are marked by violence. When he ingests the first fruits, he is supposed to "bite"; when he unites with his ritual wife, he affirms his virile power by "stabbing." He walks naked among his people, displaying himself as a creature-of-nature. When he appears in costume before his army, he engages in a veritable symbolic battle that is a guarantee of fertility. Naked or clothed, the king is "different," monstrous and indispensable to the proper functioning of the universe.

This sacred king, symbolically put to death in the form of a bullock before being reborn, is not, as René Girard would have us believe, a scapegoat upon whom the Swazi nation projects its own violence. The black color of the sacrificial bullock refers to death and witchcraft. The king dramatically assumes all the negative values of society. The nonpubescent young people who eat the accursed flesh will have to wash themselves in the river to purify themselves. The victim's remains will be burned on a purifying pyre along with the costume which the king wore when he appeared disguised as a violent spirit of nature. All these objects are polluted; the Swazi say that "the filth of the king and all the people lies here on the fire" (*ibid*.: 220). The best explanation for this is that the sacrifice of the black bullock rids the sovereign of that element of dangerous "blackness" which is one of the components of royalty. A solar being, associated with "whiteness," like all the Swazi sovereigns, the great king Sobhuza was nevertheless born "amidst black shields" and was, for this reason, "fearful," as is proclaimed in a song of praise (*ibid*.: ix).

The sacrifice of the black bullock is therefore aimed at the king, as accumulator of pollution. It represents the king on the sacrificial stage; it expels the "blackness" contained by this central focus of energy. The royal enclosure includes a "white" part, where the sovereign receives his mother and visitors, and a "black" part, strictly forbidden to the queen mother but accessible to the dignitaries who initiate him to royalty when he is young, and later on to his mistresses.

This ambivalent king, who bears the considerable responsibility of being in charge of the natural order, is the same figure as the sovereign of Léré in Adler's description of the Moundang. The latter's palace is the microcosm of which he is the sun (Adler 1978: 34). In this case, it is not an annual substitute sacrifice that assures the royalty's purification and regeneration, but a series of annual rites during which a double symbolically assumes the tragic fate of the king. A man, a "sort of scapegoat for the king," sacrifices a bullock and steals away from the palace during the night, taking with him the animal's hide; "the burden he carries soon condemns him in place of his glorious double" (*ibid*.: 36). It is strictly forbidden for the sovereign to see him. When the festival of the soul of the millet takes place at the end of the harvest, it is a servant who is substituted for the king. He goes to deposit an enormous sheaf of millet in the central granary of the palace: "Naked, his body covered with ashes, and wearing a penile case, the young man finds himself in the dress of an initiate emerging from the initiatory death." The king "throws small pebbles in his direction three times, and steals away as fast as possible into a room in order not to see him" (*ibid.*). Finally, the annual cycle is closed by the festival of the guinea fowl. This time, the sovereign himself, now naked, participates in a collective hunt to encourage the arrival of the rain. He is the object of bullying and mockery. From this group of facts, Adler concludes that, for the king, "each ritual year is worth so many units in a backwards count which will end in regicide" (*ibid.*: 37-38).

This regicide is part of a coherent symbolic structure which defines the sacred power as the site where a formidable magic force is exerted, abolishing the boundary between culture – from which the chief separates himself at the moment he becomes sacred – and nature, which he invests sovereignly.

Sacred royalty is a symbolic structure that has broken with the domestic, familial or linear order. It is a machination, a topological arrangement, which must be read as a meshing of human space and the space of the bush or forest in which the mysterious forces responsible for fecundity dwell; it can also be the bond that joins the earth and sky. The king's body, merging with the inhabited and cultivated territory, with all its richness, is also symbolically a stranger to its law. It is this paradox, this phantasmagorical plan that must be explained if one wishes to understand why the sacred king is a reducer of productive and reproductive forces on the one hand, and a dangerous creature surrounded by prohibitions and condemned to a premature death, on the other. In a number of cases, the royal body can only be used to this end as long as it is perfect, unblemished. In other cases, this essential mechanism must be replaced after an arbitrarily fixed lapse of time, unless a substitute sacrifice brings about the indispensable regeneration.

This sacrificial body is not "divine" in the strict sense of the word; this is why I chose not to use that Frazerian epithet, substituting instead the term "sacred," which harks back to the original Latin meaning of the term as defined by Benvéniste – "august and accursed, worthy of veneration and exciting horror" (Benvéniste 1969: vol. 2, 188). The divinization of the royal body, as evident as it is in Egypt, arises from another problematic, one unknown to black Africa. This new ideological structure of the ritual power, whose source is unequivocally the religious domain, is incompatible with the sacrificial execution of the magician-king. This execution is the very paradigm of the human sacrifice, the ultimate guarantor of the balance of the cosmic order. In his novel, *The Sailor Who Fell from Grace with the Sea* (Mishima, 1965: 167), Yukio Mishima perfectly expresses this exigency, as imperious as it is mysterious: "We must have blood! Human blood! If we don't get it this empty world will grow pale and shrivel up. We must drain that sailor's fresh lifeblood, and transfuse it to the dying universe, the dying sky, the dying forests and the drawn, dying land."

BIBLIOGRAPHY

Adler, Alfred, "Le pouvoir et l'interdit: Aspects de la royauté sacrée chez les Moundang du Tchad," in *Systèmes de signes: Textes réunis en hommage à Germaine Dieterlen*. Paris, 1978, pp. 25-40.

Adler, Alfred, *La mort est le masque du roi: La royauté sacrée des Moundang du Tchad*. Paris: Payot, 1982.

Benvéniste, Emile, *Le vocabulaire des institutions européennes*. vol. 1, *Economie, parenté, société*; vol. 2, *Pouvoir, droit, religion*. Paris, 1969.

Evans-Pritchard, E.E., "The Divine Kingship of the Shilluk of the Nilotic Sudan." Paper presented at the Frazer Lecture, Cambridge, 1948.

Frazer, James G., *The Dying God*. 1890. Reprint: New York: St. Martin Press, 1980.

Kuper, Hilda, *An African Aristocracy: Rank among the Swazi*. London, New York, Toronto, 1947.

Mishima, Yukio, *The Sailor Who Fell from Grace with the Sea*. Translated by John Nathan. New York: Alfred A. Knopf, 1965.

Sousberghe, L. de, "Les Pende: Aspects des structures sociales et politiques," in *Miscellanea Ethnographica*. Edited by L. de Sousberghe, B. Crine Mavar, A. Doutreloux, and J. Loose. Tervuren, 1963, pp. 1-78.

Van Everbroeck, Nestor, *Mbomb'lpoku, le seigneur de l'abîme*. Tervuren, 1961.

Veldez, F.T., *Six Years of a Traveller's Life in Western Africa*. London, 1861.

Vansina, Jan, *Le royaume Kuba*. Tervuren: Musée Royal de l'Afrique Centrale, 1964.

**Translated by Lydia Davis**

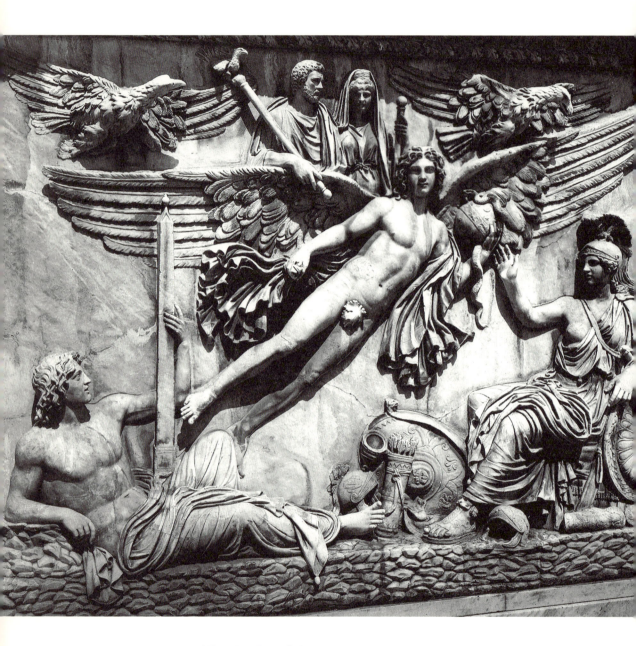

Apotheosis of Antoninus and Faustina. Bas-relief
(Cortile della Pigna, Vatican City).

# The Emperor-God's Other Body

*Florence Dupont*

> The pilot has two personas: one is common to all those who board the
> ship, the other is peculiar to him, for he is the pilot.
>
> — Seneca, *Ad Luciliam epistulae morales*

In the Christian West, the monarch has two bodies: one human, the other divine.
At his death, they are given a double funeral. The first is buried while the second is
proclaimed immortal. These two bodies express the nature of royal power exercised
by mortal man. The king is the conjunction of a private, human body and a political, divine body.

That, briefly summarized, is the thesis E.H. Kantorowicz advances in his famous
book on the king's two bodies.[1] Kantorowicz limits himself to the Christian conception of royal power, but at the end raises the issue of the archaeology of his monarchs'
divine body. He recalls the astonishing text by Herodian describing the double
funeral of the Roman emperor Septimius Severus, and closes with a description of
Septimius's apotheosis.[2] He does not develop the connections, expressing well-
founded mistrust of the temptation to seek origins. He does, however, invite researchers to transfer the analysis to Rome, a city peopled by gods, and to take a closer
look at whether the Roman emperors did not also have two bodies, one mortal,
the other immortal.

## In Rome, Divine Immortality Applies to the Body,
## Not the Soul

An article by E. Bickermann inaugurated that research fifty years ago. It created a
scandal at the time.[3] Today, Bickermann's article still stands, stronger and more imagi-

native than the critiques that have tried to refute its conclusions.[4] If Bickermann inspired so much indignation, it is because he brushed aside the reigning theory of the two funerary ideologies. According to that theory, those who cremate their dead believe in the immortality of the soul and a celestial afterlife, whereas those who bury their dead do not believe in an immortal soul but think that the dead return to their mother, the earth. This divides humanity in two: the cremating, virile, idealist, nomadic Indo-Europeans, and the burying, sedentary, materialist pre-Indo-Europeans practicing a fertility cult and worshiping a mother-goddess.

According to these presuppositions, the Romans, who cremated their dead throughout the Republican age and during the first centuries of the Empire, would have had to believe in individual immortality. If they attributed an immortal soul to man, they would have had to have seen the emperor's apotheosis as the soul's ascent to Olympus, where it would take its seat among the gods. In reality, there is no belief in an immortal soul in Roman religion. Although certain individuals in Rome, receptive to Platonic philosophy, believed in the immortality of the soul, these beliefs had nothing to do with either the gods of the city or the public deification of the emperor. Bickermann, faithful to historical reality, shows that the apotheosis of the emperor had to do with the body, not the soul. In order to attain the state of a god, the sovereign was twice burned: once in flesh and blood, and again in wax. Even if the emperor's soul was freed by the first cremation and ascended to heaven, it would only prove that it was not the soul that was deified, for in order to complete the ritual of apotheosis, the Romans fabricated a second body, in wax, for which another funeral was conducted.

For a long time ideological pressure was overpowering. Philosophical texts by Cicero and Seneca were used to obscure the cultural reality of Rome. The accounts of ancient historians were mangled or placed under suspicion, rather than admit the following truth with its scandalous implications: Antoninus Pius, Helvius Pertinax, Septimius Severus and doubtless many other emperors were cremated twice. Today the pressure has lessened. People no longer believe in the theory of the two funerary ideologies, or in the systematic opposition between burial and cremation. It cannot be denied that the two treatments of the corpse, far from being mutually exclusive, complemented each other, and that this was particularly true of Rome.

It is time, therefore, to continue Bickermann's work. We will take another path, however, toward understanding the wax body the Romans fabricated after the death of the emperor for the sole purpose of making it immediately disappear again on a second pyre, and toward understanding the cultural reality, called *imago*, that served as the emperor's second body and made his deification possible. Bickermann limits himself to demonstrating that the apotheosis ceremony was a funeral ceremony, and that beginning in the second century, a deceased emperor had to be given a double funeral in order to be deified. He does not investigate the nature of this second wax body. He merely suggests that for the system to function there had to be a contamination of the dummy by the corpse. Life (?) passed from one to the other. There is something disturbing about the idea of a "life" transmitted after death. The hypothesis does not in fact hold up, even if we take this unfortunate term to refer to the force of dissolution that transforms the body into religiously polluting, putrefied flesh. If we examine the status of the funerary *imago* in Rome, we see that this image is free from any stain the corpse might have transmitted to it.

Rather than appealing to some kind of vague magic, it is more fruitful to recall that the *imago* is a very ancient Roman reality. It is only by rediscovering the meaning and place of this tradition in Roman culture that we can understand why the cremation of a wax dummy could make a man into a god.

### The Apotheosis of the Emperor Is the Consecration of a Dead Sovereign

The emperor's apotheosis began with Augustus. After his death, the sovereign became a god, Roman fashion: he received a new given name, *divus*, a temple was dedicated to him, and priests were assigned to look after his worship. After apotheosis, an emperor became a god — wholly and entirely. However, and this is typically Roman, there was no theological speculation on his mode of existence. In Rome, religion consisted of practices, not theories.

The deification of the sovereign was called *consecratio* in Latin. In what follows, we will use the word consecration rather than apotheosis. For Greek *apotheosis* is the "transformation of a man into a god" whereas Latin *consecratio* is the "transferral from profane space to sacred space." Its meaning is broader. But above all, the practice of consecration is much older than the deification of emperors, as old as Rome itself. From time immemorial, things, people and places were consecrated on the banks of the Tiber, without necessarily being deified.[5] The Campus Martius, for example, was consecrated ground, meaning that it was prohibited to work or build a house there. When a praetor condemned a guilty man to death, he would pronounce this phrase in his presence: *Sacer esto!* In so doing, he expelled him from the human community, implicitly condemning him to death. A god could also be created by consecrating a linguistic category. For example, loyalty, *fides*, was consecrated by Atilius Catalinus and became the god *Fides*, complete with a temple, priests and observances.[6] The gods Venus and Cupid had a similar origin. Augustus deified the mistral and dedicated a temple to it,[7] just as the Romans had earlier deified the tempests they weathered off the coast of Corsica.[8] Thus, when consecration was a deification, it was the divine recognition of a linguistically designated category or natural force. This divine characteristic was called *numen*. Transcribing this sacralization in cultural terms, we may say that the newly created gods were categories constitutive of a world system, not accidents that could be warded off by trotting out a few formulas. That is why they are given the epithet "divine." The "divine tempests" were venerated in the same way *Divus Julius* would be a few centuries later.

The deification of emperors was a consecration. It meant that the sovereign was too great, too mighty, for his power not to have been the manifestation of a *numen*. Deification was a way of acknowledging the divine nature of imperial power. From a strictly politico-juridical point of view, there was no obstacle in Rome to the deification of emperors.

The procedure, of course, posed no problem. But there were religious difficulties. The consecration of the dead was spatially problematic. For consecration was the passage of the consecrated from one space to another. To consecrate someone who had died, it was thus necessary to remove him from his tomb and install him in the sacred space where his temple would stand. This was unthinkable, both from the point of view of the deceased, who would find himself without a burial place, and from the point of view of the sacred space, which would be dreadfully polluted by the presence of a corpse. Yet to consecrate the emperor before his death was equally unthinkable. The sovereign would be in the same position as someone condemned as *sacer*. He would be excluded from the world of men, and would no longer be able to exercise his power. That is why the only emperor-gods Rome ever had were dead emperors. This cultural fact inspired many a macabre joke,[9] for example Vespasian's last laugh: "Alas! I believe I am becoming a god!"[10]

The emperor's consecration, then, could only be performed after the sovereign's death, and, since the sovereign was a man, after his funeral (no religious act could take place before funeral rites had purified the community). The problem the Romans faced was to find a ritual solution that allowed them to consecrate a buried body.

## In Rome, the Deceased Was Physically Present on Earth by Virtue of His Tomb

That ritual solution could only reside in a treatment of the body. For, in Rome, the only possible treatment of the deceased was to manipulate the corpse. There is but one name for such manipulation: funeral. That is why the ritual procedures leading to the emperor's consecration could only result from the ordered transformations of the funeral rites.

What exactly was the death of a man in Rome? It was the presence on the earth's surface of a body that stained and paralyzed the community. In order to be able to act again, to sacrifice, to read auspices, the community had to purify itself and complete its mourning. But according to pontifical law, the only way this could be done was by creating a tomb, *sepulcrum*.[11] What exactly was a *sepulcrum*? It was a place outside the urban space where the remains of the deceased were buried, and which from that moment on had the legal status of a *locus religiosus*. The remains were designated by the term *ossa*. This term referred not only to the bones burned on and recovered from the pyre, but also to the corpse itself, or to a fragment of the body removed before cremation and destined for burial. The tomb was the property of the deceased, and as such was under legal protection. These property rights were based on the physical presence of the deceased, and were perpetual.

Pontifical law was strict: if the deceased's body remained above ground without being buried in whole or in part, then there was no *sepulcrum*, no *locus religiosus*, and the family was not purified.[12] Burial, total or partial, was called *humatio*, a term that does not specify any particular legal or juridical modality. The corpse was either buried intact or cremated. If it was cremated, the family would cover the pyre with earth, or, more frequently, recover the *ossa* and place them in a tomb. If the remains were kept in an aboveground urn, either the urn was covered with a thin layer of earth or a fragment of the body, called the *os resectum*, was buried.

By virtue of his tomb, the deceased remained present in the space of men – even if spatially and chronologically the mode of that presence was disjunction. The tombs were located outside the city. Ceremonies for the dead were performed on the occasion of the *Feralia* and the *Parentalia*, in February, a month set apart from the others (it came after the end of the year in December and before the beginning of the new year in the first days of March).[13] The space reserved by the living for the dead was therefore separate from the political space, from the places of power and the time of public worship.

What impeded the consecration of the deceased was precisely his burial, obligatory for any man reduced to the state of a cadaver. For the body of the deceased tied him to a religious place from which it would be impious to remove him, but where it was impossible to treat him as a god. To consecrate a buried man would be to commit a formidable confusion of spaces. That confusion is the object of Cicero's eloquent indignation in the *Philippinae*.[14] The Romans voted for public prayers for Caesar after his death. In Rome, prayers were only addressed to gods. That vote, therefore, was the first move toward a deification of the assassinated dictator. To pray to Caesar, Cicero says, is to destroy the distinction between the worship of the dead and the worship of the gods, to transform a tomb into a temple, to burden the Republic with inexpiable profanations. The places and times of *sepulcra* and *templa*, *sacra publica* and *sacra privata*, could not be mixed. That is why it was prohibited to build a tomb on public ground, where temples were dedicated. In February, the temples were closed and the priests did not wear their official insignia.

A dead man whose body had been allotted a place, and who was the object of a funerary cult there, could not have a temple or public observances dedicated to him. Unless he was divided in two.

### The Emperor-God's Imaginary Funeral

This dividing in two of the emperor's person was accomplished by the consecration ritual. The ceremonies surrounding the death of the sovereign and his deification produced two bodies. The consecration ritual took the form of a funeral rite performed after the first funeral, at which the emperor's corpse was buried in the most human of ways. Having two bodies allowed the deceased to be present in the two separate spaces of tomb and temple, in the two incompatible time frames of funerary cult and public worship. After his death, the emperor remained doubly present among men.

Consecration as we shall study it was a relatively late-developing ceremony; it first appeared with Antoninus Pius. Although it was an innovation in ritual, it was not an ideological mutation. Roman ritual in general, and in this case specifically, functioned as a collective discourse, a way of making an implicit ideology explicit through a spectacle. Roman ritual was a formulation. As we shall see, the meaning made explicit by the ritual of consecration was already present in the first deifications of emperors, from Augustus to Hadrian.

Our sources for this consecration ceremony are four texts describing the funerals of Antoninus (163), Helvius Pertinax (211) and Septimius Severus (217).[15] Herodian's text is the most complete. It outlines the functioning of the ritual, showing that the consecration constituted a second funeral performed after burial in the usual sense. Comparing Herodian's Greek text with Helvius Pertinax's *Historia Augustae* provides us with a name for the second funeral: *funus imaginarium*.[16] In translation, the expression means "funeral for an *imago*": the wax portrait of the deceased takes the corpse's place. Thus, from a certain point of view, there were two funeral rites for emperors: one for the *ossa*, culminating in the creation of a *sepulcrum*, and another for the *imago*, culminating in the creation of a *templum*.

*Imago*, image; *imaginarium*, imaginary. The English words are misleading. They could easily suggest that the second funeral is a fake, a false repetition of the first. But the Roman *imago* is not an image in the English sense, and a careful reading of Herodian's text will show that both ceremonies were equally genuine funerals and had the same mode of reality. The *imago* is not an image consisting of a signifying medium and a signified form. Both *ossa* and *imago* were parts of the emperor's body, and in the ceremonies they functioned in similar ways as figures for the whole body.

Here is the normal scenario of the ritual, as presented by Herodian. The fact that Septimius Severus died far from Rome is mere accident, and does not affect the procedure in any way, except that his body was burned on the spot and his ashes were returned to Rome in an urn. These *ossa* were ritually interred in Hadrian's mausoleum, which served as a tomb for the imperial family. The urn was brought to the mausoleum in a procession, *pompa*. Then the sacrifices completing the family's purification and concluding their mourning were performed. This brought to a close

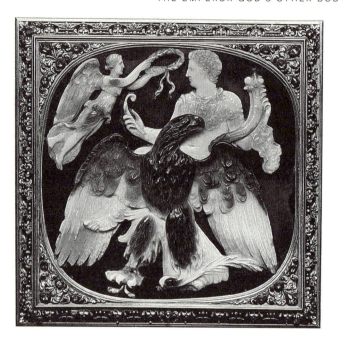

Apotheosis of Germanicus. From a Roman cameo in sardonyx
(Paris, Bibliothèque nationale).

the first part, which took place according to "human norms": *anthrōpōn nomō* is what
Herodian calls it. Septimius Severus had received his just due. For an ordinary man,
it would be all over. But for a man invested with imperial power and whose consecration had been voted by the Senate, this was only the beginning.

After the first human funeral came the "imaginary" funeral. A wax image, *eikōn*,
that according to the Greek historian "exactly resembled the deceased," had already
been made. That *eikōn*, of course, was the *imago* (a word untranslatable into Greek),
in other words a wax mask. The image was placed on the funeral bed, after having
been painted a yellowish color to give it the palor of sickness. The *imago* then experienced seven days of agony. Each day doctors would come to the sick bed; each
day their diagnosis was a little more pessimistic. The last day, they pronounced it
dead. Funeral rites were then performed for the corpse, for the *imago* was in no way
an idealized or abstract body. Saussure's word "dog" might not bark, but a dead man's
*imago* stinks. Slaves were even stationed by its sides to chase away the flies. A veritable corpse was present, and the customary ritual was necessary to rid the earth of it.

That ceremony was a *funus*. Of the different types of possible funerals, the one
chosen for the emperor's *imago* was the *funus publicum* (or *censorium*), in other words,

funeral rites in which the civic collectivity was substituted for the family, and the entire community mourned. The ceremony followed its normal course (procession, funeral oration at the forum) up to the point where people gathered on the Campus Martius, where the pyre of the imperial family was placed. A pyramidal structure for the burning of the *imago* had been erected there. On the outside, it was all sumptuousness and beauty: gold fabric, ivory statues, multicolored paintings. The pyre displayed the imperial power that ruled the entire world and to which the whole universe paid tribute. On the inside it was filled with highly flammable materials, in particular incense, that were meant to catch fire immediately and be entirely consumed in flames. The new emperor set it on fire. Huge flames rose up. An eagle flew from the top of the pyre. From that moment, the emperor was the object of a cult ranking him among the gods.

Finally, this *funus imaginarium*, this imaginary funeral, can be described as a truncated *funus publicum* that stopped at the moment of the *ossilegium*, the recovery of the remains from the pyre. Since there were no *ossa* to recover there would be no *sepulcrum* and no funerary cult – there was no place for them. But it is evident that the funeral was not fictional, otherwise there would be nothing to prevent the ritual from continuing. The *funus* treating the *imago* bore no resemblance to the *funus* treating the *ossa*, and was not defined in the same terms. The body – *imago* – was entirely consumed, and, consequently, the community did not need to be purified by a *sepulcrum*. As in cases where the deceased was lost at sea, the family was excused from having a *sepulcrum*. The consecration, like the ordinary *funus*, involved a horizontal transferral, which is the technical meaning of *funus*. It took the *imago* outside the civic space of the *urbs*. But it replaced the *ossa*'s vertical descent into the earth with a vertical climb into the sky, manifested, Herodian says, by the flight of the eagle.

We are, therefore, dealing with two types of funeral: one in which the body, *ossa*, is lowered into the earth, and one in which the body, *imago*, rises into the sky. In both cases, the *funus* serves to separate a dead body from other human bodies and to place that body in a tomb or temple.

We must now try to understand the status of the *imago* in Roman civilization. We have seen that this *imago*, like the *ossa*, functioned as a body of the dead emperor. How was this possible? Did every Roman man leave behind two bodies capable of receiving a funeral?

## The *Imago* Is Not an Image of the Body, But a Part of the Body

The *funus imaginarium*, like the consecration, was not a ritual invented specifically for the deification of emperors. It already existed, but had a different purpose and did not involve cremation. It served not to deify someone who had died, but to create a *sepulcrum* when there were no *ossa*.

The expression *funus imaginarium* occurs in an inscription dating from 133-36 A.D., thus before Hadrian's death. It is the funerary law of a college in Lanuvium.[17] It decrees that if a slave who is a member of the college dies and his master refuses to turn the body over to the college, then the college will conduct a *funus imaginarium* (unless he had a testament specifying an heir who would take care of the body). What is a *funus imaginarium* from the point of view of pontifical law? No body, no *funus*, writes Servius.[18] This is quite understandable, since the *funus* is the transferral of a body from the space of life and the city to the space of the *sepulcrum*. The *imago* takes the body's place in the *funus imaginarium*. The *imago*, still quoting Servius, makes it possible to create a *sepulcrum* by means of a *sepultra imaginaria*.[19] Technically, the word *sepultra* means the act of constituting a *sepulcrum*: *humatio* and sacrifices. The unfortunate slave thereby escapes the unenviable fate of the *inhumati*, a term designating the "unburied." The *imago* is given a *humatio*. The *funus imaginarium* allows a tomb to be dedicated and a funerary cult to be pursued in the absence of *ossa*. The aim of these funeral colleges composed of men without families was to substitute for each member's relatives after his death and during the festivals for the dead.

This inscription proves that the *imago* could play exactly the same role normally played by the *ossa*. For the substitution to be possible and effective, the *imago* had to be a part of the dead man's body. If we look at how the *humatio* of the *ossa* functioned, we do indeed see that a part of the body takes the place of the whole: either a fragment set aside before cremation, or the bones recovered after the pyre burned out. This must also be the case for the *imago*. This metonymic presence, in which the part replaces the whole, was written into Roman law. From the earliest times, civil law held that an object was equivalent to one of its parts.[20] In cases where legal proceedings had to take place in the presence of the thing under litigation, *res*, as for example in a *sacramentum in rem*, a house could be represented by one of its shingles, a field by a clod of earth, a herd by a single animal or even a tuft of hair. It must be understood that this "representation" is a real presence of the thing, not a fictional presence. The legal formula is only valid for that presence, at that moment, in the place it is pronounced, the thing being designated by the words *hanc rem*, "this thing that is here now."

We now see that we must think in terms of an *imago* and a system of images organized around metonymy rather than metaphor. This system was not understood by the Greek historians, who took the *imagines* to be "very lifelike," "the most lifelike" images of the dead — when their principle of fabrication does not in fact seem to have been resemblance to the dead, but rather the removal of a part of their bodies.

### The *Imago* Is Equivalent to the Body of the Deceased

In order to verify our hypothesis and carry our description of representational practices in Roman civilization further, we must go back to the heyday of the Republic, when the great families dedicated all their resources and ambitions to public life. A single right was granted them to attest to their nobility: the right to images, *ius imaginum*. These *imagines* were wax masks made after the death of a person with access to political power, and only nobles had the right to keep them in their atriums. It was in this way that families constituted ancestors for themselves.

Let us quickly review how these masks were made.[21] We will see that they were not modeled on the likeness of the person they represented. When someone who had attained at least the rank of curule magistrate died, his family made a wax impression of his face. That impression was in turn used to make wax masks that were then painted; these were called *imagines* or *effigies*. This second operation is an inference on our part, and is never mentioned by the ancients or taken into account in either Greek or Roman discussions of *imagines*. This operation is "forgotten," and it was this forgetting that allowed the *imagines* to be perceived as the direct result of an impression of the deceased's face. We are speaking of forgetting in the cultural sense. What we mean is that the Romans did not distinguish, did not need to distinguish, between the negative, hollow form and the positive form in relief when it was a question of wax impressions. This was true not only for death masks, but for all similar techniques.

A short digression on other *imagines* is in order here. An example is the impressions left by a seal in the wax used to sign documents in ancient times. In this context, the word *imago* designates both the impression in the wax and the seal itself, both the convex and concave forms.[22] This implies that they are equivalent. Since there is no disjunction between the initial form and the final form, they would seem to adhere to one another; the practice of taking impressions allows an infinite series of equivalences to be created, with no loss whatsoever. Returning to funeral images, nothing distinguishes the form of the dead man's face from its hundredth wax reproduction; it is always the same form that is transmitted from mask to mask.

A general characterization of the *imago* would be the following. First, no aesthetic elaboration or idealization can come between the deceased and the death mask, between the seal and the signature it leaves. That is why they could be used to mark an identity. Second, from a certain point of view the form left in wax is not distinct from the object to which the form belongs. The practice of taking impressions implies this metonymy. Pliny the Elder, for example, alternates between saying that Augustus signed official papers "using the *imago* of a Sphinx" and saying that Sulla signed "using Jugurtha's surrender," in other words using a seal with an engraving of Jugurtha's surrender on it.[23] Regarding the technique of taking impressions, what is fabricated is neither an arbitrary sign nor a metaphorical sign in which the signified resembles the referent. It is a sign that is a part of its referent. Concrete examples of this are a Roman man's name which arbitrarily signifies him; a portrait of him done by a Greek painter or sculptor which metaphorically signifies him; and finally after his death the *imago* that will preserve his imprint, in other words his person.

The word *imago* functions in Latin in the same way as the word *stamp* in English, which refers both to the instrument and the mark it leaves. But in the case of a funerary image, the first impression is left by the object itself. There is, therefore, a superimposition of and total equivalence between the face of the deceased and its *imago*. That is why Juvenal can speak of the "painted faces of the ancestors" when referring to the painted masks of the faces of the ancestors.[24] The artist who worked with the wax did not render anything "figuratively," he did not make a "beautiful dead man" a work of art inviting a different and admiring gaze.

"Beautiful dead man" is a Greek phrase pertaining to the realm of glory and the celebration of the dead. In Greece, speech or marble were used to fashion beautiful images eternally preserving the honor of a great warrior and perfect citizen. Wax was not used for that purpose. Although death masks, as we shall see, would participate in the composition of beautiful images offered in celebration of the deceased's past glory, they were not in themselves beautiful images.

### *Imago* and Aristocratic Glory

Where and how did the Romans transmit the values of war to their sons? This is the question that the Greek historian Polybius asks in the preamble to a long exposition on Roman aristocratic funeral rites.[25] This was an essential question for someone whose people had been conquered by Rome and who wanted to understand how a culture without words or marble, without heroic poetry or sculpture, could produce soldiers enamored of honor and ready to die for glory. Polybius finds the answer in a number of Roman ceremonies, in particular aristocratic funeral rites. It was these rites, he says, that celebrated courage and war exploits and gave young men the desire to imitate their ancestors. The minutely detailed description he gives of this ceremony centers on the fabrication, preservation and use of the *imago*, which Polybius calls *eikōn* also.

After the funeral, the *imago* was immediately locked away in a small chest and placed in the family atrium. It was used to trace vast genealogical trees, in which only the illustrious men of the family appeared. Ordinarily, no one saw the *imagines*, and the idea of being locked away was so closely associated with funerary *imagines* that "to open the images," *aperire imagines*, became a current expression for "to open the image boxes." The *imagines* were not seen because there was no interest in looking at them; they had no value as a spectacle. There was, however, something in the atrium that was made to be seen by visitors: the *tituli*, signs hung from the *imagines* chests. They indicated the names, *nomina*, and the magistrature, *honores*, held by the deceased. The atrium offered an awe-inspiring spectacle, a commemoration of the great men of the family — but only through the medium of reading, not through contemplation of the *imagines*.

There was nothing beautiful or glorious about the *imagines*. The way they were made reduced them to being no more than the person they represented, a singular individuality; they could not make visible collective values. Writing, on the other hand, was a way of celebrating those aspects of the dead man's life that were recognized by political institutions. This institutional glory was called *honos* in Latin, from the word for magistrature, *honores*. In addition to this political recognition, one had personal fame, called *nomen*, from the word designating the linguistic signs of identity, *nomina*, names. What the *tituli* showed were the *honores* and *nomina* of the deceased, his civic and gentilic memory. Even though the *tituli* were exposed to the gaze and the *imagines* were hidden in their chests, they were interdependent. One could not hang *tituli* in one's atrium unless one had *imagines*. Having the *ius imaginum*, the right to images, was in fact the only way one could be a noble in Rome. Thus, in order to celebrate that nobility with *tituli* showing the *honores* of one's ancestors, it was necessary to have *imagines*. Funerary images had an effect merely by virtue of their presence. The *imago* had a reality beyond that of appearance and resemblance, a reality that did not function through the recognition of a model. Once again, we are on the tracks of metonymy, representation through participation.

An examination of how the Romans used the *imagines* when they opened their boxes will take us further down this path. The *imago* was removed from its box and from the atrium for its descendants' funerals. It would finally have its hour of glory: it would be worn by an actor dressed in the costume of the highest magistrature held by the deceased. The *imago* takes its place in the *pompa funebris*, the cortege taking the newly deceased from his home to the forum for the funeral oration, then from the forum to the outskirts of the city for cremation and burial. If the man was a high-ranking noble, there was a large cortege consisting of praetors, consuls, censors and triumphant generals. Power was displayed in all its force, beauty and purity, outside of time and independent of personalities. This was an unequaled spectacle, says Polybius, for young men enamored of glory and virtue. This, then, was the object created by Roman civilization and offered for the admiration of the crowd in order to transmit, through the glory of the few, the collective values of war. We must emphasize once again that the awe-inspiring image was not made of marble or of wax, but of the material of the *honos*: the insignia of power. What was beautiful about the spectacle were the lictors bearing fasces, the ivory sedan chairs, the triumphal chariots accompanied by men in purple-fringed togas with red, star-studded sleeves. This spectacle, however, remained anonymous: although one could see the *honores* on the *tituli*, nothing showed the *nomina*, the gentilic identity of the mighty dead. Only the anonymous, silent identity of *imagines* was present.

The funeral oration is what reconstructed the gentilic identity of the deceased and celebrated his *nomina*. It was delivered from the forum, the place of public speech. Unlike the *honores*, the oration was not a part of the civic recognition, even though one had the right to deliver it before the people. The funeral cortege approached the forum, preceded by the *imagines*. The family of the deceased took the rostrum, the tribunal of political speech. It was generally a magistrate who addressed the people. A relative of the dead man, usually his son, addressed the audience from the rostrum upon which the corpse was placed, either on a litter or, occasionally, propped in a standing position. The *imagines* sat in the audience on their curule chairs.

The speech given by the deceased's relative was called an *oratio* in Latin, as were all judicial and political speeches. This term defined the status of the funeral oration, determining which of the different modes of Roman speech it belonged to: it was a speech given only once by an individual invested with the right to speak before the civic collectivity, and was anchored in the spatial and temporal context of a punctual object.

The funeral oration was also called *laudatio* in Latin. This substantive is an action noun derived from the active verb *laudare*, to praise. Taking the etymology even further, *laudare* is itself derived from the substantive *laus*. *Laus* is glory, the virtue glory confers and the open recognition of that virtue by the community. The *laudatio* is, therefore, the institutional assumption of responsibility for the practice of blame and praise, and is common to many cultures, both Indo-European and non-Indo-European. In early Latin, *laudare* also signified *nominare*, meaning both "to call by name" and to "speak someone's fame," for *nomen* was both name and fame.[26] Thus, there is a closed circuit between virtue, glory, denomination and the community's celebration of the individual, by virtue of which the *laudatio* was the oral and public equivalent of the *nomina* written on the *tituli*. The *laudatio* was a eulogy to the deceased, individualized as much as possible; he was designated by his name, and his personal exploits were related. This individualization, however, did not reach the point of singularity, in other words the level of the *imago*: the exploits and virtues praised were always gentilic, like the *nomina*. In the exceptional case where the deceased attained singular glory, his exploit was registered in an additional *cognomen* that was transmissible to his sons. Scipio became Africanus after taking Carthage, and Manlius became Torquatus after defeating a Gaul in single combat and making off with his gold torque.

Like the funeral ceremony as a whole, the *laudatio* did not outlast the celebration; it was an event, not a monument. This is implied by the term *oratio*. The *oratio* is a contextual speech, and is therefore ephemeral; since it is tailored to a particular time, place and audience, it can only be used once. The funeral oration is thus radically different from the Greek honorary poem, which retained all its efficacy, its charm, *charis*, in other times and places. Although certain conditions were placed on the enunciation of the heroic poem, its enunciation was far from unique. It was a monument, not an event. Achilles' immortality was tied to the immortality of Homer's work, to use the words of the ancients. The Greek honorary poem was, to put it in Latin, a *monumentum*, whereas the *oratio funebris* was not.

Just as a political speech or legal argument defends or attacks a man in a particular case and not in general, the funeral oration is a eulogy to the deceased in the context of his funeral, at a precise moment in history. This brings us back to the other meaning of *laudare*, "to call by name." Since *laudare* was the same as *nominare*, the person one was naming had to be present. It was not just the man being buried who was named, in other words praised, but also his noble ancestors. Polybius states explicitly that the orator, after praising the deceased, praised those present, *tōn parontōn*, in other words the *imagines* seated on their curule chairs. He also explains why the masks were placed on the forum: to guarantee the physical presence of the ancestors so that a *laudatio* could be addressed to them.

It might be assumed that in the course of the eulogy, the words of the orator would lead those in attendance to turn their gaze toward the images and contemplate their form. Nothing of the kind occurred. Far from bringing the dead man's mask into view, the funeral oration covered it with another face. This can easily be deduced from Polybius's text and from treatises on rhetoric dealing with funeral orations.[27] The funeral oration belongs to the demonstrative genre, but, contrary to what the English adjective might lead one to expect, it does not demonstrate or persuade; it brings into view the greatness and nobility of the person of whom it speaks. A speech of the demonstrative genre is not intended to lead to action, as is a political speech, but rather to produce a spectacle. Polybius says it himself when he describes the orator atop the rostrum "setting before the eyes" of the audience the illustrious past of his late family members, calling them up for review one after the other. It was, therefore, the orator who produced that image of the "beautiful dead man" without which there would be no public commemoration of glory presented for the community's admiration. The orator illustrated the *nomina*. Polybius goes on to say that the orator's art made everyone feel as though they "recognized" the exploits recounted. This was equally true, he says, for those who had not participated in the event recounted as for those who had. This enlightening formula gives us an understanding of what type of memory we are dealing with here. What the audience recognizes is not a personal remembrance based on a psychological faculty of memory, but rather a narrative schema that pertains to collective memory and that actualizes civic values attached to war, such as intelligence, constancy and strength. It is at this precise moment that admiration is inspired, and the transmission of warrior virtues is accomplished. The dead have glory, and the young have the desire to imitate them. The funeral oration effects the transformation of the singular deceased into an exemplary deceased. He becomes equal to his ancestors, and at the same time gives his own name to the admirable, exemplary deceased. The gentilic image of the "beautiful dead man" that the words produce is superimposed on the singular, insignificant mask of the dead nobleman. Laudatory speech brings something into view.

The circle is closed. We are back to our *imago*, which is the trace, not the figuration, of the deceased. The *imago* guarantees that the deceased will be present on earth after his funeral. This presence is real, and has nothing to do with the presence/absence of images that merely resemble him. In the atrium of the home as on the forum, the *imago* is not an equivalent for the deceased, but is equivalent to him. This explains why the *imago* can remain hidden, either in its chest or beneath the beautiful mask of the funeral oration. The *imago* is not the image of the deceased, but his trace, like a *vestigium*, the impression a foot leaves on the ground, which only appears when the foot is lifted.[28] This trace is a material reality, *res*, and not an impalpable equivalent for something. Whether it be the *funus imaginarium* of a slave or an aristocrat, the *imago* is a part of the deceased's body that metonymically guarantees his presence in accordance with a conception drawn from Roman law.

*Ossa* and *imago* are the two parts of the Roman body that can replace the entire body and take its place in the funeral rites. The *ossa* are constituted by the human matter not destroyed by the flames of the pyre; the *imago* is the form of the body. The *ossa* can only be disposed of by making them disappear into the earth. Even then, they are present in the tomb, to which they give the status of *locus religiosus*. The *imago* disappears during cremation, or with the corpse's dissolution in the earth — unless it is set in wax. Since the *imago* is a material form, it is not a soul, much less an immortal one. The *imago* is a religiously pure body because it can remain on the surface of the earth without staining heaven or men, but it is nevertheless a mortal form. If its wax support disappears, if the family that looks after the *imagines* dies out or loses interest, then the ancestral forms will die. Nothing is more vulnerable than an *imago*, which is even more fragile than its wax support.[29] For the *imago* is, strictly speaking, neither the wax mask nor the wax of the mask, but, as we have seen, a form detached from the corpse and transmitted to the wax.

One last remark on the choice of wax to preserve the *imagines*: wax is associated with the practice of seals, in other words with identification through signature, trace, metonymy. Wax is perfectly malleable, and short-circuits any labor of modeling — *fictio* (from the verb *fingere*: to shape, mold) — that would produce a disjunction with the model (the fiction). It avoids the destiny of flesh, to be cooked or to rot. It is on the order of materials such as wood and ivory.[30] But unlike marble and bronze, which are used to make monuments, wax is not a durable material; fire destroys it in a matter of seconds. Wax, incorruptible and mortal, renders the *imago* immortal as long as it is protected and reproduced by the *gens*. The instant it is touched by fire, it dies a rapid death.

## The Divine Immortality of the Imperial *Imago*

It was this incorruptible and mortal body of the Roman aristocrats that was to become the immortal body of the deified emperors. Let us return, then, to our imaginary funeral and the rite of consecration of the emperor. Ultimately, the ritual consists in making the sovereign's *imago* disappear from the surface of the earth. This seems like an execution of the *imago*. But it is not an execution of a mortal body, because everything mortal leaves earthly traces after its cremation. The *imago* leaves no trace, like Hercules on his Mount Oeta funeral pyre. Its departure is not the death of its materiality, but its transferral to another space, the space of the gods. In Rome, the disappearance of a mortal body is traditionally associated with fabulous deifications, such as those of Aeneas or Romulus. After having lived among men, one day they disappear from the surface of the earth, leaving nothing for a *sepulcrum*, neither *ossa* nor *imago*.[31] This facilitates the dedication of a temple to them. Diodorus recounts that when Hercules' companions gathered on Mount Oeta to recover the hero's bones, they found nothing to take. They concluded that Hercules' body had left the earth to join the gods in heaven.

Consecration is the enactment of this disappearance of the imperial *imago*, the passage of the emperor's body into the space of the gods. The imperial *imago*, like Hercules' or Romulus's entire bodies, reveals its divinity by leaving no trace on the pyre. Instead of dying during the funeral or being preserved in the atrium, it ascends to heaven, proving that it is divine and immortal.

What authorizes us to interpret the disappearance of the wax figure in terms of ascension rather than death? First, the flight of the eagle upward from the flames, which renders the *imago*'s ascent into the sky symbolically visible, if we may believe Herodian. But more importantly, we must go back to the first imperial consecrations. Before using the *funus imaginarium*, the Romans went through the following procedure: immediately after the emperor's funeral someone would testify before the Senate that he had seen the deceased's *imago* ascend into the sky. The first such witnessing occurred after Augustus's funeral. A Roman who had attended the ceremony swore that he had seen "*effigiem cremati euntem in caelum* [the image of he who had been cremated ascending into the sky]."[32] *Effigies*: the term is equivalent to the word *imago*. It is the recognizable, identifiable form of a man, the *imago* perceived from the viewpoint of resemblance, the *eikōn*. In Cassius Dionysius's account, the same man swore he saw "Augustus ascend into the sky" [*Auguston es ton ouranon anionta*].[33] If there was a moment's doubt that Augustus's *effigies* was his *imago*, it now evaporates. Augustus or his effigy: the equivalence brings us back to the ideology of impression. Only the *imago* can replace the individual. Augustus or his effigy: it is Augustus's *imago* that detaches from his *ossa* and ascends to heaven.

Thus, even before the consecration became an autonomous ritual, imaginary ascension was already indispensable to the concept of the deification of the emperor. This proves that the second-century ritual was no more than an explicit manifestation of a subjacent ideology. Beginning with Augustus, the *imago* leaves the world of men; at the same time, the deified *imagines* of the sovereigns cease to figure in the funerals of their descendants.[34] Caesar's *imago* was made to disappear when he was proclaimed Divus Julius, and did not figure in Augustus's funeral ceremony.

When the Senate voted to consecrate Augustus, it also prohibited use of his *imago*, and made that a general rule for all consecrated sovereigns. The emperor-god is thus expelled from gentilic memory.

The *iurator*, the man who would swear that he saw the *imago* above the pyre, disappeared when the *funus imaginarium* and the flight of the eagle appeared. The ritual of the imaginary funeral realized in a spectacular mode what the *iurator* had testified to. Thenceforth, the *imago* ascended to heaven in the presence of the Roman people, just as incense rose to the gods during the sacrifice. The support-form of the *imago* (the wax) was consumed in the same way as the support-odor (incense). Form and incense, both divine, rise toward the gods.

## The Emperor's Two Bodies

Thus, when the emperor died he was endowed with two bodies through the interplay of two metonymies. One of his bodies was the *imago*, divine and immortal. The other, reduced to the *ossa*, was human and mortal. These two bodies were parts of the emperor's body while he was alive; he was therefore divine in form, and human in flesh.

The *imago* was the part of the aristocratic body that was preserved and allowed it to escape its singularity, becoming an anchor for public honors and gentilic glory. It was the part of the body associated with political life. It is quite understandable that it would be perceived as the seat of the emperor's divine power, of his *numen*. Consequently, the deification of imperial power was the deification of his *imago*.

This "other body" of the emperor had a material and immortal form while he was alive. If this is so, nothing differentiates the *imago* of a citizen from that of the sovereign, just as under the Republic, the plebeian and the nobleman had the same form. Only a political decision — the right to images granted to the aristocracy; a vote of the Senate in the case of emperors — made the *imago* enduring. *Monumentum aere perennius* but as fragile as wax, the *imago* of the aristocrat would live on as long as the nobility of his *gens* shone forth.

The immortality of the emperor's *imago* was produced on the model of aristocratic survival. Two ritual procedures were combined: the funeral and consecration. The "imaginary" funeral was in fact a "time-lag" aristocratic funeral. It consummated the disappearance of the emperor's *imago* from the surface of the earth, just as the *funus* did for the *ossa*. The corpse was the aristocratic *imago* of the sovereign. What, then, in the imaginary funeral corresponds to the *imago* of the human funeral? There is only one answer: absence. An absence expressing an elsewhere. The *imago* is elsewhere. The deified sovereign does not belong to the group of his ancestors; he leaves no trace on earth, having become *sacer*. Thus, the absence of the *imago* of the emperor's divine ancestors at their funerals meant that in their case the *imago* was no longer in the space of men. At this point, the other procedure takes over — the *consecratio* that gives a content to the absence of the *imago*, a positivity to its disappearance: the material form of the sovereign is henceforth *sacra*.

On what condition is this consecration a deification? On the condition that the *imago* is not simply the trace of a singular man, a mere person; if it were, then when it was consecrated it would be expelled into the wilds, thrown into the Tiber. This would be like a *damnatio memoriae*. If it was nothing of the kind — and it was nothing of the kind — it is because the sovereign's *imago* did not have the status of a singular body, but of a category. The *imperium* of Augustus, Claudius or Hadrian does not constitute a particular modality of the general notion of monarchic power. Each is an *imperium* apart, a category, a proper power, in the same sense as we speak of a proper name as opposed to a common noun. There is an autonomous semanticization of imperial singularity; the sovereign does not owe anything to anyone. He is a *gens* unto himself. That is why as an *imago* he has no ancestors, and why he receives a new given name to signify his solitude — *divus*.

Finally, the essential thing is not the enactment of the ritual. It adds nothing to the ritual core constituted by the expulsion of the *imago* from the space of men, and the recognition of its divine character. It does, however, effect an essential qualitative leap in the domain of representation, since it appeals to fiction: the fiction of a dying then stinking *imago*, and the metaphor of the flight of the eagle. Is not the representation of what lies outside the world of men, of what is sacred, only possible through resemblance? The divine body of the emperors could subsequently be present only in Greek fashion, in a lifelike statue, a fiction.

But why, one may ask, did the Romans deify their emperors and fabricate this divine body of power? So that monarchical power would not be tied to a man, that is to say, to a tyrant, or to a man who considered himself a god and consequently became a monster; so that anyone who claimed to be more than a man would be

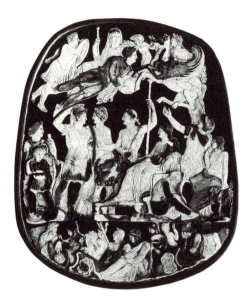

The Glorification of Germanicus.
From the large cameo at Sainte Chapelle.

seen to be less than one. Gods do not reign on earth and do not frequent men. The sovereign was attributed a body that allowed him to straddle the two spaces, human and divine. He had a double body that divided when he died, yielding two bodies, one for men, one for the gods. It was his divine body that governed, present among men by virtue of the flesh, its material support. To avoid tyranny, the Romans invented an immortal *imago*, the divine body of absolute power.

NOTES

1. E.H. Kantorowicz, *The King's Two Bodies* (Princeton: Princeton University Press, 1957).

2. Herodian 4.2.

3. E. Bickermann, "Die römische Kaiserapotheose," *A.R.W.* 27 (1929), pp. 1-34. The author backs up his point of view in "Le culte des souverains dans l'Empire romain," *Entretiens de la fondation Hardt* 19 (1972), pp. 7-37.

4. See E. Kohl, *Klio* 31 (1938), p. 169ff. More recently, see J.-C. Richard, whose latest synthesis is to be found in *Aufstieg und Niedergang der römischen Welt* 2.16.2 (1978), pp. 1122-34. In favor of Bickermann, see P. Gros, *Rites funéraires et rites d'immortalité dans la liturgie de l'apothéose impériale*, thesis for EPHE 4, abstract in *Annuaire 1965-66*, pp. 477-90.

5. John Scheid, *Religion et piété à Rome* (Paris: Editions la Découverte, 1983), p. 54.

6. Cicero, *De natura deorum* 2.61.

7. *Ibid.* 3.51.

8. Ovid, *Fastes* 6.193.

9. Tacitus, *Annales* 15.74; Tertullian, *Apologeticus* 34; *HA, V. Getae*, 2.

10. Suetonius, *Vespasian* 33.

11. Cicero, *De legibus* 2.56-57. Varro, *De lingua latina* 5.4.23.

12. Servius 1.539; Sextus Pompeius Festus 11.101.

13. Ovid, *Fastes*, 2.527-64.

14. Cicero, *Philippinae* 6.13.

15. *HA, V.M. Aurelii* 7.10-11; *V. Severi* 7.8; Cassius Dionysius 74.2; Herodian 4.2.

16. *HA, V. Pertinacis* 15; and *V. Severi* 14.

17. *CIL* 14.212; and *Fontes Juris Romani* 3.35 (1943).

18. Servius, 6.510.

19. Servius, 6.325.

20. Gaius, *Institutiones* 4.17.

21. Pliny the Elder 35.2.3.

22. Plautus, *Pseudolus* 55; Ovid, *Epistulae ex Ponto* 2.20.1.

23. Pliny the Elder 37.4.

24. Juvenal, *Satires* 8.2-9.

25. Polybius 6.53ff.

26. Sextus Pompeius Festus, ed., L, p. 105.

27. Cicero, *De inventione* 1.7; Quintilian 3.4.12ff.

28. Polybius 4.53.4.

29. Juvenal, *Satires* 12.88.

30. *HA, V. Heliogabalis* 25.9.

31. Cicero, *De republica* 3.10.17.

32. Suetonius, *De vita Caesarum: Augustus* 100.

33. Cassius Dionysius 56.46.2.

34. Cassius Dionysius 46.4, 56.34.

From "Corps des dieux," *Le temps de la réflexion*, vol. 7, Paris, Gallimard, 1986.
**Translated by Brian Massumi.**

zone

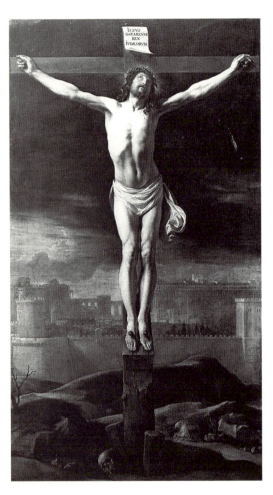

Philippe de Champaigne,
Christ on the Cross (Paris, Louvre).

Hyacinthe Rigaud,
Portrait of Louis XIV in His Majesty (Paris, Louvre).

420

# The Body-of-Power and Incarnation
# at Port Royal and in Pascal

*or*

# Of the Figurability of the Political Absolute

*Louis Marin*

> What is formulated as a rejection of the body or the world, an ascetic
> struggle or a prophetic break, is only the necessary and preliminary
> elucidation of a state of things where the work of offering a body to
> mind, of incarnating discourse and of giving place to a truth, begins.
> Contrary to appearances, lack is situated not on the side of what
> makes a break – the text – but rather on the side of what "makes
> flesh," the body.... Those who take this discourse seriously are those
> who experience the pain of an absent body. The birth they all await in
> one way or another must invent in the word a body of love.
> — Michel de Certeau, *La fable mystique*

Compare two figures of the body in order to link them to each other indissolubly:
the royal body and the divine body.

Exhibit the King's representation, the *fundamental* principle of political authority and legitimacy in its relationship to the religious, theological and spiritual
spheres, which are given as the foundation of this foundation. Convoke this relationship with a singular, horrendous image, the image of the suffering Christ, Christ
incarnate, God humiliated in agony, God in the state of death.

Give as its example and paradigm the portrait of Louis XIV in his majesty by Hya-
cinthe Rigaut, and as in a diptych – placed side by side – Christ on the Cross by
Philippe de Champaigne. Two kingly figures, the King of Earth and the King of
Heaven in a binary relationship of opposition, contrariety and contradiction.

These two images, the two volets of the diptych, when put back to back become
the front and back sides of the same painting – indeterminably hidden or revealed,

front or back. Ask yourself when you make this paradoxical gesture of closing the diptych onto itself on the outside, not face to face, but back to back — who is its spectator if not a split, cloven spectator who stands at once in front of and behind it? Ask yourself if this gesture is not Pascal's among his Port Royal friends.

The 1701 portrait of Louis XIV by Rigaut. (I cannot help thinking that the painter was the one who, at the invitation of the Duc de Saint-Simon, "stole" the portrait from M. de Rancé, abbé de La Trappe.) The crucified Christ by Philippe de Champaigne. (It predates the Rigaut by more than forty years, painted in the years when the God-given Louis Dieudonné seized power, and was for a long time at the convent of the Grande Chartreuse before it was moved to the Musée de Grenoble.)

This relationship of opposition, contrariety and contradiction is here produced, reproduced and depicted by two figures. Think of it as the intimate relationship of an indissoluble union of two represented bodies, one in the throne room, the other on the Cross: the King divine and the divine King. Attempt to see the crucified Christ *through* the King in his majesty in order to try to recognize an essential theologico-political moment in the history of power, and in the body-of-power. This movement, perceived through the spiritual religious thought of Port Royal, is Pascal's: his method, his epistemology, his ethics, his spiritual asceticism, in short, his politics as theology (or the reverse).

Place the figure and the body as closely together as possible, putting at a distance representation and image, or try to understand them differently: assume that the body-of-power, the royal body, is representation, is only representation, and, by the same movement, but reversed, that the saintly image of the Crucified Man is — *quodam modo* — the divine body, the true God incarnate. Through that double movement, signify the passage, in a moment of reversal — or catastrophe — between the political and the religious. The king (with a small k, the real individual with knees swollen by gout — the organic body), is changed entirely into his "image," and becomes "representation" — the King (capital K, dignity, Majesty and the political body). Inversely, it is by obliterating himself as a human creature that God has some chance of making himself seen. To obliterate himself is to incarnate himself, to become a body, a real individual, with his feet and hands pierced by nails, his side opened by the lance, a dead body, immobile and immobilized, presented alone on a twilit background. Here is the chance for an image to be divine presence, secret epiphany, sacred apophasis, dazzling. In both "cases," think of the figure as this process that moves from the real to the image, from representation to presence — a passage that in history sometimes verges on magic or miracle.

Or (it comes down to the same thing) think of the figure at Port Royal and in Pascal as a three- or four-way knot, whose four strands (*sens*) in turn mimic in modern times — the period of Galileo, Bacon and Descartes — the four medieval "senses" (*sens*) of the Holy Scriptures, and treat these senses as the starting points for new meanings.

How did Port Royal (the Jansenist party, the "cabal") represent the principle of political power that pursued it up until its final persecution? What images were invested in the representation of the Prince? What positions and functions did these images receive in the discourses and images produced at Port Royal, around it and against it? Thus the figure of the body-of-power, the figure of the king, would initially name the processes — metaphors, synecdoches, antonomasias and personifications — tirelessly animating the rhetorical field of language and of image — through condensations, displacements and overdeterminations — and the delicate political strategies that these processes imply.

"Figure of the king" and "figure of the body-of-power" would next name the "imaginary" of the King — that portion of imagination that the Prince's representation contains for these moralists and theologians — and the work of the "imaginary" in representation (its force, violence and fatal potential) in the effects of the authority and legitimacy of his representation. "Figure," that is to say, the processes of the image's construction that, because they have become explicit through pedagogical or ethical discourse, deconstruct it by exhibiting the psychological and sociological mechanisms — imagination and custom — that create values and essences.

The third "sense" is really a question: is the King figure? And if he is figure, of what, of whom is he the figure? Figure here understood as a process of meaning, interpretation and exegesis. If the King is figure, if the body-of-power is available only in figure, toward what meaning and toward what truth does this figure lead, providing one has eyes to see and ears to hear? And can one ever follow to its end the process of this last figure where meaning shows itself by withdrawing, exhibits itself by hiding? Is the King figure in this sense? Therefore, this third "sense" is a question. Does meaning perhaps exist at the limit of this process of figure–question in question? An indeterminability wherein recognition of the front and back sides of Rigaut-Champaigne's painting is made possible, for finally God's body is the *disfigured* body of the Crucified Man of Golgotha and not the *transfigured* body of the Son on Thabor. How can you recognize in it this last "sense" of the figure of the political body in its majesty?

The figure of the royal body — a knot of three starting points of meanings, a scenario that produces a rhetoric of the image, an anthropology of the imaginary, a hermeneutics of the symbolic — is a crossing and intersecting of pathways, or rather it is the entire structure of all these potential trajectories.

If the royal body is a triple figure in the three senses pointed out here, ask yourself if this complex figurability does not therefore interrogate the autonomy and independence of political theory in general, of the political and its hard kernel — State power.

⋆   ⋆   ⋆

*Figures*. Jesus opened their minds to understand the Scriptures.

The following are two great revelations: 1. Everything happened to them in figures — *An Israelite indeed, free indeed*, "true bread from heaven."

2. A God humiliated even unto the Cross. Christ had to suffer to enter into his glory, "that through death he might destroy death." Two comings. (487[253]-679)[1]

*Figures*. The letter kills — Everything happened figuratively — Christ had to suffer — A humiliated God — This is the cipher St Paul gives us. (502[268]-683)

*Figures*....

...It is written...that they will be without a king, without princes and without sacrifices....

It is written on the other hand that the law will last for ever, that this covenant will be eternal, that the sacrifice will be eternal, that the sceptre will never leave their midst, since it is not to go until the coming of the everlasting king. (493[259]-685)

With an immobile movement, examine the figurative relationship between a King and the Other, between one image and another, between His Majesty in the radiance of his represented body-of-power and the divine body humiliated even unto the Cross. With Pascal, understand that this perusal not only concerns the mystical exegesis of the Scriptures, but describes a universal principle of intelligibility.

424

"Everything conceals some mystery; everything is a veil that conceals God. Christians must recognize Him in everything."[2] Through a hermeneutic generalization, could not the represented body of the King be posed as figure, as the power of figurability, that is to say, as a local principle of the intelligibility of the political in rhetoric and anthropology? Like everything, the body-of-power conceals some mystery; its portrait's canvas in its majesty is a veil that conceals God. A figure. The body-of-power? A figure. The absolute Monarch? A stupifying paradox and a slanderous contrariety, the *absolutum* of political power – that is to say in its *literal* sense of "the letter that kills," power *unfettered* from all relationships that would qualify, determine or constrain it in order to "compose" it or enter it into a relationship with alterity – absolute power would thus exhaust itself in the process of the figure, a process that "includes absence and presence, pleasant and unpleasant" (499[265]-677). In the movement of alterity, *would the absolute be allegory*?

And what allegory? What alterity? Not the one that in the end is reduced by analogies of resemblance and the mimetics of proportion. But, rather, the one that is intensified by dissimilarity and insisted upon by the forces of disproportion: the allegory of absolute difference. The God who is humiliated unto the Cross and who can only be so because the *body*, flesh and blood in a state of mortal agony, the *absolute* body-of-power (no doubt because it is posed in this way) conceals the following mystery: God's Incarnation, God obliterated unto death in his redemptive union with the fallen creature. If there is a figurability of *absolute* power – a capacity of figure and meaning, a signifying potential – it must be found, with Pascal, in the absolute differentiation of the figurative process, at its end, where this process is immobilized in the mystery of the contradiction of God's body in the state of death, in mortal instance.

Champaigne's great *Crucifixion* on the other side of Rigaut's great ceremonial portrait is in this sense *strange*: it is its secret, and puts the royal representation in a state of figurability, as potential figure.

Ask yourself, then, in what way the portrait of the King, in its figurative potential, reveals or rather insinuates, communicates by "secretions" in the confines of political rhetoric and anthropology, in its desire for the absolute, the secret sense of the political at its highest power.

Then ask yourself about the reversal to difference, a difference itself absolute, of the body-of-power into divine body in a state of death. Understand or attempt to understand that for Pascal the "secret" meaning of the political would be God's death, because God "became flesh, and dwelt among us" (John 1.14).

Notice that these questions not only concern seventeenth-century theological and political relationships, but that a certain spirituality – a mysticism – of the Incarnation, of the divine body as a body of suffering, constitutes one of the strongest problematizations of the theologico-political forms of power, that is, of its very *essence*.

⋆   ⋆   ⋆

The King of France is in his reign, just like, in fact, a God in bodily form.... For what the King does, it is not as if he did it himself, but as if God did it.... Through the mouth of the prince, God speaks; and what he does, is done under God's inspiration.... And he is the spirit of the law on earth.... Likewise, he is the Minister of God on earth.... So therefore, the King is the Delegate of God.... [*Rex Franciae est in regno suo, tanquam quidem corporalis Deus.... Nam quod Rex facit, non tanquam ipse, sed ut Deus facit.... Per Principis os, Deus loquitur; et quae facit, Deo inspirante facit.... Et est lex animata in terris.... Item Minister Dei in terris.... Item Rex, est Delegatus Dei....*][3]

Finally to conclude the present discourse on the Prince, who is the Christ and the anointed one of God, it would be very useful to him to have always before his eyes Isaiah's description of the hallowed, perfect, and immaculate Christ, which cannot be wrongly attributed to Kings, of whom it is written "You are the Gods and the Sons of the Highest.... All earthly Kings are Gods."[4]

The portrait of the King in his majesty: it is not Christ on the Cross that Nicole mounts in the diptych's second volet of the profane and sacred, the worldly and supernatural, the political and religious in chapter thirteen of the third book of his *Traité des quatre fins dernières*, that we find in volume four of his *Essais de morale*;[5] it is the Christ of a republic of Kings, the Kingdom of the Blessed. A picture of contrast, of antithesis between the here-below and the beyond that denies the sign of that contrast, the articulation of that hinge which pushes the link between the opposition and the relationship of difference to its extreme, to scandal. This articulation is a link, a relationship in the form of a cross that is God's dead body; a denial, as often happens with Jansenist theologians and moralists, that promotes processes, pathways and trajectories that benefit limits, poles and *relata*.

We notice it in the first characteristic of royalty in Earth's kings: "Their power ends with their deaths.... It is attached to their lives, therefore it is as little solid and as vain as the lives of men." Simple equations and equivalences, whose evidence is initially one of Port Royal before one of faith. They are oppositions without shadow. A king's power is identified with the life of a body. The death of the body is the death of power. Death is an end, the end of power, the limit of its definition, its end in the double sense of that term: its fulfillment in finitude. In a word, power is life; life is death. A king has the same lot as all other men. Let there be no mistake: that is how the medieval theologico-political doctrine of the King's two bodies crumbles in the Christian moralist's calm assurances. The immortal body of dignity and majesty, always adult, forever removed from nature's misery, is identified with the physical, individual and singular body of the Prince. It is a man on the throne. The act of representation that Louis XIV achieves and that Rigaut stages with known success is thereby inverted: it is not the physical body that disappears in the representation of his majesty to which it is appropriated, but on the contrary, it is the body-of-power that finds its power only in the limits of the physical body that supports it, and attains its ends only with its mortal "term." Nicole outlines this movement of great ideological and theoretical magnitude only to clearly circumscribe its term:

> Sirs, the authority of Kings is sacrosanct, ordained by divinity, the principal work of His Providence, the masterpiece of His hands, the image of His sublime Majesty, proportionate to His immense greatness to the extent that a comparison can be made between the creature and the Creator, as between each Kingdom and State and the Universe, whose admirable harmony is represented by the order established here-below; for as God is by nature the first King and Prince, the King is, through creation and imitation, God in everything, and the King on earth consists of God, him alone and by himself alone, dependent on God alone who fashioned him on the pattern of his omnipotence.[6]

The second trait is as insistent as the first: after the body is the name; after the "organic" life of the individual is the sign that designates him. After the "real" is the "symbolic." If the power of the King does not transcend the mortal life of his own body, what does he identify with his title of King — that name that a crown of courtiers repeats? For as Hegel writes, he alone has a proper name, Louis, not the fourteenth of that name, King of France and of Navarre, but Louis the Great, unique by his surname in the line, with no predecessor or successor. No, for "What is the royalty of a King who sleeps?... A king is effectively King only when he enjoys his royalty and acts as King.... Now how much time in his life does a King spend not thinking of his royalty but fulfilling only base and animal functions?" When read closely, Nicole's reasoning surprises: does a king lose his title of king when he sleeps, when he thinks or acts as a man, when he suffers as an organic body? Does not the Court's as well as all of Europe's epideictic utterance of the King's name, a name that is equivalent to a title — the name of the "world's greatest King"[7] — enact the King's objective "cogito" — "*that is the King*" (not *id*, but *ille*) — by installing its substance through the community of speakers in an abstract and immutable transcendence? Nicole sets aside this curial, national and international utterance to return to the subjective, solipsistic cogito of the empirical individual: "I think (as) King, therefore I am King." This is the first moment of the cogito at which Descartes arrives, at the end of a hyperbolic doubt, a fragile, lacunary cogito, whose ontological assurance is reduced at the moment of its expression. The King's title, his name that condenses this utterance to a term and a simple, descriptive, "concrete" constant of a king's day and the life of the prince's organic body in its moments and spaces, empties this term of all objective validity.

"Sneezing absorbs all the functions of the soul just as much as the [sexual] act [*la besogne*], but we do not draw from it the same conclusions against the greatness of man, because it is involuntary..." (940[795]-160). A king sleeps; he also sneezes and satisfies (*besogner*) the queen or his mistress. "Whence then," continues Pascal,

> there is no shame in man giving in to pain, but it is shameful for him to give in to pleasure.... It is because it is not pain that tempts and attracts us; it is we ourselves who voluntarily choose it and allow it to get the better of us, so that we are masters of the occasion, and in this it is man giving in to himself. But in pleasure it is man who gives in to pleasure. Now, glory only comes from mastery and control, shame only from subjection. (940[795]-160)

Pain, pleasure; mastery, subjection; glory, shame; greatness, the misery of man; greatness, the misery of kings. Nicole inscribes these oppositional pairs that Pascal discovered in his distinction between sneezing and the sexual act in the very function of Kingship: "Even when kings enjoy their royalty and act as Kings, they are not exempt from life's miseries and Nature's infirmities." Boredom and sorrow pursue them even to the throne. That is where those "little amusements" that their Court gives them "to help them carry the weight of that crown and prevent them from thinking of themselves" come from. The body-of-power, the glory that mastery and empire guarantee it, is subject to the same analyses as the body proper, since in the end it is the *same*, but otherwise arrayed, differently situated or localized, placed on another stage: "Great and small are liable to the same accidents, the same annoyance, the same passion, but one is at the top of the wheel and the other near its centre, and thus less shaken by the same movements" (258[705]-180). Is the body-of-power the very center, the hub of *virtù* on the great wheel of fortune? Not at all: the center is itself in movement, everywhere, like the World of which it is the sun.

It is at this high place that Nicole describes the fourth characteristic of the profane body-of-power — in its very power: "To maintain authority and power, how much help and support do they need? How many people are they dependent on?... Their domination is bought only at the price of an infinity of subjection." The description shifts, resulting in the paradoxical conclusion that all domination is dependence, and all power is infinite subjection. Through retrospective anticipation, the Christian moralist replays the Hegelian dialectic of Master and slave, not in the ahistorical moment of civil society's origin and the departure from a state of nature as in Hobbes, but in the (fulfilled) moment of monarchy. Even if it is produced by the theoretical fiction of a duel to the death, the analysis does not construct a foundation for political legitimation. It is a simple phenomenology of the monarch *in situ* who, descriptively, reverses the absolute and the relative, and disseminates it in its particularities: in effect it incarnates the absolute body-of-power in an existing singular body. Reread Pascal:

> *Diversion*. Is not the dignity of kingship sufficiently great in itself to make its possessor happy by simply seeing what he is? Does he need to be diverted from such thoughts like ordinary people?... Will it be the same with a king, and will he be happier absorbed in such vain amusements than in contemplating his own greatness?... Would it not therefore be spoiling his delight to occupy his mind with thoughts of how to fit his steps to the rhythm of a tune or how to place a bar skillfully, instead of leaving him in peace to enjoy the contemplation of the majestic glory surrounding him? (270[137]-142)

But whatever the principles and means of this analysis of the royalty of profane kings are, it only really takes on meaning and value when integrated with the diptych for which it has been made when it becomes a function of the opposite volet: the Royalty of the Blessed whose characteristics permitted the selection of those of kings here-below. In the end, they are the same. Once a change of sign has occurred that converts them to their contrary — an operation so perfectly reversible that any question about its direction would be impertinent. Nicole deduces the other Kingdom "structurally": "We need only take the exact opposite of all these defects and miseries to conceive what the divine Kingdom is." It is this conversion by reversion that nullifies, erases or denies the passage or threshold, crossing or trial, that *creates* a conversion or *figure* through the disfiguration or transfiguration of the different terms. And through this transformation or transubstantiation, in which each of the "terms" is at play in their being and their reality, even their *body* is created. The passage that is, as we have said, that of the death of God in the — absolute — body-of-power; an operation of another scope — or depth — than the algebraic operation of a change in the "signs" that leaves intact, formally or substantially, the greatnesses that they determine, a simple "exact opposite," as the moralist writes, to construct the *concept* of the Kingdom. By doing this, he forgets that the Kingdom is a mystery: "unless one is be born anew, he cannot see the Kingdom of God" (John 3.3).

It is thus a "Kingdom that is eternal and that makes eternal those who possess it"; a "Kingdom that cannot be lost since there is no difficulty in keeping it"; a Kingdom that "is not enjoyed at intervals and with various interruptions"; a Kingdom that entails "neither boredom, nor sorrow, nor weariness," that is "exempt from misery and subjection of all kinds." It is a Kingdom, finally, that is possessed by an infinity of Kings, all equal, having the same mind and the same heart, because they are all together one King, Jesus Christ. All are his coheirs and brothers associated with his heritage, members of his glorious body. This last trait, the only really "positive" one, on which the echoes of 1 Corinthians resonate, expresses the identification of the Kingdom with the glorious mystical Body of Jesus Christ. The blessed, the kings that are fully kings, forever and completely kings with no temporal, material or psychic limitation on their power, are the only truly absolute body-of-power: they realize what the imperial canonists had described and built as the Emperor's majestic body, and what, following them, the jurists of the kings of England and France elaborated as their Prince's body of dignity. And yet from the paradoxical rules of the current mathematics of infinity, each of these truly absolute bodies of power in itself and for itself is only one *member* of the mystical totality, itself absolute, of the *glorious body* of Jesus Christ. "*Members. Begin there.* In order to control the love we owe to ourselves, we must imagine a body full of thinking members," writes Pascal, "[for we are members of the whole], and see how each member ought to love itself, etc." (684[368]-474). "Imagine a body of thinking members" (687[371]-473), he insists. Understand that this imagination is a universal figure whose perfect, exemplary and incomprehensible realization is the Kingdom of the Blessed: this Kingdom is a *Republic* of Kings; *it is a body full of members* that think and think of themselves in their own individuality, but that are only constituted as such because they belong to the whole. The plenitude of empire and domination is identified with total subjection: the paradox of the absolute. "We love ourselves because we are members of Christ...because he is the body of which we are members. *All are one. One is in the other*" (688[372]-483; emphasis added). Pascal, like Paul, discovers in the analogy of the body and its organs that which permits us to think about the foundation of morality, that is, to articulate a doctrine of mores and of civil society, even if this foundation forever transcends all individual and social morality and is beyond our grasp. However, with the same analogy, Nicole builds the concept of the divine Kingdom, directly contrary to the profane Kingdom – its negative image – in which, through a critique as radical as it is implicit, the theologico-political theory of the King's two bodies is exhausted. However, since, as we have suggested, in Nicole the earth's kingdoms and the Kingdom of the Blessed are caught in a structure of static equivalence through the inversion of signs, a projection of the "mystical body of Jesus Christ" in the profane political sphere – but *without its negative inversion* – would make two potential images of the political body appear. To be sure, they are not easily conceivable at that moment: either the image of a society of Nations where each one, equal to all the others, is a member of a totality whose "admirable intelligence" is obtained through "submitting this individual...to the primal will governing the whole body" (688 [374]-475); or a "democratic" society where each citizen is a thinking and deciding member of the sovereign because he is entitled to the totality of rights that all the others will have given him by a reciprocal and simultaneous contract. This is the image of a political body whose theory Rousseau will propose in the *Social Contract* through the mutation of the Unique to the Totality, from the Leviathan to the community of rights and the general will.

\* \* \*

Let the prince, therefore, question who he is: he will find himself to be by nature a man like others and his subjects equal to him.... So, consequently, when a prince begins to admire his crown, diadem, purple and royal regalia, and to flatter himself because of them, then he should promptly be reminded that his head and body, which these things pertain to outwardly, are mortal and human, and subject to the vagaries, adversities and ridicule of fortune; for those externals are not proper [to his state] but mere accidentals; so he should not harm himself by professing himself to be inferior to something external [*Querat ergo princeps quis ipse sit: inveniet se hominem similem aliis natura, et pares in ea sibi esse subditos.... Proinde si quando princeps coronam, diadema, purpuram, ornamentaque regia admirari et in his sibi complacere coeperit: statim quoque reminisci debet, quod caput et corpus, cui haec exterius accedunt mortalia, humana, morbis, lapsibus et ludibrio fortunae obnoxia sunt: quod illa extranea non propria sed accidentalia sunt: et ne injuriam sibi faciat, si se extraneo inferiorem profiteatur*].[8]

Neither in the case of princes do we look for or should we consider what they are in themselves or as men, but rather how much is conceded or allowed to them by God. Nor do we reverence princes so much as individual persons as much as we do the majesty of God and the reflection of His power, and consider how they are reassigned from the role of citizen and carry out vicarious roles on earth [*Neque in principibus, tam inspicimus vel considerare debemus quid ipsi per se et tanquam homines sunt: sed quantam illis concessum aut permissum a Deo sit. Neque in principibus tam personam singularem reveremur quantum majestatem Dei et imaginem potestatemque consideramus ex parte illius civius delegati sunt et vicarias in terra partes gerunt*].[9]

With Pascal, let us substitute for this diptych and its statics of contrasted tabular representations, the movement of the figure of the body-of-power, a matrix of simulation, on which he "experiments" through the structural variation of a characteristic trait.

In this figural model, discover, as in the shroud's weave or Veronica's cloth, the uncertain apparition of another body, the indeterminable potential of the other's face – of God at the height of His Incarnation, that is, in His suffering body, in agony, in the instance of death: the ultimate, sublime end of the royal figure's path, of the absolute body-of-power through the movement of differences, toward difference itself as absolute.

> *Imagine* [*se figurer*] any situation you [*on*] like, add up all the blessings [*biens*] with which you [*nous*] could be endowed, to be king is still the finest thing [*poste*] in the world; yet if *you* [*on*] *imagine* one with all the advantages of his rank, *but no means of diversion*, left to ponder and reflect on what he is, this limp felicity will not keep him going; he is bound to start thinking of all the threats facing him, of possible revolts, finally of inescapable death and disease, with the result that if he is deprived of so-called diversion he is unhappy, indeed more unhappy than the humblest of his subjects who can enjoy sport and diversion. (269[136]-139; emphasis added)

Pascal *constructs* the figure of the body-of-power like a model or matrix that produces effects of meaning. An epistemological subject, a pure methodological operator (marked in the text of the *Pensée* by the indefinite *on*) fashions or fictionalizes from the royal body according to a singularly determined operation, a theoretical artifact, one of its possible figures or "figurables": the "accumulation" onto one single person of "all the blessings with which you [us, *nous*] could be endowed," us, that is to say, men in general, whatever their social condition. This operation makes a figure of the body-of-power appear, a totality of appropriation and possession: "to be king is still the finest thing in the world." A second operation, just as fictitious, consists of adding to this objective, and even quantifiable construction (quantifiable because the actual royal appropriation of goods can be counted), the subjective, qualitative totality of the royal body's possible gratifications. This, then, is a double operation of filling the body-of-power until it is full.

> As for what Isocrates says regarding this subject, that the people's possessions [*biens*] are the prince's, it is understood to refer to custom, and because of the communion between the King and his subjects, who, because they are considered to form a political body, are also in charge of possessions. And just as those of the King are reputed to be public, so are those of the royal Private persons, the Prince represents the public and is able to make use of them as would a good family man [*père*].... It is true that the Prince is the dispenser of public wealth and can take it from private persons so long as necessity requires it.[10]

433

There are those who hold that Kings or Monarchs, having acquired the right to levy these great sums on their subjects, cannot arrogate or allocate the continuation of possession and tax collection, notwithstanding and regardless of how many long years it has gone on, even if it be four or five hundred years. And they endeavor to prove it with written reasons, adding that this immemorial tax collection and possession was taken and demanded by a King from his subjects, either by force or by fear if not otherwise.... Therefore concluding by this means that a King can neither usurp nor prescribe against his subjects what stands against common and natural rights, which is a freedom and immunity from all subsidies and taxes. But these or similar allegations have no place in the Kingdom of France, where Kings have been forced by the malice of the times...to continue the levy of tailles, loans and other subsidies; nonetheless, with certain resolutions to moderate the aforesaid tailles and taxes as soon as God (by his grace) will sometime give respite to their wars and other affairs.... Where our Sovereign Prince... declares himself to be the pitiable father of the country, vigilant pastor of his people... true minister or rather true image of God, the unique protector of justice, if not the living law itself; and finally the Republic's loyal guardian and defender, which is none other than a mystical body of which the Prince is the head, who seeing in himself those two fine senses, hearing and sight, which together with his intelligence govern the entire body, and which, in recompense, according to all divine and human right, gives him all right to honor and obedience, to tributes and subsidies.[11]

The simple variation of a trait of the figure thus constructed will put it in motion, into a state of action, that is to say, into the process of figurability: a variation in this case negative, achieved by removal, with "no means of diversion." But this variation is itself the negation of a negation, because diversion is defined as that which prevents the king "from ponder[ing] and reflect[ing] on what he is." This variation, or rather the process that it brings about, will have *the effect of producing his unhappiness at being* the "finest thing in the world," a figural artifact fictively constructed by the totality of *all the "having" possible*, both objective and subjective: "he is unhappy, indeed more unhappy than the humblest of his subjects." Note that the production of this effect of unhappiness is not aleatory; it is itself graduated and finalized in a series of structurally necessary potentialities or possibilities within the conditions of the experimentation on the model of the royal body: languor, threat, agony, death. A precise analysis of this series would permit us to examine the effective edges and constitutive limits of the representation of state power like a *mechanism of the legitimate monopoly of violence, but reflected onto the subject of representation*, the body-of-power itself. Indeed, the potential or real threat of death, itself possible or real, gives coercive credibility to signs that place "natural" violence in social and political representation and, moreover, indirectly operates the legitimating reinforcement of their authority on the surface or within the circumstances of the body-of-power:

> That is why our kings…have not only dressed up [*masqués*] in extraordinary clothes to show what they are, but they also have guards and scarred veterans escort them. These armed troops whose hands and strength are theirs alone, the drums and trumpets that march before them, and these legions which surround them make the most resolute tremble. (81[44]-82)

Men of war, whose role is more essential since they establish themselves by force, are in some sense the disguise of the royal body; the death that they potentially hold due to their power, their reserved force, "death is the King's mask." The legions that surround him, the Great Lord's forty thousand janissaries, are his sublime diversion. To imagine the body-of-power through the fictionalization of their disappearance is in some sense to turn over his Mask, to gorgonize omnipotence by the negative presentation of the originary violence on which it is founded; it is to reflect onto the body-of-power his own external essence, "like children taking fright at a face they have daubed themselves" (269[136]-139).

Read again:

> *Diversion*. Is not the dignity of kingship sufficiently great in itself to make its possessor happy by simply seeing what he is?… Would it not therefore be spoiling his delight to occupy his mind with thoughts of how to fit his steps to the rhythm of a tune or how to place a bar skillfully, instead of leaving him in peace to enjoy the contemplation of the majestic glory surrounding him? (270[137]-142)

This second kingly figure is similar to Rigaut's portrait in the face-to-face created by Louis XIV hanging his own picture in front of him in the throne room. The king is *happy* at just the sight of what he is, is happy to possess royal dignity; to contemplate himself, and to contemplate his own body as the support and mannequin of this accumulation of signs and insignia, from the red heels to the wig, that designate and signify the (absolute) body-of-power. The king's happiness is not to enjoy glory, but to enjoy the contemplation of the glory that is, in its species, less a quality determining the royal being than the circumstantial place of his represented body. To give himself to the Court, to offer himself to the world and the universe as a being to be contemplated, to exhaust himself, to deplete his being in this oblation: a sublime enjoyment that is ruined in the vacuity of infinite self-reflection; to enjoy is to see himself being seen. The essential being, the proper body (of power) is disseminated in a multitude of objects for the eyes that gaze upon him, a multitude of aspects and of simulacra, before being recaptured, to regain control of himself, in an eyeless gaze, the gaze that looks at all those eyes that gaze upon the body dispersed in dazzling fragments, the sight of the Monarch that cannot be situated, where his body of dignity is no longer anything but the field of a vision: the void of "seeing himself be seen."

Here is the Pascalian experimentation on this new model; here is the fictional gesture that puts it in the process of figurability:

> Put it to the test; leave a king entirely alone, with nothing to satisfy his senses, no care to occupy his mind, with no one to keep him company and no diversion, with complete leisure to think about himself, and you will see that a king without diversion is a very wretched man. (270[137]-142)

In the end, the proof, the test, is none other than a king whose unique function is to contemplate himself as King, as Monarch, as Absolute; a king reduced to his representation or completely taken over by it; a king entirely, his body and his gaze, become his own portrait; or perhaps, as courtly discourse would characterize it, *in the end a king comparable only to himself*. It is then, at that moment, at the height of representation, that the figure is absolute and the body-of-power sublime, that the "figurability" of the grandiose figure — a subliminal figure — appears in filigree, the secret mark that is its difference: "a very wretched man." A difference not yet absolute, but from which the absolute other begins to appear: "All these examples of wretchedness prove his greatness. It is the wretchedness of a great lord, the wretchedness of a dispossessed King" (220 [116]-398).

Third figure in counterpoint:

> The fact that kings are habitually seen in the company of guards, drums, officers and all the things which prompt automatic responses of respect and fear has the result that, when they are sometimes alone and unaccompanied, their features are enough to strike

respect and fear into their subjects, because we make no mental distinction between their person and the retinue with which they are normally seen to be associated. And the world, which does not know that this is the effect of habit, believes it to derive from some natural force, hence such sayings as: "The character of divinity is stamped on his features." ([25]-308)

This is the figure of counter-proof, because to build a model of the body-of-power, constructed according to the same principles as the ones above, produces a contrary effect, an effect of discourse and gaze that is a part of the world's gaze and discourse. Because through an ignorance of "cause and effect," the world reads the God of War's imprint on the monarch's face. Just as above, death is indeed the King's mask. Guards, scarred veterans, drums, trumpets, officers, legions and all the other disguises of circumstance and representation, those instruments of power put on reserve in the signs that show force at rest – that is on parade. They display the *potential* threat of death, the virtue to declare, in a simple exposition, the *legitimate* power of he who has a monopoly on force: "These armed troops whose hands and strength are theirs alone" (81[44]-82) – exhibition, show and ostentatious exposition whose effect is one of both terror and respect indissolubly bound together.

Remove them and what is the result? The king's face has acquired the effect of these external accompaniments of force. Because he is not caught in the annihilating vertigo of self-reflection, because he remains turned toward the outside, toward his court, his people, *the King's face has itself become a death mask*. Pascal gives an associationistic and mechanistic explanation for this political Medusa-effect: custom creates this astonishing surface *incorporation*; the circumstances, surroundings and accompaniments external to the king's physical body are "envisaged" on his face; they are on his body-for-others, not for the king himself, but for all those who gaze upon him. "It would take reason at its most refined to see the Grand Turk...as a man like any other" (81[44]-82), even when he is no longer surrounded, in his superb seraglio, by forty thousand janissaries. Two *secondary effects* follow from this effect of the gaze: one of belief, the other of discourse. The Prince's *sociopolitical distinction*, that he is first in the State and the nation, is *believed to be a difference of nature and force*, an ontological difference that makes him a man like others, but also a king, a superman endowed, by nature and heredity, with the might whose signs he possesses, those signs that show in him the potential threat of death. "Hence such sayings as: 'The character of divinity is stamped on his features' " ([25]-308), sayings that displace the signs' ontological natural difference in a distinction that is no longer sociopolitical, but theologico-political. This transcendent distinction not only allows the character of Divinity to be *transparent* on the King's face, the seal that marks his sacred election, but also *incarnates* God in the Monarch. Is it not indeed this expression that, in the prologue of the Epistle to the Hebrews, designates the Son of God incarnate: "He reflects the glory of God and bears the very stamp of his nature, upholding the universe by his word of power" (1.3)? But those are the words of the "world, which does not know that this is the effect of habit" ([25]-308), an ignorance of cause and effect, an ignorance of the proud profane knowledge that in its discourse claims to incarnate God in the Monarch in the name of analogies of resemblance and mimetic proportions as if guards and scarred veterans, drums and trumpets, officers and legions could be proportionate to the Divine Word incarnate.... Whereas only the absolute disproportion of absolute dissimilarity can attempt to let this nonrelation be understood, "the infinitely more infinite distance" ([308]-793) between the kings of concupiscence and the king of charity: a divine body humiliated all the way to the Cross, a suffering Christ — the Anointed One of the Lord, the King — in a state of agony *in* the portrait of the Monarch.

*   *   *

In truth, the methodological movement, the epistemological process of the "figure" disclosed in Pascal's fragments, is a characteristic of the ethical thought of the Port Royal moralists. It is a question of the (baroque?) proposition that only through surroundings, circumstances, frame, exteriority and the other is there identity as the term of a process of identification, property as the term of appropriation, face or portrait as the term of a process of incorporation. Identification of the I or of the King ("the King is me," "the State is me") exists only through a play that is ruled by gazes and discourses within the mechanism of representation.

That is why in Pascal's construction of the "figure" of the body-of-power, and especially in its functioning and the process of figurability that it exposes, the simulation of the king's solitude becomes a decisive moment — his neglect, abandonment, dereliction — for it fictitiously (methodologically), and through a mental

experiment, cancels or neutralizes all the processes of identification and incorporation by "extraneation," as Hegel would say. At the same time, it performs on the
I, just as it does on the King, one of the most radical problematizations of the (Cartesian) "metaphysical" subject, the "political" subject, the body itself – "A man is
a substance, but if you dissect him, what is he? Head, heart, stomach, veins, each
vein, each bit of vein, blood, each humor of blood?" (113[65]-115) – and finally, the
*monarchical* body-of-power.

One of the finest and most effective examples of this movement of the "figure"
in Pascal is found in the second volume of Nicole's *Essais de morale*; in the opening
of the first of the three discourses on the *Condition des Grands*[12] that the moralist
probably drafted from notes taken when they were delivered. In a way, the "figure,"
model or matrix of simulation espouses its own fictionalization and the very process of figurability by becoming a narrative – a parable "like" those that Christianity reads in evangelical texts. "To enter into a true knowledge of your condition,"
Pascal says to the young duc Charles Honoré de Chevreuse, son of the duc de Luynes,

> consider it in this image: a man is thrown by a storm onto an unknown island, whose
> inhabitants were at pains to find their king who had been lost; and, greatly resembling
> the king in body and face, he was taken for him, and recognized in that quality by the
> people. At first he did know what part to take; but he resolved at last to lend himself to
> his good fortune. He received all the respects that they wanted to pay him and let him-
> self be treated as king....

The conversion of the "figure" in the narrative-parable inverts its successive
moments and the effects of simulation. The narrative opens with the image of the
shipwrecked man "thrown by a storm onto an unknown island," a man alone,
wretched, in a state of total dereliction.

> When I see the blind and wretched state of man, when I survey the whole universe in
> its dumbness and man left to himself with no light, as though lost in this corner of the
> universe, without knowing who put him there, what he has come to do, what will
> become of him when he dies, incapable of knowing anything, I am moved to terror, like
> a man transported in his sleep to some terrifying desert island, who wakes up quite lost
> and with no means of escape. (389[198]-693)

Nonetheless, in the parable's remarkable variation, the island is not deserted but
inhabited: it is deserted by its King, a king who is lost and cannot be found. This

loss is, in the precise meaning of the term, *fundamental* (*fondamental*): it is a loss at the State's foundations (fondement), or rather it manifests the State's collapse (effondrement). The political loses its foundations. This island's king, "who had been lost," is, upon consulting the dictionaries of the time, "out of reach of the senses" of his people, is invisible – whether he has gone astray, has drowned, or has been engulfed (*abysmé*). On the one hand, there is a man alone and wretched, "thrown by the storm" and, on the other, there is a King, the King *en abysme*, invisible, *lost*: the front and back sides of a single mechanism that is referred to in one narrative structure. Front and back sides: the shipwrecked man on the front side and the king on the back side, between the two, the island's people are placed in a state of destitution.

Experimentation on the parabolic narrative figure can then begin: a new and strange element is introduced into the narrative from the outside, a fluke that is a "coincidence," as we say, but that focuses on the mimetic structure, on the relationship of resemblance: "greatly resembling the king in body and face, he was taken for him...." The physical body, the singular face of the shipwrecked man; and the King's body, his majestic face. The first is the whole portrait of the other, its identical figure, the portrait identified *by chance*, in the fluke of the narrative, the accident of fiction, the chance of the figure, not by metaphysical necessity or ethico-political obligation. In the system of variety and variation, in the field of diversity and difference, in bodies ready for infinite differentiation, it could well be that analogies of mimesis and proportions of resemblance, far from being manifestations of the *law* of the world and of being, are only flukes, erratic "coincidences." But the necessity of the effects clings to this "fluke" and, retroactively, makes it destiny. Through the effects of recognition and belief, through political effects, the people recognize in him the quality of King and he receives their respects. He "let himself be treated as king." Instantly, through the simple fortuitous "play" of resemblance, the dignity of a King ceases to be a transcendent essence and becomes a pure quality adrift and in search of a body that suits it. And the chain of respects and subjections that cling to it exposes – after the fact – that the foundation of the political is a "semblance," a "lure."

However, in a new and surprising effect, the situation of the initial loss, shipwreck and deviation is renewed, this time in the body-of-power itself thus reconstituted, and in the subject of political representation thus reinstituted, *in the form of that body's fission — a split in that subject*:

> as he could not forget his natural condition, he reflected at the same time as he received those respects that he was not the king that the people sought, and that that kingdom did not belong to him. He had therefore a double thought: one by which he acted as king; the other by which he recognized his true state.... He hid the latter thought and exposed the other. It is by the first that he dealt with the people, and by the latter that he dealt with himself.

A fission of the body-of-power in public and in private; a split in the subject of representation into an exposed side and a hidden side, into an external mask and an internal face.

This new figure of the King that Pascal constructs at the beginning of his discourse on the condition of the Greats, new in its parabolic form, but new also in the virtual processes of figurability that it opens up, unleashes — we might say — a sort of crisis in the body-of-power: the split between the King who is of representation and in representation and the "real-true" man is such that the former only finds his legitimacy through a *transcendent* principle of authorization that has no natural foundation: it is perfectly arbitrary. "I do not want to say that [all those goods that you possess]," says Pascal to the young duc de Chevreuse,

> do not legitimately belong to you and that another is permitted to strip them from you; for God who is their Master has permitted societies to make laws to share them; and once these laws are established it is unjust to violate them. This is what distinguishes you *a little* from the man who would possess his kingdom only by the error of the people.... But what you have *entirely* in common with him is that the right that you have to them is not *founded*, no more than his, *on some quality and on some merit that be in you....* *Your soul and your body* are of themselves indifferent to the estate of a boatman or of a duke; and there is *no natural tie* that attaches them to one condition rather than to another.... (emphasis added)

Besides, the figure of the King thus drawn and set in motion covers a secret: the King is a man like the others; his royalty is not real greatness founded in nature. Like his secret, the figure of the King hides the split that that very figure (such as Pascal has constructed it) reveals by uncovering its secret. However, the figurative narrative, because it is narrative and parable, and through the very secret that it reveals in the figure of the body-of-power, conceals another secret, the secret of the secret, which is not and cannot be the object of a *revelation*, but that Pascal's text lets escape by *insinuation*. This narrative, like the evangelical parable or biblical text, is a "cipher with a double meaning" (494[260]-678): the second meaning or secret is the one that hides the legitimate King of the island "who had been lost."

The loss that is named and figured in this narrative fiction, the deviation, the abyss, is none other than "the strange secrecy into which God has withdrawn, *impenetrable to the sight of men*"; a strange secrecy that is "a great lesson for bringing us to solitude, far away from the sight of men,"[13] the solitude that all of Port Royal will describe as the place antithetical to the Court.

But this loss is equally man fallen from his primal state: " 'I have created man holy, innocent, perfect,' " cries God's wisdom, through Pascal's pen, " 'I filled him with light and understanding, I showed him my glory and my wondrous works. Man's eye then beheld the majesty of God.' " King of creation, " 'he could not bear such great glory without falling into presumption' " (309[149]-430). "Who cannot see from all this that man is lost, that he has fallen from his place, that he anxiously seeks it, and cannot find it again?" (394[430]-431). The man, a king who is lost, a king "dispossessed" of his kingdom, "obviously gone astray; he has fallen from his true place" (312[400]-427) by his original sin.

Therefore, the figure of the King thus constructed insinuates a double figurability of the body-of-power: according to the first, it is a body-of-power but in retreat, God's impenetrability far away from the sight of men; and second, it is "figurable" man, the king of creation fallen from his place, astray in a corner of the universe... God, man: the first, unfathomable in his transcendence; the second, an abyss of "impenetrable darkness" (312[400]-427). Here again, there is a body-of-power but in a loss and a fall. It is the truly legitimate and founded body — the engulfed body of foundation. God has withdrawn and man is engulfed; and in the locus and place of the first the latter returns, its representative by fortuitous mimesis and recognized as such by others, in "extraneation." A man wretched and alone, returns to his place, to his true locus where he had once resembled and been the image of the King and now, by chance, because he, in his exteriority re-sembles that King, he becomes its semblance, its double, its replica. He is the *usurper of the Kingdom*, no longer its legitimate proprietor. To be sure, he is a "truthful" usurper, but this authenticity is very singular, for it is truthfulness for himself alone, existing in the interior of a subject that denies itself the body and the face that it has received from the people, all while acting externally and publicly as a foreign body-of-power: "Just as Jesus remained unknown among men, so the truth remains among popular opinions with no outward difference. Thus the Eucharist and ordinary bread" (432[225]-789). The infinite difference, the "without-rapport" is thus "mysteriously" what is "with no outward difference."

In other words, the figurative place that the double figurability of the wretched shipwrecked man whom the inhabitants "falsely" recognized as *their* King draws in relief, is, through *dissimilarity* and *difference in the identification of the same*, at once that of God who "has withdrawn, impenetrable to the sight of men," and a God who "when it was necessary for him to appear, he hid himself all the more by covering himself with humanity," so that "he was much more recognizable when he was invisible than when he made himself visible."[14] But it is also that of sinning man in the abyss of his wretchedness: God incarnate. The Incarnation — which I understand in the theological and spiritual sense of the term — the *mystery* of the Incarnation, of a *God become flesh*, insinuates, within the ambiguous figurability of the body-of-power, by an infinitely more infinite difference, the secret-of-the-political, of a presence *and* an absence, of a disappearance *and* a return, of a loss *and* a gain, precisely what Pascal calls a figure or a portrait:

> A picture includes absence *and* presence, pleasant and unpleasant. Reality excludes absence and unpleasantness.
>
> *Figures....*
>
> ...They [Jesus and the apostles] have taught us...that the redeemer will be spiritual and his kingdom of the spirit, that there will be two comings, one in wretchedness to humble the proud, the other in glory to exalt the humble, that Jesus is God and man. (494[260]-678)

The secret of the political is that the King, the body-of-power, is a portrait, but a portrait in which the true convert will discern in the King, in the exposition of his majesty, the dying Christ hung on the Cross.

The secret meaning of the political — this "theologeme" like the infinite difference between the absolute and the body-of-power — is the divine body in his mortal and redemptive humiliation. When Nicole opposed the kingdoms of the here-below with the Kingdom of the Blessed, the glory of his diptych anticipated the Second Coming. The Christ of suffering, God incarnate, the divine body is the necessary and invisible hinge between the two volets of "earth" and "heaven," their "mystical" articulation, like the mechanism of a spiritual and theological dialectic, an *itinerarium mentis in Deum* (to speak like the Seraphic Doctor), which, in the political field, is the place of conversion, the passage of reversal from the king of concupiscence to the King of charity. The "spring" of this "dialectic" of the suffering Christ, the dynamic that the pious call the "sufferings" of Jesus, is a movement of retreat, withdrawal, a movement that is, in a way, the difference of the social bond, the paradoxical bond of a community's nonrelation, a movement that we will have to think of and grasp in the "infinitive" of its neutral status, between active and passive, at once the gesture of God *withdrawing* into his secrecy or the saint retreating into the desert or the just going into solitude, and the movement of Adam falling from his true place, the original model of the others, of almost all the others who pull away from only one, the Unique, and who leave, desert and abandon him, separating themselves from him: "And so Jesus was abandoned to face the wrath of God alone" (739[919]-553); "I have cut myself off from him, shunned him, denied him, crucified him.... Sweet and total renunciation" (737[913]). "What makes solitude *boring* to most of the world is that *being separated from the sight of men*, they are also *separated* from their judgment and their thoughts. Thus, their hearts remain *empty and starving*, being *deprived* of that ordinary food":[15] a double tearing away that is inscribed as wounds and humiliation, as mortifying instance on the body-of-power as on the divine body.

A God abandoned, whose bodily wounds and tortures even unto execution are the "historical" manifestations and "spiritual" signs of that abandonment, dissipates the illusions of the "finest thing of the world," that of the King as paradigm of each I: it is inscribed in it as the invisible "figurable" of defiguration.

A God deserted, torn from a society of friends and disciples, demonstrates figuratively the essential ordeal of the soul, a prey to self-love, loving itself in all things, making itself the center and wanting to subjugate all others. Read about this desertion within a state of concupiscence as Nicole has "imaged" it:

> Imagine then a universal scourge or rather a mass of wounds, plagues and carbuncles with
> which the body of a man is covered.... That is the image of the state in which we are

born and that we are by nature. Our love of ourselves which is the center and course of all our ills....[16]

But if the divine body abandoned in its tortures and agony can be negatively inscribed in the King's portrait and the soul of the I, it is because it retains and exposes through its humiliations the *wickedness* that makes of each "I" a king of concupiscence, that is to say, a tyrant, an illegitimate, unjust king, an executioner of the King of charity. The motive is one of "mystical" meditation as much as it is of a theologico-political character, but it is one in which the theological and the political are put at an infinitely more infinite distance. The convert of the *Mystère de Jésus* writes:

> I see the *depths* of my pride, curiosity, concupiscence. *There is no link between me and God or Jesus Christ the righteous.* But he was made sin for me. All your scourges fell upon him. He is more abominable than I, and, far from loathing me, feels honored that I go to him and help him.... *I must add my wounds to his, and join myself* to him....
> (739[919]-553; emphasis added)

The union is made through the wounds of two bodies, the body-of-sin and the body-of-God, between which the relationship is nonetheless abysmal. Here the *end* is declared — in the two senses of the term — in the great theme of the King's two bodies: proportionate indeed to his divinity, the body of suffering of the Christ is the end of the body of dignity of the profane and profanatory King because it is his secret: the body of a man full of misery. But it indicates just as mysteriously the passage through conversion, that is to say through annihilation, infinite difference, toward the Kingdom.

That is what the end of the third discourse on the *Condition des Grands* signals, where Pascal again picks up the contradiction between concupiscence and Charity: "To be King is to be the Master of many objects of the concupiscence of men, and thus to be able to satisfy the needs and desires of many. It is these needs and desires that attract them to your side." Such is the essential social bond. Pascal continues:

> It is concupiscence that provides the force of the earth's greatest kings, that is to say the possession of things that men's cupidity desires.... It is not your natural force or power that subjects all these people to you. Do not claim to dominate them by force....

For, if we may comment, that would be *tyranny*: do not claim to reign by a path other than that which makes you king, but maintain yourself in the *essential injustice of the body-of-power, to be central to the desires of others*, because you are master of the wealth that they covet. "If you remain there," adds Pascal,

> you will not fail to ruin yourself, but as *honnête homme*. But it is always great folly to damn oneself. You must despise concupiscence and its kingdom and aspire to that kingdom where God is king and where all subjects breathe only charity and desire only the blessings of charity. Others than myself will tell you the way.

One of these paths is the process of figurability of the body-of-power: contemplate the divine body of suffering that, by its very dereliction, is the infinite body of love; contemplate it *in* the profane body of represented royal majesty, its portrait; contemplate, that is, examine *on the spot* the infinite distance of the difference of the one in the other.

NOTES

1. Blaise Pascal's *Pensées* are cited from Louis Lafuma's edition (Paris: Delmas, 1967); the second number is from Léon Brunschvicg's edition. Translator's note: I have used A.J. Krailsheimer's excellent translation of the *Pensées* (New York: Penguin Books, 1966), occasionally adding the original French in brackets to clarify Louis Marin's textual argument; the alternative Lafuma numbers Krailsheimer uses are in brackets.

2. Pascal, fourth letter to Mlle de Roannez, end of October 1656. Translator's note: See *Oeuvres complètes* (Paris: Editions du Seuil, 1963), p. 267.

3. Charles de Grassaille, *Regalium Franciae, libri duo: Jura omnia et dignitates christianissimi Galliae regis continentes* (Lyon, 1538), pp. 63-64. Translator's note: All translations from the Latin are by George Greenia.

4. David du Rivault, *Les Etats, esquels il est discouru du prince, du noble et du tiers Etat, conformément à notre temps* (Lyon, 1596), pp. 136-37, 139.

5. Translator's note: Pierre Nicole, *Essais de morale*, 13 vols. (Paris, 1723-35).

6. Jacques de La Guesle, "Harangue de 1595," *Les remontrances* (Paris, 1611).

7. Translator's note: Pierre Pellisson-Fontanier, *Oeuvres diverses*, 3 vols. (Paris, 1735), vol. 2, pp. 323-28.

8. Pierre Grégoire, *De Republica, libri sex et viginti* (Lyon, 1609), bk. 6, ch. 3, no. 7.

9. *Ibid.*, bk. 6, ch. 2, no. 9.

10. François de Gravelles, *Politiques royales* (Lyon, 1596), pp. 202-03.

11. Jean Combes, *Traité des tailles et aultres charges, et subsides tant ordinaires que extraordinaires qui se lèvent en France* (Paris, 1576), pp. 18a-19b.

12. Translator's note: See Pascal's "Trois discours sur la condition des Grands," *Oeuvres complètes*, pp. 366-68.

13. Fourth letter to Mlle de Roannez.

14. Fourth letter to Mlle de Roannez.

15. *Logique de Port-Royal*, pt. 1, ch. 10. Translator's note: Antoine Arnauld and Pierre Nicole, *La logique ou l'art de penser*, intro. Louis Marin (Paris: Flammarion, 1970), p. 114, emphasis added.

16. "Traité de la connaissance de soi-même," vol. 3, *Essais de morale*, pt. 2, ch. 3.

**Translated by Martha M. Houle.**

# Mapping the Body

*Mark Kidel and Susan Rowe-Leete*

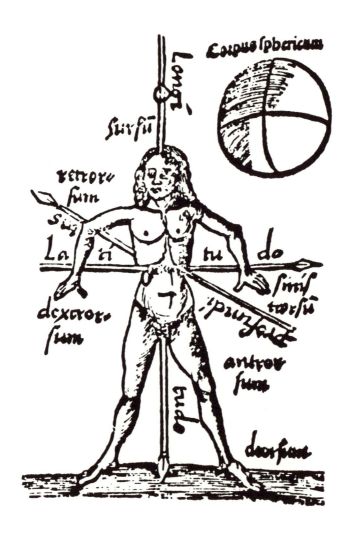

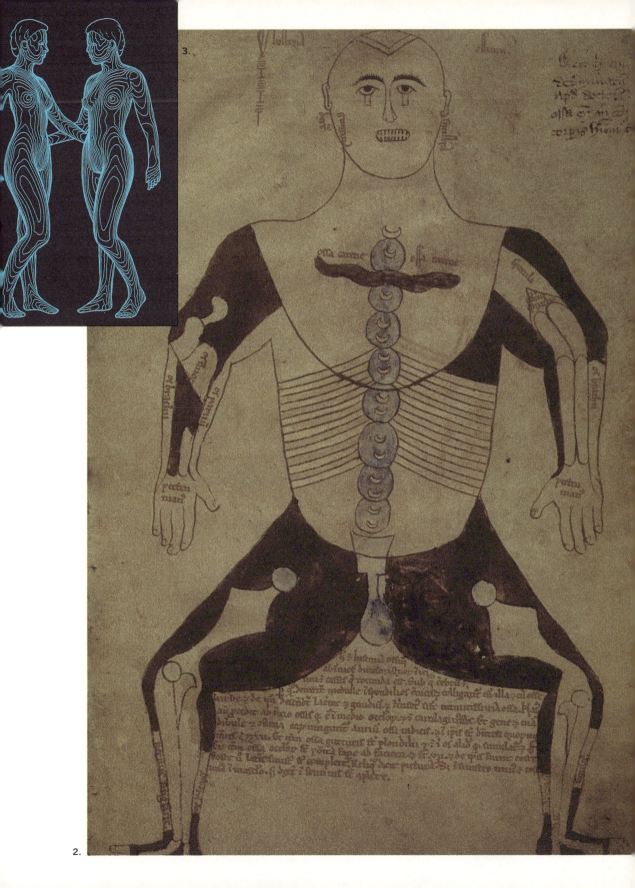

4.

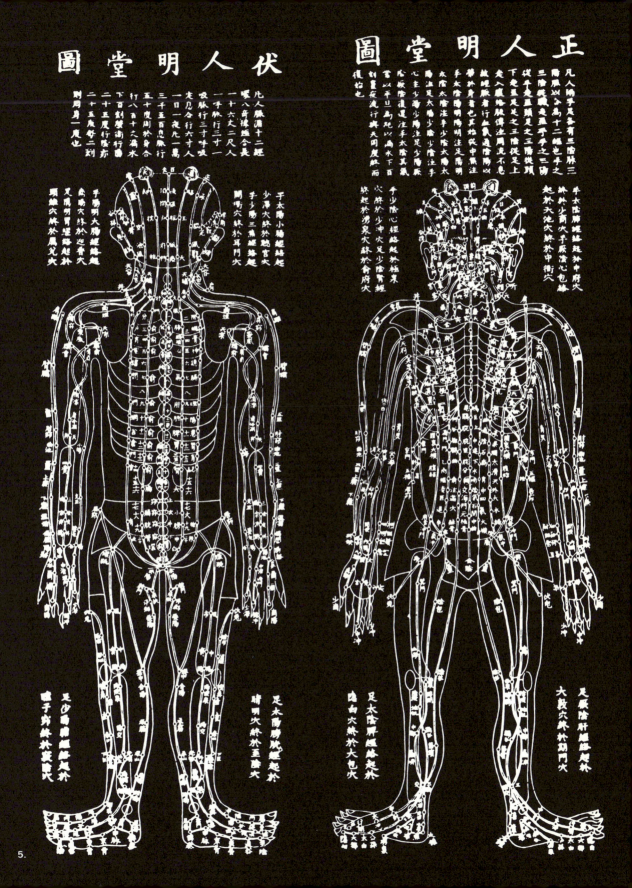

5.

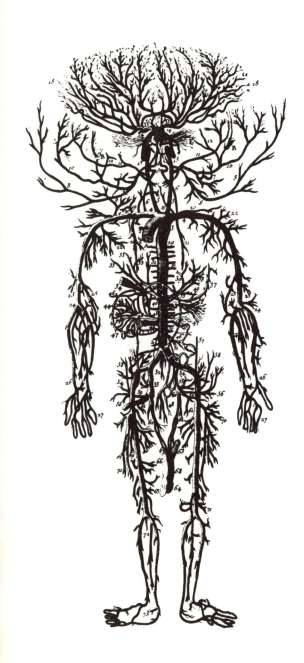

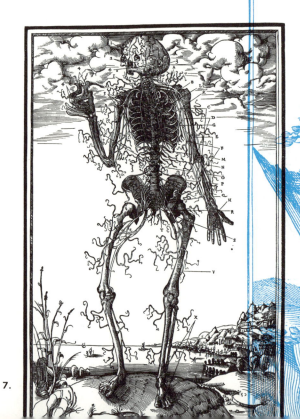

6.          7.

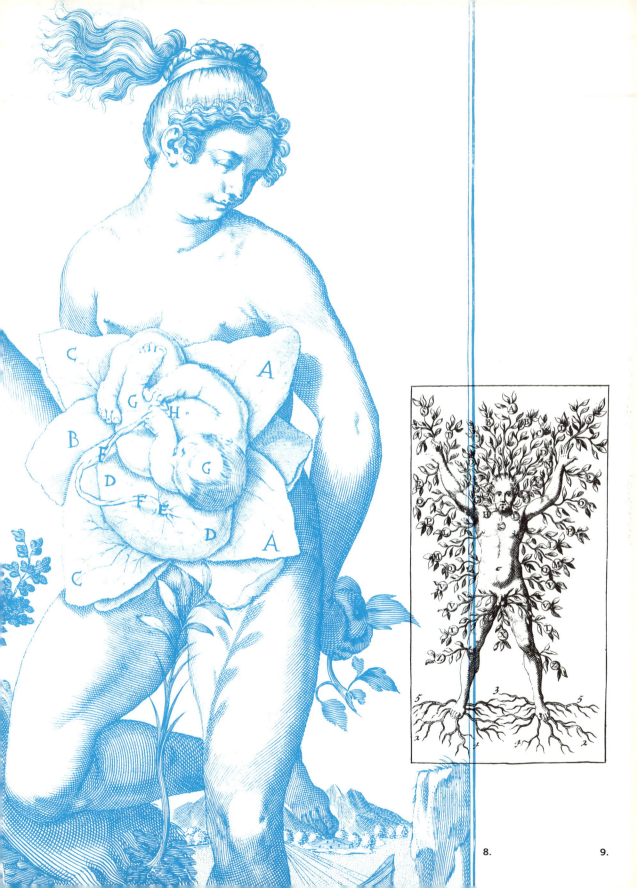

8.

9.

Man is called by the ancients a world in miniature and certainly this name is well applied, for just as man is composed of earth, water, air and fire, so is the body of the earth. If man has in him bones which are the support and armor of the flesh, the world has rocks which are the support of the earth; if man has in himself the sea of blood, in which the lungs rise and fall in breathing, so the body of the earth has its oceanic sea which also rises and falls every six hours for the world to breathe. If from the said sea of blood spring veins which go on ramifying throughout the human body, similarly the oceanic sea fills the body of the earth with infinite veins of water. — Leonardo da Vinci

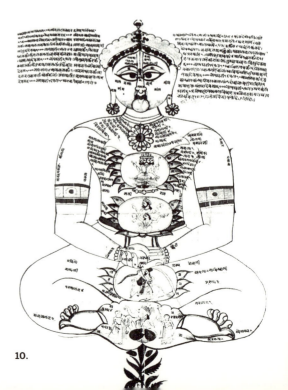

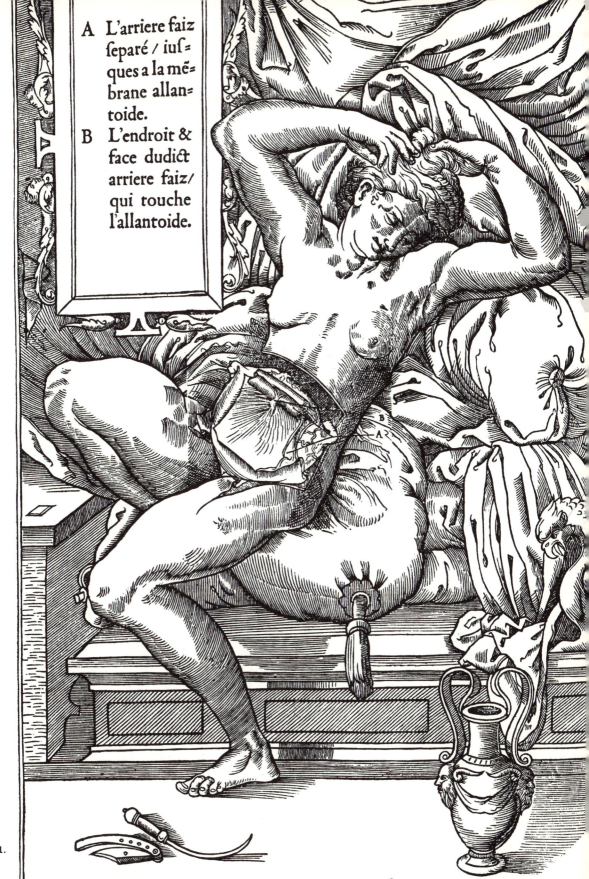

A L'arriere faiz
separé / iuſ=
ques a la mē=
brane allan=
toide.
B L'endroit &
face dudict
arriere faiz/
qui touche
l'allantoide.

11.

I think the physician...is to look upon the patient's body as an engine that is out of order, but yet so constituted that, by his concurrence with the endeavors or rather the parts of the automaton itself, it may be brought to a better state. (Robert Boyle, *Works*, 1772, vol. 5, p. 236.)

12.

Might it be, perhaps, that the body can only be thought of as a reality in terms of categories which negate life...that its nature is only 'thinkable' through the death-dealing structures of reason? (Paul Gerôme, *Les anatomies fantastiques*, Geneva, Editions D3, 1983.)

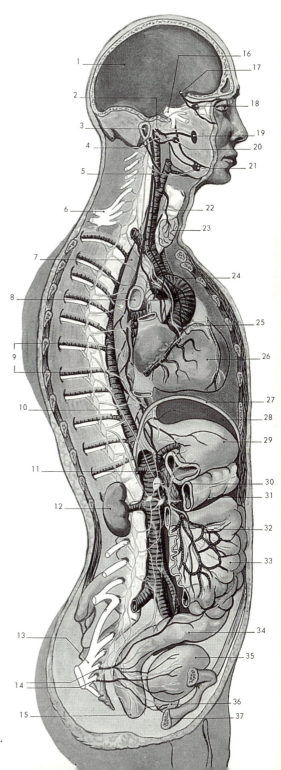

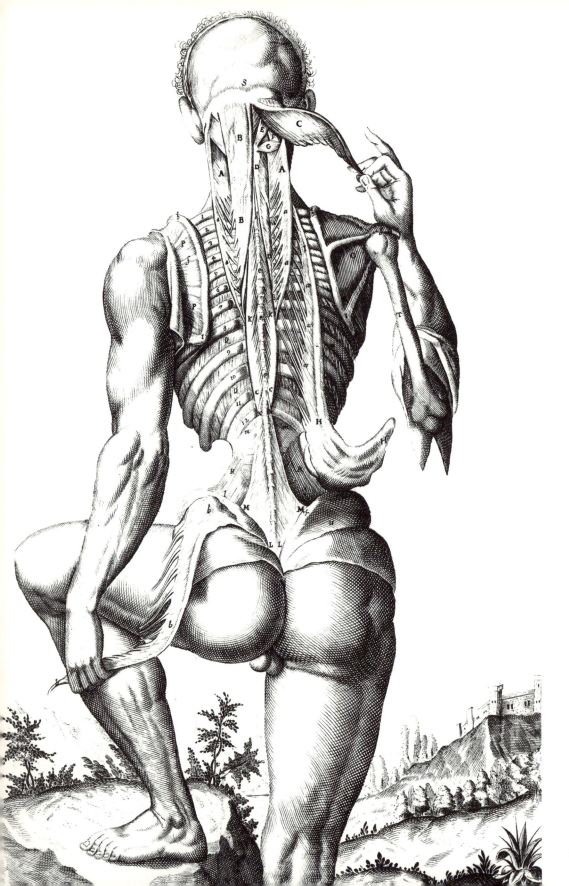

14.

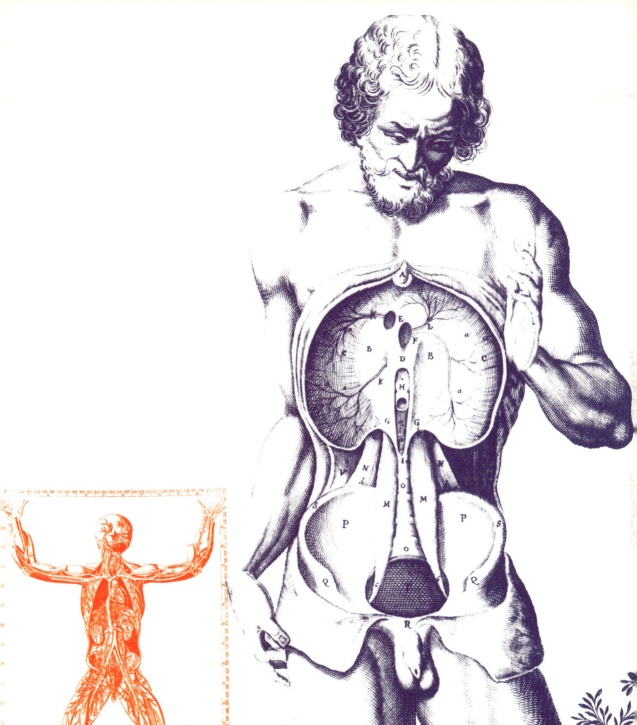

Knowledge of life is given only through a cruel, reductive and cursed form of knowing, which wants life only as dead. The way of looking which envelops, caresses, minutely details and fragments that most personal flesh, picking out its secret wounds, is an attentive, fixed and somewhat inflated gaze which has, from the vantage point of death, already condemned life. (Michel Foucault, *Birth of the Clinic*, New York 1974.)

16.

...of two physicians, the one who deserves most trust is always, in my opinion, the one who is better versed in physics or the mechanics of the human body, and who, leaving the soul and all the anxieties which this illusion causes in the foolish and ignorant, occupies himself earnestly with pure naturalism. (La Mettrie, *L'Homme Machine*, 1748.)

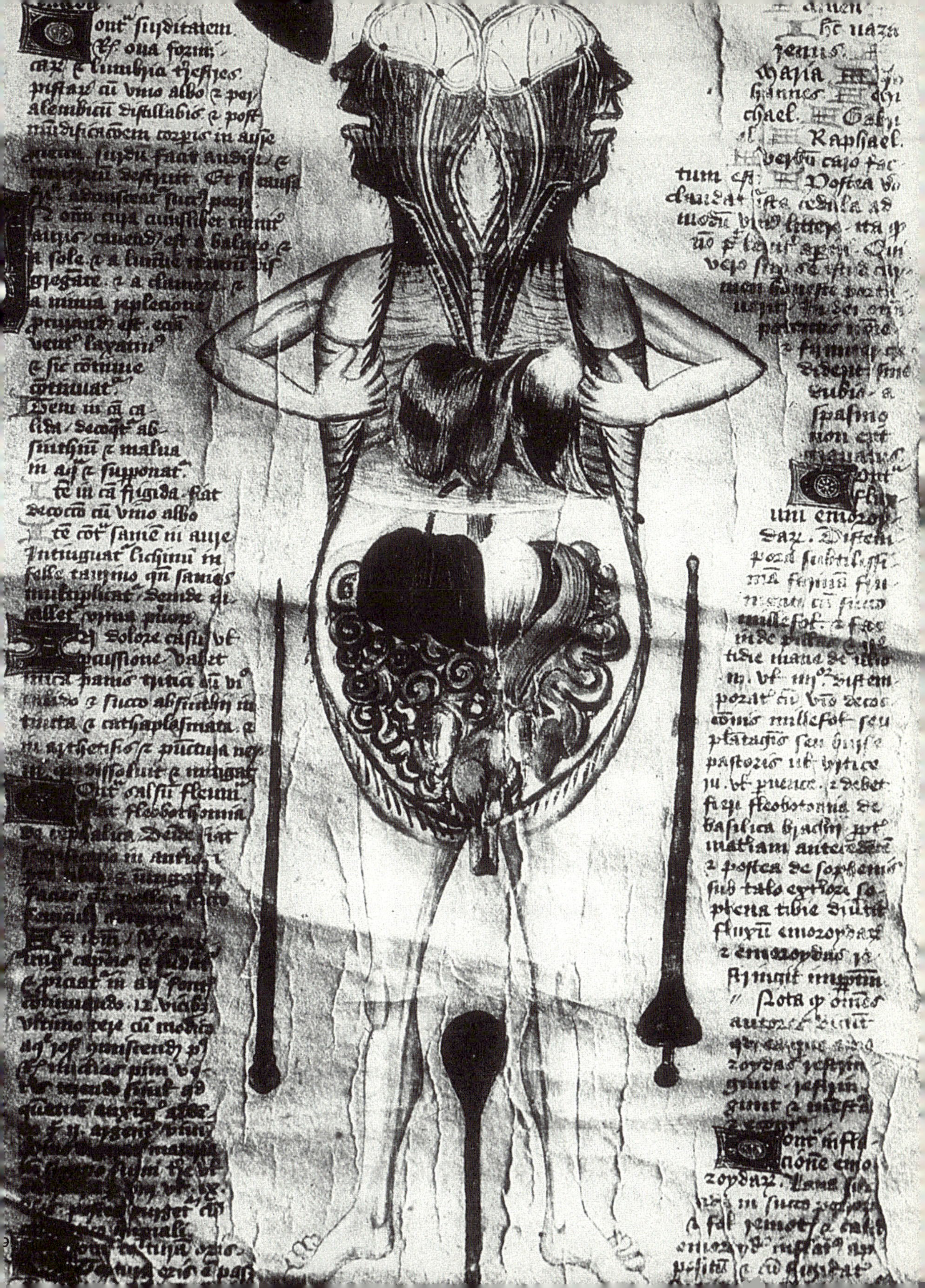

The quality of 'humanity,' incidentally, has nothing to do with happiness; we are, here, very far from any idea of charity: the most horrifying experiences and the cruelest of pleasures are entirely valuable if they contribute to the development of a real understanding of what it is to be human. Only a puritan would disagree, seeing in the body only gross matter and a despicable magma of viscera, rather than a mysterious theater which provides a stage for all exchange — whether of matter, mind or the senses — between inner and outer worlds. (From Michel Leiris, "Le corps enjeu," Musée d'Ethnographie, Neuchâtel, 1983. Originally published in *Documents*, 1930.)

20.

21.

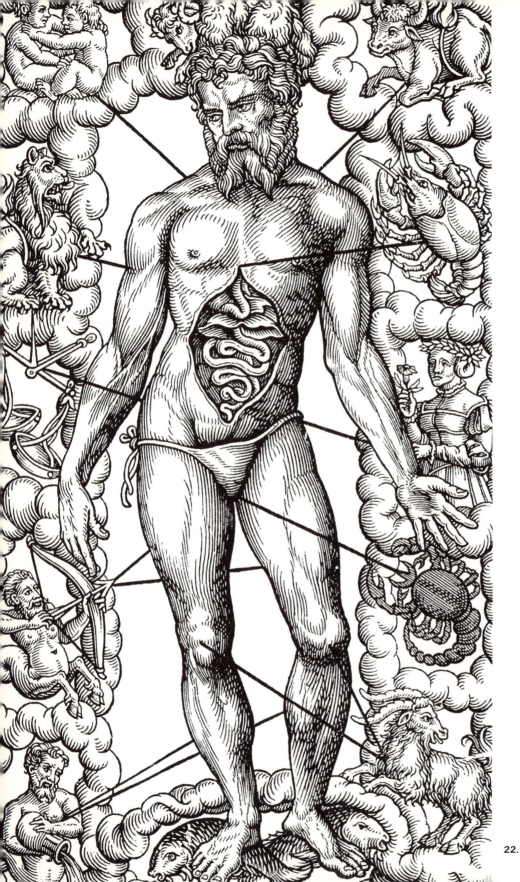

22.

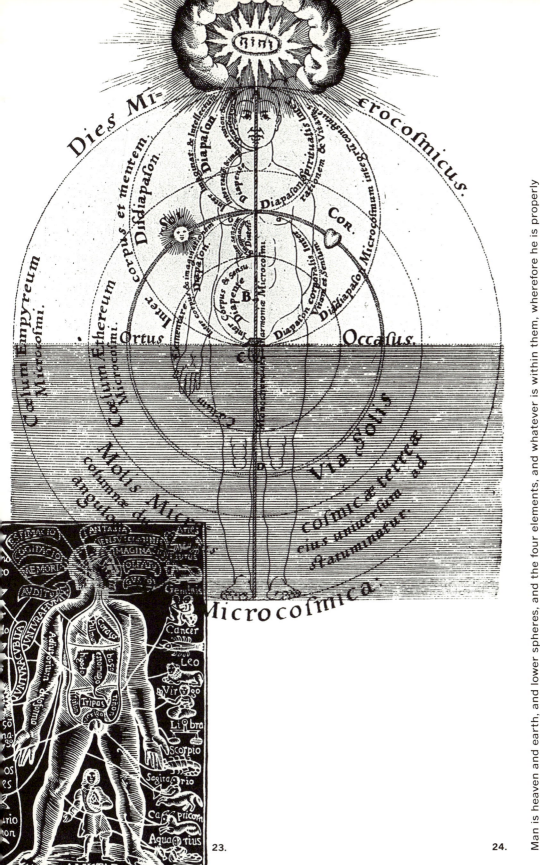

23.

24.

Man is heaven and earth, and lower spheres, and the four elements, and whatever is within them, wherefore he is properly called by the name of microcosmos for he is the whole world.... Know then that there is also within man a starry firmament with a mighty course of planets and stars that have exaltations, conjunctions and oppositions. The heart is the sun; and as the sun acts upon the earth and upon itself, so also acts the heart upon the body and upon itself. — Paracelsus

The essence, the content, the qualitative unity of a thing, can never be grasped by a 'step-by-step' process of measurement, but only by a comprehensive and immediate experience or 'vision'.... A science based on quantitative analysis...must of necessity be blind to the infinitely fruitful and many-sided essence of things. For such a science, what the ancients called the 'form' of a thing (i.e., its qualitative content) plays virtually no role. This is the reason why science and art, which in the prerationalistic age were more or less synonymous, are now completely divorced from one another, and also why beauty, for modern science, offers not the smallest avenue toward knowledge. (Burkhardt, *Alchemy*, London, Stuart and Watkins, 1967, p. 61.)

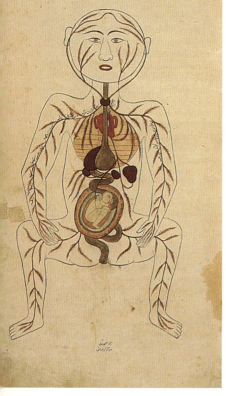

25.

26.

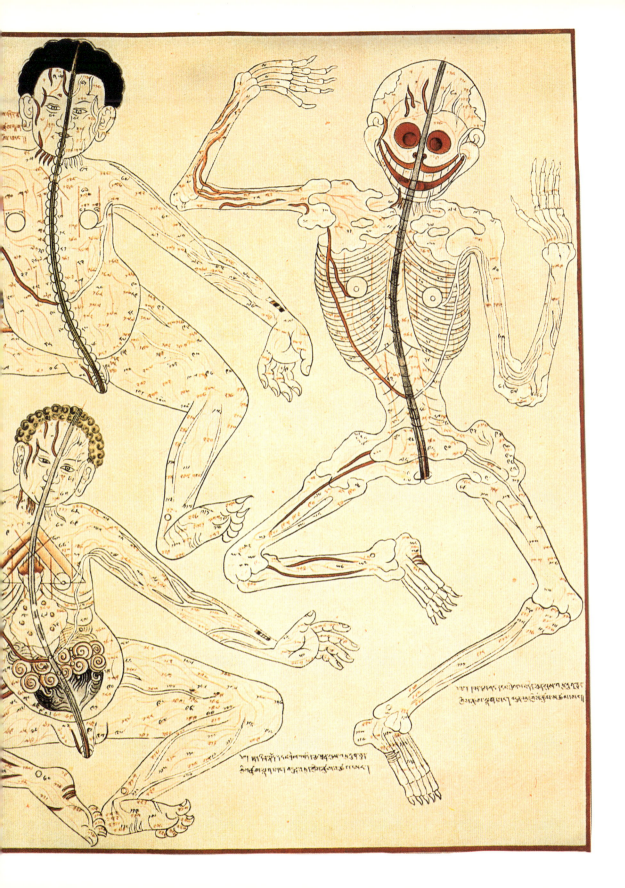

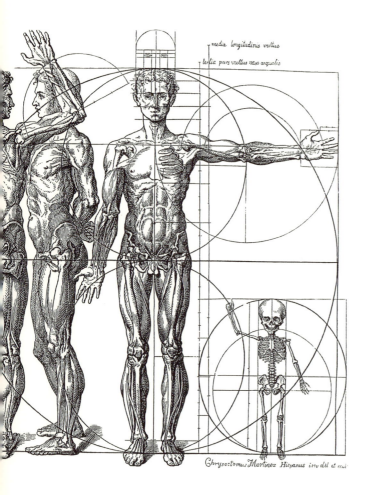

media longitudinis vultus

tertia pars vultus naso aequalis

Chrysostomus Martinez Hispanus inv del et sculp

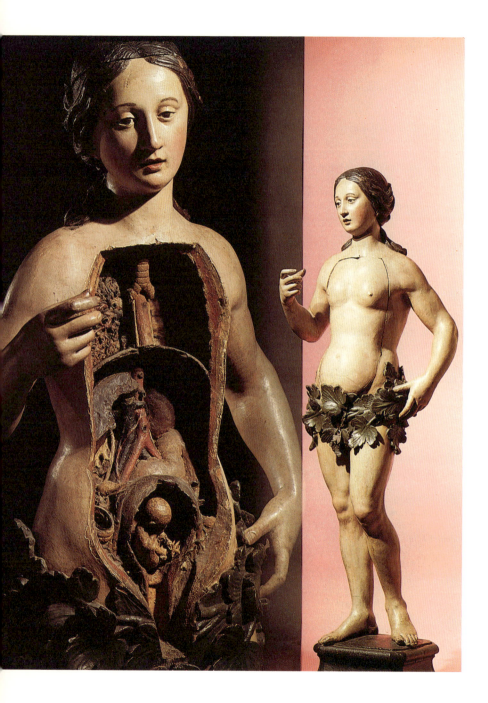

Anatomical Statue, 1600. Roudillon Collection.

# A Repertory of Body History

*Barbara Duden*

## Introduction

This repertory lists books and articles that have been discussed during the last five years in a conversation with Ivan Illich and other participants in a circle which continues to grow. The conversation grew out of my attempt to interpret the "Weiberkrankheiten" ("Diseases and Infirmities of Women") of Dr. Johann Storch. In his seven-volume text, this small-town physician from Thüringen recorded the complaints of hundreds of women whom he met in his practice between 1719 and 1742. To understand these complaints I had to grasp the meaning these women gave to their aches and pains, and the more I grappled with their sufferings the more I myself began to feel strange. The sense of existence which their recorded complaints express, is foreign to the bodily identity as a woman that I have been taught to "have." My training as a historian had not equipped me with methods with which I could grasp the lived body recorded in these documents as a subject for historical study. The search for these methods sparked the conversation whose bibliographic result is gathered in this repertory.

As the conversation continued, now with an iconographer and semanticist, then with an Indologist, psychologist, Chinese historian or medievalist, it became evident that the history of the lived body was a new territory, crossed by many roads. I assumed the responsibility of establishing criteria for the exclusion of literature, including bibliographic suggestions sent by colleagues and friends, keeping the files that were piling up, and working on comments on the items.

The items listed do not necessarily have as their subject our main theme, namely the *historicity of the human body*. However, they have all been helpful to one or more of us in dealing with the *perceived body* and with the *perceptual milieu*, both subjects that deserve historical study. Almost everything ever written can be understood as an embodiment of its time and as related to body perception. But sources that concentrate directly on the *Gestalt* of women's and men's bodies in a given epoch are rather scarce. Books and articles written during the last hundred years and dealing more or less directly with the everyday experience of the body in past times constitute the bulk of my list. I draw on the history of medicine, religion, alchemy, philosophy and architecture when I judge it relevant to the everyday experience and meaning of bodies. It was particularly difficult to draw a line in medical history; most authors dealing with medical concepts, themes or images touch on body experience only in tangential ways. It was even more difficult for me, as a social historian, to distinguish body history from some of the subjects with which I am most familiar: the enclosure of women into the domestic sphere; the gender-specific definition of industrial work; the new kinds of violence experienced by women, soldiers, inmates and prostitutes since the mid-nineteenth century; the history of violence in the family; the marginalization of the aged and the experience of the raped in our time. From studies in these areas I could only pick and choose. The history of the industrial milieu and of its social or technical aspects which have shaped the body experience we now "have" is, in my opinion, a territory so vast, that it calls for separate treatment. So this list is weak on recent social history, and on feminist social history. Access to materials in these fields, much of which pertains to body experience, is already provided by the pertinent journals.

This list is also weak in studies on contemporary body perception in psychology, psychoanalysis, motivational research and proxemics. Some of these empirical studies might be useful for historians to shape their concepts and perspectives, but I would need advice to make the right selections. Also, I decided to exclude the vast literature on contemporary reproductive technologies and their impact on women, because, while it is relevant, it also is more generally accessible.

This list focuses on the body in Western societies. I often regretted that for the moment this decision precluded my including valuable studies in non-European cultural anthropology. I do cite sources from archeology, Near Eastern philology and Islamic, Hebrew and Christian biblical studies when they seem relevant to the sociogenesis of the characteristically Western body. Studies of some topics are included primarily because of their methodological value, like Van Gulik's great monograph on Chinese sexual techniques, Malotki's study of the linguistic representation of Hopi space or Pinxten's work on Navajo directions. For the same reason, items from word field studies (semantics) reaching beyond the Western realm are occasionally included.

This is still a working paper: I request corrections and suggestions for additions and omissions. The annotations which are taken from notes written to each other, especially need further editing. Further, this repertory has been prepared as part of a larger project: although in parts published first, it is the third part of a Guide to Body History, whose first part will be an introduction on which I am collaborating with Ivan Illich and whose second will be bibliographical essays prepared by a dozen colleagues, essays on body history in relation to their fields of specialization.

The research leading to this repertory, the time and space that made it possible, were aided by the United Nations University, Tokyo, with the support of its rector Dr. Soetjatmoko; the California Institute of Technology, Pasadena, with the support of Prof. John Beton and the multilingual competence of Rosy Meiron; and the Pennsylvania State University Women's Studies and Science, Technology and Society Program, with support from Drs. Lynne Goodstein and Rustum Roy.

# Bibliography

A

**ABLEMAN, Paul.**
*Anatomy of Nakedness.* London: Orbis Publ., 1982.

**ACCATI, Louisa.**
"Lo spirito della fornicazione: Virtù dell'anima e virtù del corpo in Friuli: Fra '600 e '700." *Quaderni storici* 41 (1979): 644-72. Based on an inquisition on the parish level in Friuli around 1645 against women practicing age-old magical rituals. Women's bodies appear as the source of communal self-understanding and power.

**ACKERKNECHT, Erwin H.**
"Death in the History of Medicine." *Bulletin of the History of Medicine* 42 (1968): 19-23. Death has been a marginal problem in medical literature since the time of the ancient Greeks. Discussion centered in artisan-like fashion around "prediction" ("facies"), "moment" and "signa." During the eighteenth century discussion on signa grew to extraordinary proportions, starting with Lancisi 1707. Apparent death became a major evil feared by the Enlightenment. "Rettungsgesellschaften" became important. This hysteria ends abruptly around 1800.

____. "Medical Practices." In *Handbook of South American Indians*, ed. by Julian Haynes STEWARD, vol. 5, 621-43. Washington: U.S. Govt. Print. Off., 1957.

____. *Medicine and Ethnology: Selected Essays*, ed. H.v.WALSER and H.M.KOELBING. Bern: Hans Huber, 1971. "Medicine has much more the character of a function of the culture pattern than of 'biology'." An important collection of early articles by a pioneer in medical ethnology.

____. "Midwives as Experts in Court." *Bulletin of the New York Academy of Medicine* 52, no. 10 (1976): 1224-28. Midwives were not recognized as a guild, yet necessary as court experts in case of rape. In the attempt to make them unnecessary "medical authorities for centuries denied the existence of the hymen."

____. *Therapie von den Primitiven bis zum 20 Jahrhundert*. Stuttgart: Enke, 1970 (*Therapeutics from the Primitives to the 20th Century*). New York: Macmillan, 1973.

**ADLER, Alfred.**
"Les jumeaux sont rois." *L'Homme* 13, nos. 1-2 (1973): 167-92. Synthesis of African perception of and belief about twin births.

**ADLER, Hans.**
*Lebensdrang und Todesverlangen in der deutschen Literatur 1850-80*. Dissertation. Heidelberg, 1932.

**ADOLF, Helene.**
*Wortgeschichtliche Studien zum Leib/Seele-Problem: Mittelhochdeutsch* lîp *'Leib' und die Bezeichnungen für* corpus. Vienna: Intern. Religionspsychol. Gesellschaft, 1937 (Zeitschrift für Religionspsychologie, Sonderheft 5). In German, as in French, two bodies can be expressed. The author traces the history of "Leib" and "Körper." 1100-50 the wordfield takes shape in which "lîp" meant "body." Much later the Latin "corpus" could denote both living and dead bodies.

**AGUIRRE BELTRAN, G.**
*Medicina y magia: El proceso de aculturación y el curanderismo en México*. Mexico, 1955. Extensive examination of inquisitorial proceedings in Mexico for references to folk medical practice and magic. Respondents are very often indians or black slaves.

**AHRENS, Heinrich Ludolf.**
*Die griechischen und lateinischen Benennungen der Hand: Etymologische Untersuchung*. Leipzig: Teubner, 1879. Both etymological and semantic treatment of the stem corresponding to "hand."

**AIGREMONT (pseud).**
"Beiträge zur Hand- und Fingersymbolik und Erotik." *Anthropophyteia* 10 (1913): 314-29.

____. (pseud. SCHULTZE-GALLERA, S.).
*Volkserotik und Pflanzenwelt: Eine Darstellung alter wie moderner erotischer und sexueller Gebräuche, Vergleiche, Benennungen, Sprichwörter, Redewendungen, Rätsel, Volkslieder, erotischen Zaubers und Aberglaubens, sexueller Heilkunde, die sich auf Pflanzen beziehen*. 2 vols. Halle: Hallescher Verlag für Literatur und Musik, 2d ed. 1919.

____. *Fuss- und Schuhsymbolik und Erotik: Folkloristische und sexualwissenschaftliche Untersuchungen*. Leipzig: Deutsche Verlagsanstalt, 1909.

**ALBERT, Christine Ottilie H.**
*Leiderfahrung und Leidüberwindung in der deutschen Lyrik des 17. Jhs.* Dissertation. Munich, 1956.

**ALCHIAN, Armen A., ed.**
*The Economics of Charity: Essays on the Comparative Economics and Ethics of Giving and Selling with Applications to Blood.* London: Inst. of Economic Affairs, 1973.

**ALIMENTI, Alessandro, FALTERI, Paola.**
"Donna e salute nella cultura tradizionale delle classi subalterne." *Donna-Woman-Femme* (Rome) 5 (1977): 75-104.

**ALLAN, N.**
"I santi thaumaturghi." *KOS* 1, no. 7 (1984): 55-68.

**ALLEN, Catherine J.**
"Body and Soul in Quechua Thought." *Journal of Latin American Lore* 8, no. 2 (1982): 179-96.

**ALLEN, Sally G., HUBBS, Joanna.**
"Outrunning Atalanta: Feminine Destiny in Alchemical Transmutation." *Signs* 6, no. 2 (1980): 210-21. Investigates the emblems of alchemical texts and the likening of alchemical "cooking" to the creative capacities of the womb.

**ALLEN, Suzanne.**
"Plus outre." *Revue des sciences humaines* 44, no. 168 (1977): 503-15. "Outre" in French has two meanings: "tube," "pipe" or "bag" and "beyond all measure." The vocabulary of anatomical descriptions of one seat of female pleasure discloses ways in which the female body has been fantasized, especially in orgasm.

**ALLERS, Rudolf.**
"Microcosmus: From Anaximandros to Paracelsus." *Traditio* 2 (1944): 319-407.

**ALP, S.**
"Zu den Körperteilnamen im Hetitischen." *Anatolia* 2 (1957): 1-48.

**ALSTON, Mary Niven.**
"The Attitudes of the Church toward Dissection before 1500." *Bulletin of the History of Medicine* 16 (1944): 221-38. Prospero Lambertini, later Pope Benedict XIV, stated in 1737 that the Church, always in favor of arts and sciences, would never have opposed anything as beneficial as dissection. Alston reviews conflicting opinions of historians and of late medieval evidence.

**ALTIERI-BIAGI, Maria Luisa.**
*Guglielmo Volgare: Studio sul lessico della medicina medievale.* Bologna: Forni, 1970.

**AMES, R.S.**
"The Meaning of Body in Classical Chinese Thought." *International Philosophical Quarterly* 24 (1984): 39-53.

**ANCHIETA CORREA, José de.**
"L'évolution de la notion de 'corps' à la notion de 'chair' chez Maurice Merleau-Ponty." *Kriterion* (Belo Horizonte, Brazil) 19 no. 66 (1966-72): 75-115. In the posthumously published writings of MERLEAU-PONTY (1964) Freudian categories are used to move from the phenomenological analysis of the "visible" body ('corps') to a quasi-ontological "flesh" ('chair') -the pre-predicative, "wild" state of being, comparable to the pre-Socratic "elements."

**ANDRAE, W.**
*Die ionische Säule: Bauform oder Symbol?* Berlin: Verlag für Kunstwissenschaft, 1933 (Studien zur Bauforschung 5). Some references on body symbolism.

**ANDRESEN, Karl Gustav.**
*Ueber Volksetymologie.* Heilbronn, 1876 (7th enl. ed. Leipzig: Reisland, 1919). A standard reference work on folk etymology that went through many editions. Two of more than a dozen sections deal explicitly with folk etymology related to body parts, illness and remedies.

**ANNALES DE BRETAGNE.**
86, no. 2 (1979). Special issue, "La médicalisation en France du XVIIIe au début du XXe siècle."

**ANNALI di MEDICINA NAVALE e TROPICALE.**
"Pagine di storia della scienza e della tecnica." Roma: Ministerio della Difesa Marina, 1952. Special issue dedicated to the Leonardo anniversary (1452-1952). Excellent survey of the pictorial evolution of anatomic representation: LIBER, STROPPIANA, TAVONE, PASSALAQUA, GALEAZZI, MOELLER.

**ANTHROPOPHYTEIA.**
*Jahrbücher für Folklorist: Erhebungen und Forschungen zur Entdeckungsgeschichte der gesellschaftlichen Moral*, ed. by Friedrich Salomon KRAUS, vols. 1-10 and: "Beiwerke zum Studium der Anthropophytie" vols. 1-7. Leipzig: Ethnologischer Verlag, 1904-14.

**ANZIEU, Didier.**
*Le moi-peau.* Paris: Dunod, 1985. Reflections on the analogy between "ego" and the "skin" by a practicing psychoanalyst. Valuable for the historian mainly for the clarification of *skin* as an experience.

**ARANO, Luisa Cogliati, ed.**
*The Medieval Health Handbook Tacuinum Sanitatis.* New York, 1976. (German: *Tacuinum Sanitatis*: ed. L.C.ARANO, with an intro. by H.SCHIPPERGES and W.SCHMITT, Munich, 1976).

**ARCHIVES DES SCIENCES SOCIALES DES RELIGIONS.**
54, no. 1 (1982). Special issue, "Guérisons et faits religieux."

**ARDENER, Shirley, ed.**
*Women and Space: Ground Rules and Social Maps.* New York: St. Martin's, 1981. Contributions by British anthropologists on the social and symbolic use

of space and settings in England, Peru, Iran, Greece and Africa.

____, ed. *Defining Females: The Nature of Women in Society*. London: Croom Helm, 1978.

____,ed. *Perceiving Women*. London: Dent, 1982.

**ARIES, Philippe.**

*L'Homme devant la mort*. Paris: Seuil, 1977 (*The Hour of Our Death*. New York: Knopf, 1981). See especially ch. 8: "The dead body." Mainly a commentary on L.Chr.F. GARMANN, "De miraculis mortuorum," Leipzig, 1709. During this period the dead body itself (without any attention paid to the cause of demise) becomes an object of study for medicine. The corpse, though dead, is conceived as still partially ensouled (by the vegetative part of the *anima*-as-*forma corporis*). Even in the mummy there is still some "life" which now falls into the purview of the physician as researcher.

____. and BEJIN, André, eds. *Western Sexuality: Practice and Precept in Past and Present Times*. London: Basil Blackwell, 1985 (orig.: "Sexualités occidentales." *Communications* 35, 1982). The outcome of a seminar led by Ariès and the last of his books. "Few books are so detached, so informative, so alive with the intellectual interest and importance of the Western forms and traditions of sexuality" (P.LASLETT).

**ARMOROLI, M., ed.**

*Le cere anatomiche Bolognesi del settecento: Catalogo della mostra organizzata Sett.-Nov. 1981*. Bologna: Università degli Studi di Bologna, Accademia delle Scienze, 1981. Catalogue for an exposition of eighteenth-century anatomical wax models.

**ARMSTRONG, David.**

*Political Anatomy of the Body: Medical Knowledge in Britain in the Twentieth Century*. New York: Cambridge Univ. Press, 1983. The Goodenough commission which reorganized medical education in England after WW II barely mentions the patient; only twenty years later the Todd report challenged medical schools to focus this education on the doctor-patient relationship. The fabrication of the patient as a subject became the goal of good practice. First, medicine became concerned with the patient's "compliance." The clinical examination that had been used as a mere device for constituting the body as an object of treatment turned into the medical interview for analyzing and thereby fabricating idiosyncratic patients. Insistence on compliance, sensitivity, meaning and subjectivity had the effect of constituting the patient's subjectivity as the object of the medical enterprise. Together with ARNEY this is one of the important reminders that we might be living at the hinge-time of body history.

**ARNEY, William Ray.**

*Power and the Profession of Obstetrics*. Chicago: Univ. Chicago Press, 1982.

____, BERGEN, Bernard J. *Medicine and the Management of Living: Taming the Last Great Beast*. Chicago: Univ. Chicago Press, 1984. Points toward a major transformation in American attitudes toward the body - if not a new way of perceiving it. At the end of WW II the major criticism of mainline medicine was that its professional perspective objectified and alienated the patient's body, forcing the patient to look at himself through the physician's eye. By 1980 the substance of medical discourse has shifted: the patient is wooed as a partner of his therapist - and the therapist often presents himself in an ancillary function in the maintenance or recovery of the patient's body. This transformation might be hailed by pupils of Szacz or Balint as the transition from a model of passive to one of active interactions, thus obscuring the unprecedented newness of the ways in which patients now objectify themselves. The authors claim that it would be more fruitful to follow Foucault's analytic model and speak of a successful discourse that has created the body as object, analogous to the nineteenth-century discourse that created "sexuality."

**ARNOLD, Odile.**

*Le corps et l'âme: La vie des religieuses au XIXe. siècle*. Paris: Seuil, 1982.

**ARNOLDSON, Torild Washington.**

*Parts of the Body in Older Germanic and Scandinavian*. Repr. New York: AMS Press, 1971 (orig. Chicago, 1915). Examines the "ideas" behind the formation of words for body parts. A history of Gothic and Old English ideas about the body's capacities.

**ARON, Jean Paul, KEMPF, Roger.**

*Le pénis et la démoralisation de l'occident*. Paris: Grasset, 1978.

____. *La Bourgeoisie, le sexe et l'honneur*. Paris: Ed. Complexe, 1984.

**ARTELT, Walter.**

*Studien zur Geschichte der Begriffe 'Heilmittel' und 'Gift': Urzeit-Homer-Corpus Hippocraticum*. Darmstadt: Wissenschaftliche Buchgesellschaft, 1968 (orig. Leipzig, 1937).

____. "Bemerkungen zum Stil der Anatomischen Abbildungen des 16 und 17 Jahrhunderts." In *Acta del XV Congresso internacional de historia de la medecina Madrid-Alcala 1956*, vol. 1, 393-961. Madrid, 1958. A sequence of aperçus on the artistic intent in anatomical paintings, especially mannerism.

**ASPIZ, Harold.**

*Walt Whitman and the Body Beautiful*. Urbana: Univ. Illinois Press, 1980. Whitman repeatedly stated that poetry involves the reciprocal relationship between language and the human body. The study concentrates on the physiological ideas and connotations of Whitman's poetry and explores their provenance. Whitman was a keen observer of nineteenth-century medical practice, hospitals and American healing cults. He transmutes decade-specific lore and scientific opinion (chs. 4, 5: phrenology, physiognomy, electrical biology, magnetism, spiritism and ch. 6: sexual, eugenic themes related to motherhood) into a gestic gospel of the body.

**ATKINSON, Clarissa W.**
"Precious Balsam in a Fragile Glass: The Ideology of Virginity in the Later Middle-Ages." *Journal of Family History* 8, no. 2 (1983): 131-43.

**ATKINSON, J.W.**
"E.G.Conklin on Evolution: The Popular Writings of an Embryologist." *Journal of the History of Biology* 18, no. 1 (1985): 31-50.

**AUER, A.**
*Leidenstheologie des Mittelalters: Das geistige Oesterreich.* Vol. 3. Salzburg: Igonta, 1947.

**AUGE, Marc.**
"Introduction." *History and Anthropology* 2 (1985): 1-15 (special issue, "Interpreting Illness").

____, HERZLICH, Claudine. *Le sens du mal: Anthropologie, histoire, sociologie de la maladie.* Paris: Editions des Archives Contemporaines, 1984.

**AZOUVI, François.**
"Woman as a Model of Pathology in the Eighteenth Century." *Diogenes* 115 (1981): 22-36. The ancient tradition imagining gender differences in the body disappears in the eighteenth century. AZOUVI asks about the destiny of difference: "The weakness of woman, the softness of her tissues remain the constants among doctors of the seventeenth and eighteenth centuries, even if they cease to attribute them to a cold and humid constitution....but this theme acquires, in the medical systems of the eighteenth century, a completely new meaning: her 'delicateness' makes woman no longer a species perfect in herself, distinguished by a different constitution, but a being in which the principles of all life and all illness are eminently manifested."

____. "Le rôle du corps chez Descartes." *Revue de Métaphysique et de Morale* 83 (1978): 1-23.

# B

**BAADER, Gerhard, KEIL, Gundolf, eds.**
*Medizin im mittelalterlichen Abendland.* Darmstadt: Wissenschaftliche Buchgesellschaft, 1982 (Wege der Forschung 363). An excellent reader that gathers hith-

erto dispersed articles, which reflect on centuries' progress in the history of medieval medicine.

____. "Die Entwicklung der medizinischen Fachsprache im hohen und späten Mittelalter." In *Fachprosaforschung*, ed. by G.KEIL and P.ASSION, 88-123. Berlin: E. Schmidt, 1974. In classical Rome medical terminology was derived from popular speech, not from high Latin, notwithstanding Cicero's efforts. The medical Latin taken for granted by humanists is of twelfth-century origin. Constantinus Africanus, a north African drug merchant and later monk at Monte Cassino, who had studied in Baghdad and who translated Galen from Arabic into the best then available Latin, began to create the abstract technical language capable of rendering the strongly "Aristotelian" Arabic Galen. The physician's response was soon doubly removed from the patient's complaint: it was in a foreign and also in a new language.

**BACHELARD, Gaston.**
*La Poétique de l'espace.* Paris: Presses Universitaires de France, 1985 (*The Poetics of Space*, with a foreword by E.GILSON, Boston: Beacon Press, 1969).

____. *La Terre et les rêveries du repos: Essai sur les images de l'intimité.* Paris: J. Corti Publ., 1984.

____. *L'eau et les rêves: Essai sur l'imagination de la matière.* Paris, 1942 (*Water and Dreams: An Essay on the Imagination of Matter.* Dallas: Institute for Humanities and Culture, 1983).

____. *L'air et les songes: Essai sur l'imagination du mouvement.* Paris: J. Corti Publ., 1983 (*Air and Dreams: An Essay on the Imagination of Movement.* Dallas: Institute for Humanities and Culture, 1987). An odd yet influential epistemologist concerned with the perception of "elements" (earth, water, space, fire) as "stuff," and the history of this stuff as imagined. The approach to body history taken by the author of this bibliography has been influenced decisively by this author.

**BACHOFEN, Johann.**
"Fortsetzung der Betrachtung der Sümpfe und Sümpfpflanzen: Ihre Gleichstellung mit den menschlichen Haaren und beider Beziehung zu hetärischer Geschlechtermischung." In *Gesammelte Werke*, ed. by Karl MEULI, vol. 4, 380-84. Basel: Schwabe, 1954.

**BAEUMKER, Clemens, ed.**
*Des Alfred von Sareshel-Alfredus Anglicus-Schrift De motu cordis.* Münster, 1923 (Beiträge zur Geschichte der Philosophie 23.1-2). Alfred's prescholastic treatise became known due to Thomas Aquinas's refutation of its thesis, that the heart is the seat of the soul. It also seems to have been known to Harvey. "Motus" here explicitly refers to a spinning movement, not to a beating or pumping.

**BAKAN, David.**
*Disease, Pain and Sacrifice: Towards a Psychology of*

*Suffering*. Chicago: Univ. Chicago Press, 1968. The practice of clinical psychology, the study of the history of religion and philosophical acumen make this an important text for the phenomenology of the body. It is mostly pain or discomfort which attracts attention to body perception. The distinction between pain and disease, stimulus and response is based on the rather clear-cut distinction between organism and environment - while it is precisely this distinction which breaks down when we have pain. Pain has no other locus but the conscious ego - it is literally the price for the "possession of a conscious ego."

**BAKHTIN, Mikhail.**
*L'Oeuvre de François Rabelais et la culture populaire au Moyen Age et sous la Renaissance*. Paris: Gallimard, 1970.
____. *Rabelais and His World*. Cambridge, Mass.: MIT Press, 1965.

**BALAN, B.**
*L'ordre et le temps: L'anatomie comparée et l'histoire des vivants au XIXe siècle*. Paris: Vrin, 1979.

**BALDWIN, Robert.**
*An Interdisciplinary Bibliography of Body Movement and Body Symbolism*. Harvard University, Fine Arts Department. December 1979 (mimeographed typescript 9th ed.). Two thousand entries, many on gestures in different historical periods, on "actions" (breathing, crying, praying), on expressions of emotions (grief, despair, shame, fidelity) and on anatomical parts, mostly taken from art history.

**BALLAUF, Theodor.**
*Die Wissenschaft vom Leben: Eine Geschichte der Biologie*. Freiburg i. Br.: Alber, 1951.

**BALTHASAR, Hans Urs von.**
*Theodramatik*. 4 vols. Einsiedeln: Johannes Verlag, 1976. Vol. 2, pp. 289-305 deals with body metaphors used by Church Fathers in their exegesis of the history of salvation.

**BALTRUSAITIS, Jurgis.**
*Aberration: Quatre essais sur la légende des formes*. Paris: Olivier Perrin, 1957. Pp. 8-46 give a brilliant and learned history of the analogies between human and animal physiognomy in postmedieval Europe; what these similarities or analogies tell about nativity, destiny, character and the world's destiny. Bibliography, pp. 127-28.

**BAMBERG, Corona.**
"Der Leib des Menschen nach dem Zeugnis der Väter." *Anima* 9 (1954): 117-30. The appearance of bridal symbolism among early Church Fathers.
____. *Was Menschsein kostet: Aus der Erfahrung des früchristlichen Mönchtums gedeutet*. Würzburg: Echter, 1971. A modern Benedictine nun's meditations on the texts of early Christian monks who find keen self-awareness in asceticism.

**BARAKAT, Robert A.**
*The Cistercian Sign Language: A Study in Non-Verbal Communication*. Kalamazoo, Mich.: Cistercian Publ., 1975.

**BARASCH, Moshe.**
*Gestures of Despair in Medieval and Early Renaissance Art*. New York: New York Univ. Press, 1976.

**BARB, A.A.**
"Diva Matrix: A Faked Gnostic Intaglio in the Possession of P.P. Rubens and the Iconology of a Symbol." *Journal of the Cortauld and Warburg Institutes* 16 (1953): 193-238. Exhaustive iconographic documentation of gems representing the womb.

**BARDY, G.**
"Catherine, Sainte," *Dictionnaire d'histoire et de géographie ecclésiastique*. Paris: Letauzey, 1912ff. Catherine of Alexandria is supposed to have bled milk when decapitated.

**BARGHEER, Ernst.**
*Eingeweide: Lebens- und Seelenkräfte des Leibesinneren im deutschen Glauben und Brauch*. Berlin, 1931. The major encyclopedia of European lore, folk and medical, religious, superstitious and scientific beliefs about the human guts: heart and brains, urine and blood, gall and excrement serve as the seat of life, mantic device, magic tool, remedy or the seat of illness.

**BARKAN, Leonard.**
*Nature's Work of Art: The Human Body as Image of the World*. New Haven: Yale Univ. Press, 1975. "An attempt to define a habit of thought...the cause [of which] is to be found in the history of ideas and the effect in poetic imagery and metaphor" (p. 7). The habit in question is that of thinking of the body as a microcosm relative to the cosmos, the commonwealth and the domain of aesthetics and architecture. The study examines the Fairie Queene, and the idea that men are multiple rather than single beings.

**BARKER-BENFIELD, G.J.**
*The Horrors of the Half-Known Life: Male Attitudes Toward Women and Sexuality in Nineteenth-Century America*. New York: Harper & Row, 1976. Describes the social construction of American sexuality in the discourse of mid-nineteenth-century American gynecological discourse. Careful exegesis of the changing metaphors in these texts.

**BARREAU, S.**
"Essai d'écologie des métamorphoses de l'alimentation et des fantasmes du goût." *Informations sur les sciences sociales* 18, no. 3 (1979): 421-35. A sociological study of the change (and loss) of taste as a result of the homogenization and standardization of food.

**BARREL, John.**
*The Idea of Landscape and the Sense of Place, 1730-1840: An Approach to the Poetry of John CLAIRE.*

478

Cambridge: Cambridge Univ. Press, 1972. A recognized masterpiece of literary criticism: the best introduction to the complexities of this subject.

**BARTH, Suse.**
*Lebensalter-Darstellungen im 19. und 20. Jahrhundert: Ikonographische Studien.* Inaugural dissertation, Ludwig Maximilian Universität, Munich, 1971. Akademischer Photodruck, Bamberg. Iconography of the Ages of Man, aging and the difference of its appearance in men and women in the nineteenth and early twentieth centuries. Mostly German art.

**BASKETT, William Denny.**
*Parts of the Body in the Later Germanic Dialects.* Chicago: Univ. Chicago Press, 1920 (Linguistic Studies in Germanic 5). How words came to have their present meanings rather than their original meaning. Beside each word the author places related words from the same and other dialects in order to exhibit the primary meaning. Extremely rich in varieties, e.g., "penis," pp. 106-11, contains seventeen different fields of meaning, which are not all even related to scrotum or testicles.

**BASTIEN, Joseph W.**
*Qollahuaya-andean Body Concepts: A Topographical, Hydraulic Model of Physiology.* Paper, Univ. Texas at Arlington, 1984.

**BATAILLE, Georges.**
L'Erotisme. Paris: Minuit, 1957 (*Eroticism.* London, New York: Marion Boyars 1987). Pp. 45ff. gives a short, clear summary of an idea that runs through the author's work: only in the act of transgressing taboos which inspire horror, nausea and anguish can the flesh be experienced as the border that is trespassed.

**BATHE, Johannes.**
*Die Bewegungen und Haltungen des menschlichen Körpers in H. von Kleists Erzaehlungen.* Dissertation. Tübingen: Laupp, 1917. One in every thirty-six words in KLEIST's opus designates a movement or posture of the human body - more so in his early work. Compared with C.F.MEYER, G.KELLER. Heinrich Kleist stresses gesture over posture and describes it to tell a story rather than to express the feelings of his protagonist.

**BATTISTI, Carlo.**
"Les dénominations de la luette dans les dialectes calabrais." *Mélanges de linguistique...offert à M. Roques.* Vol. 1, 33-37. Paris: Didier, 1952. Luette = the "uvula" in the throat.

**BAUDINET, Marie-José.**
"L'incarnation, l'image, la voix." *Esprit* (Paris, Febr. 1982): 188-94 (special issue on the body). Reflections on the characteristics of the body as such in icons of the Eastern church.

**BAUDRILLARD, Jean.**
*Pour une critique de l'économie du signe.* Paris: Gallimard, 1972 (*For a Critique of the Political Economy of the Sign.* New York: Telos Press).

____. *L'échange symbolique et la mort.* Paris: Gallimard, 1976 (esp. ch. 4: "Le corps ou le charnier du signe").

**BAUER, Gerhard.**
*Claustrum animae.* 3 vols. Munich: Fink, 1971. Thorough semantic study of the medieval topos, "the soul's cloister," the retreat within.

**BAUER, Joseph.**
*Geschichte der Aderlässe.* Repr. Munich: W. Fritsch, 1966 (orig. Munich, 1870). Dated, but still the broadest and most reliable history of medical ideas on induced "bleeding."

**BAUER, Veit Harold.**
*Das Antonius-Feuer in Kunst und Medizin.* Berlin: Springer, 1973 (Heidelberg: Akademie der Wissenschaften. Math. naturw. Klasse, Supplement 1973). A social history of the crippling epidemic resulting from ergot poisoning. What was known in Antiquity and the Middle Ages about its aetiology. The main part of the book is a detailed analysis of paintings by Matthias Grünewald, Hieronymus Bosch and Pieter Brueghel. The Altar of Isenheim was commissioned by the "Order of St. Anthony," a religious foundation originating in 1049, which specialized in the care of ergot victims and for long periods maintained more than three hundred and fifty hostels. Sixty-one excellent reproductions.

**BAUERREISS, Romuald.**
*Pie Jesu: Das Schmerzensmann-Bild und sein Einfluss auf die Mittelalterliche Frömmigkeit.* Munich: Widmann, 1931.

**BAXANDALL, Michael.**
*Painting and Experience in Fifteenth-Century Italy: A Primer in the Social History of Pictorial Style.* Oxford 1972. Gestures in preaching and praying; see pp. 45ff.

**BAZIN, Nancy Topping.**
"The Concept of Androgyny: A Working Bibliography." *Women's Studies* 2 (1974): 217-35.

**BEATRICE, Pier Franco.**
"Continenza e matrimonio nel cristianesimo primitivo (sec. 1-2)." In *Etica sessuale e matrimonio nel cristianesimo dalle origini,* ed. by Raniero CANTALAMESSA. Milano: Vita e Pensiero, 1976 (*Studia Patristica Mediolanensia* 5).

**BECHTEL, Fritz.**
*Ueber die Bezeichnungen des Magens im Griechischen.* Berlin: Weidmann, 1903.

____. *Ueber die Bezeichnung der sinnlichen. Wahrnehmungen in den indogermanischen Sprachen: Ein Beitrag zur Bedeutungs-Geschichte.* Weimar: H. Böhlau, 1879. The study deals with the etymology of words that designate experience rather than with the field of words that refer to an experience. Author concludes that in Indo-Germanic languages the words designating sensual experience take their origin from those which designate the experienced object rather than the act of experience: the smell, taste, sound of the object leads to the designation of the sense perception. Frequently in Indo-Germanic languages, the experience of hearing and sight are expressed with the same word.

**BECK, Brenda.**
"The Symbolic Merger of Body, Space and Cosmos in Hindu Tamilnad." *Contributions to Indian Sociology* 10 (1976).
____. "The Anthropology of the Body." *Current Anthropology* 16, no. 3 (1975).

**BEDALE, Stephen.**
"The Meaning of 'Kefale' in the Pauline Epistles." *The Journal of Theological Studies* 5 (1954): 211-15. In St. Paul's days, according to popular physiology, both Greek and Hebrew, a man reasoned and purposed not with his "head" but in his "heart" (or diaphragm). Why does Paul use "kefale" in his epistles to speak of Christ as the "Head of the Church"?

**BEER, Ellen, J.**
*Die Rose der Kathedrale von Lausanne und der kosmologische Bilderkreis des Mittelalters.* Bern: Benteli Verlag, 1952. An iconographic study of the rosette window of the Cathedral of Lausanne in which early Christian doctrine, geometrical semantics and medieval exegesis unite: four elements, seasons, rivers in Paradise, eight winds and monsters combine with trinitarian symbolism to give the twelve months which project the mysteries of the liturgical year into the zodiac. All this is reflected in the geometrical rules according to which the human figure is constructed (pp. 47ff.).

**BEHLING, Lottlisa.**
*Zur Morphologie und Sinndeutung kunstgeschichtlicher Phänomene: Beiträge zur Kunstwissenschaft.* Köln, Vienna: Böhlau, 1975.
____. "Zur Engeldarstellung in der deutschen Kunst um 1000." *Beiträge zur christlichen Philosophie* 6 (1950): 25-37.

**BEHM, Johannes.**
"Koilia" (i.e. "belly" etc.). In *Theologisches Wörterbuch zum Neün Testament,* ed. by Gerhard KITTEL. Vol. 3, 786-89. Stuttgart, 1938 (*Theological Dictionary of the New Testament,* ed. by G.FRIEDRICH). The perception of the belly in the New and Old Testament.

**BEIDELMANN, T.O.**
"The Blood Covenant and the Concept of Blood in Ukaguru." *Africa* 33 (1963): 321-42.

**BEINHAUER, Werner.**
"Ueber 'Piropos' (Eine Studie über spanische Liebessprache)." *Volkstum und Kultur der Romanen* 7, nos. 2-3 (1934): 111-62. A rich and varied collection of those exclamations that Spanish men cultivated when passing a woman on the street. The metaphors used to suggest body type and carriage are manifold and surprising.

**BEISSEL, Stephan.**
*Die Verehrung der Heiligen und ihrer Reliquien* in *Deutschland im Mittelalter.* 2 vols. Freiburg: Herder, 1880, 1882. Repr. with an intro. by Horst APPUHN. Darmstadt: Wissenschaftliche Buchgesellschaft, 1976. Still unsurpassed synthesis of medieval devotion to the Catholic saints, particularly their bodies (relics). The author was guided by surviving popular rituals in the sanctuaries of the late nineteenth century.

**BELL, Rudolph.**
*Holy Anorexia.* Chicago: Univ. Chicago Press, 1985.

**BELMONT, Nicole.**
*Les signes de la Naissance: Etude des représentations symboliques associées aux naissances singulières.* Paris: Plon, 1971. A major attempt to gather interpretations of two exceptional forms of birth: cowl and feet-first. The first part deals with European folklore and medical tradition, first descriptive then interpretive. The second analyzes African and Oceanic materials. A comparison leads the author to assign a worldwide central mythopoetic function to these strange births, and to compare the inductive-folklorist approach with the systemic approach of the enlightened mythologist who has learned where to look for relevant details in folklore.

**BENEDEK, Thomas G.**
"Beliefs about Human Sexual Function in the Middle Ages and Renaissance." In *Human Sexuality in the Middle Ages and Renaissance,* ed. by Douglas RADCLIFF-UMSTEAD, 97-119. Pittsburgh: Center for Medieval & Renaissance Studies, 1978. A judicious choice of a few illustrations and texts. The difference between men's and women's anatomies is established primarily through symbolic reference to such dualities as warm/cold, right/left.

**BENEDICENTI, A.**
*Malati, medici e farmaciste, storia dei rimedi traverso i secoli e delle teorie che ne spiegano l'azione sull'organismo.* 2 vols. Milan, 1925. An early social history of drugs and what their use allows one to surmise about lay and medical body perception.

**BENSON, R.G.**
*Medieval Body Language: A Study of the Use of Gestures in Chaucer's Poetry.* Copenhagen: Rosenkilde and Bagger (Anglistica 21) 1980. Scholars have, in the main, overlooked Chaucer's innovative use of gesture, which he developed in Troilus and in the Canterbury Tales into a complex and flexible artistic device.

**BENTHALL, J., POLHEMUS, T., eds.**
*The Body as a Medium of Expression.* New York: Dutton, 1976.

**BENTON, John F.**
"Trotula, Women's Problems, and the Professional-ization of Medicine in the Middle Ages." *Bulletin of the History of Medicine* 59 (1985): 30-53.

**BENVENISTE, Emile.**
"Termes gréco-latins d'anatomie." *Revue de Philologie* 39 (1965): 7-13. Several of the most common body terms in later Latin are the result of medical transla-tions from the Greek, e.g., "stomachus," "colon."
____. "Med\*- et la notion de mesure." In *Le vocabu-laire des institutions Indo-Européennes*, vol. 2, 123-32. Paris: Minuit, 1969 (*Indo-European Language and Society*. Coral Cables,Fl.: Univ. Miami Press, 1973). See for the etymological relationship between mea-sure, moon and medicine.

**BENZ, Ernst.**
*Die Vision: Erfahrungsformen und Bilderwelt.* Stuttgart: Klett, 1969. The author taught religious sci-ences and was firmly rooted in the Eranos-Circle (Zürich), yet criticized the psychological interpretation of visions current in C.G.JUNG's school because of its methodology. It is unhistorical to assume that the "imaginings" of pictures and symbols of all epochs and religions can be deciphered by referring them to the same set of archetypes. Hence the author stresses the specificity in form and content which distinguishes and characterizes visions - very often those of bodies - in different cultures.
____. *Urbild und Abbild: Der Mensch und die mythis-che Welt.* Leiden: E.J. Brill, 1974 (Gesammelte Beiträge zum Eranos Jahrbuch).

**BERG, Alexander.**
*Der Krankheitskomplex der Kolik- und Gebärmutterleiden in der Volksmedizin und Medizingeschichte.* Berlin: Ebering, 1935. The per-ceived similarity between "stomach" and "womb," between digestion and gestation, finds its expression in three ways: the pain in the two organs is designated by the same terms; the same herbs are used in therapeutic practice and votive offerings of the same shape are made. Ethnological testimonies (mainly from Eastern Prussia and the Baltic) are interpreted by ample refer-ence to earlier medical tradition.

**BERGER, John.**
*Ways of Seeing.* London: British Broadcasting Corpo-ration and Penguin Books, 1972.

**BERGER, Kurt.**
*Die Ausdrücke der Unio Mystica im Mittelhoch-deutschen.* Berlin: Ebering, 1935 (Germanische Studien 168). Great variety of verbal expressions almost all of which refer to bodily movements, feel-ings, activities.

**BERGHOFF, Emanuel.**
*Entwicklungsgeschichte des Krankheitsbegriffes.* Vienna: Maudrich, 1947 (Wiener Beiträge zur Geschichte der Medizin 1).

**BERGMANN, Karl.**
"Kulturgeschichtliche Wortbetrachtungen: Der men-schliche Körper, seine Krankheiten, sein Bau und die Aufgaben gewisser körperlicher Organe." *Zeitschrift für Deutschkunde* 41 (1927): 387-94.

**BERLINER, Rudolph.**
"Der Logos am Kreuz." *Das Münster* 11 (1958).
____. "Bemerkungen zu einigen Darstellungen des Erlösers als Schmerzensmann." *Das Münster* 9, nos. 3-4 (1956): 1-21. Important contributions to the iconog-raphy of Christ's crucified body, which is first repre-sented as that of a dead man in the twelfth century.

**BERNARD, Michel.**
*Le corps.* Paris: Editions Universitaires, 1974.

**BERNARDS, Peter.**
"Die rheinische Mirakelliteratur im 12. Jahrhundert." *Annalen des historischen Vereins für den Niederrhein* 138 (1941): 1-78, 140 (1942): 112-16.

**BERNHEIMER, Richard.**
*Wild Men in the Middle Ages: A Study in Art, Sentiment, and Demonology.* Cambridge, Mass.: Harvard Univ. Press, 1952.

**BERNITT, Paul Friedrich.**
*Lateinisch "caput" und "capum" nebst ihren Wortsippen im Französischen: Ein Beitrag zu franz. bzw. romanischen Wortgeschichte.* Dissertation. Kiel: R. Cordes, 1905.

**BERRY, Patricia.**
*Echo's Subtle Body: Contributions to an Archetypal Psychology.* Dallas: Spring, 1982.

**BESTOR, T.W.**
"Dualism and Bodily Movement." *Inquiry* 19, no. 1 (1976).

**BETEROUS, Paule-V.**
"A propos d'une des légendes mariales les plus répan-dues: Le 'lait de la Vierge.'" *Bulletin de l'association Guillaume BUDE* 4 (1975): 403-11. Miracles per-formed by the breastmilk of the Virgin Mary are wide-ly reported during the thirteenth century. Reports are contained in eight collections examined here.

**BETTELHEIM, Bruno.**
*Symbolic Wounds: Puberty Rites and the Envious Male.* New York: Macmillan, 1954 (German: *Die symbolis-chen Wunden: Pubertätsriten und der Neid des Mannes.* Munich: Kindler, 1975).

**BEYERLE, Franz.**
"Sinnbild und Bildgewalt im älteren deutschen Recht." *Zeitschrift d. Savigny Stiftung f. Rechtsgeschichte* 71, Germ. Abt. 58 (1938): 788-807.

**BIALE, David.**
"The God with Breasts: El Shaddai in the Bible." *History of Religions* 21, no. 3 (1982): 240-56.

**BILZ, Rudolf.**

*Studien über Angst und Schmerz*. Frankfurt: Suhrkamp Taschenbuch Wissenschaft, 1971 (Palaeoanthropologie 1/ 2).

**BIRCHLER, U.B.**

"Die Rolle der Frau bei der Liebeskrankheit und den Liebestränken." *Sudhoffs archiv* 59 (1975): 311-20.

**BIRKE, Lynda I.A., BEST, Sandy.**

"Changing Minds: Women, Biology and the Menstrual Circle." In *Biological Woman - The Convenient Myth: A Collection of Feminist Essays and a Comprehensive Bibliography*, ed. by Ruth HUBBARD, Mary Sue HENIFIN, Barbara FRIED, 161-79. Cambridge, Mass.: Schenkmann, 1983.

**BISILLIAT, Jeanne.**

"Village Diseases and Bush Diseases in Songhay: An Essay in Description and Classification with a View to Topology." In *Social Anthropology and Medicine*, ed. by J.D.LOUDON, 553-93. London, 1976.

**BLACKING, John, ed.**

*The Anthropology of the Body*. London, New York, San Francisco: Academic Press, 1977. Outcome of a gathering of British social anthropologists who began to react against a trend within anthropology to monopolize the body as a subject of a new physical anthropology, esp. ethnology and social biology. The one common aim of the nine contributors is a focus on the symbolic dimension: the interface between body and society.

____. "Towards an Anthropology of the Body." In *The Anthropology of the Body*, ed. by J.BLACKING, 1-28.

**BLACKMAN, Janet.**

"Popular Theories of Generation: The Evolution of Aristotle's Works: The Study of an Anachronism." In *Health Care and Popular Medicine in Nineteenth-Century England*, ed. by J.WOODWARD, D.RICHARDS, 56-88. New York: Holmes & Meier, 1977. A pamphlet that has often been titled "The Works of Aristotle" was widely read from the fifteenth century until well into the twentieth. Its text changed from edition to edition and arguably it "provides a barometer of ideas on sexual relations and childbirth." This vernacular pamphlet was certainly one agent that kept alive long-obsolete beliefs. At the turn of the nineteenth century, references to the seat of lust are omitted when the womb is described and also this organ ceases to be pictured as a phallus turned inside out.

**BLAICHER, Günther.**

*Das Weinen in mittelenglischer Zeit: Studien zur Gebärde des Weinens in historischen Qüllen und literarischen Texten*. Dissertation. Phil. Fak. Universität des Saarlandes, 1966. Mainly concerned with the analysis of the occasions at which tears are shed, and the words with which weeping is expressed; contains many passages in which the bodily expression of sorrow in Middle English has been described.

**BLANK, Walter.**

"Mikro- und Makrokosmos bei Konrad von Megenberg." In *Geistliche Denkformen in der Literatur des Mittelalters*, ed. by K.GRUBMULLER et al., 83-100. Munich: Fink Verlag, 1984. Konrad is doubly important to understanding the transformation of hermetic tradition during the fourteenth century: he adapted it to German expression, and to late-scholastic concern about "free will," distinguishing between cosmological correspondence and deterministic influence.

**BLASIUS, D.**

"Geschichte und Krankheit: Sozialgeschichtliche Perspektiven der Medizingeschichte." *Geschichte und Gesellschaft* 2, no. 3 (1976): 386-415.

**BLEKER, Johanna.**

"Von der medizinischen Volksbelehrung zur Popularisierung der medizinischen Wissenschaft." *Medizinhistorisches Journal* 13 (1978): 112-19.

**BLERSCH, K.**

*Wesen und Entstehen des Sexus im Denken der Antike*. Stuttgart: Kohlhammer, 1937 (Tübinger Beiträge zur Altertumswissenschaft 29).

**BLOCH, Iwan, ed.**

*Handbuch der gesamten Sexualwissenschaft in Einzeldarstellungen*. 3 vols. Berlin: L. Marais, 1912-25. Encyclopedia of sexual practices; historical.

**BLOCH, Marc.**

*Les rois thaumaturges: Etude sur le caractère surnaturel attribué à la puissance royale*. Paris: A. Colin 1961 (*The Royal Touch: Sacred Monarchy and Scrofula in England and France*. London: Routledge & Kegan Paul, 1973). Pioneer study in the history of mentality: the inherited power of French and English kings to heal scrofula by touch.

**BLOND, Georges, BLOND, Germaine.**

*Histoire pittoresque de notre alimentation: Les grandes études historiques*. Paris: Fayard, 1960.

**BLUMENBERG, Hans.**

"Licht als Metapher der Wahrheit: Im Vorfeld der philosophischen Begriffsbildung." *Studium Generale* 10 (1957): 432-47. A philosophical-historical "metaphorology" of light; pp. 441-43 contain a section on the eye and the ear in metaphors.

**BODEMER, Charles.**

"Embryological Thought in Seventeenth-Century England." In *Medical Investigations in Seventeenth-Century England*, by Charles BODEMER, Lester KING, 3-25. Los Angeles: Univ. California Press, 1968.

____. "Historical Interpretations of the Human Uterus and *Cervix Uteri*." In *The Biology of the Cervix*, ed. by R.BLAND, K.MOGHBISSI, 1-11. Chicago: Univ.

Chicago Press, 1973. The historical contribution to a symposium on the cervix. The contemporary certainties about the uterus and its functions derive from many thoroughly modern concepts, methods and techniques, mostly beyond the conceptual frame even of late-nineteenth-century anatomists.

**BOEHME, Gernot.**
"Wissenschaftliches und lebensweltliches Wissen am Beispiel der Verwissenschaftlichung der Geburtshilfe." In *Wissenssoziologie*, ed. by N.STEHR and V.MEJA, 445-63. Opladen, 1981 (*Kölner Zeitung für Soziologie und Sozialpsychologie* 22). The author is a sociologist of knowledge and historian of science concerned with a critique of the current scientific model. Eighteenth-century midwives are his example for a different, albeit declining mode of knowledge.

**BOESPFLUG, François.**
*Dieu dans l'art: "Sollicitudini Nostrae" de Benoît XIV (1745) et l'affaire Crescence de Kaufbëren.* Paris: Cerf, 1980. Detailed history of the repression of a trend in popular iconography to represent the Holy Spirit (third person of the Trinity) embodied as a man rather than a dove.

**BOLELLI, Tristano.**
"Il valore semasiologico delle voci...nell'epos omerico." *Annali della Scuola Normale Superiore di Pisa* 17 (1948): 65-75.

**BOLLEME, Geneviève.**
"L'enjeu du corps et la bibliothèque bleue." *Ethnologie française* 6, nos. 3-4 (1976): 285-92. Examines French popular literature from the late seventeenth to the early nineteenth century to reflect on the way the body appears.

**BOLTANSKI, Luc.**
*La découverte de la maladie: La diffusion du savoir médical.* Paris: Centre de Sociologie Européenne, 1968 (mimeographed typescript). Based on empirical data the author supports the thesis of the class-specific diffusion of modern medical civilization in France. Argues that the origin of the poorer man's "hardiness" toward suffering is economic, and contrasts it with the growing middle-class struggle to eliminate pain.
____. *Consommation médicale et rapport au corps.* Paris: Centre de Sociologie Européenne, 1970 (mimeographed typescript). The author uses an analysis of class-specific levels in consumption of medical services to reach conclusions about their symbolic effect on the construction of a class-specific body percept.
____. "Les usages sociaux du corps." *Annales E.S.C.* 26 (1971): 205-33.
____. *Prime éducation et morale de classe.* La Haye, Paris: Mouton, 1969 (Cahiers du Centre de Sociologie Européenne 5). The author studies the class-specific retardation in the spread of eighty manuals on infant care. Any important manual reaches working-class homes when the upper classes have already discarded it. The cumulative tendency of these tracts is the transformation of "infants" into "babies."

**BONFANTE, Giulio.**
"Nota sui nomi indoeuropei delle parti del corpo in latino." In *Hommages à Max Niedermann*, 71-81. Brussels: Berchem, 1956 (Coll. Latomus 23). Studies Indo-European wordfields of body parts and their route into Romance languages.
____. "Note sui nomi della 'guancia' e della 'mascella' in Italia." *Biblos* 27 (1951): 361-96. In Corsica there still existed seven different types of words for "cheek." The author maps two of these expressions in the Italian verbal landscape.
____. "Sull'animismo delle parti del corpo in indoeuropeo." *Ricerche linguistiche* 4 (1958): 19-28. The author starts with the observation of linguists that the active organs of the body in Indo-European have either masculine or feminine names, while the organs considered as immobile are neuter. The uterus was an active, moving organ, but the "liver", the penis, the testicles, the entrails and other inner body parts were also conceived of as "animated." Author lists ancient and modern slang words testifying to an age-old belief.

**BONNE, J.C.**
"Depicted Gesture, Named Gesture: Postures of the Christ on the Autun Tympanum." *History and Anthropology* 1, no. 1 (November 1984): 77-96. A comparison between Christ's posture depicted in sculpture and the description of this same pose in written contemporary texts. The sculpture shows at one glance, simultaneously, what linear descriptions can report only as a succession. "The depicted gesture is ambivalent because it is polymorphic: this gesture can even stand up to contradiction consistently."

**BONNET, Marie-Jo.**
*Un choix sans équivoque: Recherches historiques sur les relations amoureuses entre les femmes, XVI-XXième s.* Paris: Denoel, 1981. Discovery, rediscovery and public discourse on the seat of female pleasure since the sixteenth century.

**BORD, B.**
"Les grossesses à enfant visible dans l'art chrétien." *Aesculape* n.f. 23 (1933): 50-55, 81-88, 105-22, in BOROVICZENY, Ch.G., SCHIPPERGES, H., SEIDLER, E., eds. *Einführung in die Geschichte der Hematologie.* Stuttgart: Thieme, 1974. A serious introduction to the history of hematology rather than a guide to further research. Contributions by H.SCHRENK (pp. 1-16) on the ritual use of blood; by K.E.SCHIPPERGES (pp. 17-30) on the perception of blood in Antiquity and the Middle Ages; by E.ROTHSCHUH (pp. 31-46) on the discovery of

blood corpuscles; and by E.SEIDLER (pp. 44-47) on the state of knowledge around 1800.

**BOSCHUNG, Urs.**
"Geburtshilfliche Lehrmodelle: Notizen zur Geschichte des Phantoms und der Hysteroplasmata." *Gesnerus* 1, no. 2 (1981): 59-68. "Phantoms," later "pelviarium" then "hystero-plasma" are terms to designate increasingly complex models of woman's organs used in the training of midwives since the eighteenth century.
____. and STOIBER, E. *Wachsbildnerei in der Medizin.* Zürich, 1979.

**BOSWELL, John.**
*Christianity, Social Tolerance and Homosexuality.* Chicago: Univ. Chicago Press, 1981. With broad scope and immense learning the author documents but does not explain the appearance of an unprecedented image of the "homosexual" toward the end of the twelfth century, reflected in the rise of universal intolerance toward him.

**BOTTOMLEY, Frank.**
*Attitudes to the Body in Western Christendom.* London: Lepus Books, 1979. A survey of the contributions of Christianity toward the perception of the body culled from secondary sources.

**BOUCE, Paul-Gabriel, ed.**
*Sexuality in Eighteenth-Century Britain.* New York: Manchester Univ. Press, 1982.

**BOUGHALI, Mohammad.**
*La représentation de l'espace chez les marocains illettrés: Mythes et traditions orales.* Préface de Germaine Tillion. Paris: Ed. Anthropos, 1974. Thoughtful interpretation of oral testimony about space perception given by illiterate Moroccans: distinct layers of qualitatively different "space" lead from the home, the neighborhood, the town into the Muslim universe. Gender-specifically different postures and gestures are exacted in each of these spaces.

**BOULLOSA, Virginia H.**
"La concepción del cuerpo en la Celestina." In *La idea del cuerpo en las letras españolas*, ed. D. CVITANOVIC. Bahía Blanca (Argentine): Instituto de Humanidades, Univ. Nacional del Sur, 1973. The anonymous "tragicomedia de Calisto y Melibea" (1499-1502) places the demonic go-between, Celestiña, at the center of interest. Widely translated. Had an immense influence on Spanish, but also generally European literature. Four situations in which Celestina reflects on the body. Parmeno and its suitability for love are studied.

**BOURDIEU, Pierre.**
"La maison ou le monde renversé." In *Esquisse d'une théorie de la pratique, précédée de trois études d'ethnologie kabyle*, 45-69. Geneva: Droz, 1972 (*Outline of a Theory of Practice.* Cambridge: Cambridge Univ.

Press, 1977). The classical structuralist work on gender-specific perception and the use of domestic space. The construction of the house reflects the logic of mythical and ritual opposition between men's and women's orientation in space, expressed in gesture, posture and movement: in the way of sitting, speaking, feeling and thinking.
____. "Remarques provisoires sur la perception sociale du corps." *Actes de la Recherche en Sciences Sociales* 1, no. 14 (1977).
____. *Un art moyen: Essai sur les usages sociaux de la photographie.* 2d ed. Paris: Minuit, 1970. Contains some of the most influential observations on the sociological conditions through which a class-specific body is shaped.
____. *Le sens pratique.* Paris: Minuit, 1980. See ch.4: "La croyance et le corps" (pp. 3-134). Claudel said "con-naître c'est naître avec" (p. 112). The "hexis" or state of the body is the realization of a political mythology: the embodiment of what the man or the woman does. The most elementary movements of everyday "gymnastics" inculcate the equivalence between physical and social space.
____. *La distinction: Critique sociale du jugement.* Paris: Minuit, 1979 (*Distinction: A Social Critique of the Judgment of Taste.* Cambridge, Mass.: Harvard Univ. Press, 1984). Ch. 3 develops a theory about posture and gesture (*les pratiques corporelles*) as objectifications and incorporations of social space.

**BOURGEOIS, A.**
*Lépreux et maladreries du Pas-de-Calais du Xe au XIIIe s: Psychologie collective et institutions charitables.* Mémoires de la commission départementale des Monuments historiques du Pas-de-Calais, Tome XVI. Arras, 1972.

**BOURKE, John Gregory.**
*Der Unrat in Sitte, Brauch, Glauben und Gewohnheitsrecht der Völker*, ed. by F.KRAUSS, H.IHM. With a foreword by Sigmund FREUD. Leipzig: Ethnologischer Verlag, 1913.

**BOUTEILLER, Marcelle.**
*Médecine populaire d'hier et d'aujourd'hui.* Paris: Ed. Maisonneuve & Larose, 1966. The author is curator of an important religious-ethnological collection, and most of the examples are drawn from Anjou.
____. *Chamanisme et guérison magique.* Paris: Presses Universitaires de France, 1950.
____. *Sorciers et jeteurs de sorts.* Foreword by Claude LEVI-STRAUSS. Paris: Plon, 1958.

**BOWMAN, Frank Paul.**
"La circulation du sang religieux à l'époque romantique." *Romantisme* 31 (1981): 17-36.

**BRAIN, Robert.**
*The Decorated Body.* London: Hutchinson, 1979.

**BRANCA, Patricia, ed.**
*The Medicine Show: Patients, Physicians and the Perplexities of the Health Revolution in Modern Society.* New York, 1977.

**BRANDL, Leopold.**
*Die Sexualethik des Heiligen Albertus Magnus: Eine moralgeschichtliche Untersuchung.* Regensburg: Pustet, 1955 (Studien zur Geschichte der Katholischen Moraltheologie 2).

**BRAUER, Ernst Hannes.**
*Studien zur Darstellung des Schmerzes in der antiken bildenden Kunst Griechenlands und Italiens.* Dissertation. Breslau: R. Nischkowsky, 1934.

**BRAUN, R.**
"Zur Geschichte des Wortes 'Kopf' in der Sieben-bürgischen Sprachlandschaft." *Forschungen zur Volks- und Landeskunde* 9, no. 2 (1966): 91-98.

**BREMER, Dieter.**
"Licht als universales Darstellungsmedium. Materialien und Bibliographie." *Archiv für Begriffsgeschichte* 18 (1974): 185-206. An ample yet selective bibliography of historical studies on the representation of light and of darkness in art, literature, philosophy, theology (pp. 197-202), on theories about vision and the eye's function (pp. 203-05) and on the nature of color. Preceded by a dense survey of those traditions that interpret light and space as two aspects of the same experience.

**BRISSON, L.**
"Bisexualité et médiation en Grèce ancienne." *Nouvelle revue de psychanalyse* 7 (1973): 27-48.

**BRODY, Saul Nathaniel.**
*The Disease of the Soul: Leprosy in Medieval Literature.* Ithaca, New York: Cornell Univ. Press, 1974.

**BROOKS, Chandler McC., CRANEFIELD, Paul F. eds.**
*The Historical Development of Physiological Thought: A Symposium Held at the State University of New York Downstate Medical Center.* New York: Hafner, 1959.

**BROOKS-DAVIES, Douglas.**
"The Mythology of Love: Venereal and Related Iconography in Pope, Fielding, Cleveland, and Sterne." In *Sexuality in Eighteenth-Century Britain*, ed. by Paul-Gabriel BOUCE, 176-97. New York: Manchester Univ. Press, 1982.

**BROWE, Peter S.**
*Beiträge zur Sexualethik des Mittelalters.* Breslau: Müller, 1932.
____. *Zur Geschichte der Entmannung. Eine religions- und rechtsgeschichtliche Studie.* Breslau: Müller, 1936. The author's primary concern is the attitude of the Western and Eastern churches to castration. But the careful quotations from sources which are often unre-lated to the Church make this a valuable reference. The Church pronounced itself formally against ascetic self-castration, but explicitly accepted penal and thera-peutic forms. It also tolerated - and in the Renaissance promoted de facto - the castration of sopranos.

**BROWN, E. A.**
"Death and the Human Body in the Later Middle Ages: The Legislation of Boniface VIII on the Division of the Corpse." *Viator* 12 (1981): 221-70. Since Charles the Bald died in 877 crossing the Alps, the practice of dividing and boiling the body had come into use. Barbarossa's boiled remains accomplished the pilgrimage which his death had threatened to inter-rupt. In 1299, Boniface VIII in the Bull "De testandae feritatis" with horror forbids the practice - but with little success. The powerful became increasingly con-cerned with dividing their body in various burial places, a practice rooted in belief that the body contin-ues to live, desires to be near relatives, to obtain their prayers, to rise with them, etc.

**BROWN, Frank C.**
*The Frank C. Brown Collection of North Carolina Folklore.* 7 Vols. Vol. 1: *Games and Rhymes, Beliefs and Customs, Riddles, Proverbs, Speech.* Vols. 6, 7: *Popular Beliefs and Superstitions from North Carolina.* Durham, N.C.: Duke Univ. Press, 1952-64.

**BROWN, Peter.**
"Society and the Supernatural: A Medieval Change." *Daedalus* 104 (1975): 153-75.
____. *The Cult of the Saints: Its Rise and Function in Late Antiquity.* Chicago: Univ. Chicago Press, 1982 (The Haskell Lectures on the History of Religion 2). Together these constitute a sensitive study on the change of attitudes toward the body as a relic from Roman Antiquity into the Middle Ages.
____. "The Saint as Exemplar in Late Antiquity." *Representations* 1-2 (Spring 1983).
____. "Antiquité tardive." In *Histoire de la vie privée*, ed. by Philippe ARIES, Georges DUBY, vol. 1, 225-99. Paris: Seuil, 1985. A contribution to the five-vol-ume *History of Private Life* (trans.: Cambridge, Mass., Harvard Univ. Press) launched at the initiative of P.ARIES This essay deals mainly and directly with the convergence of late imperial and Christian trends in Italy by which an entirely new perception of "flesh" came into existence. Insists on the different evolutions in Byzantine Christianity.

**BROWN, Theodore K.**
"From Mechanism to Vitalism in Eighteenth-Century Physiology." *Journal of the History of Biology* 7, no. 2 (1974): 179-216.

**BRUAIRE, Claude.**
*Philosophie du corps.* Paris: Seuil, 1968. An important French attempt to recognize the "body" as a central philosophical theme, speculative rather than historical,

epistemological rather than phenomenological. Valuable for body history, especially the historical steps by which the "body" becomes the object of a silent gaze (pp. 193-230) and of a language which makes the body into "something" rather than somebody (ch. 3, pp. 231ff.).

**BRUECH, Josef.**
"Die Wörter für 'Haar' im Latein und ihr Fortleben im Romanischen." *Wiener Studien* 70 (1957): 44-77.

**BRUECKNER, Wolfgang.**
*Bildnis und Brauch: Studien zur Bildfunktion der Effigies.* Berlin: E. Schmidt, 1966.
____. "Hand und Heil im Schutzbehälter und auf volkstümlicher Graphik." *Anzeiger des Germanischen Nationalmuseums* (1965): 60-109. Well-illustrated and documented study by an outstanding religious ethnologist of the representation of the hand (especially of drawings which show nothing else) since the Middle Ages. The hand is a symbol of God, integral to gesture. But the left hand has also been used widely and intensively as a mnemotechnic device.
____. "Das Bildnis in Rechtlichen Zwangsmitteln." In *Festschrift für Harald KELLER*, 111-29. Darmstadt: Röther, 1963. Well into the Renaissance public enemies and criminals were ridiculed or punished through the debasing exposition of their effigies. In this juridical use of (frequently naked) pictures, old magical belief about the presence of the real body in the image continues.

**BRUEGELMANN, Jan.**
*Der Blick des Arztes auf die Krankheit im Alltag 1779-1850: Medizinische Topographien als Quelle für die Sozialgeschichte des Gesundheitswesens.* Dissertation. Berlin F.U.,1982. A history of the medical gaze taking as a source the medical topographies written by physicians and medical administrators.
____. "Observations on the Process of Medicalization in Germany 1770-1830 Based on Medical Topographies." *Historical Reflections - Réflexions historiques* 1, 1982.

**BRUN, Jean.**
*La main et l'esprit.* Paris: Presses Universitaires de France, 1963. Phenomenological reflections on the hand.

**BRUNNER, Hellmuth.**
"Die Hieroglyphen für 'räuchern,' 'bedecken,' 'Handfläche' und die ihnen entsprechenden Wörter." *Nachrichten der Akademie der Wissenschaften in Göttingen: Philologisch-historische Klasse* 1965, no. 3: 80-96.
____. *Das Herz im aegyptischen Glauben.* 1967. Two key words refer in Egypt to the heart; it is the seat of life, the source of movement and feeling, and also a divine entity that reigns over man, unless he loses it -

and with it his afterlife. This is the up-to-date monograph by a recognized egyptologist.

**BRYK, Felix.**
*Circumcision in Man and Woman: Its History, Psychology and Ethnology.* Repr. of the 1934 ed. New York: AMS Press, 1972 (Orig. publ. in German, 1931). Very dated, and still a good survey. Among the literature on body markings wherein circumcision (of the Western body) holds a special place: it is vast and mostly interpretive of Jewish self-image, Christian theological legitimation, psychoanalytic significance of a sexist ritual, etc. For bibliographic guidance see the major specialized encyclopedias. Among these, note: G.KITTEL, *Theological Dictionary*, "Peritemno"; for biblical archeology, *Dictionnaire de Théologie Catholique* (vol. 2.2, 1938, pp. 2519-27); for Christian theological metaphors, the four articles in *Religion in Geschichte und Gegenwart* (1957). For recent bibliography *The Encyclopedia of Islam*. Vol. 5, "khitan".

**BUCHER, Bernadette.**
*La sauvage aux seins pendants.* Paris: Hermann, 1977 (*Icon and Conquest: A Structural Analysis of the Illustrations of de Bry's Great Voyages.* Translated by Basia Miller GULATI. Chicago: Univ. Chicago Press, 1981). Members of the Dutch Protestant de Bry family published a monumental series of books on the New World while in exile in Germany. Bucher examines the human figure in the illustrations of the first volumes, which appeared at the beginning of the seventeenth century. She applies the theories of E.LEACH and M.DOUGLAS in a structural analysis of the unconscious, symbolic thinking that develops in these images when ideas about the body have to be graphically expressed, ideas which fail to fit into the preconceived order of a northern Protestant.

**BUCK, Carl Darling.**
*A Dictionary of Selected Synonyms in the Principal Indo-European Languages: A Contribution to the History of Ideas.* Chicago: Univ. Chicago Press, 1949. Ch. 4, pp. 196-325: parts of the body, bodily functions and conditions.

**BUECHNER, F.**
"Vom Wesen der Leiblichkeit." *Beuroner Hochschulwochen* 1948 (1949): 77-109.

**BUETTNER, Ludwig.**
*Fränkische Volksmedizin. Ein Beitrag zur Volkskunde Ostfrankens.* Erlangen: Palm & Enke, 1935. See ch. 2: popular expressions of illness, pp. 24-61.

**BUGNER, Ladislas, gen. ed.**
*The Image of the Black in Western Art.* Vol. 1: *From the Pharaohs to the Fall of the Roman Empire* (J.VERCOUTTER, J.LECLANT, F.M.SNOWDEN, J.DESANGES). Vol. 2: *From the Early Christian Era to the "Age of Discovery."* Sec. 1, "From the Demonic Threat to the Incarnation of Sainthood" (J.DEVISSE),

486

Sec. 2, "Africans in the Christian Ordinance of the World" (J.DEVISSE, M.MOLLAT). Vol. 3: *From Europe to America*. New York: Morrow; and French version Fribourg: Office du Livre, 1976ff. (Publications of the Menil Foundation). Still unfinished magnificently produced multivolume iconography of the black man in Western art. Lengthy articles by an international team, profuse illustrations and wide-ranging bibliography.

**BUHAN, Christine.**
*La mystique du corps: Jalons pour une anthropologie du corps. Les Yabyan et les Yapeke, Bakoko...au Sud-Cameroun*. Paris: L'Harmattan, 1979. A major study of a previously unrecorded language. Analyzes its symbolic universe primarily through body- and movement-related designations.

**BULLOUGH, Vern L.**
"Medieval Medical and Scientific Views of Women." *Viator* 4 (1973): 485-501.

____, BRUNDAGE, James, eds. *Sexual Practices and the Medieval Church*. Buffalo, New York: Prometheus Books, 1982. Collection of essays that touch on themes related to the body in the Middle Ages: transvestism, asceticism, homosexuality, impotence. Canon law and scholastic disputes are used as sources.

____, VOGHT, M. "Women, Menstruation and Nineteenth-Century Medicine." *Bulletin of the History of Medicine* 47 (1973): 62-82.

**BUNGE, Mario.**
*The Mind-Body Problem: A Psycho-Biological Approach*. New York: Pergamon, 1980. "The psychophysical dualism embedded in European languages" renders them inept to examine the intersection of mental and body experience. The author constructs a formal and abstract "space-state language" to explore this intersection of science and philosophy.

**BUNIM, Miriam Schild.**
*Space in Medieval Painting and the Forerunners of Perspective*. New York: Columbia Univ. Press, 1940.

**BURROW, T.**
"Dravidian Studies 4: The body in Dravidian and Uralian." *Bulletin of the School of Oriental and African Studies* 11 (1943/46): 328-56.

**BURTON, Ernest de Witt.**
*Spirit, Soul and Flesh: The Usage of Pneuma, Psyche and Sarx in Greek Writings and Translated Works from the Earliest Period to 225 A.D. and Their Equivalents in the Hebrew Old Testament*. Chicago: Univ. Chicago Press, 1918. The use of words for these three fields in the ancient Greek and Judaic writers up to and including the New Testament, but not in later Christian writers. Not a history of the psychology or anthropology of Semites or Greeks, but narrowly a lexical study, to make further research into cultural history more solid and precise.

**BUSCH, Theodor.**
*Der leibliche Mensch im Leben der Sprache: Teil I: stehen, sitzen, liegen*. 1912-13. (Beilage zum Jahresbericht d. Kgl. Gymnasiums zu Muenstereifel Progr. Nr. 643.) What do those action words which primarily refer to the human body say about the rest of the world? The author examines what "goes" or "stands" in analogy to the human body, but since he does not attend to the historical change in such attributions, his article is of limited value.

**BUYTENDIJK, Frederik Jacobus Johannes.**
*Allgemeine Theorie der menschlichen Haltung und Bewegung: als Verbindung und Gegenuberstellung von physiologischer und psychologischer Betrachtungsweise*. Berlin: Springer, 1956. A central theme: the distinction between "the" body that science constructs and the body of one concrete person in that person's perception. See pp. 46-63 for specific aspects: invisibility of the experienced body; the body as record of personal past.

____. *Mensch und Tier: Ein Beitrag zur vergleichenden Physiologie*. Reinbek: Rowohlt, 1958.

____. *Prolegomena einer anthropologischen Physiologie*. Salzburg: O. Muller, 1967 (*Prolegomena to an anthropological physiology*. Pittsburgh: Duchesne, 1974).

____. "Zur Phänomenologie der Begegnung." *Eranos Jahrbuch* 19 (1950): 431ff.

____. *Über den Schmerz*. Trans. from Dutch by H.PLESSNER. Bern: Huber, 1948 (*Pain: Its Modes and Functions*. Repr. Westport, Conn.: Greenwood, 1973).

**BYDLOWSKI, Monique.**
"Essai sur les coutumes entourant l'accouchement." *Revue de médecine psychosomatique et de psychologie médicale* 18, no. 1 (1976): 9-18 (special issue on "La naissance").

**BYLEBYL, Jerome J.**
"The Medical Side of Harvey's Discovery: The Normal and the Abnormal." In *William Harvey and His Age*, ed. by Jerome J.BYLEBYL, 28-102. Baltimore: Johns Hopkins, 1979. Social circumstances had to change to enable Harvey to create a new conception of the body's interior mostly out of elements which had been known and described already before 1600.

**BYLOFF, Fritz.**
"Nestelknüpfen und -lösen." *Archiv für Geschichte der Medizin* 19 (1927): 203-08.

**BYNUM, Caroline Walker.**
*Jesus as Mother: Studies in the Spirituality of the High Middle Ages*. Los Angeles: Univ. California Press, 1982.

____. *Holy Feast and Holy Fast, the Religious Significance of Food to Medieval Women*. Berkeley: Univ. California Press, 1987.

zone

**BYNUM, William.**

"The Anatomical Method, Natural Theology, and the Functions of the Brain." *Isis* 64 (1973): 445-68. Like W.PAGEL the author underlines the importance of not "modernizing" seventeenth-century thinking when commenting on their texts that deal with the soul's relation to the body. For two centuries the medical researcher tended to assign physiological functions to the theological soul. "The resolution of the (consequent) dilemma was ultimately effected in the nineteenth century not by the fusion of mind and body, but by the separation of mind from soul."

**BYRDE, Penelope.**

*The Male Image: Men's Fashion in Britain 1300-1970*. London: Batsford, 1979. The most striking fact about men's clothes in the modern West is that they are quite different from women's: reports on the sociogenesis of this unique polarization of body perception through dress.

**CABANES, Augustin.**

*Esculape chez les artistes*. Paris: Le François, 1928.

**CABASSUT, André.**

"Coeurs..., changement des, échange des." In *Dictionnaire de spiritualité*, 11, 1046-51. 1948. Solid orientation for the study of a medieval motif: "the exchange of hearts" - in the perspective of ascetic theology.

**CABRAL, Oswaldo.**

*A medicina teologica e as benzeduras*. São Paulo, Brazil, Departamento de Culturas, 1958. "Benzeduras" are the therapeutic and preventive prayers addressed to specific saints, very common in rural Brazil, that survive within urban cultures. One-hundred and eighty-six texts from the southern state of St. Catarina are compared with ninety of other origin. These prayers are inherited secrets of certain families, though some have become public domain. Author establishes structural correlations between saints, body parts and objects used in the ritual concomitant with the recitation of the prayer.

**CAHEN, Maurice.**

"'Genou,' 'adoption' et 'parenté' en germanique." *Bulletin de la Société de Linguistique de Paris* 27, no. 81 (1927): 56-67.

**CAILLOIS, Roger.**

"Préface." In *Masques*. Exposition Musée Guimet. Paris: Perrin 1960.

____. *Au coeur du fantastique*. Paris: Gallimard, 1965.

**CALAIS, M.**

*Répertoire bibliographique des manuels de savoir-vivre en France*. Conservatoire National des Arts et Métiers, Institut National des Techniques de la Documentation, exemplaire dact., 1970.

**CALLAWAY, H.**

"The Most Essential Female Function of All: Giving Birth." In *Defining Females*, ed. by S.ARDENER, 163-85. London: Halsted, 1978.

**CALLOT, Emile.**

*La Renaissance des sciences de la vie au XVIe s.* Paris: Presses Univ. de France, 1951. Anatomy is a science which constitutes its object: an *organization* which is at the same time analytic and synthetic. It separates constituent parts of the organism and creates liaisons between the entities thus manufactured. Callot deals with the evolution of this methodological approach to body description rather than with the facts which resulted from it.

**CALVI, Giulia.**

*Storie di un anno di peste: Comportamenti sociali e immaginario nella Firenze barocca*. Milan: Bompiano, 1984.

____. "A Metaphor for Social Exchange: The Florentine Plague of 1630." *Representations* 13 (Winter 1986): 139-63.

**CAMBIANO, G.**

"Patologia e metafora politica: Alcmeone, Platone e corpus Hippocraticum." *Elenchos* 2 (1982): 219-36.

**CAMERON, Sharon.**

*The Corporeal Self: Allegories of the Body in Melville and Hawthorne*. Baltimore: Johns Hopkins Press, 1981. A major contribution of American literary scholarship. This many-layered, short and lucid text sets new standards for the critical techniques by which the body as percept, analogue and metaphor can be studied in an author. (Moby Dick takes monster bodies apart in order to examine what they are made of. Hawthorne takes human bodies apart in order to reveal what they are made of.)

**CAMPESI, Silvia, Paola MANULI, Giulia SISSA.**

*Madre Materia, Sociologia e biologia della donna greca*. Boringhieri: Turin, 1983.

**CAMPORESI, Piero.**

*Il sugo della vita: Simbolismo e magia del sangue*. Milano: Saggiatore, 1984. Through commentaries of Italian sources of the sixteenth through eighteenth century (medical, literary, religious and poetic) the author reconstructs in great detail and in a most readable way the symbolic meaning and power of the blood. Memorable pages on the exhibition of blood at executions, the miracles involving Christ's blood, the changing perception of life-blood under the influence of New Philosophy.

____. *La carne impassibile*. 2d ed. Milano: Saggiatore, 1983.

____. *Le officine dei sensi: il corpo, il cibo, i vegetali: La cosmografie interiore dell' uomo...iconologia e antropologia*. Milan: Garzanti, 1985.

**CANGUILHEM, Georges.**

*La formation du concept de réflexe aux 17e et 18e siècles*. Paris: Presses Univ. de France, 1955.

____. "L'homme et l'animal du point de vue psychologique selon Charles Darwin." *Revue d'histoire des sciences et de leur application* 13, no. 1 (1960): 81-94.

____. *Le normal et le pathologique*. Paris: Presses Univ. de France, 1972 (*On the Normal and the Pathological*. With an introduction by M.FOUCAULT) (New York: Zone Books, 1989). A doctoral thesis on the history of the idea of "normalcy" in nineteenth-century pathology (1943) with a lengthy postscript (1966) by the author.

**CARDINI, Franco.**

"Magia e stregoneria nella Toscana del trecento." *Quaderni medievali* 5 (1978): 121-48. A Florentine synodal decree of the early fourteenth century induces the author to speculate on the dissociation of witchcraft from magic, as Church authorities effectively claim competence over the control of certain age-old practices, define these in a new way, and thereby dissociate witchcraft from magic.

**CARNOY, Albert J.**

"Symbolisme des mains et noms de nombres en Indo-Européen." *Le Museon* 59 (1946): 557-70.

**CARO, Francis A. de.**

*Women and Folklore: A Bibliographic Survey*. London: Greenwood Press, 1983.

**CASH, Arthur.**

"The Birth of Tristram Shandy, Sterne and Dr. Burton." In *Sexuality in Eighteenth-Century Britain*, ed. by Paul-Gabriel BOUCE, 198-224. New York: Manchester Univ. Press, 1982.

**CATTERMOLE, Tally Frances.**

*From the Mystery of Conception to the Miracle of Birth: a Historical Survey of Beliefs and Rituals Surrounding the Pregnant Woman in German Folk Tradition, Including Modern American Folklore*. Dissertation. Univ. California Los Angeles, 1978 (Los Angeles Univ. Micro. RPC 78-20302).

**CAVANAUGH, G. S. T.**

"A New View of the Vesalian Landscape." *Medical History* 27, no. 1 (1983): 77-79. Attention is centered on the landscape in relation to the original figures of Vesal's Muscle Man.

**CAYROL, Jean.**

*De l'espace humain*. Paris: Seuil, 1968.

**CEARD, Jean.**

*La Nature et les prodiges: L'insolite au XVIe siècle en France*. Genève: Droz, 1977.

____. ed. *La folie et le corps*. Paris: Presses de l'Ecole Normale Superieure, 1985.

**CERTEAU, Michel de.**

"Des outils pour écrire le corps." *Traverses* nos. 14-15 (April 1979): 3-14.

____. "Surin's Melancholy." In *Heterologies: Discourse on the Other*, by M.de CERTEAU, 101-15. Minneapolis: Univ. Minnesota Press, 1985. First published as "Mélancolique et/ou mystique: J.J.Surin," in *Analytiques* 2 (Oct. 1978): 35-48.

**CERULLI, Ernesta.**

*Vestirsi-spogliarsi-travestirsi. Come, quando, perché*. Palermo: Sellerio Editore, 1981. The activity of dressing and undressing rather than dress itself captures the attention in these essays.

**CHARLTON, Donald.**

*New Images of the Natural in France: A Study in European Cultural History 1750-1800*. Cambridge: Cambridge Univ. Press, 1985. The outlook on landscape, the sea, mountains, wildlife, the "sublime" and the concept of wilderness and "the wild" underwent profound changes at the end of the ancien régime. This new attitude transformed the attitude to "nature" and to man within it.

**CHARMASSON, Thérèse.**

*Recherches sur une technique divinatoire: La divination dans l'occident médiéval*. Paris: Droz, 1980.

**CHATELET, Noelle.**

*Le corps à corps culinaire*. Paris: Seuil, 1977. References to a relationship between certain foods and their preparation, on the one hand, and the body percepts, on the other, are frequent in this study on French kitchen folklore.

**CHENU, Marie Dominique.**

"Disciplina: Notes de lexicographie philosophique médiévale." *Revue des sciences philosophiques et théologiques* 25 (1936): 686-92.

____. "Spiritus: Le vocabulaire de l'âme au XIIe siècle." *Revue des sciences philosophiques et théologiques* 41 (1957): 209-32. During the twelfth century the term "spiritus" acquires new shades of meaning in psychology and cosmology. It now can stress the coherence between macro- and microcosm (pp. 220-23). Ample quotations and further citations.

____. "Situation humaine: Corporalité et Temporalité." In *L'homme et son destin d'après les penseurs du Moyen Age*, 23-49. Louvain: Vander Oyez, 1960. In the Augustinian and Thomist traditions, man's nature is historically determined, because it consists in the embodiment of spirit. Augustine emphasizes the aspect of the temporal element of the incarnation, Thomas on embodiment.

**CHOAY, F.**

"La ville et le domaine bâti comme corps dans les textes des architectes théoriciens de la première

Renaissance italienne." *Nouvelle Revue de Psychanalyse* 9 (1974): 239-51.

**CHOLLET, A.**

"Corps glorieux," article in *Dictionnaire de Théologie Catholique* vol. 3, 1879-1906. The resurrection of the body is a fundamental Christian belief. This particular article from a vast early twentieth-century encyclopedia reports on eighteen hundred years of writings about the appearance, faculties, characteristics of the body after the end of time. Many major quotations - even from unpublished sources - make it into a useful source.

**CHOULANT, Johann L.**

*History and Bibliography of Anatomic Illustration.* Trans. and ed. by Mortimer FRANK. Chicago: Univ. Chicago Press, 1920. Enl. repr. New York: Hafner, 1962.

_____.*Geschichte und Bibliographie der anatomischen Abbildung nach ihrer Beziehung auf anatomische Wissenschaft und bildende Kunst.* Leipzig: Rudolph Weigel, 1852.

**CHRISTIAN, Paul.**

*Das Personenverständnis im modernen medizinischen Denken.* Tübingen: Mohr, 1952.

**CHRISTIAN, W.A.**

*Apparitions in Late Medieval and Renaissance Spain.* Princeton: Princeton Univ. Press: 1981. A careful analysis of bodily apparitions of divine or saintly persons to children, peasants and others, based on the textual analysis of records by Church authorities. The texts are limited to the fifteenth century and the first quarter of the sixteenth, since after that time - probably out of fear of the inquisition - "real" apparitions disappear or go unrecorded in Spain until the early twentieth century.

**CHURCHILL, F.B.**

"The History of Embryology as Intellectual History." *Journal of the History of Biology* 3, no. 1 (1970): 155-81. Review of five important books on the subject.

**CIAVARELLI, Marica Elise.**

*El tema de la fuerza de la sangre: Antecedentes europeos: Siglo de oro español: Juan de la Cueva, Cervantes, Lope, Alarcon.* Madrid: Porrua-Turranzas, 1980. Without understanding the nature of "blood," neither the concept of "honor" nor the bonds tying people to each other can be understood. Both are basic in Spanish literature 1500-1700.

**CLAES, Jacques.**

"Metabletica or a Psychology of History." *Humanitas* 7 (1971): 269-78. Karl MANNHEIM asks: "Why did completely different types of people emerge in the Middle Ages than at the time of the Renaissance?" And answers: "Up to now we have never had historical psychology." VANDENBERG followed HUSSERL's advice to inquire into "the reality of the diversity of things" and concentrated his attention on "discovering words and deeds before they have been smoothed out by the events that followed." By engaging in "historical psychology" rather than "psychological history" he called attention to epoch-specific reality - above all, that of the body.

**CLARK, Kenneth.**

*The Nude: A Study in Ideal Form.* New York: Pantheon, 1959. A delightful reformulation of lectures accompanied by three hundred excellent reproductions of paintings and sculpture since early Greece. The naked figure in this European tradition always evokes a connection with garment (contemporary, or, as often in the late sixteenth century, the drapery of past epochs).

**CLARKE, Juanne N.**

"Sexism, Feminism and Medicalism: A Decade Review of Literature on Gender and Illness." *Sociology of Health and Illness* 5, no. 1 (1983): 62-82.

**CLAVERIE, E.**

"Temporal Sickness, Spiritual Healing: Therapeutic Remedies and Itineraries in Margeride, Lozère," *History and Anthropology* 2 (1985): 155-72. Margeride is a mountainous province in Southern Central France. When people feel ill they simultaneously pick therapeutic offerings from three distinct curative systems: physicians, healers and "Heaven" (esp. pilgrimages). The author believes that this expresses the peasant's view of the body's place simultaneously in three spheres. It would be inconceivable to entrust "oneself in illness" to just one of these, least of all medicine alone.

**CLERCQ, C. de.**

"'Ordines unctionis infirmi' des IXe et Xe siècles." *Ephemerides liturgicae* 44 (1930): 100-22. The last rites administered by the Catholic church to its dying members consist of an anointing of various body parts with consecrated olive oil. The prayers that accompany these symbolic actions have changed over the centuries, and reflect the changing symbolism of the frontal body, hands, feet, eyes, ears and lips.

**COCCHIARA, Giuseppe.**

*Il linguaggio del gesto.* Turin: Bocca, 1932. Attempts neither to develop a complete theory of gesture, nor to provide a vocabulary or dictionary, but to provide an "introduction to the grammar of gesture."

**COHEN, G.**

*Le thème de l'aveugle et du paralytique dans la littérature française.* Paris: Mélanges Picot, 1913.

**COHEN, Marcel.**

"Genou, famille, force dans le domaine chamito-sémitique." In *Memorial Henri Basset: Nouvelles Etudes nord-africaines et orientales.* Vol. 1, 203-10. Paris: Geuthner, 1928 (Publ. de l'Inst. des Hautes Etudes Marocaines 17).

**COLE, F.J.**

*A History of Comparative Anatomy.* London: Macmillan, 1944. So far the only attempt at a monographic global treatment of the theme.

**COLEMAN, William.**

"Health and Hygiene in the *Encyclopédie*: A Medical Doctrine for the Bourgeoisie." *Journal of the History of Medicine and Allied Sciences* 29 (1974): 399-421. The Encyclopedia appears to readers in a "world where each man must make his own way" and proposes "an applicable, not an abstract, guide to the first of man's needs - health." The ancient doctrine of the so-called nonnaturals changes its meaning profoundly.

_____.*Death Is a Social Disease: Public Health and Political Economy in Early Industrial France.* Madison: Univ. Wisconsin Press, 1982. The emerging scientific approach to public health in early nineteenth-century France through men committed to biological inquiry and the tenets of political economy. The intellectual development of the foremost hygienic investigator (L.R.VILLERME) and his contribution to the concept "population" is discussed. The concept of "population" is essential for understanding the new body-perception. It results - originally - from a pathological approach to society. The clinical gaze engages in the anatomy from which the individual patient emerges, and the hygienic synthesis integrates the patients first in an analogy with eighteenth-century physiological organisms, then, collectively, into a population.

_____."The People's Health: Medical Themes in Eighteenth-Century French Popular Literature." *Bulletin of the History of Medicine* 51 (1977): 55-74. From popular tracts, especially calendars, astrological forecasts and the *secreta mulierum*, the author culls passages incorporating certain themes: micro/macrocosm; herbal remedies; prayers; astrological precautions. Anatomy and physiology as such are not mentioned; neither the pursuit of health nor its preservation is represented as a goal. And yet these text-fragments abound with references to the body and its botanical, meteorological and culinary correlates.

**COLLINET-GUERIN, Marthe.**

*Histoire du nimbe des origines aux temps modernes.* Paris: Nouvelles Editions Latines, 1961. The record of an amateur's lifelong collection of evidence about the luminous extension of the body, called "nimbus."

**COMMUNICATIONS.**

35 (1982). Special issue, "Sexualités occidentales."

**COMMUNIO.**

54 (1980). Special issue, "Il Corpo." Very orthodox modern Catholic journal.

**CONGAR, Yves M.-J.**

"Cephas, céphale, caput." *Revue du Moyen Age Latin* 8 (1952): 5-42. The fascinating story of the political use of folk etymology: in the synoptic gospels Peter is called Cephas (the rock) on which the Church will be built. The claim to the pope's primacy is built substantially on this passage. Through Isidore the Hebrew "kefas" (Rock-Petra-Petrus) and the Greek "kefale" (head) are semantically identified.

**CONGER, Georgie Perrigo.**

*Theories of Macrocosms and Microcosms in the History of Philosophy.* New York: Columbia Univ. Press, 1922.

**CONKLIN, H.C.**

*Folk Classification: A Topically Arranged Bibliography of Contemporary and Background References through 1971.* New Haven: Yale Univ. Press, 1972.

**CONTENEAU, G.**

*La déesse nue babylonienne: Etudes d'iconographie comparée.* Paris: P. Geuthner, 1914. The evolution of the most common representation of the naked goddess in the Middle East. Merely descriptive.

**COOPER, Wendy.**

*Hair: Sex, Society, Symbolism.* New York: Stein & Day, 1971.

**COOTER, Roger.**

"The Power of the Body: The Early Nineteenth-Century." In *Natural Order: Historical Studies of Scientific Culture,* ed. by B.BARNES and S.SHAPIN, 73ff. London, Beverly Hills: Sage, 1979.

_____. *The Cultural Meaning of Popular Science. Phrenology and the Organization of Consent in Nineteenth-Century Britain.* Cambridge: Cambridge Univ. Press, 1984.

**COPEMAN, W.S.C.**

"The Evolution of Anatomy and Surgery under the Tudors." *Annals of the Royal College of Surgeons of England* 32 (January 1963): 1-21.

**CORBIN, Alain.**

"Le péril vénérien au début du 19ème siècle: prophylaxie sanitaire et prophylaxie morale." In *L'haleine des Faubourgs,* ed. by Lion MURARD and Patrick SYLBERMAN, 245-84. Paris: Recherches, 1977.

_____. *Le miasme et la jonquille: L'odorat et l'imaginaire social XVIIIe-XIXe siècles.* Paris: Aubier, 1982 (*The Foul and the Fragrant: Odor and the French Social Imagination.* Cambridge, Mass.: Harvard Univ. Press, 1986). A pioneer study on the history of odor-perception in France, during the late eighteenth century, written in a popular style and well documented. Attitudes toward the bodily presence of the dead within the city; toward the disposal of excrement; toward the body's exhalations and odors, are here interpreted by a competent social historian.

**COULTER, Harris L.**

*Divided Legacy: A History of Schism in Medical Thought.* Washington D.C.: McGrath, 1973. The major social history of homeopathy in America. A vast and amply documented history of empirical medicine in the U.S. and its conflict with the rationalist tradition, written by a contemporary practitioner. An excellent introduction to authors who are rarely mentioned and hardly ever quoted in other studies of health in the U.S.

**COURCELLES, D.**

"Le corps des saints dans les cantiques catalans de la fin du Moyen Age." *Médiévales* 8 (1985): 43-53.

**COUSIN, B.**

"L'ex-voto, document d'histoire, expression d'une société." *Archives des sciences sociales des religions* 48, no. 1 (1979).

**CRANDON, Libbet.**

"Why Susto?" *Ethnology* 22, no. 2 (1983): 153-67. Survey of the anthropological and psychological literature and review of methods of approach.

**CRAWFORD, Patricia.**

"Attitudes to Menstruation in Seventeenth-Century England." *Past and Present* 91 (1981): 47-73. During the seventeenth century menstruation takes on a new meaning in medical thought: it gets upgraded by being turned into a sign of the female's procreative and domestic destination. First traces of this reevaluation are discussed. Detailed summary of traditional views of women's blood, monstrous births, corrupted conceptions and herbal concoctions.

**CRELIN, J.K., HELFAND, W.H.**

*Medical Care in the Twentieth Century: Facets of Change Illustrated by American and British Postcards.* Durham: Duke Univ. Medical Centre, 1982.

**CREMENE, A., ZEMMAL, Françoise.**

*Mythologie des vampires en Roumanie.* Paris: Editions du Rocher, 1981.

**CROIX, Alain.**

"L'homme et son corps dans l'Au-delà." In *Leib und Leben in der Geschichte der Neuzeit*, ed. by A.E.IMHOF, 155-64. Berlin, 1983.

**CUNNINGTON, C. Willett, CUNNINGTON, Phillis.**

*The History of Underclothes.* London: M. Joseph, 1951.

**CUSHING, Harvey.**

*A Bio-Bibliography of Andreas Vesalius,* New York: Schumans, 1943.

**CVITANOVIC, Dinko, et al.**

*La idea del cuerpo en las letras españolas (Siglo XIII a XVII).* Bahía Blanca, Argentina: Instituto de Humanidades. Univ. Nac. del Sur, 1973.

____. "De la 'disputa' medieval al 'pleito' calderoniano." In *La idea del cuerpo en las letras españolas,* 11-45. Bahía Blanca, Argentina, 1973. A new literary genre was born under Innocent III: the conversation between Body and Soul. It began as an ascetical exercise, in which the soul belittles the body. By the end of the thirteenth century it increasingly became macabre. In the seventeenth century in Spain the original

scholastic dispute and gory wrangle under CALDERON became "el pleito matrimonial [the marital squabble] del cuerpo y del Alma."

____. ed., *El sueño y su representación en el baroco español.* Bahía Blanca, Argentina: Instituto de Humanidades, Univ. Nac. del Sur, 1969.

# D

**D'ALVARENGA, Aida Sa V.**

"Algumas designações da cabeça humana na linguagem popular e no calão." *Boletim de Filologia* (Lisbon) 13 (1952): 257-72.

**D'ALVERNY, Marie-Thérèse.**

"Comment les théologiens et les philosophes voient la femme." *Cahiers de civilisation médiévale* 20 (1977): 105-29.

____. "Le Cosmos symbolique du XIIe siècle." *Archives d'histoire doctrinale et littéraire du Moyen Age* 20 (1953): 31-81. Exegesis of text and miniatures on the Clavis Physicæ of Honorius AUGUSTODUNENSIS (early twelfth century).

____. "L'homme comme symbole: Le microcosme." *Settimana di studio del centro italiano del Alto Medioevo* 23, no. 1 (1976): 123-83. While all civilizations have a set of beliefs about the correspondence man/universe, only the Greeks imagined man as a "résumé" of the cosmos. The idea, expressed in Plato's *Timaeus,* was transmitted by Boetius, Macrobius and Calcidius. The author examined the texts, especially those which support an "anatomical" correspondence between macro- and microcosm from early hermetic authors down to Honorius AUGUSTODUNENSIS. The analogy between the *imago mundi* and the human body, pp. 179ff.

**DANIELOU, Jean.**

"Question d'anthropologie." In *Message evangélique et culture hellénistique aux IIe et IIIe siècles,* by Jean DANIELOU, esp. pp. 355-90. Paris: Desclée, 1961.

____. *Platonisme et théologie mystique: Doctrine spirituelle de saint Gregoire de Nysse.* Paris: Aubier, 1944. See pp. 27ff. for the topos: "skin as dress."

**DARMON, Pierre.**

*Le Tribunal de l'impuissance: Virilité et défaillances conjugales dans l'ancienne France.* Paris: Seuil, 1979 (*Damning the innocent.* New York: Viking, 1986).

____. *Le mythe de la procréation â l'âge baroque.* Paris: Seuil, 1984.

____. *Mythologie de la femme dans l'ancienne France (XVIe-XIXe s.).* Paris: Seuil, 1983. An easily readable, broadly documented history of French misogynist discourse since the sixteenth century.

**DARNTON, Robert.**

"Workers Revolt: The Great Cat Massacre of the Rue Saint-Séverin," in *The Great Cat Massacre and other Episodes in French Cultural History*, by R.DARNTON, pp. 75-104. New York: Random House, 1985. Darnton uses his training in archival research to tell credible stories that stand up to the criticism of his colleagues, who are historians. And he angers literary critics by incorporating methodological sections into his racy stories that read like fiction. This procedure allows him to place the direct speech and action of illiterates into the center of his stories, rather than using them as illustrations for statements made about them. As a result, the almost unbearable otherness of past attitudes to cats or to people is made very clear.

**DAUZAT, Albert.**

"Les noms populaires de la pointe du coude: La sucette ou suzette et le petit juif." *Le français moderne* 11 (1943): 174. Modern French children's words for the "bone of the elbow."

**DAVID-DANEL, Marie-Louise.**

*Iconographie des Saints médecins Côme et Damien.* With a foreword by M. Louis Réau. Lille: Morel & Corduant, 1958. St. Cosmas and St. Damian, always mentioned in one breath, have inherited the mythical function of the Twins as Healers; since the late Middle Ages they are represented explicitly as physicians, often as medical men from the East. Their iconography allows many inferences about each epoch's peculiar view of the body.

**DAVIDOFF, L.**

"Class and Gender in Victorian England: The Diaries of Arthur J. Munby and Hannah Cullwick." *Feminist Studies* 5, no. 1 (1979): 86-140.

**DAVIDSON, J.R.**

"The Shadow of Life: Psychosocial Explanations for Placenta Rituals." *Culture, Medicine and Psychiatry* 9 (1985): 75-92. Most societies have established rituals for the disposal of the placenta, which figures prominently in folk belief and practice (Africa and Peru are studied). The author interprets these procedures as the anxiety-releasing delimitation of an important aspect of reality.

**DAVIS, Natalie Zemon.**

"The Sacred and the Body Social in Sixteenth-Century Lyon." *Past and Present* 90 (1981): 40-70.

**DAWSON, Warren.**

*The Custom of Couvade.* Manchester: Manchester Univ. Press, 1929.

**DEBONGNIE, P.**

"Essai critique sur l'histoire des stigmatisations au Moyen Age." *Etudes carmélitaines* 21 (1936): 22-59. The stigma (bleeding wounds on hands, feet and sometimes above the heart) become a widely reported and frequently verified bodily phenomenon during the later Middle Ages. The appearance correlates with a change in iconography: the appearance of Christ's wounded and dead body on the Cross.

**DEBUS, Allen G., ed.**

*Science, Medicine and Society in the Renaissance: Essays to Honor W. Pagel.* 2 vols. London: Heinemann, 1972.

**DE CARO, Francis A., comp. and ed.**

*Women and Folklore: A Bibliographic Survey.* London: Westport, 1983.

**DEGLER, Carl H.**

"What Ought to Be and What Was: Women's Sexuality in the Nineteenth-Century." *The American Historical Review* 79, no. 5 (1974): 1467-90. Searches medical literature 1870-80 for a new entity: the female "orgasm." Finds a very first mention in 1866.

**DEICHGRAEBER, Karl.**

"Zur Milchtherapie der Hippokratiker." In *Medizingeschichte in unserer Zeit: Festgabe fur Edith Heischkel-Artelt und W. ARTELT*, ed. by H.H.EULNER, et al., 36-53. Stuttgart: Enke, 1971.

**DEIMEL, Anton P.**

"Zur Erklaerung sumerischer Wörter und Zeichen." *Orientalia* 14 (1945): 70-82 und 259-272. Note especially para. 17 for "blood" and in relation to it para. 21 for "water" and 26 for "spook."

____. *Zur Etymologie der Namen der Körperteile.* Helsinki: Soc. Orientalis Fennica, 1946 (Studia Orientalia 13, 6).

**DELAMARRE, X.**

*Le vocabulaire indo-européen: Lexique étymologique thématique.* Paris: Maisonneuve, 1984. Pp. 96-112: reconstruction of the Indo-Germanic terminology for the human body and for dress.

**DELANEY, Janice, LUPTON, Mary Jane, TOTH, Emily.**

*The Curse: A Cultural History of Menstruation.* New York: Dutton, 1976. Menstruation in myth, poetry, fiction, drama, folkstyle and history - anecdotal rather than historical.

**DELAPORTE, François.**

*Nature's Second Kingdom: Explorations of Vegetality in the Eighteenth-Century.* With an introduction by G. CANGUILHEM. Cambridge, Mass.: MIT Press, 1982. A historical epistemology of research on plants from the late sixteenth through the eighteenth century. Suggests many parallels to changing perceptions of the human body.

**DELCOURT, Marie.**

*Pyrrhos et Pyrrha: Recherches, sur les valeurs du feu dans les légendes helléniques.* Paris: Belles Lettres, 1965.

____. *Stérilités mystérieuses et naissances maléfiques dans l'antiquité classique.* Paris: Droz, 1938.

____. "Le complexe de Diane dans l'hagiographie chrétienne." *Revue de l'histoire des religions* 153 (1958): 1-33.

____. *Hermaphrodite: Mythes et rites de la bisexualité dans l'antiquité classique*. Paris: Presses Universitaires de France, 1958 (*Hermaphrodite: Myths and Rites of the Bisexual Figure in Classical Antiquity*. London: Studio Books, 1961).

____. *Hermaphroditea: Recherches sur l'être double promoteur de la fertilité dans le monde classique*. Brussels: Berchem, 1966 (Collection Latomus 86).

**DELON, Michel.**
"Le prétexte anatomique." *Dix-huitième siècle* 12 (1980): 35-48. "Strangeness" (l'étrangeté corporelle) emerges as an ethnological theme during the eighteenth century and prepares anatomists for the social construction of racist categories.

**DELORME, Fr. A.**
"La morphogénèse d'Albert le Grand dans l'embryologie scolastique." *Revue Thomiste* 36, no. 65 (1931): 352-60. Commentary on *De animalibus* 16.1.16. Only when the "virtus formativa" of the male seed has nourished the female seed and all the members of the future human being have taken their form, is the human soul infused.

**DELPORTE, Henri.**
*L'image de la femme dans l'art préhistorique*. Paris: Picara, 1979. Contains 136 splendid reproductions of mostly neolithic female figures. Analyzes the style and techniques used. Reviews former interpretations of their meaning, and develops a new theory: the consciousness about a specific otherness of humans in relation to all animals has developed through the opposition between figures of women and animals.

**DELUMEAU, Jean.**
*La Peur en Occident XIVe-XVIIIe siècles*. Paris: Fayard, 1978. The author sets out to go beyond L. FEBVRE in constituting the experience of anguish and fear into an object of historical research. The social communitary aspects of both feelings (which psychology usually distinguishes only on the level of individual expression) and different ways they were experienced by the literate few and by the great masses are the subject of this book. Both fear and anguish create new images of the flesh - primarily the flesh of others: women, demons, poor souls, ghosts, outsiders, Jews and Muslims.

____. *Le péché et la peur. La culpabilisation en Occident (XIII-XVIIIe s.)*. Paris: Fayard, 1983. The entire community's concern with sin - as distinct from guilt - is a characteristic feature of the period that goes from the declining Middle Ages to the Enlightenment. And public concern with sin is equivalent with an intense and scrupulous, deeply ambiguous and constant presence of "God" in everyday life: worries about his

goodness, justice and hatred. Sin and God shape body experience: macabre (98-128), evil and monstrous (143ff.) make the body the place of imagined torture (331ff.), not only in this but in the next world (416ff.).

**DEMAITRE, L., TRAVILL, A.A.**
"Human Embryology and Development in the Works of Albertus Magnus." In *Albertus Magnus and the Sciences*, ed. by J.A.WEISHEIPL, 405-40. Toronto: Pontifical Institute of Mediaeval Studies, 1980.

**DEMANDT, Alexander.**
*Metaphern für Geschichte: Sprachbilder und Gleichnisse im historisch-politischen Denken*. Munich: C.H. Beck, 1978. Contains various sections on the use of the body and its transformations as a metaphor for society and for history.

**DEMISCH, Heinz.**
*Erhobene Hände: Geschichte einer Gebärde in der bildenden Kunst*. Stuttgart: Urachhaus, 1984. The artistic representation of one gesture, that of uplifted hands, is studied in thirteen "situations" in which it occurs from prehistory to the twentieth century, and an interpretation is attempted.

**DEMUTH, Franz.**
"Dermatologische Bezeichnungen in der luxemburgischen Mundart." *Vierteljahresblaetter fur Sprachwissenschaft, Volks und Ortsnamenkunde* 2 (1936): 90-99 and 200-02.

**DEONNA, Waldemar.**
"La légende de Pero et de Micon et l'allaitement symbolique." *Latomus* 13 (1954): 140-66 and 356-75. Exhaustive archeological and philological documentation of a motif: the adult being breast-fed by the goddess, the daughter and later, the Virgin Mary.

____. "Aphrodite à la coquille." *Revue archéologique*. 5 ser., vol. 6 (1957). Like the shell Venus arises from the waves. The shell represents the female organs and is used as an amulet in analogy of the prophylactic and apotropaic phallus. The footnotes provide guidance to the semantic of "shell."

____. *Le Symbolisme de l'oeil*. Paris: Ed. Broccard, 1965 (Ecole française d' Athènes, fasc. 15).

____. "Manus oculatae." In *Hommages à Léon Herrman*. 292-300. Brussels: Berchem, 1960 (Collection Latomus 44).

**DEROUET-BESSON, Marie Claude.**
"Inter Duos Scopulos, Hypothèses sur la place de la sexualité dans les modèles de la représentation du monde au XIe siècle." *Annales E.S.C.* 36, no. 5 (1981): 922-45.

**DESAIVE, Jean-Paul, et al.**
*Médecins, climat et Epidémies à la fin du XVIIIème siècle*. Paris: Mouton, 1972.

**DESHAIES, Gabriel.**
*L'Esthétique du Pathologique*. Paris: Presses Universitaires de France, 1947. Frequently an artist

z o n e

494

who tries to represent disease, suffering or pain has as his object something which in his society is considered ugly. In the aesthetic representation of the ugly (pathological) three cases ought to be distinguished: its beautiful representation, its sickening (morbid) representation and its representation as a "beautiful medical case." The author deals with the aesthetics of this third case.

**DEVEREUX, George.**
"A Typological Study of Abortion in 350 Primitive, Ancient and Pre-Industrial Societies." In *Abortion in America*, ed. by Harold ROSEN. Boston: Beacon Press, 1967.

**DEWEZ, Léon, ITERSON, Albert.**
"La lactation de Saint Bernard: Légende et iconographie." *Citeau in de Nederlanden* 7 (1956): 165-89. Origin of the legend and of the devotion, evolution of the iconography.

**DE ZORDI, Guido.**
*Die Wörter des Gesichtsausdruckes im heutigen Englisch*. Bern: Francke, 1972. A terminological and semantic study of modern British words that refer to facial expression.

**DHORME, Edouard.**
*L'emploi métaphorique des noms de parties du corps en hébreu et en accadien*. Paris: Gabalda, 1923. Repr. Paris: Paul Geuthner, 1963. An important and beautifully written study that stresses the several layers of reference from organs to passions, desires, souvenirs; from these organs to the physiognomy (eyes, nose, mouth, neck, front, feet) and to the external world. The heavens have a heart, a face, a skull, horns, which can be seen at sunrise, and a tongue which flashes as lightning; they open their eyes at dawn. Excellent conclusion, pp. 161ff.

**DICKISON, S.**
"Abortion in Antiquity." *Arethusa* 6 (1973): 159-66. A review article on E.NARDI on abortion. Exposes NARDI's "pro-life" prejudice and complements his bibliography.

**DI CORI, Paola.**
"Rosso e bianco: La devozione al Sacro Cuore di Gesù nel primo dopoguerra." *Memoria* 5 (1982): 82-107.

**DIDI-HUBERMAN, Georges.**
*Invention de l'hystérie. Charcot et l'iconographie photographique de la Salpêtrière*. Paris: Macula, 1982. More than four hundred women were kept in the Paris hospital where CHARCOT invented hysteria through observation, description and demonstration, but above all through the new technique of psychiatric photography. Here the photographic plate became for the first time the "true retina of the scientist."

**DIELS, Hermann.**
*Beiträge zur Zuckungsliteratur des Okzidents und Orients* (Photomech. reproduction). Leipzig: Zentral-

antiquariat, 1970. Cramps and the fits have always attracted attention and called for interpretation. The author thoroughly reviews classical opinion and its survival in folklore - especially religious.

**DIEPGEN, Paul.**
"Die Lehre von der Leibseelischen Konstitution und die spezielle Anatomie und Physiologie der Frau im Mittelalter." *Scientia* 84 (1949): 97-103 and 132-34.
____. "Eine volkstümliche Darstellung des Todes vom Oberrhein." *Zeitschrift fur Volkskunde* n.f. 2, nos. 1-2 (1930): 189-92.
____. *Medizin und Kultur: Gesammelte Aufsätze*. ed. by W.ARTELT, E.HEISCHKEL, J.SCHUSTER. Stuttgart: Enke, 1938.
____. *Studien zur Geschichte der Beziehungen zwischen Theologie und Medizin im Mittelalter*. Berlin: Grünewald, 1922.
____. *Ueber den Einfluss der autoritativen Theologie auf die Medizin des Mittelalters*. Mainz: Verlag der Akademie der Wissenschaften, and Wiesbaden: Steiner, 1958 (Akademie der Wissenschaften u.d. Literatur. Abhandlungen. Geistes- und Sozialwiss. Klasse Jg. 1958, 1).
____. "Zum Einfluss der Theologie auf die ärztliche Ethik und Pflichtenlehre im Mittelalter." In *Jahrbuch für das Bistum Mainz* (Festschrift STOHR) 5 (1950): 195-206.
____. *Zur Frauenheilkunde im byzantinischen Kulturkreis des Mittelalters*. Mainz, Verlag der Akademie der Wissenschaften, and Wiesbaden: Steiner, 1950. (Akademie der Wissenschaften u.d. Literatur. Abhandlungen. Geistes- und Sozialwiss. Klasse Jg. 1950, Nr.1).
____. *Frau und Frauenheilkunde in der Kultur des Mittelalters*. Stuttgart: Thieme, 1963.

**DIEPGEN, P., GRUBER, G.B., SCHADEWALDT, H.**
"Der Krankheitsbegriff, seine Geschichte und Problematik." In *Altmanns Handbuch der allgemeinen Pathologie*, vol. 1, 1-50. Berlin: Springer, 1969.

**DIERAUER, U.**
*Tier und Mensch im Denken der Antike*. Amsterdam, 1977. The zoological tradition within which PLINY wrote.

**DIESTER, Manfred.**
*Koerpergeschichten: eine Untersuchung zum Mythos-Begriff am Beispiel der Darstellung von Mann und Frau in der Kriegsliteratur von 1939-43*. Bern: Lang, 1980. Based mostly on an analysis of Nazi propaganda, posters and journalism.

**DIETRICH, Franz Ed. Christoph.**
*Abhandlungen für semitische Wortforschung*. Leipzig: Vogel, 1844. Pp. 99-258 deal with upper and lower limbs in the Semitic vocabulary.

**DOCKES, Pierre.**
*L'espace dans la pensée économique du 16e au 18e siècle.*
Paris: Flammarion, 1969. A theory of spatial economy
constructed as a history of economic reflections on the
value of space and distance since the late sixteenth
century.

**DOEHNER, O.**
"Historisch-soziologische Aspekte des Krankheits-
begriffs und des Gesundheitsverhaltens im 16.-18.
Jahrhundert." In *Leichenpredigten als Quelle historischer Wissenschaften,* ed. by Rudolf LENZ. Köln,
Vienna: Böhlau, 1975. Epilogues and funeral sermons
from the sixteenth to the eighteenth century abound in
details about the last illness, the suffering and comportment of the deceased.

**DOELGER, F.J.**
"Das Lebensrecht das ungeborenen Kindes und die
Fruchtabtreibung in der Bewertung der heidnischen
und Christlichen Antike." *Antike und Christentum*
(Münster) 4, nos. 1-2 (1933): 1-51.

**DOERRER, Anton.**
"St. Kümmernis in Oesterreich: Zur Verkörperung
eines Menschheitsmotivs als Volksfigur." *Archiv für
Kulturgeschichte* 44 (1962): 120-29. The volto Santo
legend gave rise in the northern Alps around 900 to
the embodiment of a "crucifixa." Guide to the literature.

**DOLCH, Martin.**
"Schöpferische und entwickelnde Sprachkräfte in den
deutschen Bezeichnungen für Augenbraue, Lid und
Wimper." *Zeitschrift für Mundartforschung* 20 (1952):
146-84.
____. *Wortgeographie von Augenbraue, Lid und
Wimper.* Dissertation. Marburg, 1947.

**D'ONOFRIO, Cesare.**
*La papessa Giovanna: Roma e papato tra storia e
leggenda.* Rome: Romana Società Editrice, 1979. A
detailed study of the legend of a woman-pope.
D'Onofrio believes that he can find the origins of this
legend in early medieval liturgy: the newly elected
pope was seated on a birthstool in the Lateran, and in
a solemn gesture widely spread his legs - Mother
Church renewing herself in the birth of a new pontifi-
cate. Pp. 24ff. deal with the explicit collaboration
between Urban VIII, Barberini and Bernini on the St.
Peter Baldachine; on the stone bases of the bronze
baldachine over Peter's tomb the same birth is represented.

**DONTENVILLE, Henri.**
*Histoire de géographie mythique de la France.* Paris:
Maisonneuve et Larose, 1973. In various chapters
materials on the appearances of supernatural bodies
such as fairies, melusine, demons.

**DOOB, Penelope B.R.**
*Nebuchadnezzar's Children: Conventions of Madness in
Middle English Literature.* New Haven: Yale Univ.
Press, 1974. Covers drama, romance, lyric, theological
and medical debate in the Middle Ages that deal with
the madman and the bodily signs by which he is recognized. Nebuchadnezzar is the prototype for the sinner
who is punished through madness like Herod, the
tyrant; the man who is part of wilderness like Merlin;
and the holy man, like Sir Orfeo who goes out into
wilderness. The lovelorn man like Ywain or the wise
fool does not fit the pattern.

**DORFLES, G.**
"'Innen' und 'aussen' en Architecture et en Psychanalyse." *Nouvelle revue de psychanalyse* 9 (Spring,
1974): 229-38.

**DORNSEIF, Franz.**
*Der deutsche Wortschatz nach Sachgruppen,* 7th ed.
Berlin: De Gruyter, 1970. Bibliography for the study
of German. Words referring to the body can be found
in sect. 2.16-2.27 and 2.41-2.45.

**DOUGLAS, Mary, ed.**
*Food in the Social Order: Studies of Food and
Festivities in Three American Communities.* New
York: Sage, 1984.
____. *Purity and Danger: An Analysis of the Concepts
of Pollution and Taboo.* London: Routledge and Kegan
Paul, 1984.
____. *Natural symbols. Explorations in Cosmology.*
New York: Random House, 1972. (German: *Ritual,
Tabu und Körpersymbolik: Sozialanthropologische
Studien in Industriegesellschaft und Stammeskultur.*
Frankfurt: Suhrkamp, 1981).
____. "Do Dogs Laugh? A Cross-Cultural Approach
to Body Symbolism." *Journal of Psychosomatic
Research* 15 (1971): 387-90.
____. "The Healing Rite," *MAN* n.s. 5 (1970):
302-08.

**DRESSEN, Wolfgang.**
"Infame Körper: Widerstand im Erziehungsprozess."
In *Der andere Körper,* ed. by C.WULF, 67-83. Berlin:
Edit. Corpus, 1984. Reflection on the production line
as a metaphor for the body.

**DUBOIS, P.**
"Phallocentrism and Its Subversion in Plato's
*Phaedrus.*" *Arethusa* 18 (1985): 91-101. In the
*Phaedrus,* in a passage on friendship, reproduction
seems ascribed exclusively to men, who inseminate
each other with philosophy in an act in which women
have no place. Against DERRIDA, the author sees
here not phallocentrism but a mimesis of the female
and maternity.

**DUBOS, René, DUBOS, Jean.**
*The White Plague: Tuberculosis, Man and Society.*
Boston: Little, Brown, 1953. A seminal work on the
social construction of one disease (tuberculosis) that
has been consistently misread as nothing but a study

of the social consequence of its incidence.

**DUDEN, Barbara.**

*Geschichte unter der Haut: Ein Eisenacher Arzt und seine Patientinnen um 1730.* Stuttgart: Klett-Cotta, 1987. Forthcoming from Harvard Univ. Press.

**DUDLEY, Edward, NOVAK, Maximilian, eds.**

*The Wild Man Within: An Image in Western Thought from the Renaissance to Romanticism.* Pittsburgh: Univ. Pittsburgh Press, 1972. The book focuses on the importance of wildness and wildman during the period of Western experience which came to hold up ideals of culture and civilization as its finest accomplishments. While madness at this time became something to be cast out, the savage became something to come to terms with, to be discovered beneath clothes and possibly below the skin. In the mirror of the wildman the historical nature of civilized flesh and blood was reflected.

**DUERR, Hans Peter.**

*Traumzeit: Ueber die Grenzen zwischen Wildnis und Zivilisation.* Frankfurt: Syndikat 1978. (*Dreamtime: Concerning the Boundary between Wilderness and Civilization.* London: Basil Blackwell, 1985).

**DUEWEL, Klaus.**

"Das Bild von den 'Knien des Herzens' bei Heinrich von Kleist." *Euphorion* 68 (1974): 185-97. This article introduces the history of the metaphor with biblical references. The metaphor is renewed by Winkelmann, Goethe and finally by Kleist.

_____. "Kleiner Beitrag zu einer verkannten Herz-Metapher des Wilden Mannes." *Germanische-Romanische Monatsschrift* 14 (1964): 421-23. In middle-high German literature the "heart" is imagined sometimes as having not only eyes but other senses and members of its own.

**DUFFIN, Lorna.**

"The Conspicuous Consumptive: Woman as an Invalid." In *The Nineteenth-Century Woman: Her Cultural and Physical World*, ed. by Sara DELAMONT and Lorna DUFFIN, 26-56. London: Croom Helm, 1978.

**DUMORTIER, Jean.**

*Le vocabulaire médical d'Eschyle et les écrits hippocratiques.* Dissertation. Paris, 1935.

**DURAFFOUR, A.**

"Notules sur les dénominations du mollet, et quelques termes connexes dans le Sud-Est de la France." In *Sache, Ort und Wort: Festschrift für J. Jud. Romanica Helvetica* 20, 378-88. Geneva: Droz, 1943. Traces the many expressions for "mollet," the fleshy, meaty or fatty portions of the (female) body in southeast French folk usage.

**DURAND, J. L.**

"Le faire et le dire: Vers une anthropologie des gestes iconiques." *History and Anthropology* 1, no. 1 (November 1984): 29-48 (special issue on gestures).

**DYBWIG, Magne.**

"Zur Ontologie der Körperlichkeit des Menschen." *Ratio* 2, no. 1 (1979): 13-30.

# E

**EASLEA, Brian.**

*Witch-Hunting, Magic and the New Philosophy: An Introduction to Debates of the Scientific Revolution 1450-1750.* Brighton: Harvester-Humanities Press, 1980. Changes in descriptive (scientific) paradigms can be understood only when they are placed into the much wider-ranging environment of contemporary changes in basic social themes. If and how a "scientific" paradigm is accepted and repeated depends on how it fits into this wider milieu of simultaneously evolving everyday perceptions. For Easlea the phenomenon of witchcraft in the seventeenth century is representative of this context for new science. Aristotelian cosmology (hulemorphism) finds in witchcraft its last embodiment.

**EBERS, G.**

*Die Körperteile, ihre Bedeutung und Namen im Altaegyptischen.* Munich: G. Franz, 1897.

**EBIN, Victoria.**

*The Body Decorated.* London: Thames & Hudson, 1979.

**ECCLES, Audrey.**

*Obstetrics and Gynaecology in Tudor and Stuart England.* Kent, Oh.: Kent State Univ. Press, 1982.

**ECKERT, R.**

"Litauisch 'antis' etc. 'Brust, Busen' und hethitisch hant 'Vorderseite, Stirn'." *Baltistica* 6, no. 1 (1970): 33-41.

**EDELSTEIN, Emma, EDELSTEIN, Ludwig.**

*Asclepius: A Collection and Interpretation of the Testimonies.* 2 vols. Baltimore: Johns Hopkins Press, 1945.

**EDELSTEIN, Ludwig.**

"The Dietetics of Antiquity." In *Ancient Medicine: Selected Papers of L. Edelstein*, ed. by O.TEMKIN and L.TEMKIN, 303-16. Baltimore: Johns Hopkins Press, 1967.

**EDHOLM, F., YOUNG, K., HARRIS, O.**

"Conceptualizing Women." *Critique of Anthropology* 3, nos. 9-10 (1977): 103-30.

**EDSMAN, C.M.**

*Ignis, Divinus: Le feu comme moyen de rajeunissement*

*et d'immortalité: contes, légendes, mythes et rites.* Lund: Gleerup, 1949.

**EHRENREICH, Barbara, ENGLISH, Deirdre.**
*For Her Own Good: 150 Years of Experts' Advice to Women.* Garden City, N.Y.: Anchor Press, 1978.

**EHRHARD, Peter.**
*Anatomie de Samuel Beckett.* Basel, Stuttgart: Birkhäuser, 1976 (Schriftenreihe der Eidg. Technischen Hochschule Zurich. Abt. f. Geistes- und Sozialwissenschaften). For Samuel Beckett "anatomy" is more than a simple theme: it is the constitutive element, the very substance of an imaginary world and of a language out of which his opus is constructed. In successive chapters quotations from Beckett about fingers, hands, feet, eyes, mouth, ears, nose, genitals, skin are densely interwoven - Beckett appears to be analogous to Rabelais.

**EHRISMANN, Gustav.**
"Psychologische Bezeichnungen in Ottfrieds Evangelienbuch." In *Beiträge zur Germanischen Sprachwissenschaft. Festschrift O. BEHAGEL*, 324-38. Heidelberg: C. Winter, 1924.

**EICH, Paul.**
*Die Maria Lactans: Eine Studie ihrer Entwicklung bis in das 13. Jh. und ein Versuch ihrer Deutung aus der mittelalterlichen Frömmigkeit.* Dissertation. Phil. Fak. Frankfurt am M., 1953.

**EINHORN, Jürgen Werinhard.**
"Der Begriff der 'Innerlichkeit' bei David von Augsburg und Grundzuege der Franziskanermystik." *Franziskanische Studien* 48 (1966): 336-76. Semantic analysis of writings in Latin and middle-High German by David of Augsburg (d. 1272). A large and differentiated vocabulary refers to the "inner" or "interior" life. This new dimension of experience can be traced to St. Francis of Assisi.

**EIS, Gerhard.**
*Medizinische Fachprosa des späten Mittelalters und der frühen Neuzeit.* Amsterdam: Rodogsi, 1982. An attempt to identify the terminology actually used by practitioners during the late Middle Ages, rather than that characteristic for academic discussion.

**EISENBERG, Leon.**
"Disease and Illness: Distinctions between Professional and Popular Ideas of Sickness." *Culture, Medicine, and Psychiatry* 1 (1977): 9-23.

**EISLER, Colin.**
"The Athlete of Virtue: The Iconography of Asceticism." In *Essays in Honor of E. Panofsky*, ed. by M.MEISS. Vol. 1: 82-97. New York: New York Univ. Press, 1961.

**EISLER, Georg.**
*From Naked to Nude: Life Drawing in the Twentieth Century.* London: Thames & Hudson, 1977.

**ELIAS, Norbert.**
*Ueber den Prozess der Zivilisation: Wandlungen des Verhaltens in den weltlichen Oberschichten des Abendlandes.* 2 vols. Basel, 1939 (*The History of Manners: The Civilizing Process.* 2 vols. New York: Pantheon, 1982-83).

**ELLEN, Roy.**
"Anatomical Classification and the Semiotics of the Body." In *The Anthropology of the Body*, ed. by John BLACKING, 343-73. New York, 1977. Recent literature on the cognitive and cultural uses of classificatory structures related to the body.

**ELSAESSER, Gunter.**
*Ausfall des Coitus als Krankheitsursache in der Medizin des Mittelalters.* Berlin: Ebering, 1934 (Abhandlungen zur Geschichte der Medizin und der Naturwissenschaften, Heft 3).

**ELWIN, Verrier,**
"The Vagina Dentata Legend." *British Journal of Medical Psychology* 19 (1941): 439ff.

**ELWORTHY, Fredrick Thomas.**
*The Evil Eye: An Account of an Ancient and Widespread Superstition.* Orig. ed. 1895. Repr. Secaucus, N.J.: Citadel Press, 1982.

**ENCYCLOPEDIA OF WORLD ARTS.**
"Human Figure." Vol. 7, 654-702 and pls. 351-92. New York: McGraw Hill, 1971. Excellent short introduction with selective bibliography: art and anatomy; visualization (col. 665ff.); proportion, schematization; pose, color, physiognomy; idealization, expression, symbolism and projection. Finally: deformation of the figure by painting, tattooing and hairdressing (col. 698).

**ENGLERT, Ludwig.**
"Konstitution und Leibesuebung bei Hieronymus Mercurialis." *Archiv für Geschichte der Medizin* 24 (1931): 131-49.

**ERICH, Oswald A.**
*Die Darstellung des Teufels in der christlichen Kunst.* Berlin: Deutscher Kunstverlag, 1931. (Kunstwissenschaftliche Studien 8.)

**ERNOUT, Alfred.**
"Les noms des parties du corps en latin." *Latomus* 10 (1950): 3-12. Notes the large percentage of Latin names for body parts which either have no clearly established etymology (*femur, ren, sanguen, digitus, frons, tergus*) or are derived from the Greek.

**ERTZDORFF, X. von.**
"Das 'Herz' in der lateinisch-theologischen und frühen volkssprachigen religiösen Literatur." *Beiträge zur Geschichte der Deutschen Sprache und Literatur* (Halle) 84 (1962): 249-301.

_____. "Die Dame im Herzen und das Herz bei der Dame: Zur Verwendung des Begriffes 'Herz' in der höfischen Liebeslyrik des 11. und 12. Jh." *Zeitschrift für deutsche Philologie* 84 (1965): 6-46. During the twelfth century the "heart," as of then the innermost locus that is open to the encounter with God, becomes also the place in which the experience of courtly love is located as well.

____. *Studien zum Begriff des Herzens und seiner Verwendung als Aussagemotiv in der höfischen Liebeslyrik des 12. Jhs.* Dissertation. Phil. Fak. Freiburg, 1958.

**L'ESPERANCE, J.L.**

"Doctors and Women in Nineteenth-Century Society: Sexuality and Role." In *Health Care and Popular Medicine in Nineteenth-Century England*, ed. by J.WOODWARD and D.RICHARDS. New York: Holmes & Meier, 1977.

**EWING, Elizabeth.**

*Underwear: A History*. New York: Theatre Arts Books, 1972. The underclothing, neither dress nor skin, reveals attitudes and feelings about the body in a poignant way.

____. *Dress and Undress: A History of Women's Underwear*. New York: Drama Book, 1978.

F

**FABRICANT, Caroline.**

"Binding and Dressing Nature's Loose Tresses: The Ideology of Augustan Landscape Design." *Studies in 18th Century Culture* 8 (1979): 109-33. Women and gardens are refined out of wilderness, fenced in, shaped and created as paradise, until both, being carefully watered and tended, begin to flower. The language of English landscape gardening is a forerunner of the gynecological pornography that appeared in the next century; less rude, but with more conscious intent.

____. "Pope's Portrait of Women: The Tyranny of the Pictorial Eye." In *Women and Men: The Consequences of Power*, ed. by Dana V.HILLER and Robin Ann SHEETS, 74-91. Cincinnati: Univ. Cincinnati Office of Women's Studies, 1977.

____. *Swift's Landscape*. Baltimore: Johns Hopkins Press, 1983.

**FAHRAEUS, Robin.**

"Basic Facts Concerning Humoral Pathology and Relicts of These in the Language and in Folk Medicine." *ARV Tidskrift för Nordisk Folkminnesforskning* 18/19 (1962-63): 165-79 (German: "Grundlegende Fakten über die Pathologie der Körpersäfte und ihre Relikte in Sprache und Volksmedizin." In *Volksmedizin*. Ed. by E.GRABNER,

444-58. Darmstadt: Wissenschaftliche Buchgesellschaft, 1975).

**FALK, Pasi.**

"Corporeality and Its Fates in History." *Acta Sociologica* 28, no. 2 (1985): 115-36. Reflections on a possible theory to deal, in sociology, with the "historicalness" of body and corporeality (reference to BATAILLE).

**FALLER, A.**

*Die Entwicklung der makroskopisch-anatomischen Praeparierkunst von Galen bis zur Neuzeit*. New York, Basel: Karger, 1948.

**FARGE, Arlette.**

"Accouchement et naissance au XVIIIe s." *Revue de médecine psychosomatique et de psychologie médicale* 18, no. 1 (1976): 19-28.

____. "Signes de vie, risques de mort: Essai sur le sang et la ville au 18e siècle." *URBI* 2 (1979). Literally deals with the blood flowing on eighteenth-century streets: from murder, slaughter, wounds. Also speaks about perceptions of menstruation.

____. "Comment vieillir, d'après les guides de conservation de la santé au XVIIIe siècle." In *Le vieillissement: Implications et conséquences de l'allongement de la vie humaine depuis le XVIIIe siècle*, publ. sous la direct. de A.BIDEAU et al., 161-66. Lyon: Presses Universitaires de Lyon, 1982.

____. ed. *La bibliothèque bleue: Le miroir des femmes*. Paris: Montalba, 1982.

____. "Work Related Diseases of Artisans in Eighteenth-Century France." In *Medicine and society in France*, ed. by R.FORSTER and O.RANUM, 89-103. Baltimore: Johns Hopkins Press, 1981 (orig. *Annales E.S.C.* 32 (1977): 993-1006).

**FAVRET, Jeanne.**

"Le malheur biologique et sa répétition." *Annales E.S.C.* 26, no. 3-4 (1971): 873-88.

**FEATHERSTONE, Mike.**

"The Body in Consumer Culture." *Theory, Culture and Society* 1 (1982): 12-34.

**FEE, Elizabeth.**

"The Sexual Politics of Victorian Social Anthropology." In *Clio's Consciousness Raised*, ed. by Mary S.HARTMAN and Lois BANNER, 86-103. London, New York: Harper: 1974.

____. "Nineteenth-Century Craniology: The Study of the Female Skull." *Bulletin of the History of Medicine* 53, no. 3 (1979): 415-33. Phrenology and craniology were taken for scientific specialties well into the nineteenth century. Craniologists invented techniques for measuring angles and dimensions of the skull to correlate them to supposedly "real" differences in mind and capacity between men and women. Amply documented.

**FEHR, Hans.**

*Das Recht im Bild.* Zürich, Erlenbach: E. Rentsch, 1923. Two hundred twenty-two reproductions, mostly of miniatures, each annotated and interpreted in detail. Shows the use of the gesture, posture and physiognomy associated with three dozen legal categories - mostly in Germany from the Middle Ages to the Enlightenment.

**FERGUSON, John.**

*The Place of Suffering.* Cambridge: James Clarke & Co. 1972. A dense history of the classical and Judaic background against which the Christian attitudes toward pain and the Christian conception of suffering have developed.

**FERRANTE, Joan M.**

*Woman as Image in Medieval Literature: From the Twelfth Century to Dante.* New York: Columbia Univ. Press, 1975. In twelfth-century literature women are presented not as persons but as symbols that personify those cosmological forces that govern man's life. The fictional world is dominated by women: historical figures, particularly Eve, and interpretations of the bride of the Song of Songs: if they are portrayed as "good" they inevitably are symbols for the Church, if "bad" for carnal desire and inconsistency (both masculine), and later the threat of heresy (which like woman attracts with superficial beauty). Dante picks up these strains, both positive and negative symbolism, and particularly sees both good and bad aspects of himself as female (p. 141ff.). In the *Commedia* Dante creates a world of "bodies" that are shadows and develops, based on Thomist theory, the intellectual framework for the reality of disembodied flesh.

**FEUDALE, Caroline.**

"The Iconography of the Madonna del Parto." *Masyas* (New York) 7 (1957): 8-26.

**FICHTNER, Gerhard.**

"Das verpflanzte Mohrenbein - Zur Interpretation der Kosmas-und-Damian-Legende." In *Medizin im mittelalterlichen Abendland*, ed. by G.BAADER and G.KEIL, 324-44. Darmstadt: Wissenschaftliche Buchgesellschaft, 1982.

**FICKEL, Maria Erika.**

*Die Bedeutung von 'sêle,' 'lîp' und 'herze' in der frühmittelhochdeutschen Dichtung und in den Texten der mittelhochdeutschen Klassik.* Dissertation. Tübingen, 1949.

**FIELD, David.**

"Der Körper als Träger des Selbst." Materialien z. Soziologie des Alltags. *Kölner Zeitschrift f. Soziologie u. Sozialpsychologie* 20 (1978): 244-64.

**FIELHAUER, P.**

"Volksmedizin-Heilkulturwissenschaft." *Mitteilungen der anthropologischen Gesellschaft in Vienna* 102 (1973): 114-36. A proposal formulated by a medical folklorist to abandon the analytic division now separating his field from that of medical social science and to recognize "healing" as an overarching cultural category. Based on observations from agrarian eastern Austria.

**FIERZ, J.**

*Die pejorative Verbildlichung menschlicher Korperbautypen im Schweizerdeutschen.* Zürich: Lang, 1943.

**FIGLIO, Karl M.**

"The Historiography of Scientific Medicine: An Invitation to the Human Sciences." *Comparative Studies in Society and History* 19 (1977): 262-86.

____. "The Metaphor of Organization: An Historiographical Perspective on the Biomedical Sciences of the Early Nineteenth Century." *History of Science* 14 (1976): 17-53.

____. "Theories of Perception and the Physiology of Mind in the Late Eighteenth Century." *History of Science* 12 (1975): 177-212.

____. "Chlorosis and Chronic Disease in Nineteenth-Century Britain: The Social Constitution of Somatic Illness in a Capitalist Society." In *Women and Health: The Politics of Sex in Medicine*, ed. by Elizabeth FEE, 213-41. New York: Baywood, 1983.

In these articles Figlio views "science" as the label for an activity that pursues the naturalization of both experience and ideology by expressing this achievement in ordinary language. Science, thus, is a collage whose persuasiveness rests on the assertion that what has been formulated is natural - and just could not be otherwise. Rather than being concerned with the social construction of reality, Figlio explores the social origin of those nineteenth-century axioms that generate twentieth-century mental topologies. The idea of "organization" and even more so that of "life" are such axioms.

**FINUCANE, Ronald C.**

"Sacred Corpse, Profane Carrion: Social Ideals and Death Rituals in the Later Middle Ages." In *Mirrors of Mortality: Studies in the Social History of Death*, ed. by Joachim WHALEY, 40-60. New York: St. Martin's, 1981.

____. *Miracles and Pilgrims: Popular Beliefs in Medieval England.* Totowa, N.J.: Rowman & Littlefield, 1981. See pp. 59-112: medicine and miracles; shrine cures and home cures; posthumous miracles.

**FIRTH, Raymond.**

*Symbols: Public and Private.* Ithaca, N.Y.: Cornell Univ. Press, 1973.

____. "Hair as Private Asset and Public Symbol." In *Symbols: Public and Private*, ed. by R.FIRTH, 262-98. Ithaca, N.Y.: Cornell Univ. Press, 1973.

**FISCHER-HOMBERGER, Esther.**

"Krankheit Frau - aus der Geschichte der Menstruation in ihrem Aspekt als Zeichen eines Fehlers." In

*Krankheit Frau,* by E.FISCHER-HOMBERGER, 49-84. Bern: Huber Verlag, 1979.

____. *Medizin vor Gericht: Gerichtsmedizin von der Renaissance bis zur Aufklärung.* Bern: Huber Verlag, 1983. A treasure trove of carefully interpreted medico-legal texts (sixteenth to eighteenth century). Fundamental for understanding that medical opinions of the past often yield entirely new insights when they are challenged in court, thereby allowing the historian to reconstruct the meaning given in everyday life to pregnancy and its termination, death and its onset, wounds and their effect.

____. "Zur Geschichte des Zusammenhangs zwischen Seele und Verdauung." *Schweizerische mediz. Wochenschrift* 103 (1973): 1433-41. Since Antiquity a close correlation between psychic well-being and a good digestion has been taken for granted. This correlation is firmly believed in by physicians well into the nineteenth century. The author explores the possibility that a "disease" is actually created by a firm medical tradition.

____. "Krankheit Frau." In *Leib und Leben in der Geschichte der Neuzeit,* ed. by A.E.IMHOF, 215-30. Berlin, 1983.

____. "Zwerchfellverletzung und psychische Störung. Zur Geschichte der Körpermitte." *Gesnerus* 35, nos. 1-2 (1978): 1-19. How the midriff, the center of the body, the Greek "phren" (which means both the anatomical diaphragm and also sense, consciousness, sensibility) was transformed by anatomy into the divider between two spaces within the body, which is called the "diaphragm."

**FLANDRIN, J.-L.**

"La diversité des goûts et des pratiques alimentaires en Europe du XVIe au XVIIIe siècle." *Revue d'histoire moderne et contemporaine* 30 (1983): 66-83.

____. *Un temps pour embrasser: aux origines de la morale sexuelle occidentale.* Paris: Seuil, 1983. Christian moral theology abounds with reflections and rules on "times to embrace" and "times of continence." The author describes the rise of this literature from the sixth through the eleventh centuries, and its impact on the demography of married life. Ample examples of women's impurity during bleeding, pregnancy and confinement.

____. *Le sexe et l'occident: Evolution des attitudes et des comportements.* Paris: Seuil, 1981. A collection of most of the author's contributions to the history of "love," sexual comportment and morals, ideas about conception, contraception and wet-nursing.

____. *Les amours paysannes: Amour et sexualité dans les campagnes de l'ancienne France (XVI-XIXe s.).* Paris: Gallimard (Collection Archives), 1975. The first attempt by a cultural historian to survey sexual behavior in rural France in early modern times.

**FLASCHE, Hans.**

"Der Begriff 'coeur' bei Guez de Balzac: Eine Untersuchung zur Vorgeschichte des Pascalschen Denkens." *Romanisches Jahrbuch* 2 (1949): 224-54.

____. "Similitudo templi: Zur Geschichte einer Metapher." *Deutsche Vierteljahrschrift für Literatur-wissenschaft und Geistesgeschichte* 23 (1949): 81-125. The temple as metaphor especially for body and soul; survival of classical themes; influence of the Pauline simile; the use of the metaphor in European literature.

**FLECK, Ludwik.**

*Entstehung und Entwicklung einer wissenschaftlichen Tatsache: Einführung in die Lehre vom Denkstil und Denkkollektiv.* Basel: Benno Schwabe, 1935 and Frankfurt, 1986 (*Genesis and Development of a Scientific Fact,* ed. by Th.TRENN, and R.K.MERTON, with a foreword by Thomas KUHN, Chicago: Univ. Chicago Press, 1979).

**FLEISCHHAUER, Wolfgang.**

"Zur Geschichte des Wortes 'innig' und seiner Verwandten." *Monatshefte für Deutschen Unterricht: Deutsche Sprache und Literatur* 27 (1945): 40-52. Author believes that the suffix *-ig,* and *-ig-lich* became important only during the twelfth century. Combined with the term referring to the interior "in" they were cultivated by mystics and spread to popular speech. Current lexica (1945) underrepresent the usage of the term.

**FLOHR, Heiner.**

"Geschichtswissenschaft und Biologie. Ueberlegungen zur biowissenschaftlichen Orientierung des Historikers." *Saeculum* 36, no. 1 (1985): 80-97 (special issue on the relevance of biology for a historical anthropology).

**FLOREZ, L.**

*Lexico del cuerpo humano en Colombia Bogota.* Bogota, 1969 (Publicaciones del Instituto Caro y Cuervo 27).

**FOA, Anna.**

"Il ventre sterile: Religione e medicina tra XVI e XVII secolo." *Memoria* (Turin) 3 (March 1982): 50-60. Sterility has forever been frightening and interpreted as either divine punishment or magical aggression. During the sixteenth century two new ideas become prevalent in medical writing: the barren womb brings forth monsters and the "mother" is blamed.

**FOSTER, B.**

"English 'Jaw': A Borrowing from French." *Neuphilo-logische Mitteilungen* 71 (1970): 99-101.

**FOSTER, George M.**

*Culture and Conquest: America's Spanish Heritage.* Chicago: Quadrangle, 1960.

____. "Relationship between Spanish and Spanish-American Folk Medicine." *Journal of American Folklore* 66 (1953): 201-17. Foster has strongly influenced historical anthropology

zone

of Latin America by focusing attention on two processes: only by colonizing the huge areas of this continent could the various ethnocentric cultures of the Iberian peninsula generate the image of a "Spanish" culture that came into existence in the colonies (1960). The evolution of Spanish-American patterns was complicated further through contact with local traditions (1953 on "medicine"). Though dated, this article remains valuable because of its wisely chosen references.

**FOUCAULT, Michel.**

*Birth of the Clinic: An Archeology of Medical Perception.* New York: Pantheon, 1973.

____. "Les déviations religieuses et le savoir médical." In *Hérésies et sociétés dans l'Europe pré-industrielle (XI-XVIIIe s.),* ed. by J.LE GOFF, 19-29. Paris, La Haye: Mouton, 1968. Explores the analogy between three "rationales" for ostracism: incest, madness and religious status. At the beginning of the sixteenth century a new, intense concern with the third ostracizes those who have contact with the devil.

____. *L'histoire de la sexualité.* Vol. 1: *La volonté de savoir.* Paris: Gallimard, 1976 (*The History of Sexuality.* Vol. 1: *An Introduction.* New York: Pantheon, 1978).

____. *L'usage des plaisirs: Histoire le la sexualité.* Vol. 2. Paris, 1984 (*The Use of Pleasure: History of Sexuality.* New York: Pantheon, 1985).

____. *Le souci de soi: Histoire de la sexualité.* Vol. 3. Paris, 1984. (*The Care of the Self: History of Sexuality.* New York: Pantheon, 1987).

____. *Surveiller et punir: Naissance de la prison.* Paris, 1975 (*Discipline and Punish: The Birth of the Prison.* New York: Random House, 1979).

**FOUQUET, Catherine.**

"Le détour obligé, ou l'histoire des femmes passe-t-elle par celle de leur corps?" In *Une histoire des femmes est-elle possible?* ed. by Michelle PERROT, 71-84. Paris; Marseille: Rivages, 1984.

**FOWKES, Robert.**

"On the etymology of NHG 'Eingeweide'." *Journal of English and Germanic Philology* 52 (1953): 96-98.

**FRANCASTEL, Pierre.**

*La figure et le lieu.* Paris: Gallimard, 1967. Orientation of figures within painted "space" in medieval art. Excellent illustrations.

**FRANKL, Viktor E.**

"Metaklinische Sinndeutung des Leidens." In *Homo patiens: Versuch einer Pathodizee,* by Viktor E.FRANKL. Vienna: F. Deuticke, 1950.

**FRANKLIN, K.L.**

"Kewa Ethnolinguistic Concepts of Body Parts." *Southwestern Journal of Anthropology* 19 (1963): 54-63.

**FRASER, Nancy.**

"Foucault's Body Language: A Post-Humanistic Political Rhetoric." *Salmagundi* (Sarasota, N.Y.) 61 (Fall 1983): 55-70.

**FRENK ALATORRE, Margit.**

"Designaciones de rasgos fisicos personales en el habla de la ciudad de México." *Nueva revista de filología Hispánica* 7 (1953): 134-56.

**FREVERT, Ute.**

"Frauen und Aertzte im späten 18. und frühen 19. Jahrhundert - Zur Sozialgeschichte eines Gewaltverhältnisses." In *Frauen in der Geschichte II,* ed. by A.KUHN and J.RUESEN, 117-210. Düsseldorf: Schwann, 1982.

**FREYTAG, Fredericka F.**

*The Body Image in Gender Orientation Disturbances.* New York: Vintage Press, 1977.

**FRICKE, Gerhard.**

*Die Bildlichkeit in der Dichtung des Andreas Gryphius: Materialien und Studien zum Formproblem des deutschen Literaturbarock.* Berlin: Juncker und Dünnhaupt, 1933. Andreas Greif, the Baroque poet of the thirty years war, has been credited with the first bourgeois tragedies in German. Fricke examines a wealth of imagery and metaphors (also explicitly those relating to the human body) from two perspectives: Where do the images originate? And to what kind of experience do they refer?

**FRIEDRICH, J.**

"Zu den hetitischen Wörtern für 'Stern' und 'Hand.'" *Athenaeum* (Pavia) 49 (1969): 116-18.

**FRISK, Hjalmar.**

*Quelques noms de la tempe en indo-européen.* Göteborg: Wettergren & Kerber, 1951.

____. "Zu einigen Verba des Hörens im Indogermanischen." In *Symbolae Philologicae Göteburgenses,* 1-22. Göteborg: Wettergren & Kerber, 1950.

**FRÜHSORGE, G.**

*Der politische Körper: Zum Begriff des Politischen im 17. Jh. und in den Romanen Christian Weises.* Stuttgart: Metzler, 1974.

**FUERST, L.**

"Das Pathologische auf der Bühne." *Bühne und Welt* 5 (1903).

**FUMAROLLI, M. et al.**

"Rhétorique du geste et de la voix à l'âge Classique." *XVIIe siècle* 132, no. 3 (1981): 235-55 (special issue on gesture and rhetoric).

**FURTH, Charlotte.**

"Blood, Body and Gender: Medical Images of the Female Condition in China, 1600-1850." *Chinese Science* 7 (1986): 43-66.

**FUSCO, Laurre Smith.**

*The Nude as Protagonist: Pollaiolo's Figural Style*

*Explicated by Leonardo's Study of Static Anatomy.*
Dissertation. New York: New York University.

**GABKA, Joachim.**
*Die erste Zahnung in der Geschichte des Aberglaubens, der Volksmedizin und der Medizin: ein Beitrag zur Transformation eines Krankenbildes.* Berlin: Die Quintessenz, 1970. Though written to promote visits to the dentist in early childhood and the medicalization of teething, this book contains good illustrations about folk traditions.

**GAETJE, Helmut.**
"Philosophische Traumlehren im Islam." *Zeitschrift der deutschen Morgenländischen Gesellschaft* 109 (1959): 258-85.

**GALANT-PERNET.**
"'Genou' et 'force' en berbère." In *Mélanges Marcel Cohen*, ed. by David COHEN, 254-62. The Hague: Mouton, 1970 (Janua Linguarum Series Maior 27 ).

**GALIMBERTI, Umberto.**
*Il corpo: antropologia, psicanalisi, fenomenologia.* Milano: Feltrinelli, 1983.

**GALLAGHER, Catherine, LAQUEUR, Thomas, eds.**
*The Making of the Modern Body: Sexuality and Society in the Nineteenth Century.* Berkeley: Univ. California Press, 1987.

**GAMILLSCHEG, Ernst.**
"Dorsum-renes." In *Romanica Festschrift G. Rohlfs*, 159-65. Halle: Niemeyer, 1958.

**GANDOLFO, Francesco.**
*Il "dolce tempo." Mistica, ermetismo e sogno nel Cinquecento.* Preface by Eugenio BATTISTI. Rome: Bulzoni, 1978. The representation of dreams and of dreamers from fifteenth-century Florence, Giorgione's Venice, to the Counter-Reformation. A history of bodies as they appear when they are represented as the content of dreams. Attempts to relate these to epoch-specific courtly ritual and literary iconology.

**GANUZA, Maria Christina.**
"El sensualismo y la dificultad del equilibrio en 'El Esclavo del Demonio.'" In *La Idea del cuerpo en las letras españolas* ed. by D.CVITANOVIC, 181-201. Bahía Blanca, Argentina: Instituto de Humanidades, Univ. Nac. del Sur., 1973. In Baroque art the artist is aware that the part of the lover's body which brings the beloved body into existence is the lover's eyes. From the description of the lover's eyes the beloved body can be known.

**GAOS, Jose.**
*Dos exclusivas del hombre: la mano y el tiempo.* Mexico: Universidad Nacional de México, 1945. A phenomenological essay which connects the hand with the awareness of time.

**GARCIA BALLESTER, Luis.**
*Galeno en la sociedad y la ciencia de su tiempo.* Madrid: Edit. Guadarrama, 1972. "The most recent comprehensive book on Galen's life and work" O.TEMKIN).

**GARDETTE, P.**
"Trois anciens mots francoprovençaux." In *Verba et vocabula: Festschrift. E.GAMILLSCHEG*, ed. by H.STIMM and J.WILHELM, 241-50. Munich: Fink, 1968.

**GARDINER, Edward N.**
*Athletics of the Ancient World.* Oxford: Oxford Univ. Press, 1930.

**GARRISON, Fielding H.**
"The Romantic Episode in the History of German Medicine." *Bulletin of the New York Academy of Medicine* 7 (1931): 841-64. Describes both the influence of Romantic literature on German physicians during the first half of the nineteenth century and the literary works by noted German physicians under the influence of Romanticism.

**GAUPP, R.**
"Das Pathologische in der Kunst und Literatur." *Deutsche Rundschau* (Berlin) 36 (1911).

**GAY, Jules.**
*Bibliographie des ouvrages relatifs à l'amour, aux femmes, au mariage et des livres facétieux pantagruéliques, scatologiques, satiriques etc.* 6 vols. San Remo: J. Gay & Fils, 1871-73.

**GEBHARDT-WAEGER, Gusti.**
*Die Dichtung des 18. Jhs. in ihrem Verhältnis zur körperlichen Krankheit.* Dissertation. Erlangen, 1948.

**GEBSATTEL, Victor E. von.**
*Imago hominis: Beiträge zu einer personalen Anthropologie.* 2. Aufl. Salzburg: Otto Müller.
____. *Prolegomena einer medizinischen Anthropologie. Ausgewählte Aufsätze.* Berlin: Springer, 1954.

**GEERTZ, Clifford.**
"The Impact of the Concept of Culture on the Concept of Man." In *New Views of the Nature of Man*, ed. by John R.PLATT. Chicago: Univ. Chicago Press, 1965. Men unmodified by the customs of particular places do not, did not and cannot exist. If we want to avoid searching with evolutionists for Man with a capital M behind his customs, or to dissolve Man with relativists into his culture, we arrive at the following idea: culture is best seen not as a complex of behavior patterns but as a set of rules, symbolically mediated programs (for producing artifacts, organizing social life, expressing emotions) by which men or women determine and achieve their biological destiny.

zone

**GEFFRIAUD, J.**
*Montesquieu et la femme*. Pisa: Libreria Goliardica Editrice, 1977. Useful introduction to recent French literary studies on the contributions made by literature to "gynecomythie": the perception of "femininity," "feminine destiny" and new myths about the female body.

**GELIS, Jacques.**
"De la mort à la vie: Les sanctuaires à répit." *Ethnologie française* 11 (1981): 211-24. In Catholic France a perinatal death saddened parents for two reasons: the loss of the "fruit" and of the unbaptized soul unable to enter heaven. At certain sanctuaries, some Saints specialized since the fifteenth century in the resurrection of such infants for just the few moments necessary to baptize them. Church authorities looked askance at the rituals.

____. "L'accouchement au XVIIIe siècle: pratiques traditionelles et contrôle médical." *Ethnologie française* 6, nos. 3-4 (1976): 325-39.

____. *L'Arbre et le fruit: La naissance dans l'occident moderne (XVIe-XIXe siècle)*. Paris: Fayard, 1984.

____. "Refaire le corps: Les déformations volontaires du corps de l'enfant à la naissance." *Ethnologie française* 14, no. 1 (1984): 7-28. The infant's body is plastic. Evidence of its routine deformation by bandaging, massage and manipulation is studied by anthropologists through observation or through the statistical analysis of skeletal remains. GELIS studies deformation as a historian in contemporary France, dealing with techniques (pointed skull, crusted ears, pulled nose, shaped breasts, disarticulated fingers, "circumcised" tongue), their geographic distribution in France and the evolution of medical opinion on the subject. Illustrated with contemporary photographs.

____. LAGET, M., MOREL, M.-F. *Entrer dans la vie: Naissances et enfances dans la France traditionelle*. Paris: Gallimard, (Collection Archives), 1978.

____, REDON, Odile, eds. *Les miracles miroirs des corps*. Paris, 1983.

**GENZEL, Peter.**
*Die Lebensfunktionen der Menschen und Sauegetiere im Spiegel der englischen Sprache*. Halle: VEB Niemeyer, 1959. Based on the study of dictionaries, medical literature new and old, literary texts since the Middle Ages to contemporary newspapers. The theme is designations for body functions and the body parts related to them. The author selects some eighty subjects (which can be indicated by one or several German words) and then searches for the English designations, and their historical evolution. Dialects are excluded, but all language-levels, including the most vulgar, are documented, primarily with words that refer to the human body but not excluding those referring to domestic animals or venery. Individual terms

are contrasted not only with synonyms in English but with their equivalents in German.

**GERHARDT, C.**
"Kröte und Igel in schwankhafter Literatur des späten Mittelalters." *Medizinhistorisches Journal* 16, no. 4 (1981): 340-57.

**GERLACH, Wolfgang.**
"Das Problem des 'weiblichen Samens' in der antiken und mittelalterlichen Medizin." *Sudhoffs Archiv* 30, nos. 4-5 (1938): 177-93. Though weak on interpretation, useful as a collection of texts evidencing the tradition of semen in women.

**GERNSHEIM, Alison.**
*Victorian and Edwardian Fashion: A Photographic Survey*. New York: Dover, 1981.

**GEYER-KORDESCH, Johanna.**
"Cultural Habits of Illness: The Enlightened and the Pious in Eighteenth-Century Germany." In *Patients and Practititioners*, ed. by Roy PORTER, 177-204. Cambridge: Cambridge Univ. Press, 1985.

**GHISALBERTI, Allessandro.**
"Il pensiero medievale di fronte al corpo." In *Il corpo in scena*, ed. by V.MELCHIORRE and A.CASCETTA, 55-69. Milan: Vita e Pensiero, 1983.

**GIEDKE, Adelheid.**
*Die Liebeskrankheit in der Geschichte der Medizin*. Dissertation. Med. Düsseldorf, 1983.

**GIEGERICH, Wolfgang.**
"Die Bedeutung des Körpers in Psychologie und Psychotherapie." *Analytische Psychologie* 14 (1983): 264-84.

**GILBERT, Helen.**
"Pregnancy Cravings as a Motif in Folktale." *Folklore Forum* 5, no. 4 (October 1972): 129-42. A short, cross-cultural survey of the literature, valuable because of the bibliography assembled.

**GILMAN, Sander L.**
"Black Bodies, White Bodies: Toward an Iconography of Female Sexuality in Late Nineteenth-Century Art, Medicine and Literature." *Critical Inquiry* 12 (1985).

____. *Seeing the Insane: A Cultural History of Madness and Art in the Western World*. New York: J. Wiley, 1982.

**GINZBURG, Carlo.**
*Indagini su Piero: Il battesimo, Il ciclo di Arezzo, La flagellazione di Urbino*. Turin: Einaudi, 1981 (*The Enigma of Piero*. London: Verso, 1981).

**GITTER, Elisabeth G.**
"The Power of Women's Hair in Victorian Imagination." *Proceedings of the Modern Language Association* 99, no. 5 (1984): 936-54. From novels and poetry, scientific texts and the observation of figurative art the author weaves a tight account of the importance and ambiguity of hair in the Age of Rossetti and

504

Baudelaire. The aureole of the woman as angel and the glittering snare, web or noose of woman as demon.

**GIVRY, Gillot de.**
*Witchcraft, Magic and Alchemy.* New York: Dover, 1971 (orig. 1931). See ch. 3: "Astrology and the Microcosm."

**GLACKEN, C.L.**
*Traces on the Rhodean Shore: Nature and Culture in Western Thought from Ancient Times to the End of the Eighteenth Century.* Berkeley: Univ. California Press, 1967.

**GLATIGNY, M.**
"Le champ sémantique des parties du corps dans la poésie amoureuse de 1550." *Le français moderne* 37 (1969): 7-34. First the author establishes which of the terms referring to the body in RONSARD, BAIF, du BELLAY and contemporaries are used idiosyncratically - and which forms of usage reflect the epoch's standard. Particularly for the latter, patterns of associations are identified.

**GLOCKNER, H.**
"Der eigene Leib." *Kantstudien* 53 (1961-62): 289-308.

**GLOOR, B.**
*Die künstlicherischen Mitarbeiter an den naturwissenschaftlichen und medizinischen Werken Albrecht von Hallers.* Berner Beiträge z. Geschichte der Medizin und der Naturwissenschaften, No. 15. Bern: Paul Haupt Verlag, 1958. Haller dissected and prepared anatomical specimens at Göttingen 1736-53. Three of his craftsmen are studied, and four of the artists who etched his famous plates. This allows us to distinguish three stages at which the epoch's perceptions and taboos shaped the style of representation in the copper plates. Many plates remained normative for medical studies for over a century.

**GOBERT, E.G.**
"Le pudendum magique et le problème des cauris." *Revue africaine* 95 (1951): 5-62.

**GOEDEL, Eckhard.**
"Die aegyptische Terminologie um Herz und Magen in medizinischer Sicht." *Wissenschaftliche Zeitschrift der Universität Leipzig* 7 (1957-58): 643-50.

**GOESSMANN, Elisabeth.**
"Anthropologie und Soziale Stellung der Frau nach Summen und Sentenzenkommentaren des 12. Jahrhunderts." *Miscellanea Medievalia* 12, no. 1 (1979): 281-97. The early Franciscan theologians maintain a markedly greater distance from the Aristotelian doctrine of the "mas occasionatus" than their Dominican contemporaries, especially Thomas Aquinas.
____. *Metaphysik und Heilsgeschichte: eine theologische Untersuchung der Summa Halensis.* Munich: Max Huber, 1964. Pp. 215-29 ("Der Mensch als Mann und Frau") are outstanding not only for the commentary on the text but for the balanced introduction to thirteenth-century thought on gender difference.
____. "Mass- und Zahlangaben bei Hildegard von Bingen." In *Mensura: Mass, Zahl, Zahlensymbolik im Mittelalter*, ed. by Albert ZIMMERMANN, 2. Halbbd. 294-309. Berlin: De Gruyter, 1984.

**GOFFMAN, Erving.**
*Gender Advertisements.* Cambridge, Mass.: Harvard Univ. Press, 1979.
____. *Relations in Public Places: Microstudies of the Public Order.* New York: Basic Books, 1971. From patient and careful observation and frequent reference to creative literature the author creates a taxonomy of interactions that forces the historian to pay more attention to the gestures of past times.

**GOLDBECK, Ingeborg.**
"Die Jungfrau." *Muttersprache* (1953): 50-55. A collection of phrases, composed words and names in which equivalents for "virgin" appear in French, German and English; in geography, botany, culinary arts, etc.

**GOLDSCHMID, Edgar.**
*Entwicklung und Bibliographie der pathologisch-anatomischen Abbildung.* Leipzig: Hiersemann, 1925. Though dated as a history of medical illustrations, still invaluable because of its bibliography of more than six hundred illustrated medical texts since 1517.

**GOLDSTEIN, Jan.**
"'Moral contagion': A Professional Ideology of Medicine and Psychiatry in Eighteenth- and Nineteenth-Century France." In *Professions and the French State, 1700-1900*, ed. by G.L.GEISON, 181-222. Philadelphia: Univ. Pennsylvania Press. As witchcraft trials were abandoned a new secular theory about the dangers of moral contagion developed which was clearly formulated by early nineteenth-century French psychiatrists. A Dr. Bouchut wrote in 1857: "There ought to be in society a sort of moral lazaretto where mental and nervous disorders whose contagious properties have been established could be hidden away as soon as they manifest themselves. The trained eye easily recognizes the 'pathognomic signs'...of persons susceptible to reciprocal inflammation" (pp. 214ff.).

**GOLTZ, Dietlinde.**
"Krankheit und Sprache." *Sudhoffs Archiv* 53, no. 3 (1969): 225-69.

**GOMBRICH, E. H.**
*The Image and the Eye: Further Studies in the Psychology of Pictorial Representation.* Oxford: Phaidon, 1982.

**GONDA, J.**
*Eye and Gaze in the Veda.* Amsterdam: Noord-Hollandsche Uitgevers Mij, 1969 (Verhandelingen van de Koniglijke Nederlandse Akademie van Wetenschappen Afdeling Letterkunde).

**GOTTLIEB, Carla.**

"The Pregnant Woman, the Flag, the Eye: Three New Themes in Twentieth-Century Art." *Journal of Aesthetics and Art Criticism* 21 (1961): 177-87.

____. *The Window in Art: From the Window of God to the Vanity of Man: A Survey of Window Symbolism in Western Painting*. New York: Abaris Books, 1981. The major iconography of the "window" theme. Relevant to body perception: the eyes as windows - and the window as an eye.

**GOTTSCHALK, Walter**

*Die bildlichen Sprichwörter der Romanen.* Vol 2: *Der Mensch im Sprichwort der romanischen Völker.* Heidelberg: Winter, 1936. Proverbs in Romance languages. On the body pp. 1-45.

**GOUBERT, J. P.**

"L'art de guérir: Médecine savante et médecine populaire dans la France de 1790." *Annales E.S.C.* 32, no. 5 (1977): 908-26. (In *Medicine and Society in France*, ed. by R.FORSTER and O.RANUM, 1-23. Baltimore: Johns Hopkins Press, 1980).

____. *Malades et médecins en Bretagne 1770-1790.* Paris: Klincksieck, 1974.

____. "Réseau médical et médicalisation en France à la fin du XVIIIe siècle." *Annales de Bretagne* 86, no. 2 (1979): 221-29.

**GOUDSBLOM, J.**

"Zivilisation, Ansteckungsangst und Hygiene." In *Materialien zu Norbert Elias' Zivilisationstheorie*, ed. by P.GLEICHMANN, et al., 215-53. Frankfurt: Suhrkamp, 1977.

**GOULEMOT, Jean Marie.**

"Prêtons la main à la nature: II. Fureurs utérines." *Dix-huitième siècle* 12 (1980): 97-111.

**GOUREVITCH, Danielle.**

*Le mal d'être femme: La femme et la médecine à Rome.* Paris: Belles Lettres, 1984.

____. *Le triangle hippocratique: Le malade, sa maladie et son médecin aux époques hellénistique et romaine.* Rome, Paris: Broccard, 1983.

**GRABNER, Elfriede.**

"Der 'Wurm' als Krankheitsvorstellung: Süddeutsche und Südeuropäische Beiträge zur allgemeinen Volksmedizin." *Zeitschrift für deutsche Philologie* 81, no. 2 (1962): 224-40. Worms can originate within the body. They settle especially in the heart or in the brain. They also eat away at hollow teeth, in the scalp and under inflamed nails. Evidence from Austrian ethnology.

____. "'Menschenfett' und 'Mumie' als Heilmittel: Volksmedizin, Volksglaube und Schauermärchen um die medizinische Verwertung menschlicher Leichen." *Neue Chronik zur Geschichte und Volkskunde der innerösterreichischen Alpenländer* 64 (1961). The touch of the executioner was ascribed healing power throughout the Middle Ages; fat from a beheaded criminal was used for otherwise incurable conditions. Later, powdered mummy was commercialized.

____. "'Rotes Haar und Roter Bart...' Redensart, Volksmedizin und Volksmeinung um die Rothaarigen." *Schweizer Volkskunde* 53 (1963): 10-20.

____. "Das 'Umgürten' als Heilbrauch. Kulturhistorisches und Volksmedizinisches um die Gürtung menschlicher Körperteile." *Carinthia 1* (Mitteilungen des Geschichtsvereins für Kärnten) 155, nos. 1-3 (1964): 548-68. Symbolism of the cincture and its apotropaic and healing powers in folklore, mostly alpine, Austria.

____. "Der Mensch als Arznei. Alpenländische Belege zu einem Kärntner Schauermärlein." In *Festgabe für Oskar Moser: Beiträge zur Volkskunde Kärntens,* 81-95. Klagenfurt: Habelt, 1974 (Kärtner Museumsschriften 55). Anthropophagy as therapy in folklore (Alps) and in medical opinion. Powdered mummy was particularly appreciated and led to advice on pharmaceutical embalming.

____. "Die 'transplantatio morborum' als Heilmethode in der Volksmedizin." *Oesterreichische Blätter für Volkskunde* 21 (1972): 178-95. 'Transplantatio' of disease is an important magical tradition in Western medicine. It consists in the 'implantation' of a part of the sick body into the cosmologically appropriate element of the environment. According to Pliny, the glance of an *Amsel* (Latin *icterus*) suffices to heal a person afflicted with hepatitis. A fresh catskin worn around the chest until it decomposes draws consumption out of the lungs. The tradition is surveyed.

____. "'Schnurziehen' und 'Fontanellensetzen': Künstliche Wunden als Krankheitsableitung im Wechselspiel von Schul- und Volksmedizin." *Schweizerisches Archiv für Volkskunde* 62 (1966): 133-50. Since Antiquity artificial wounds have been inflicted to allow evil to drip out of the body. The practice remained a standard procedure in European folk medicine into our days. The various methods for keeping incisions "letting" are discussed.

____. "Verlorenes Mass und heilkräftiges Messen: Krankheitsforschung und Heilhandlung in der Volksmedizin." *Zeitschrift für Volkskunde* 60 (1964): 23-34.

____. ed. *Volksmedizin: Probleme und Forschungsgeschichte.* Darmstadt: Wissenschaftliche Buchgesellschaft, 1974. Selections reflecting the historiography of folk medicine as a discipline.

____. "Volkstümliche Fiebervorstellungen: Ein Beitrag zur steirischen Volksmedizin." *Oesterreichische Zeitschrift für Volkskunde* n.s. 15 (1961): 81-97. Alpine folk beliefs about fever are frequently connected with number symbolism and magic; transfer of fevers (of which there are sixty-six or seventy-seven or ninety-nine kinds) onto certain plants and objects; fever is imagined as a being that takes possession of the person and must be exorcised.

____. "Gallensteine als Heiligenattribut: Clara von Montefalco in Ikonographie und Legende." In *Dona Ethnologica. Beiträge zur Vergleichenden Volkskunde, Leopold KRETZENBACHER zum 60. Geburtstag*, ed. by H.GERNDT and G.R.SCHRAUBEK, 172-84. Munich: Oldenbourg, 1973. The study of gallstones as iconographic attributes of a seventeenth-century nun leads to documents in which contemporary lay attitude toward the opening of the body (p. 179ff.) become manifest.

____. *Grundzüge einer ostalpinen Volksmedizin.* Vienna: Verlag der Akademie der Wissenschaften, 1985.

**GRABOWSKI, S.J.**
"St. Augustine and the Doctrine of the Mystical Body of Christ." *Theological Studies* 7 (1946): 72-125. The paper deals with the theological content of the body metaphor - only indirectly relevant in understanding Augustine's perception of the human body.

**GRAF, H.**
*Bibliographie zum Problem der Proportionen: Literatur über Proportionen, Mass und Zahl in Architektur, bildender Kunst und Natur.* Speyer: Pfälzische Landesbibliothek, 1958. Teil I: Von 1800 bis zur Gegenwart. (Pfälzische Arbeiten zum Buch- und Bibliothekswesen und zur Bibliographie 3.) An unusual bibliography which contains many items that link body proportion (or the perception of these proportions) to nature and Architecture. Part 2 on earlier literature seems never to have been published.

**GRANQUIST, Hilma.**
*Birth and Childhood Among the Arabs: Studies in a Muhammadan Village in Palestine.* Helsingfors: Söderström, 1947. Customs of childbirth now observed among Middle Eastern Arabs may shed light on the origin of medical views brought to Europe during the Crusades. For the interpretation of body symbolism through customs see esp. "cohabitation/conception," pp. 29-51.

**GREIVE, A.**
"Die lexikalische Differenzierung des Begriffs 'Fleisch' im Französischen." *Archiv für das Studium der neueren Sprachen und Literaturen* 204 (1967-68): 426-29.

**GREVERUS, Ina-Maria.**
*Der territoriale Mensch: ein literaturanthropologischer Versuch zum Heimatphänomen.* Frankfurt: Athenaeum, 1972. A thorough study on the role that the theme "Heimat" has had on the portraiture of main figures in modern German literature.

**GRIMES, Larry M.**
*El tabú lingüístico: su naturaleza y función en el*
*español popular de México.* Cuernavaca: CIDOC, 1971 (CIDOC Cuaderno 64). From field notes by Oscar Lewis and his own observations in the slums of Mexico City, Grimes assembles the vocabulary used to designate body orifices and their functions. His special interest focuses on euphemisms and their symbolism.

**GRINELL, R.**
"The Theoretical Attitudes Towards Space in the Middle Ages." *Speculum* 21 (1946): 141-57.

**GRMEK, M.D.**
"Le concept d'infection dans l'Antiquité et au Moyen Age." *Rad Jugoslavenske Akademije Znanosti i Umjetnosti* 384 (1980): 5-55.

____. *Les maladies à l'aube de la civilisation occidentale.* Paris: Payot, 1983.

**GROEN, K.**
"Lepra in Literatur und Kunst." In *Handbuch der Haut- und Geschlechtskrankheiten*, Bd. 10, Teil 2. Berlin: Springer, 1930.

**GRUMAN, Gerald J.**
*A History of Ideas about the Prolongation of Life: The Evolution of Prolongevity Hypotheses to 1800.* Philadelphia, 1966 (Transactions of the American Philosophical Society n.s. 56, pt. 9, 1966).

**GRUTTMANN, Felicitas.**
*Ein Beitrag zur Kenntnis der Volksmedizin in Sprichwörtern, Redensarten und Heilsegen des englisches Volkes, mit besonderer Berücksichtigung der Zahnheilkunde.* Greifswald, 1939.

**GUENTERT, Hermann.**
"Weiteres zum Begriff 'Winkel' im ursprünglichen Denken." *Wörter und Sachen* 11 (1928): 124-42.

**GUENTHER, Louis.**
"Die Ausdrücke unserer Sprache für das weibliche Geschlecht im Wandel der Zeiten." In *Von Wörtern und Namen*, by L.GUENTHER, Berlin: F. Dümmler, 1926.

**GUERRINO, Antonio A., KOHN-LON-CARICA, Alfredo G.**
"La uroscopía en la edad media." *Episteme* 7 (1973): 289-97.

**GUGGENHEIM, K.**
"Soranus of Ephesus on Obesity." *Internat. Journal of Obesity* 1, no. 3 (1977): 245-46. Quotes the passages in which Soranus discusses obesity as a form of "marasmic wasting" rather than as a sign of plentiful health.

**GUICCIARDI, Jean Pierre.**
"L'hermaphrodite et le prolétaire." *Dix-huitième siècle* 12 (1980): 49-77. Observes in some French authors of the mid-eighteenth century two things: an obsessive interest in the hermaphrodite and the lack of a vocabulary and concepts fit to express this fascination with "otherness."

**GUILLAUMONT, Antoine.**
"Les sens des noms du coeur dans l'Antiquité." *Etudes*

*Carmélitaines* 29 (1950): 41-81. The entire issue of this journal is dedicated to the perception of the "heart" in Christian mysticism.

**GUILLERME, Jacques.**

"Le malsain et l'économie de la nature." *Dix-huitième siècle* 9 (1977): 61-72.

____. "Sur l'esthétique du décharnement." *Revue d'Esthétique* 12 (1970): 139-54. Analysis of the aesthetics of the skinned body in VESAL.

**GULDAN, Ernst.**

*Eva und Maria: Eine Antithese als Bildmotiv.* Köln, Graz: Böhlau, 1966. The major iconography of Mary as the second Eve.

____. " 'Et verbum caro factum est.' Die Darstellung der Inkarnation Christi im Verkündigungsbild." *Römische Quartalschrift für christliche Altertumskunde und Kirchengeschichte* 63 (1968): 145-69.

**GUTH, Klaus.**

*Guibert von Nogent und die hochmittelalterliche Kritik an der Reliquienverehrung.* Ottobeuren: Kommissionsverlag Winifried Werk, 1970. A doctoral thesis that attempts to clarify the place and function of relics within a history of piety during the twelfth century, which, in turn, is perceived as just one aspect of the century's reality perception. Abbot Guibert and his unprecedented historical and critical attitude toward the authenticity of relics is at the center of study.

# H

**HABICHT, Werner.**

*Die Gebärde in englischen Dichtungen des Mittelalters.* Munich: Verlag der Bayer. Akademie der Wissenschaften, 1959. Still the major monograph on gesture in Old and Middle English poetry: expressive gesture which translates emotion into behavior; demonstrative gesture which is intentional movement or pose and ceremonial or liturgical gesture. The word gesture does not come into use before the fifteenth century, and even then meant bearing, carriage, deportment and pose in addition to some of its still current definitions.

____. "Zur Bedeutungsgeschichte des englischen Wortes 'countenance'." *Archiv für das Studium der neueren Sprachen und Literaturen* 203 (1966): 32-51. 'Countenance' in Middle English means bearing, conduct 'Haltung,' 'Gebaren' or occasionally a gesture ("with his hands made countenance"). Its current meaning emerges late in the Renaissance.

**HAGEN, H.**

*Die physiologische und psychologische Bedeutung der*

*Leber in der Antike.* Dissertation. Bonn, 1961.

**HAGER, Gertrud.**

*Gesundheit bei Goethe: Eine Wortmonographie.* Berlin: Akademie-Verlag, 1955. Goethe's lifespan coincides with the discovery of "health" as a goal, as a public concern and finally as a pursuit which ought to be regulated by policy. This study of Goethe's use of the word "gesund" might therefore give further clues to the history of "health" and the body that needs it. The author assembles thirteen hundred passages in Goethe where the word occurs, examines the field the word covers, its content and context, as opposite to disease, its positive aesthetic value. It is a key word in Goethe.

**HAHN, Ingrid.**

*Raum und Landschaft in Gottfried's Tristan: Ein Beitrag zur Werkdeutung.* Munich, 1963 (Medium Aevum 3). Valuable for understanding the correlations between the medieval perception of space and posture, carriage and gesture.

**HAIRE, Doris.**

"The Cultural Warping of Childbirth." *Environmental Child Health* (June 1973), 172-91.

**HALE, David George.**

*The Body Politic: A Political Metaphor in Renaissance English Literature.* The Hague: Mouton, 1971.

**HALL, Edward.**

*The Silent Language.* Greenwich, Conn.: Fawcett World Library, 1957. "The clumsy ethnographic illustrations" and "tendentious misleading hunches" (E.LEACH) with which this and subsequent volumes by the author are filled have had a strong influence on general readers, and the adoption of stereotypes about "proxemics" have created an obstacle to the interdisciplinary discussion of body and space perceptions.

**HALLPIKE, C. R.**

"Social Hair." *MAN* n.s. 4 (1969): 256-64. Symbols can be studied as being "about" the unconscious or as being "about" the world and man's place in it. Opposing E.R. Leach's approach the author tries to explain the social symbolism of hair in relation to society and the physical environment.

**HAMBLY, W.D.**

*The History of Tattooing and Its Significance: With Some Account of Other Forms of Corporal Marking.* London: Witherby, 1925 (Repr. Gale Research Corp., 1974).

**HAMBURGH, Harvey E.**

*Aspects of the Descent from the Cross from Lippe to Cigoli.* 2 vols. Dissertation. The Graduate College, Univ. Iowa, July 1978.

**HAMILTON, Mary.**

*Incubation: The Cure of Disease in Pagan Temples and Christian Churches.* London: Henderson, 1906.

**HAMMER, Felix.**

*Leib und Geschlecht: Philosophische Perspektiven von*

*Nietzsche bis Merleau-Ponty*. Bonn: Bouvier, 1974.

**HAMP, Eric P.**

"Latin 'Poples,' 'Back of the Knee.'" *The American Journal of Philology* 75 (1954): 186-89.

____. "On the Paradigm of 'Knee.'" *Glotta* 48 (1970): 72-75.

**HAMPP, Irmgard.**

*Beschwörung, Segen, Gebet: Untersuchungen zum Zauberspruch aus dem Bereich der Volkskunde.* Stuttgart, 1961 (Veröffentlichung des Staatl. Amtes für Denkmalpflege Stuttgart, Reihe C. Volkskunde).

**HAND, Wayland.**

*Magical Medicine: The Folkloric Component of Medicine in the Folk Belief, Custom and Ritual of the Peoples of Europe and America.* Foreword by Lloyd G.STEVENSON, Berkeley: Univ. California Press, 1980. A rich collection of selected essays.

____. "American Analogues of the Couvade." In *Studies in Folklore in Honor of Stith Thompson*, 213-29. Bloomington: Univ. Indiana Press, 1957.

____. "'Measuring' with String, Thread, and Fibre: A Practice in Folk Medical Magic." *Schweizerisches Archiv für Volkskunde* 68 (1972-73): 240-51.

____. *Popular Beliefs and Superstitions: A Compendium of American Folklore*, ed. by Wayland HAND, A. CASETTA and S.B. THIEDERMAN. From the Ohio Collection of Newbell Niles PUCK-ETT, vol. 1, Boston: Hall, 1981. Volume 1 introduces the beliefs about body parts (from cane, p. 53, to skin, dimples, p. 64); functions (from crying, p. 64, to yawning, p. 67); attributes (pp. 67-74). The corresponding documentation (pp. 161-253).

**HANDLEY, E.W.**

"Words for 'Soul,' 'Heart' and 'Mind' in Aristophanes.' *Rheinisches Museum für Philologie* 99 (1956): 205-25. The words used for "soul," "heart" and "mind" used by Aristophanes enter very little into the ordinary vocabulary of fifth-century B.C. everyday life. For the young Aristophanes they are - with the possible exception of "heart" - words to play with.

**HANSMANN, Liselotte, KRISS-RETTENBECK, Lenz.**

*Amulett und Talisman: Erscheinungsform und Geschichte.* Munich: Callwey, 1966.

**HARAWAY, Donna.**

"Animal Sociology and a Natural Economy of the Body Politic." *SIGNS* 4, no. 1 (1978): 21-60.

____. "The Biological Enterprise: Sex, Mind and Profit from Human Engineering of Sociobiology." *Radical History Review* 20 (1979): 206-37.

**HARRELL, Barbara.**

"Lactation and Menstruation in Cultural Perspective." *American Anthropologist* 83 (1981): 796-823.

**HARRIS, C.R.S.**

*The Heart and the Vascular System in Ancient Greek Medicine: From Alcmaeon to Galen*. New York, Oxford: Oxford Univ. Press, 1973.

**HARTE, N.B., PONTING, K. G., eds.**

*Cloth and Clothing in Medieval Europe: Essays in Memory of Professor E.M. Carus-Wilson*. Heinemann Educational Books, 1983. Essays on the history of European clothing, dress, textile finishing and the clothing trade.

**HARTLAUB, G. F.**

*Zauber des Spiegels: Geschichte und Bedeutung des Spiegels in der Kunst.* Munich: Piper, 1951. On the mirror, mainly as the painter has dealt with it. Iconography of several motifs: man and woman as they look into the mirror; what the mirror reflects; the magical mirror; the mirror as a tool and the mirror as a symbol. For the historical evolution of body perception chapter four is particularly valuable: it deals with the gesture, posture and expression of the person seeing what the mirror reflects - the flesh, the background, the viewer's own bones or the devil.

____. "Die Spiegel-Bilder des Giovanni Bellini." *Pantheon* 15, no. 2 (November 1942): 235-41.

**HARTMANN, Fritz.**

*Aerztliche Anthropologie: Das Problem des Menschen in der Medizin der Neuzeit.* Bremen: Schünemann, 1973.

____. "The Corporeality of Shame: Fx and Hx at the Bedside." *The Journal of Medicine and Philosophy* 9, no. 1 (1984): 63-74. In order to appreciate the role of the phenomenon of shame in the context of medical treatment, a philosophical, anthropological description of shame is offered. The author takes up biblical metaphors and more recent phenomenologico-psychological description from Max Scheler and others. The corporeality of shame is constituted as "what envelopes the body."

____. "Homo patiens: zur ärztlichen Anthropologie von Leid und Mitleid." *Sudhoffs Archiv*, Beiheft (Supplement) 24 (1984): 35-44.

**HARTOG, François.**

*Le miroir d'Hérodote: Essai sur la représentation de l'autre.* Paris: Gallimard, 1980.

____. "Les Amazones d'Hérodote: Inversion et tiers exclu." In *Le racisme: Mythes et sciences. Pour Léon POLIAKOV*, ed. by M.OLENDER, 177-85. Paris: Editions Complexe, 1981.

**HASKELL, Frances, HASKELL, Penny Nicholas.**

*Taste and the Antique: The Lure of Classical Sculpture 1500-1800.* New Haven: Yale Univ. Press, 1981.

**HATTENHAUER, Hans.**

"Das Herz des Königs in der Hand Gottes: Zum Herrscherbild in Spätantike und Mittelalter." *Zeitschrift für Rechtsgeschichte* 98 Kan. Abt. 67-68 (1981): 1-35.

**HAULOTTE, Edgar S.J.**

*Symbolique du vêtement selon la bible.* Paris: Aubier, 1964. Pp. 237-71 deals with women's veil and the inability of Christian tradition to recognize it as a sign of authority. The book is full of surprises.

**HAUSCHILD, Thomas.**

"Abwehrmagie und Geschlechtssymbolik im Mittelmeerraum." *Curare* 7 (1984): 205-22 (special issue in honor of Georges Devereux). Contains information on the significance of body-shaped amulets to protect against the evil eye.

_____. "'Weiblicher Schamanismus' und 'wilde Frauen': Bemerkungen zu Muhlmann und Devereux." *Curare* 5 (1982): 75-80.

_____. *Der böse blick: Ideengeschichtliche und Sozialpsychologische Untersuchungen.* 2d rev. ed. Berlin: Verlag Mensch und Leben, 1982.

**HAUSENSTEIN, Wilhelm.**

*Die Kunst und die Gesellschaft.* Part 1: *Die Gestalt des Menschen und die Gesellschaft.* Part 2: *Die kulturellen Voraussetzungen des Nackten.* Munich: Piper, 1916.

_____. *Der Körper des Menschen in der Geschichte der Kunst.* Munich: Piper, 1916.

**HAYES, Francis.**

"Gesture: A Working Bibliography." *Southern Folklore Quarterly* 21 (December 1957): 218-317. Well over a thousand items, one sixth are annotated. However, first of all the author calls gesture any nonvocal expression (folk or "technical"), even if it is not meant to tell another (autistic), and second, literature dealing with these expressions is listed, academic (social sciences or humanities), journalistic and amateurish.

**HECKSCHER, William S.**

*Rembrandt's Anatomy of Dr. Nicolaas Tulp: An Iconographical Study.* New York: New York Univ. Press, 1958.

**HEIN, Wolfgang-Hagen.**

*Christus als Apotheker.* Frankfurt: Govi Verlag, 1974.

**HEINE, Susanne.**

*Leibhafter Glaube: Ein Beitrag zum Verständnis der theologischen Konzeption des Paulus.* Vienna: Herder, 1976.

**HEINTEL, Helmut, ed.**

*Quellen zur Geschichte der Epilepsie.* Berlin, Stuttgart, Vienna: Huber, 1975 (Hubers Klassiker der Medizin und der Naturwissenschaften 14). Thirty-seven European texts since Antiquity (two-thirds since 1783) dealing with the perception of epilepsy. Most translations were prepared for this publication.

**HELGELAND, John.**

"The Symbolism of Death in the Later Middle Ages." *Omega* 15, no. 2 (1984-85): 145-60. Starts from the assumptions that previous authors have failed to explain the gruesome images of death occurring during the late Middle Ages. The author interprets

Mary Douglas as saying that the human body is the most natural symbol for describing social institutions. By means of gruesome images the artists and poets symbolized the disintegration of medieval institutions by analogy with the decomposition of bodies.

**HELLERMANN, Fritz.**

*Mienenspiel und Gebärdenspiel in Conrad Ferdinand Meyers Novellen: Die Ausdrucksbewegungen mit besonderer Berücksichtigung der Augen.* Hamburg: Fremdblatt Druckerei Broschek & Co., 1912. The Swiss-German novelist C.F. Meyer was a contemporary of Darwin (the author of "The Expression of Emotions in Man and Animal," 1872). Hellermann indicates an analogy in body perception in both authors. Meyer pioneered German symbolist techniques by avoiding the description of emotions, letting them be expressed in the gesture, facial expression and - especially - the play of the eyes.

**HELM, Rudolf.**

*Skelett- und Todesdarstellungen bis zum Auftreten der Totentänze.* Dissertation. Marburg, 1927. The "Dance of the Dead" is a very common motif in paintings during the later Middle Ages. A careful study of the skeletons, represented in many dancing postures, reveals that many of the bones do not at all look like those with which the painter must have been acquainted from cemeteries: sometimes the pelvis is missing, and Holbein even doubles the thigh bone. Helm argues that before Vesalius there was insufficient terminology for the skeleton to be able to reason about it, and that artists often painted what they could neither name nor see as an entity apart.

**HELMAN, Cecil G.**

"'Feed a Cold, Starve a Fever' - Folk Models of Infection in an English Suburban Community and Their Relation to Medical Treatment." *Culture, Medicine and Psychiatry* 2 (1978): 107-37. Some folk beliefs survived almost intact until the Health Act (1949) in England. Some of them, since then, have been actually reinforced by modern biomedical treatment and are now presented by physicians to gain the trust of patients.

**HELTEN, W.L. von.**

"Zu einigen germanischen Benennungen für 'cunnus' und 'veretrum'." *Zeitschrift für deutsche Wortforschung* 10 (1908-09): 195-97. A careful examination of the oldest and most traditional terms for these organs.

**HENISCH, Bridget Ann.**

*Fast and Feast: Food in Medieval Society.* University Park: Pennsylvania State Univ. Press, 1976.

**HENTIG, Hans von.**

*Vom Ursprung der Henkersmahlzeit.* Tübingen: Mohr, 1958. Instead of being given a last cigarette, people condemned to death were feasted. In this unusual monograph on this last meal the author records many details on the victim's body in this liminal stage, especially in postmedieval Europe.

**HERMANN, Alfred.**
"Das steinharte Herz: Zur Geschichte einer Metapher." *Jahrbuch für Antike und Christentum* 4 (1961): 77-107. The author pursues explicitly only the history of the hard or stony heart, up to and in Augustine, in whom that tradition culminated and from which later, Western heart metaphors derive. Classical, biblical and Egyptian sources are identified. The 186 notes, however, make this article into a bibliography on this theme.

**HERMANN, Hans Volkmar.**
*Omphalos.* Münster: Aschendorfsche Verlagsbuchhandlung, 1959. The navel in Greek myth, ritual and art, especially its relation to altar and grave. Also a history of archeologists' interpretations of the stone objects representing the navel.

**HERRLINGER, Robert.**
"Die frühesten embryologischen Abbildungen in der Geschichte der Medizin." *Zeitschrift für Anatomie und Entwicklungsgeschichte* 116 (1951-53): 1-13. Splendid reproductions.

____. *Körperproportionen im 14. Jahrhundert.* Marburger Jahrbuch für Kunstwissenschaft. Marburg, 1949.

____. "Zur Frage der ersten anatomisch richtigen Darstellung des menschlichen Körpers in der Malerei." *Centaurus* 2 (1951-53): 283-88.

____. *Geschichte der medizinischen Abbildung.* Vol. 1: *Von den Anfängen bis um 1600.* Munich: Heinz Moos, 1972. Vol. 2: Marielene PUTSCHER. *Von 1600 bis zur Gegenwart.* Munich: Heinz Moos, 1972. (Vol. 1: *History of Medical Illustration from Antiquity to 1600.* London: Pitman Medical Publ., 1970.)

**HERSANT, Y.**
"Figures des passions: la pathognomie de Charles Le Brun." *History and Anthropology* 1, no. 1 (November 1984): 163-74.

**HERSHMAN, P.**
"Hair, Sex and Dirt." *Man* n.s. 9, no. 2 (1974): 274-98.

**HERTER, Hans.**
"Die Haaröle der Berenike." In *Medizingeschichte in unserer Zeit: Festgabe für Edith Heischkel-Artelt und Walter Artelt zum 65. Geburtstag,* ed. Hans-Heinz EULNER, et al., 54-187. Stuttgart: Enke, 1971.

**HERTZ, Robert.**
"La prééminence de la main droite: Etude sur la polarité religieuse." In *Mélanges de sociologie religieuse et de folklore.* Paris, 1928 ("The Preeminence of the Right Hand: A Study in Religious Polarity." In *Right and Left,* ed. by R. NEEDHAM, 3-29. Chicago: Univ. Chicago Press, 1973).

**HERZLICH, Claudine, PIERRET, Janine.**
*Malades d'hier, malades d'aujourd'hui: de la mort collective au devoir de guérison.* Paris: Payot, 1984 (*Illness and Self in Society.* Baltimore: Johns Hopkins Press 1987).

**HESSELING, Dirk Christian.**
"Les mots désignant le palais de la bouche en grec et en hollandais." *Laographia* 7 (1923): 422-25.

**HEWSON, Anthony.**
*Giles of Rome and the Medieval Theory of Conception: A Study of "De formatione corporis humani in utero."* London: Athlone Press, 1975.

**HILDBURGH, W,L.**
"Images of the Human Hand as Amulets in Spain." *Journal of the Cortauld and Warburg Institutes* 18 (1955): 67-89. Christian and Moslem representations of fists, figs and open hands, mostly amulets: their history, meaning and use.

____. "Some Spanish Amulets Connected with Lactation." *Folklore* 106 (1951): 430-48.

**HILL, Christopher.**
"William Harvey and the Idea of Monarchy." In *The Intellectual Revolution of the Seventeenth-Century,* ed. by Charles WEBSTER, 160-81. London: Routledge and Kegan Paul, 1974.

**HILLMAN, James.**
*The Thought of the Heart.* Dallas: Spring, 1984. The American director of studies at the C.G. Jung Institute in Zürich writes with erudition and clarity, developing Jung's thought on the heart as it is imagined, as distinct from the heart that scientists describe. "The scientific outlook requires a heart that it sees. The act of demonstration creates what it demonstrates." As Harvey reached into the body of his dogs, he noticed that the heart "may be felt to become harder during its action." Even today it is difficult to imagine a good heart as "hard" or "divided."

**HINTNER, Valentin.**
*Benennungen der Körperteile in Tirol, besonders im Isel-Tale: Ein Beitrag zur Tiroler Dialektforschung.* Vienna: Hoelder, 1879.

**HINTZE, Fritz.**
"Zu den Wörtern für 'Herz' und 'Magen' im Aegyptischen." *Veröffentlichungen des Instituts für Orientforschung.* (Festschrift Grapow) 29 (1955): 140-42.

**HINTZSCHE, Erich.**
"Die Entwicklung der Teratologie seit dem 17. Jahrhundert und ihr Einfluss auf die klinische Medizin." *Clio Medica* 7 (1972): 55-68.

**HIRSCH, Ernst.**
"Der Aberglaube vom guten und bösen Blute in den Waldenserdörfern." In *Forschungen und Berichte zur Volkskunde in Baden-Württemberg, 1971-1973,* ed. by J.HAMPP und P.ASSION, 87-88. Stuttgart: Müller & Gräff, 1973.

zone

**HIRSCHBERG, Julius.**

*Entwicklungsgeschichte der augenärztlichen Kunstausdrücke.* Berlin: Springer, 1917.

**HOEFLER, Max.**

*Deutsches Krankheitsnamenbuch.* Munich: Piloty & Loehle, 1899. The author was a provincial practitioner and avid collector of folk medicine. Here he gathered vernacular, dialectical expressions for body organs, functions and illnesses in humans and animals. A monumental and indispensable route to the "body" in popular culture in the nineteenth century.

____. *Die volksmedizinische Organotherapie und ihr Verhältnis zum Kultopfer.* Stuttgart: Union, 1909. A supplement to the former, contains seventy-one names for plants and herbs.

____. *Volksmedizinische Botanik der Germanen.* Vienna: R. Ludwig, 1908 (Quellen und Forschungen zur Deutschen Volksmedizin 5).

**HOFER, Philip.**

"Some Little-Known Italian Illustrations of Comparative Anatomy, 1600-26." In *Essays in Honor of E. Panofsky,* ed. by M.MEISS, vol. 1, 230-37. New York: New York Univ. Press, 1961.

**HOFFMANN, Gerda.**

"Beiträge zur Lehre der durch Zauber verursachten Krankheiten und ihrer Behandlung in der Medizin des Mittelalters." *Janus* 37 (1933): 129-44, 179-92, 211-17. Medieval medical sources are examined for diseases that are caused by magic.

**HOFFMANN, Karl**

"JB. vanakaksah." *Indo Iranian Journal* 9 (Dordrechts, Netherlands, 1965-66): 99-101. Refers to the etymology of the armpit.

**HOFFMANN, Paul.**

"Féminisme Cartésien." *Travaux de linguistique et de littérature* 7, no. 2 (1969): 83-105.

____. *La femme dans la pensée des lumières.* Strasbourg: Association Publ. Université de Strasbourg, 1976.

**HOFFMANN, Siegfried.**

"Professor Franz Anton Stobler als Gutachter für die Wunderheilungen in Apperdorf: Ein Repräsentant des Barocks im Spannungsfeld von kritischer Diagnose und unkritischer Volksfrömmigkeit." In *Medizinische Diagnostik in Geschichte und Gegenwart.* Festschrift H. GOERKE, ed. by Christa HABRICH, et al. Munich: Fritsch, 1978. A physician and professor of medicine in Ingolstadt retained by church authorities as an expert reports on 366 miraculous healings at the Sanctuary he is supervising, 1742-50.

**HOFFMANN, Walter.**

*Schmerz, Pein, Weh: Studien zur Wortgeographie deutschmundartlicher Krankheitsnamen.* Giessen: Schmitz Verlag, 1956. On pp. 16-29 analysis of words for pricking, cutting, tearing, pressing, biting, cramping pain.

**HOFMANN, Fritz.**

*Der Kirchenbegriff des Hl. Augustins in seinen Grundlagen und in seiner Entwicklung.* Munich: Huber, 1933.

**HOFSTAETTER, Hans H.**

*Symbolismus und die Kunst der Jahrhundertwende.* Köln: Du Mont Schauberg, 1975.

**HOLLANDER, Anne.**

*Seeing Through Clothes.* New York: Viking Press, 1978. Formulates and supports a decisive insight: the experience of one's naked body inevitably implies a reference to clothes. Historically the "inner eye" is pleased only when the clothed self fits the epoch's pictorial convention. Equally, the self-perception of the naked body is based on the pictorial canon of the moment, which in turn is based on the pictorial ideal of the period. For the history of body perception this thesis leads to two insights: first, the percept of the body always implied its wrappings; and second, Hollander distinguishes distinct epochs in the history of clothing: the drapes of Antiquity; the stitched-together rectangles typical, for instance, for the early Middle Ages, and the tailored dress, which first appears in the twelfth century. Distinct kinds of self-perception correspond to these stages in the history of clothing.

**HOLMA, Harry Gustav.**

*Die Namen der Körperteile im Assyrisch-Babylonischen: Eine lexikalisch-etymologische Studie.* Dissertation. Helsinki: Sumalainnen, 1911.

**HOLZINGER, Ernst.**

"Von Körper und Raum bei DUERER und GRUNEWALD." In *Essays in Honor of E. Panofsky,* ed. by M.MEISS, vol. 1, 238-53. New York: New York Univ. Press, 1961. "Bei einem extremen Grad des Körperhaften Sehens kann der Körper ... verschlossen gegenüber dem Raum erscheinen, als stosse er ihn ab." Two models of seeing and representing the body: DUERER creates it as an isolated object, GRUNEWALD as a figure which emerges from and merges in the medium.

**HONEGGER, Claudia.**

"Ueberlegungen zur Medikalisierung des weiblichen Körpers." In *Leib und Leben in der Geschichte der Neuzeit,* ed. by A.E.IMHOF, 203-14. Berlin, 1983.

**HONNINGS, Bonifacio.**

"L'aborto nei libri penitenziali irlandesi: Convergenza morale e divergenze pastorali." In *Una componente della mentalità occidentale: i penitenziali nell' alto medioevo,* ed. by M.G.MUZZARELLI, 155-84. Bologna: Patron, 1980. Useful only as an up-to-date compilation of references to abortion in penitential books.

**HOROWITZ, M.C.**

"Aristotle and Women." *Journal of the History of Biology* 9 (1976): 183-213. "Aristotle's biological, psychological ideas about women parallel his political and ethical ideas about women. Together, these ideas are circular, self-supporting and antifeminist to the core" (p. 210).

**HUBBARD, Ruth, HENIFIN, Mary Sue, FRIED, Barbara, eds.**

*Biological Woman - The Convenient Myth: A Collection of Feminist Essays and a Comprehensive Bibliography.* Cambridge, Mass.: Schenkman, 1982.

**HUBSCHMID, Johannes.**

"Auffällige Ubertragungen von Gegenstaenden und Körperteilen auf Geländeformen." *Revue internationale d'onomastique* 12 (1960): 85-91. Body parts can be used not only as a metaphor for geographic entities, but also as their names.

**HUDSON, I.**

*Bodies of Knowledge: The Psychological Significance of the Nude in Art.* London: Weidenfeld & Nicholson, 1982.

**HUIZINGA, J.**

*The Waning of the Middle Ages: A Study of the Forms of Life, Thought and Art in France and in the Netherlands in the Late Fourteenth and Fifteenth Centuries.* 1924. Repr. New York: St. Martin's, 1984. See ch. 11: "The Vision of Death." The wistfulness of remembrance and the thought of frailty cultivated during the High Middle Ages now demand a new embodiment in the macabre body.

**HUMPHREY, David C.**

"Dissection and Discrimination: The Social Origins of Cadavers in America 1760-1915." *Bulletin of the New York Academy of Medicine* 49 (1973): 819-27.

**HUNZIKER, Heinrich Martin.**

*Die bleiche Hautfarbe in der Sicht des Schweizerdeutschen: Versuch einer sprachinhaltlichen Interpretation von Material aus dem schweizerischen Idiotikon.* Dissertation. Zürich: Juris-Druck, 1966. The material analyzed by the author is the dialect of one region in Switzerland. The meanings, emotions and value judgments involved in the reference to *light skin* are examined, both positive and negative.

**HUTTMANN, Arnold.**

"Eine imaginäre Krankheit: Der Polyp des Herzens." *Medizinhistorisches Journal* 18, nos. 1-2 (1983): 43-51.

**HYRTL, J.**

*Die alten deutschen Kunstworte der Anatomie: Gesammelt und erlaeutert mit Synonymenregister.* Vienna: W. Braumuller, 1884. Repr. Munich: W. Fritsch, 1966. Dictionary of more than 150 German terms, synonym register giving approximate modern equivalents, and a careful discussion of each term.

Many otherwise submerged associations and metaphors come to light in these etymological mini-essays.

# I

**ILLICH, Ivan.**

*Limits to Medicine: Medical Nemesis, the Expropriation of Health.* London: Penguin Books, 1976 (*Die Nemesis der Medizin: Von den Grenzen des Gesundheitswesens.* Reinbek: Rowohlt, 1977).

____. *Gender.* London: Marion Boyars, 1982 (*Genus: Zu einer historischen Kritik der Gleichheit.* Reinbek: Rowohlt, 1983).

____. *H$_2$O and the Waters of Forgetfulness: Reflections on the Historicity of 'Stuff.'* Berkeley: Heyday, 1987. (*H$_2$O und die Wasser des Vergessens.* Reinbek: Rowohlt, 1987).

**IMHOF, Arthur E., ed.**

*Biologie des Menschen in der Geschichte: Zwölf Beiträge zur Sozialgeschichte der Neuzeit aus Frankreich und Skandinavien.* Stuttgart: Frommann-Holzboog, 1978.

____, ed. *Der Mensch und sein Körper: Von der Antike bis heute.* Munich: Beck Verlag, 1983.

____, ed. *Leib und Leben in der Geschichte der Neuzeit.* Berlin: Friedrich Meinecke Institut, 1983 (Berliner Historische Studien. Einzelstudien 2, Bd. 9).

____, ed. *Mensch und Gesundheit in der Geschichte.* Husum: Mathiessen, 1979 (Abhandlungen z. Geschichte d. Medizin u. Naturwissenschaften, 39).

**IMMELMANN, Klaus, IMMELMANN, Thomas.**

"Historische Antropologie aus biologischer Sicht." *Saeculum* 36, no. 1 (1985): 70-79.

# J

**JABERG, Karl.**

"Zu den italienischen und rätoromanischen Namen des Muttermals." *Miscelanea filologica ded. a. A.GRIERA,* 355-66. Barcelona: CSICI, 1955. Notions of (Latin) *macula, signum* and *pica* ( envy or craving) enter into the meaning of "birthmark."

____. "The Birthmark in Folk Belief, Language, Literature and Fashion." *Romance Philology* 10 (1956-57): 307-42. Not only the words used for the "birthmark" but also their spread and meaning are touched upon: superstition, designation, literary function (323ff.) and the artificial beauty spot.

_____. "Krankheitsnamen: Metaphorik und Daemonie." *Schweizerisches Archiv für Volkskunde* 47 (1951): 77-113. Combines linguistic and ethnological method in the analysis of central European expressions or words for body experience that imply a "supernatural" aetiology for the phenomenon: Hexenschuss, Boestier, Grille, Haarwurm, ingrillito, etc.

_____. "Sprache als Aeusserung und Sprache als Mitteilung: Grundfragen der Onomasiologie." *Archiv für das Studium der Neueren Sprachen und Literaturen* 136, no. 71 (1917): 84-123.

**JACKSON, Michael.**
"Thinking Through the Body: An Essay on Understanding Metaphor." *Social Analysis* 14 (1983): 127-49.

_____. "Knowledge of the Body." *MAN* n.s. 18 (1983): 327-45.

**JACOB, Wolfgang.**
*Medizinische Anthropologie im 19. Jahrhundert: Mensch-Natur-Geist. Beitrag zu einer theoretischen Pathologie; zur Geistesgeschichte der sozialen Medizin und allgemeinen Krankheitslehre von Virchow.* Stuttgart: Enke, 1967. Virchow, remembered as a pathologist, statesman and by historians as a revolutionary in 1848, referred to the 'cells' in his own tissue as "tiers état." Many of the analogies now seen between society and human organism have grown from his texts. Jacob focuses on Virchow to explore the transformation in the concept of "nature" during the latter part of the nineteenth century. In his opinion DIEPGEN, SUDHOFF, SIGERIST and even PAGEL have not noticed how far from contemporary conception nature was around 1850 (see p. 11ff.) and therefore have been unable to grasp how the object of modern medicine was brought into being.

**JACOBS, M.**
"Geometry, Spirituality, and Architecture in Their Common Historical Development as Related to the Origin of Neuroses: A Summary." In *The Changing Reality of Modern Man: Essays in Honor of Jan Hendrik VAN DEN BERG*, ed. by Dreyer KRUGER, 62-86. Pittsburgh: Duquesne Univ. Press, 1985.

**JACQUART, Danielle.**
*Le Milieu médical en France au XIIe et au XVe siècle* Geneva: Droz, 1981.

_____ and THOMASSET, C. "Albert le Grand et les problèmes de la sexualité." *History and Philosophy of the Life Sciences* 3 (1981): 73-93.

**JAEGER, W.**
*Diokles von Karystos: Die griechische Medizin und die Schule des Aristoteles.* 2d ed. Berlin: De Gruyter, 1963.

_____. "Greek Medicine as Paideia." In *Paideia: The Ideals of Greek Culture*, by Werner JAEGER, vol. 3,

3-45. New York: Oxford Univ. Press, 1971.

**JAGER, Bernd.**
"Body, House and City: The Intertwinings of Embodiment, Inhabitation and Civilization." In *The Changing Reality of Modern Man: Essays in Honour of Jan Hendrik VAN DEN BERG.* ed. by Dreyer KRUGER, 51-58. Pittsburgh: Duquesne Univ. Press, 1985.

_____. "Of Mouth and Mind: A Psychology of Foundations." In *The Changing Reality of Modern Man: Essays in Honor of Jan Hendrik VAN DEN BERG, ibid.*, 150-60

**JAKOBOVITS, Immanuel.**
*Jewish Medical Ethics: A Comparative and Historical Study of the Jewish Religious Attitude to Medicine and Its Practice.* New York: Bloch, 1959.

**JANNE, Henri.**
"La Lettre de Claude aux Alexandrins et le Christianisme." In *Mélanges F. Cumont*, 273-95. Brussels: Secrétariat de l'Institut, 1936 (Annuaire de l'Institut de philologie et d'histoire orientales et slaves 4). Commentary, calling attention to the early Christian (or Jewish) influence on disease metaphors.

**JANSON, H.W.**
"The Image of Man in Renaissance Art." In *Sixteen Studies*, by H.W.JANSON. New York: Abrams, 1973.

_____. "Observations on Nudity in Neo-classical Art." In *Sixteen Studies.*

_____. *Apes and Ape Lore: In the Middle Ages and the Renaissance.* London: Warburg Institute, 1952.

_____. "The 'Image Made by Chance' in Renaissance Thought." In *Essays in Honor of E. Panofsky*, ed. by M. MEISS, vol. 1, 254-66. New York: New York Univ. Press, 1961.

**JARECKI, Walter, ed.**
*Signa Loquendi: die cluniazensischen Signa-Listen.* Baden-Baden: Korner, 1981 (Saecula Spiritualia 4 ). A detailed comparison of the sign language lists originating in Cluny during monastic silence.

**JAX, Karl.**
*Die weibliche Schönheit in der griechischen Dichtung.* Innsbruck: Wagner, 1933. Images and comparisons with the stars, flowers, morphology of landscape and artifacts.

**JAYNE, Walter Addison.**
*The Healing Gods of Ancient Civilizations.* New Hyde Park, N.Y.: Univ. Books, 1962 (1st ed. 1925).

**JEAY, Madeleine.**
"Albert le Grand entre Aristote et Freud: La femme est-elle un acte manqué?" In *Le racisme: Mythes et sciences: pour Léon POLIAKOV*, ed. by Maurice OLENDER, 1-13. Paris: Editions Complexe, 1981.

**JEGGLE, Utz.**
"Im Schatten des Körpers: Vorüberlegungen zu einer

Volkskunde der Körperlichkeit." *Zeitschrift für Volkskunde* 76, no. 2 (1980): 169-88.

____. *Der Kopf des Koerpers. Eine volkskundliche Anatomie.* Weinheim: Quadriga, 1986.

**JEHL, Rainer.**
*Melancholie und Acedia: Ein Beitrag zu Anthropologie und Ethik BONAVENTURAS.* Paderborn: Schöningh, 1984. pt. 1, sec. 1., pp. 15-90 deals in great detail with Bonaventura's ideas about the "order of the body" and the mixture of elements within it.

**JENSEN, Ad. E.**
"Die mythische Vorstellung vom halben Menschen." *Paideuma* 5 (1950): 23-43.

**JEVREINOV, Nicolai.**
*Die Körperstrafen in der Russichen Rechtspflege und Verwaltung. Beiträge zur Sittengeschichte des vorrevolutionären Russland.* Leipzig,-Vienna: Verlag für Sexualwissenschaft Schneider, 1931. A large sadistic congery of detailed but not properly documented descriptions of bodily punishment throughout Russian history.

**JEWSON, N.D.**
"Medical Knowledge and the Patronage System in Eighteenth-Century England." *Sociology* 8 (1974): 369-85.

____. "The Disappearence of the Sick-Man from Medical Cosmology." *Sociology* 10 (1976): 225-44.

**JOFFE, Natalie F.**
"The Vernacular of Menstruation." *Word: Journal of the Linguistic Circle of New York* 4, no. 3 (1948): 181-86. It appears that where the fact of menstruation is concealed, as among the Irish, the vocabulary is meager. In France and today's U.S. it is vivid and luxuriant, except among groups like Orthodox Jews. P. 185ff. list of expressions.

**JOHNSON, Davis.**
*Blood Policy: Issues and Alternatives.* Washington, D.C.: Institute for Public Policy Research, 1976. Report on a symposium held at a Republican think tank, countering the arguments marshalled by TIT-MUS (1971) against the gathering of human blood on the free market.

**JONAS, Hans.**
*The Phenomenon of Life: Toward Philosophical Biology.* New York: Harper & Row, 1966. Eleven previously published philosophical essays all use the tools of phenomenological description and critical analysis on the originally obscure and implicit knowledge of the author's own "inwardness." Jonas revives and critically reconstructs the Aristotelian idea that existence can be arranged in a hierarchy with nonliving matter at the bottom; merely living "plants" that metabolically interact above this; topped by "animals" free to move through distance and perceive from a distance, but also compelled to do so; and finally man, capable of pur-posely constructing a likeness of reality which then is viewed as a likeness, and not as reality. A careful, critical and lucid philosophy of biology.

**JONES, George Fenwick.**
"The Function of Food in Medieval German Literature." *Speculum* 35 (1960): 78-86.

____. "The Kiss in Middle High German Literature." *Studia Neophilologica* 38, no. 2 (1966): 192-210.

**JORDANOVA, Ludmilla.**
"La donna di cera." *KOS* 1, no. 4 (1984): 82-89. Historical interpretation of anatomical wax models.

____. "Earth Science and Environmental Medicine: The Synthesis of the Late Enlightenment." In *Images of the Earth: Essays in the History of Environmental Sciences*, ed. by L.JORDANOVA and R.PORTER, 121-46. Chalfont, St. Giles: British Society for the History of Science, 1979.

____. "Guarding the Body Politics: Volney's Catechism of 1793." In *Reading Writing Revolution: Proceedings of the Essex Conference on the Sociology of Literature, July 1981*, 12-21. Essex: Univ. Essex, 1982.

____. "Natural Facts: A Historical Perspective on Science and Sexuality." In *Nature, Culture, Gender*, ed. by Carol P. MCCORMACK and Marilyn STRATHERN, 42-69. Cambridge: Cambridge Univ. Press, 1980.

____. "Gender, Generation and Science: William Hunter's Obstetrical Atlas." In *William Hunter and the Eighteenth-Century Medical World*, ed. by W.F.BYNUM and R.PORTER, 385-412. Cambridge: Cambridge Univ. Press, 1985. Mid-eighteenth-century English gynecologists express a new desire with naturalistic visualization and representation of their specimen.

**JOUSSE, Marcel.**
*Le style oral rythmique et mnémotechnique chez les verbo-moteurs.* Paris: Beauchesne, 1925. A Jesuit scholar who spent most of his life in Middle Eastern villages studying the speech of illiterates was the first who sharply differentiated between oral composition and any written arrangement of texts. By his recognition of the "verbo-motoric" origin of pre-alphabetic speech and remembrance he preceded - and probably influenced - the discoveries of Milman PERRY. (Alphabetization of cultures literally leads to a disembodiment of speech, a disembedding from its bodily verbo-motor matrix.)

____. *L'anthropologie du geste.* Paris: Gallimard, 1974. A manuscript finished in 1955, just before the author was struck by a disease from which he died seven years later, published with a twenty-year delay. The author studies the Aramaic *Targum*, Hellenistic and contemporary sayings in order to develop his earlier theory of the verbo-motor (body-based) nature of speech and

z o n e

remembrance. He argues persuasively that pre-alphabetic speech flows essentially from body rhythms which by their very nature (breathing, gestures) are bilateral.

**JUCQUOIS, G.**
"Sur un des mots signifiant 'parler' et 'bouche' en indo-européen." *Museon* 76 (1963): 215-17.

**JUD, Jakob.**
"Acerca de 'ambuesta' y 'almuerza.'" *Revista de filología española* 7 (1920): 339-50. Etymological controversy about words that in Spanish (and Raetho-Roman) designate the cupped or partially folded hands.

**JUILLARD, A., LUNEAU, R.**
"La medicine populaire dans les campagnes françaises aujourd'hui: Bibliographie thématique." *Archives des sciences sociales des religions* 54, no. 1 (1982): 77-83.

**KAEMMERER, Ernst-Wilhelm.**
*Das Leib-Seele-Geist Problem bei Paracelsus und einigen Autoren des 17. Jahrhunderts.* Wiesbaden: Franz Steiner, 1971.

**KAESEMANN, Ernst.**
*Leib und Leib Christi: Eine Untersuchung zur paulinischen Begrifflichkeit.* Tübingen: Mohr, 1933 (Beiträge zur Historischen Theologie).

**KAHANE, Heinrich.**
*Bezeichnungen der Kinnbacke im Galloromanischen.* Dissertation. Berlin, 1932 (Berliner Beiträge zur Romanischen Philologie 2 ).

____. "Die Margariten." *Zeitschrift für Romanische Philologie* 76 (1960): 185-204. "Margarita" - the small finger in Spanish - has a fascinating wealth of other meanings.

____. "Designations of the Cheek in the Italian Dialects." *Language* 17 (1941): 212-22. The ethnographic atlas of Italy and southern Switzerland records 447 equivalents for the Italian 'guancia' ("cheek"), representing twenty types.

**KAISER, Holger.**
*Die Bedeutung des leiblichen Daseins in der paulinischen Eschatologie.* 1974.

**KAMPER, D., WULF, Ch., ed.**
*Der andere Körper.* Berlin: Verlag Mensch und Leben, 1984.

**KANTOROWICZ, Ernst Hartwig.**
*The King's Two Bodies: A Study in Medieval Political Theology.* Princeton: Princeton Univ. Press, 1957.

**KAPFERER, R.**
"Heilentzündung und Heilfieber in den Hippokratischen Schriften." *Hippokrates* 13 (1942): 233-36.

**KASSING, Altfrid Th.**
*Die Kirche und Maria: Ihr Verhaeltnis im 12. Kapitel der Apokalypse.* Düsseldorf: Patmos-Verlag, 1958. Deals with the iconography of the birth-pangs of the woman of the Apocalypse (Revelations 13).

**KAULBACH, F.**
"Leibbewusstsein und Welterfahrung beim frühen und späten Kant." *Kantstudien* 54 (1936): 464ff.

**KEES, H.**
"Herz und Zunge als Schöpferorgane in der aegyptischen Götterlehre." *Studium generale* (1966): 124-26. Heart and tongue respectively are the organs by which Thoth and Horus created the world.

**KELLER, Hans.**
"Lachen und Weinen: Ein Versuch anthropologischer Literaturbetrachtung." *Germanisch-Romanische Monatsschrift* 38 (1957): 309-28.

**KELLERSMANN, Edward.**
*Die geschichtlichen Annahmen über Schwangerschaftsgelüste.* Dissertation. Med. Fak., Kiel 1966.

**KELLY, Henry Ansgar.**
*Love and Marriage in the Age of Chaucer.* Ithaca, New York: Cornell Univ. Press, 1975. Pt. 4 deals with the conflict between norms and practice in relation to lust and passion.

**KEMPF, Roger.**
*Sur le corps romanesque.* Paris: Seuil, 1968.

**KERN, E.**
"Zur Kulturgeschichte des Schmerzerlebnisses." *Hefte zur Unfallheilkunde* 138 (1979): 9-22. Medical reflections on pain and its representation in the past.

**KERN, S.**
*Anatomy and Destiny: A Cultural History of the Human Body.* Indianapolis: Bobbs-Merrill, 1975.

**KESTENBERG, Judith.**
"Outside and Inside, Male and Female." *Journal of the American Psychoanalytic Association* 3 (1968): 457-520.

**KIEFER, Karl.**
*Körperlicher Schmerz auf der attischen Bühne.* Dissertation. Heidelberg: Carl Winters Universitätsbuchhandlung, 1908.

**KILMER, M.**
"Genital Phobia and Depilation." *Journal of Hellenic Studies* 102 (1982): 104-12.

**KING, Lester S.**
"Some Basic Explanations of Disease: A Historian's Viewpoint." In *Evaluation and Explanation in Biomedical Sciences,* ed. by H.T.ENGELHARDT and S.SPICKER, 11-27. Dordrecht, Boston: Reidel, 1975.

**KIRCHNER, Joseph.**
*Die Darstellung des ersten Menschenpaares in der*

*bildenden Kunst von der älteren Zeit bis auf unsere Tage*. Stuttgart: Enke, 1903.

**KIRIGIN, Martin.**
*La Mano Divina nell'iconografia Cristiana*. Rome: Città del Vaticano, 1976 (Studi di Antichità Cristiana: Pontificio Istituto di Archeologia Cristiana 31).

**KLEINMAN, Arthur.**
"The Meaning Context of Illness and Care: Reflections on a Central Theme in the Anthropology of Medicine." In *Science and Cultures*, ed. by E.MENDELSOHN and Y.ELKANA, 161-76. Dordrecht, Boston: Reidel, 1981.
____. "Medicine's Symbolic Reality: On a Recent Problem in the Philosophy of Medicine." *Inquiry* 16 (1973): 206-13. "A cross-cultural perspective on the symbolic, language-centered character with emphasis on the biophysical reality characteristic of Western academic medicine" (RATHER).

**KLIBANSKY, R., SAXL, F., PANOFSKY, E.**
*Saturn and Melancholy: Studies in the History of Natural Philosophy, Religion, and Art*. London: Thomas Nelson, 1964.

**KNETSCHKE, Edeltraut.**
*Genick und Knöchel in der deutschen Wortgeographie: Untersuchungen zur Wortbildung*. Dissertation. Marburg, 1956.

**KNIBIEHLER, Yvonne.**
"Le discours médical sur la femme: constantes et ruptures." *Romantisme* 13-14 (1976): 41-56 (special issue, "Mythes et représentations de la Femme au XIXe siècle").
____. "Les médecins et la 'nature féminine' au temps du Code Civil." *Annales E.S.C.* 31, no. 4 (1976): 424-45. Examines medical encyclopedias and manuals 1780-1830 for the image of women that emerges. The result: by the end of the epoch concerns with "female nature" overshadow all discussion of woman's body; *tota mulier in utero* now means that female nature determines the body, the soul and the person. Finally medical authority can be used to determine the sphere into which woman by nature fits.
____, and FOUQUET, Catherine. *La femme et les médecins*. Paris: Hachette, 1983. The authors are competent historians specializing in the fate of women's image during the eighteenth and nineteenth century. In this volume the authors relate sequentially medical perception of women since the early Egyptian empire in an evolutionist, progressive perspective. Basically the history of the female body that issued from male fears and the demise of these fears.

**KNIGHT, G. Wilson.**
"Soul and Body in Shakespeare." In *Shakespearian Dimensions*, by G.W.KNIGHT, 3-21. Sussex: Harvester Press, 1984.

**KNORTZ, Karl.**
*Der menschliche Körper in Sage, Brauch und Sprichwort*. Würzburg: C. Kabitzsch, 1909.

**KOBUSCH, H.**
*Der Zahnwurmglaube in der deutschen Volksmedizin der letzten zwei Jahrhunderte*. Dissertation. Frankfurt am M., 1955.

**KOCH, Richard.**
*Das Als-Ob im ärztlichen Denken*. Munich: Roesl, 1924 (*Bausteine zu einer Philosophie des Als-Ob*, ed. by Hans VAIHINGER, Raymund SCHMIDT, vol. 8).

**KOEHLER, Reinhold.**
"Die Erde als jungfräuliche Mutter Adams." *Germania* 7 (1862): 476-80. Collection and comparison of texts from Greek, Latin and Middle High German sources establishing the parallel Mary/Jesus = virginal earth/Adam. The earth was a virgin before she had been soaked by rain, tilled by man; before she had swallowed Abel's blood and harbored the first corpse. Adam was shaped by the Creator from this virgin mother.

**KOELBING, H., BIRCHLER, U., ARNOLD, P.**
"Die Auswirkung von Angst und Schreck auf Pest und Pestbekämpfung nach zwei Pestschriften des 18. Jahrhunderts." *Gesnerus* 36 (1979): 116-26.

**KOERNER, Joseph Leo.**
"The Mortification of the Image: Death as a Hermeneutic in Hans Baldung Grien." *Representations* 10 (Spring 1985): 52-101. Death and knowledge are linked in Western tradition, death and the Fall. In Baldung Grien this is central: his images of death are commentaries on the status of the human experience.

**KOLLER, Hermann.**
"Aima." *Glotta* 45 (1967): 149-55. A semiological study of Homeric texts dealing with blood (*haima*) as the juice of life and with the spilling of blood. Greek has no common Indo-Germanic word for blood.
____. "Melos." *Glotta* 43 (1965): 24-38. Etymological ruminations on parallels between the Greek terms for the limbs and music.

**KOTY, J.**
*Die Behandlung der Alten und Kranken bei den Naturvölkern*. Stuttgart: Kohlhammer, 1934. Still the most comprehensive collection of materials reporting on the ways and circumstances in which, throughout history, the old, the sick and the dying have been killed.

**KRANEMANN, Niels.**
"Krüppel und Kropf: eine Wortinhaltsbetrachtung." *Wirkendes Wort* 17 (1967): 12-21.

**KRANZ, Walther.**
"Kosmos." *Archiv für Begriffsgeschichte* 2 ( 1958): 7-113 and 115-282. Report on the state of historical research on the idea of "cosmos."

**KRISS, Rudolf.**

*Das Gebärmuttervotiv: Ein Beitrag zur Volkskunde nebst einer Einleitung über Arten und Bedeutung der deutschen Opfergebräuche der Gegenwart.* Augsburg: Filser, 1929. A toadlike object has been (and is) offered frequently as a votive gift imploring relief or expressing acknowledgment for it. It consistently represents the womb - as the womb and its functions are frequently imagined in the image of a toad. The metamorphoses of this "womb" can be followed, as it torments men and becomes a "crab" (cancer) and as men seek to rid themselves of it by a ritual wedding to a toad.

____, KRISS-HEINRICH, Hubert. "Amulette, Zauberformel und Beschwörungen." In *Volksglaube im Bereich des Islam*, by R.KRISS, and H.KRISS-HEINRICH, vol. 2. Wiesbaden: Otto Harrasowitz, 1962. A major reference for Muslim parallels or origins of post-medieval European superstitions and folk practice.

**KRISS-RETTENBECK, Lenz.**

*Bilder und Zeichen religiösen Volksglaubens.* Munich: Callwey, 1963.

____. "Vorbemerkungen zu einer volkskundlichen Gebildelehre." *Bayerische Blätter für Volkskunde* 7 (1980): 26-40. Following CASSIRER and WEISS-GERBER, KRISS-R. formulates in his lecture the hypotheses that have been adopted by the authors of this bibliography: understanding and perception of the flesh is the result of self-embodiment in expressions and signs, which corresponds to the embodiment of the time- and place-specific environment. Elaborating on A.SCHUETZ and T.LUCKMANN, the author proposes a schema for the ethnological study of physiognomy, posture and gesture that includes neuromotoric activities such as goose pimples, red face, sweat, tears or sneezing and *turgor*.

____. "Probleme der volkskundlichen Gebärdenforschung." *Bayerisches Jahrbuch für Volkskunde* (1964-65): 14-46. This introduction to the ethnography of gesture is unparalleled for two reasons: first, the exceptional philosophical grounding enables the author to define the almost unexplored territory of ethnopsychological research on gesture integrating phenomenological and behavioristic approaches; second, his formation in religious anthropology enables him to map the contributions of over a century to the analysis of meaningful gestures and their representations.

____. *"Feige." Wort-Gebärde-Amulett: ein Volkskundlicher Beitrag zur Amulettforschung.* Dissertation. Phil. Fak. Munich, 1953.

____. *Ex Voto: Zeichen, Bild und Abbild im christlichen Votivbrauchtum.* Freiburg: Atlantis, 1972.

**KRISS-RETTENBECK, Ruth.**

"Am Leitfaden des weiblichen Leibes." *Bayerische Blätter für Volkskunde* 8, no. 3 (1981): 163-82.

**KRISS-RETTENBECK, Ruth, KRISS-RETTENBECK, Lenz.**

"Reliquie und ornamenta ecclesiae im Symbolkosmos der Kirche." In *Ornamenta Ecclesiae: Kunst und Künstler der Romanik*, ed. by A.LEGNER, vol. 3, 19-24. Köln, 1985. Introduction to the magnificently illustrated catalogue of an exposition of Christian cult-related objects. The authors find the key to the understanding of these "sacred objects" of a now bygone age in "the Christian commitment to a mimetic process" - namely resurrection in the body of the incarnate God.

**KRITZMAN, Lawrence.**

"My Body, My Text: Montaigne and the Rhetoric of Sexuality." *Journal of Medieval and Renaissance Studies* 13, no. 1 (1983): 75ff. Montaigne carefully avoids divorcing language from the reality he purports to describe: he seeks to give body to this thought in clear language: to regenerate his flesh through the pleasure of the text.

**KROELL, Heinz.**

"Termes désignant les seins de la femme en portugais." *Orbis* 2 (1953): 19-32.

**KRUECKE, Adolf.**

*Der Nimbus und verwandte Attribute in der frühchristlichen Kunst.* Strasbourg: Heitz, 1905.

**KRUGER, Dreyer, ed.**

*The Changing Reality of Modern Man: Essays in Honor of Jan H. VAN DEN BERG.* Pittsburgh: Duquesne Univ. Press, 1985.

**KUCHENBUCH, Ludolf.**

"Bäuerliches Genus im Frühmittelalter." In *Wider den Turmbau zu Babel*, ed. by Stephan PFUERTNER, 131-146. Reinbek: Rowohlt, 1985.

**KUDLIEN, Fridolf.**

"Antike Anatomie und menschlicher Leichnam." *Hermes* (1969): 78-94.

____. *Der griechische Arzt im Zeitalter des Hellenismus.* Wiesbaden: Steiner, 1979.

____. "The Seven Cells of the Uterus: The Doctrine and Its Roots." *Bulletin of the History of Medicine* 39 (1965): 415-23.

**KUEHN, J.H., ed.**

*Die Diätlehre im frühmittelalterlichen lateinischen Kommentar zu den hippokratischen Aphorismen.* Neustadt A. W., 1981.

**KUEN, H.**

"Beobachtungen an einem kranken Wort." In *Festschrift für Ernst Tappolet*, 185-212. Basel: Schwabe, 1935. Words for "breast" in Ladinic, the dialect spoken in a secluded valley of the Dolomiti.

**KUGELMANN, Robert.**

*The Windows of Soul: Psychological Physiology of the Human Eye and Primary Glaucoma.* London: Associated Univ. Presses, 1982 (Studies in Jungian Thought). For the author twentieth-century culture's image of the body is expressed in the descriptive language of anatomy and physiology. Kugelmann listens to the metaphors of scientific language - "by seeing the world with glaucomatous eyes...he peers into the blind spots of the flesh"; by quoting from medical texts as if they were myths he reconstructs the myth of Glaucos in a new dress.

**KUNTNER, Liselotte.**

*Die Gebärhaltung der Frau: Schwangerschaft und Geburt aus geschichtlicher, völkerkundlicher und medizinischer Sicht.* Munich: H. Marseille, 1985.

**KUNZE, Wolfgang B.F.**

*Krankheitsdaemonen: Daemon und Daemonie. Agents of Disease in German Oral Literature, Custom and Belief.* Dissertation. Los Angeles: Univ. California, 1977.

**KURDZIALEK, Marian.**

"Der Mensch als Abbild des Kosmos." In *Der Begriff der Repräsentatio im Mittelalter: Stellvertretung, Symbol, Zeichen, Bild*, ed. by A.ZIMMERMANN, 35-75. Berlin: De Gruyter, 1971. The definition, taken from Holy Scripture, that man is "omnis creatura" enables medieval philosophers and theologians to interpret the human being along the lines of 'Neoplatonic conceptions: in the whole of man, in his soul as much as in his body, and in his actions, the cosmos is mirrored with its order, its proportions and its harmonies.

**KUSCHE, Brigitte.**

"Zur 'Secreta mulierum'-Forschung." *Janus* 62, nos. 1-3 (1975): 103-23. Text, title, author and reception of this influential treatise.

**KUTZELNIGG, Arthur.**

"Die Verarmung des Geruchswortschatzes seit dem Mittelalter." *Muttersprache* 94, nos. 3-4 (1983-84): 328-45. "Ware," that is commodity, was a term which in German, well into the nineteenth century, referred mainly to merchandise brought from distant places, mostly the colonies. The author of this unusual paper, who died in 1984, was professor of "use-oriented commodity sciences" (Waren-kunde) and concentrated on the historical terminology of commodity designations. The aroma of the commodity until recently was one of its decisive characteristics. Author identifies 158 words in Middle German that designate different smells (and often tastes) which fall into about sixty-two major categories. At best thirty-two of these categories are still recognized, many of them only in local dialects.

**LA BARRE, Weston.**

"The Cultural Basis of Emotions and Gestures." *Journal of Personality* 16 (1947): 49-68 (Repr. in *The Body Reader*, ed. by T.POLHEMUS, 50-68, New York: Pantheon 1978).

**LABISCH, A.**

"Zur Sozialgeschichte der Medizin: Methodologische Ueberlegungen und Forschungsbericht." *Archiv für Sozialgeschichte* 20 (1980): 431-69.

**LACHAL, J.-Cl.**

"Infirmes et infirmités dans les proverbes italiens." *Ethnologie française* 1-2 (1972): 67-96. Proverbs fix and transmit over generations a concrete experience of life: they sometimes originate as quotations from learned sources and more often rise from popular roots, but, once current, they become a mainstay of collective representation. The author culls 367 proverbs referring to illness from forty collections and ten other sources, some in dialects. The list of original quotations is in the appendix.

**LADNER, Gerhart B.**

"The Gesture of Prayer in Papal Iconography of the Thirteenth and Early Fourteenth Centuries." In *Didascaliae: Studies in the Honor of Anselm M. Albareda*, ed. by Sesto PRETE, 245-75. New York: B.M. Rosenthal, 1961.

____. "Medieval and Modern Understanding of Symbolism: A Comparison." *Speculum* 54 (1979): 223-56.

____. "The Concept of the Image in the Greek Fathers and the Byzantine Iconoclastic Controversy." *Dumbarton Oaks Papers* 7 (1953): 1-34.

____. *Ad Imaginem Dei: The Image of Man in Medieval Art.* (Wimmer Lecture 1962) Latrobe, Pa.: Archabby Press (1965).

**LAGET, Mireille.**

"La césarienne, ou la tentation de l'impossible." *Annales de Bretagne* 68, no. 2 (1979): 177-89. During the sixteenth century the cesarean operation emerges from myth into controversial practice, but is performed only after the woman's death. First to baptize the "fetus" while it still might be alive, then to "save" the child. During the seventeenth century it is especially attempted on living women; during the eighteenth century documented instances multiply. A lengthy 1746 description (pp. 184-87) of an operation is discussed. Guide to the scarce secondary literature.

____. *Naissances: L'accouchement avant l'âge de la clinique.* Paris: Seuil, 1982.

zone

____. and LUU, Claudine, eds. *Médecine et chirurgie des pauvres au XVIIIe siècle : d'après le livret de Dom Alexandre.* Toulouse: Privat, 1984.

____. "Childbirth in Seventeenth- and Eighteenth-Century France: Obstetrical Practices and Collective Attitudes." In *Medicine and Society in France*, ed. by R.FORSTER and O.RANUM, 137-76. Baltimore: Johns Hopkins Press, 1981 (orig. *Annales E.S.C.* 1977).

**LAIN ENTRALGO, Pedro.**

*La historia clínica: Historia y teoría del relato patográfico.* Madrid: Consejo superior de investigaciones cientificas, 1950. At the suggestion of TEMKIN the author gathered medical case histories from Hippocrates to von WEIZSAECKER. His primary interest is in the history of the literary genre, he also stresses the changing perception of disease mirrored in these texts.

____. *The Therapy of the Word in Classical Antiquity.* ed. by L.J.RATHER, J.M.SHARP. Foreword by W.ONG, New Haven: Yale Univ. Press, 1970.

**LAMBRECHTS, P., VAN DEN BERGHE, L.**

"La divinité-oreille dans les religions antiques." *Bulletin de l'institut historique belge de Rome* 29 (1955): 177-97. Attempts to interpret the antique steles in North Africa representing an ear.

**LANDY, David, ed.**

*Culture, Disease and Healing: Studies in Medical Anthropology.* New York: Macmillan, 1977.

**LANGAGES (Paris).**

"Pratiques et langages gestuels." 10 (special issue on gesture. June 1968). Note particularly the selective and annotative bibliography by J.KRISTEVA and M.LACOSTE, pp. 132-49.

**LANGE, Klaus.**

"'Geistliche Speise': Untersuchungen zur Metaphorik der Bibelhermeneutik." *Zeitschrift für deutsches Altertum und deutsche Literatur* 95 (1966): 81-122.

**LAPLANTINE, François.**

"La maladie, la guérison et le sacré: Médecines populaires et savantes de la France Contemporaine." *Archives des sciences sociales des religions* 54, nos. 1-2 (1982): 63-83.

**LAQUEUR, Thomas.**

"Bodies, Death, and Pauper Funerals." *Representations* 1, no. 1 (February 1983): 109-31. "How the commemoration of the soul's departure from the body and the body's return to dust became an occasion to represent...the possibility of social worthlessness, earthly failure, and profound anonymity [1750-1850]" (109). The pauper's funeral is analyzed as a "looking glass in which a person's life and his relationship to society could be viewed with a certainty and finality that only death could bring" (120).

____. "Orgasm, Generation, and the Politics of Reproductive Biology." *Representations* 14 (April

1986). Until the Renaissance the anatomical understanding of gender difference was vertical: woman was a less perfect male, having a smaller amount of bodily heat. Her internal organs were an inverted version of the male's. Author follows the demise of this view, prior to new scientific discoveries and attests for the inherently political function of bodily description. The new horizontal polarization of sex differences in the bodies mirrors a social polarization between men and women.

**LAROQUE, F.**

"Images et figurines du grotesque à l'Epoque Elisabéthaine: calendrier, corps, cuisine." *Cahiers Charles V*, no. 2 (1980): 29-39. Methodological reflections on the epistemology of historical body perceptions, based on BAHKTIN.

**LASH, Scott.**

"Genealogy and the Body: Foucault, Deleuze, Nietzsche." *Theory, Culture and Society* 2, no. 2 (1984): 1-17. A social-theoretical analysis of the body. Criticizes FOUCAULT's genealogy of the body as one-sided: by neglecting "desire" which DELEUZE, following Lacan, had stressed, Foucault's "body" becomes a passive result of "discourse."

**LASLETT, Peter.**

"Age at Menarche in Europe since the Eighteenth Century." *Journal of Interdisciplinary History* 2, no. 2 (1971): 221-36.

**LA TORRE, Felice.**

*L'utero attraverso i secoli da erofilo ai giorni nostri: storia, iconografia, struttura, fisiologia.* Città di Castello: Unione Arti Grafiche, 1917. A voluminous (800 page), amply illustrated historical iconography of the womb, mostly but not exclusively from medical sources, especially Italian.

**LAUER, Richard.**

"Ontology and the Body: A Reflection in Organism, Medicine and Metaphysics." In *Organism, Medicine, and Metaphysics: Essays in Honor of Hans JONAS*, ed. by Stuart F.SPICKER. Dordrecht, Boston: Reidel, 1978 (Philosophy and Medicine 7).

**LAWRENCE, C.**

"The Body Culture and Society in Eighteenth-Century Scotland." In *Natural Orders: Historical Studies of Scientific Culture*, ed. by S.SHAPIN and B.BARNES, 19-40. London, Beverly Hills: Sage, 1979.

**LEACH, E.R.**

"Magical Hair." *Journal Royal Anthropological Institute* 88 (1958): 147-61. The seminal paper on hair in social anthropology. Starts from the psychoanalytic assumption of a basic equivalence between hair and male genitals, which makes hair-cutting into an analogue of castration. Though the ethnographer's subject is of a different type than that of the psychoanalyst, the latter can contribute to his understanding of the rituals that are his subject.

**LE BRETON, David.**

"Corps et symbolique sociale." *Cahiers internationaux de sociologie* 73 (1982): 223-32. To be aware is equivalent to transforming the environment into socially coded gestures, and the translation of the sensations thus provoked into meanings. The other person's gestures are experienced as an echo of one's own sensations. If, however, the other is a fool, cripple or monster this correspondence is upset and, with it, one's own bodily balance.

_____. "La symbolique corporelle." *Ethnologie française* 15, no. 1 (1985): 73-78.

**LEBRUN, François.**

*Les Hommes et la mort en Anjou aux 17e et 18e siècles: Essai de démographie et de psychologie historique.* Paris: Mouton, 1971. Ch. 11 (pp. 391-415) deals with the meaning attributed to disease (God's will, result of magic), recourse to faith and/or superstition, the sanctuary, conjurer or witch. Only during the eighteenth century, and then only for a minority, the local church tries to enlighten the prevalent magical view, which can only be overcome at the cost of an abolition of most of the church's own beliefs and practices.

**LECHNER, Gregor Martin.**

*Maria Gravida: zum Schwangerschaftsmotiv in der bildenden Kunst.* Munich: Schnell-Steiner, 1981 (Münchner Kunsthistorische Abhandlungen 19). An exhaustive and well-illustrated study of the Virgin Mary represented as a pregnant woman, with many references to the representation of pregnancy and a large bibliographic apparatus.

**LECLERCQ, Jean.**

"La dévotion médiévale envers le Crucifié." *La maison Dieu* 75 (1964): 119-32.

_____. "Le Sacré Coeur dans la tradition bénédictine au Moyen Age." *Cor Jesu Roma* 11 (1959): 3-28.

_____. "S. Bernard et la dévotion médiévale envers Marie." *Revue d'Ascétique et de Mystique* 30 (1958): 361-75.

Monastic (especially Cistercian) piety in the twelfth century expressed itself unashamedly in metaphors, analogies and expressions recalling the body. Arguably the ascetic, mystical and epistolary literature of that age is a much richer source for the history of body perceptions than the contemporary medical texts. Jean Leclercq's almost innumerable contributions to monastic history of that period provide trustworthy guidance.

**LEDER, D.**

"Medicine and Paradigms of Embodiment." *Journal of Medicine and Philosophy* 9 (1984): 29-43.

**LEFEVRE, A.**

"La blessure du côté." *Etudes Carmélitaines* (special issue: "Le coeur"). Paris, 1950.

**LE GOFF, J., LE ROY LADURIE, E.**

"Mélusine maternelle et défricheuse." *Annales E.S.C.* 26, no. 3-4 (1971): 587-622.

**LEGRAIN, Michel.**

*Le corps humain: Du soupçon à l'évangélisation.* Paris: Centurion, 1978.

**LEGROS, Elisée.**

"Les maladies portant le nom du saint guérisseur." *Enquêtes du Musée de la Vie Wallone* 5 (1948): 90-119. In France of the ancien régime, doctors were known to be powerless in the face of certain diseases (màs d'sints) which were the domain of specific saints. Three dozen patron saints, sanctuaries and attributes are discussed.

**LEMAY, Helen Rodnite.**

"Human Sexuality in Twelfth- through Fifteenth-Century Scientific Writings." In *Sexual Practices and the Medieval Church*, ed. V.L.BULLOUGH and J. BRUNDAGE, 187-205. Buffalo, New York: Prometheus Books, 1982. Discussion of "virginity," "sexual proclivities," "illegitimate progeny," "sterility," "coitus" and "orgasm" as they are treated in Latin texts which are mainly translations from Arabic medicine.

_____. "The Stars and Human Sexuality: Some Medieval Scientific Views." *Isis* 71 (1980): 127-37. Astrology was an integral part of that Arabic scientific corpus that shaped Western intellectual and medical thought during the thirteenth century. According to the authoritative *centiloquium* (Cairo, ninth century) the stars determine each man's attraction (to black women), proclivity (woman to woman), preference (on coarse blanket of goat's hair), destiny (man changes into woman), behavior (adulterous inclination). Western astrologers were extremely wary of falling into the trap of determinism (unlike a mule, man is free under the reign of the stars). Thus philosophers and physicians could look for "cures" of sexual predisposition.

**LENHARDT, Friedrich.**

"Zur Ikonographie der Blutschau." *Medizinhistorisches Journal* 17, no. 1-2 (1982): 63-77.

**LEPENIES, Wolf.**

*Das Ende der Naturgeschichte: Wandel kultureller Selbstverständlichkeiten in den Wissenschaften des 18. und 19. Jahrhunderts.* Frankfurt: Suhrkamp, 1976.

_____. "Naturgeschichte und Anthropologie im 18. Jahrhundert." *Historische Zeitschrift* 231 (1980): 21- 41.

**LERCH, Eugen.**

"Die sprachliche Sexualisierung der Sachen: Eine sprachphilosophische Betrachtung." *Westermanns Monatshefte* 85 (1941): 286-288.

**LEROI-GOURHAN, André.**
"Les mains de Gargas: Essai pour une étude d'ensemble." *Bulletin de la société préhistorique française* 64 (1967): 107-22.

____. *Le geste et la parole*: Vol 1: *Technique et Langage*, Vol. 2: *La mémoire et les rythmes*. Paris: Albin Michel, 1964-65.

____. *Evolution et techniques: Milieu et techniques*. Rev. ed. Paris: Albin Michel, 1973.

**LE ROY LADURIE, Emmanuel.**
"L'aiguillette." In *Le territoire de l'historien*, by E. LE ROY LADURIE, vol. 2, 136-49. Paris: Gallimard, 1977 ("The Aiguillette: Castration by Magic." In *The Mind and Method of the Historian*, 84-96. Chicago: Univ. Chicago Press, 1981). Through the symbolic tying up of natural powers, impotence or sterility can be magically inflicted. Spread and forms of this belief, and apotropaic measures.

____. *Montaillou, village occitan de 1294-1324*. Paris: Gallimard, 1975 (*Montaillou: The Promised Land of Error*. New York: Random House, 1979). See especially ch. 8 (gestures and sex), chs. 11-13 (marriage, childhood and aging) and ch. 20 (magic).

____. "Famine Amenorrhoea (17th-20th century)." In *Biology of Man in History. Selections from the Annales E.S.C.*, ed. by R.FORSTER and O.RANUM, 163-78. Baltimore: Johns Hopkins Press, 1975.

**LESCHHORN, Maria-Lisa.**
*Die syntaktische Darstellung von Körperteilen im Englischen: Studien zum Grenzgebiet von Syntax und Semantik*. Frankfurt: Peter Lang, 1973.

**LESKY, Erna.**
*Die Zeugungs- und Vererbungslehren der Antike und ihr Nachwirken*. Wiesbaden: Steiner, 1950 (Akademie der Wissenschaften u. d. Literatur. Abhandlungen der Geistes-und Sozialwissenschaftlichen Klasse 19. 1950).

**LEVY, A.**
"Evaluation étymologique et sémantique du mot 'secret'." *Nouvelle revue de psychanalyse* 14 (1976).

**LEVY, Mervin.**
*The Moons of Paradise: Some Reflections on the Appearance of the Female Breast in Art*. London: Arthur Barker, 1962.

**LHERMITTE, Jacques J.**
*L'image de notre Corps*. Paris, 1939.

**LIDEN, Evald.**
"Zur alten tieranatomischen Terminologie." *Zeitschrift für vergleichende Sprachforschung* 61 (1934): 14-28. Traditional terms for animals' innards and afterbirths.

**LINEBAUGH, Peter.**
"The Tyburn Riots against the Surgeons." In *Albion's Fatal Tree: Crime and Society in Eighteenth Century England*, ed. by Douglas HAY et al., 65-111. New York: Pantheon, 1975. A respectful treatment of the dead was a profound and explicit concern of early eighteenth-century crowds, also when the corpse was that of a criminal. The Crown (which granted the bodies of the condemned felons to anatomy) regarded their dissection not from the viewpoint of science but as a means to dishonor the "scum of the people." In a lively way the article documents the attitudes toward the corpse and survival which underlay this conflict.

**LIPPE, Rudolf zur.**
*Naturbeherrschung am Menschen*. Vol. 1: *Körpererfahrung als Entfaltung von Sinnen und Beziehungen in der Aera des Italienischen Kaufmannskapitals*. Vol. 2: *Geometrisierung des Menschen und Repräsentation des Privaten im französischen Absolutismus*. 2d rev. ed. Frankfurt: Syndikat, 1981. One part of this thesis makes a significant and original contribution to body history: the section which treats the methods used under French Absolutism to interiorize the perception of the Cartesian three-dimensional, totally visual space: a new kind of fencing, in which opponents conceive of their movements as circumscribed within an imaginary globe, a new kind of dancing, and, for the commoners, a new kind of military drill, in which the loading and shooting of the recruit's rifle is broken down into 168 successive movements

____. "Wiederbegegnung der Industriegesellschaft mit dem Körper." *Neue Sammlung* 20, no. 4 (1980).

**LLOMPART, Gabriel.**
"Longitudo Christi Salvatoris: una aportación al conocimiento de la piedad popular catalana medieval." *Analecta sacra tarraconensia* 40 (1967): 1-23. Focuses on Catalan instances of a devotional practice that is widespread in all of Europe: the cutting of a belt or string to the length of a sacred object, which is worn by pregnant women as a belt (cintura, en-cinta). The name of this object is "length of Christ" and Llompart explores the meaning given to it: involvement of the pregnant woman in the "Incarnation."

**LLOYD, G.E.R.**
"Right and Left in Greek Philosophy." *Journal of Hellenic Studies* 82 (1962): 56-66. Also in *Right and Left: Essays on Dual Symbolic Classification*, ed. by Rodney NEEDHAM, 167-86. Chicago: Univ. Chicago Press, 1973.

____. *Magic, Reason and Experience: Studies in the Origin and Development of Greek Science*. Cambridge: Cambridge Univ. Press, 1979.

____. *Polarity and Analogy: Two Types of Argumentation in Early Greek Thought*. Cambridge: Cambridge Univ. Press, 1966. A large number of the theories in early Greek thought belong to one of two simple logical types: first, objects are classified by being likened or assimilated to something, and second, objects are explained by their relation to one or another of a pair of opposite principles. Lloyd studies the steps which led to the formulation of the principle of contradiction, the law of excluded middle, the recognition of degrees of similarity. This evolution coincides historically with the dis-embedding of the "soma" in contrast with the world.

____. *Science, Folklore and Ideology: Studies in the Life Sciences in Ancient Greek*. Cambridge: Cambridge Univ. Press, 1983.

____. "The Hot and the Cold, the Dry and the Wet in Greek Philosophy." *Journal of Hellenistic Studies* 84 (1964): 92-106. Explores the stages in which binary oppositions came to correspond to preconceived notions of value - especially in Aristotle. The view that males are hotter than females depends on the notion that semen and menses are the end products of strictly comparable processes. Aristotle's view that males are hot depends on his arbitrary value judgment decision that woman is a deformed man, and semen the natural product of concoction while menses are the impure residue.

**LOCK, Margaret.**
"L'homme machine et l'homme microcosme: l'approche occidentale et l'approche japonaise des soins médicaux." *Annales E.S.C.* 35, no. 2 (1980): 1116-36.

**LOCKER, David.**
*Symptoms and Illness: The Cognitive Organization of Disorder*. London, New York: Tavistock, 1981. Argues that illness is a social phenomenon constituted by the meaning actors employ to make sense of observed or experienced events. Thesis explored by means of case studies. An approach to the sociology of illness that tries to move beyond Parson's theory of the sick-role, the study of illness behavior and labelling theory.

**LOCKER, Ernst.**
"Etre et avoir: Leurs expressions dans les langues." *Anthropos* 49 (1954): 481-510. This article is important for body history, because subtle but important changes have been observed in the use of possessive expressions in regard to the body ("my" body). Locker suggests cultural and anthropological differences that are expressed and supported by the register of possibilities which language affords to express the "copula" (i.e. the "is"-statement) of the sentence. Some languages can do without a special word - the tone of voice indicates it. Others can express the copula with (something akin to) a personal pronoun. The predominance of the verbal copula is a characteristic of Indo-Germanic languages, which makes the distinction between the "have" and "is" sentence so important. Locker (p. 501ff.) suggests the evolution of "imperialist tendencies" in relation to all reality based on this verbal copula and its evolution.

**LODOLO, Gabriella.**
"Il segno della Donna nel medioevo." *Aevum* (Milan) 3-4 (1976): 348-56.

**LOEFFLER, Joseph.**
*Die Störungen des geschlechtlichen Vermögens in der Literatur der autoritativen Theologie des Mittelalters: Ein Beitrag zur Geschichte der Impotenz und des medizinischen Sachverständigenbeweises im kanonischen Impotenzprozess*. Wiesbaden: Steiner, 1958 (Akademie der Wissenschaften und der Literatur. Abhandlungen der Geistes- und Sozialwissenschaftlichen Klasse Jg. 6 1958).

**LOEFSTEDT, Bengt.**
"Bemerkungen zum Problem Genus: Sexus im Lateinischen." *Symbolae Osloenses* (Oslo) 38 (1963): 47-68.

**LOHFF, Brigitte.**
"Zur Geschichte der Lehre von der Lebenskraft." *Clio Medica* n.s.16, 2-3: 101-12. Discusses how the notion of "Lebenskraft" disappears from scientific physiology and terminology in the beginning of the nineteenth century.

**LOPEZ AUSTIN, Alfredo.**
*Cuerpo humano e ideología: Las concepciones de los antiguos Nahuas*. 2 vols. México: Instituto de Investigaciones Antropológicas, 1980. All preserved Nahuatl (Aztec) texts that refer to the body are gathered and examined and their metaphorical use is explored. However, the author gives the impression that the Nahuas spoke essentially about the tables of our anatomical atlas, even though its organs and functions carried a different meaning.

**LORAUX, Nicole.**
*Tragic Ways of Killing a Woman*. Cambridge, Mass.: Harvard Univ. Press, 1987.

**LOT BORODINE, Myrrha.**
"Le mystère du 'don des larmes' dans l'orient chrétien." Supplément à la *Vie Spirituelle* (1936): 65-110.

**LOTTIN, Odon.**
*Psychologie et Morale aux XIIe et XIIIe siècles*. Louvain: Abbaye du Mont César, 1942-1960. A monumental study of largely unpublished sources: learned controversies on psychological and moral issues in the late twelfth century. Vol. 2/1 deals largely with the ethical status of involuntary or unintentional "movements of the flesh" (*motus primo primi*).

**LOUDON, G.B. ed.**
*Social Anthropology and Medicine*. New York: Academic Press, 1976.

**LOUDON, J.S.L.**
"Leg Ulcers in the Eighteenth and Early Nineteenth Century." *Journal of the Royal College of General Practitioners* 31 (1981): 263-73 and 32 (1982): 301-09.

**LOUX, Françoise, ed.**
*L'homme et son corps dans la société traditionelle: Catalogue d'une exposition, Musée national des arts et traditions populaires*. Paris, 1978.

____. *Le corps. Pratiques et savoirs populaires dans la*

z o n e

*société traditionelle*. With a foreword by
J.CUISINIER. Paris: Berger-Levrault, 1979.

____. "Pratiques médicales préventives et recours
religieux." *Archives des sciences sociales des religions* 44,
no. 1 (1977): 45-58.

____, and PETER, Jean-Pierre. "Présentation:
Langages et images du corps." *Ethnologie française* 6,
nos. 3-4 (1976): 215-18.

____, and RICHARD, Ph. "Alimentation et maladie
dans les proverbes français: un exemple d'analyse de
contenu." *Ethnologie Française* 2, 3-4 (1972): 267-86.
Based on seven thousand regional proverbs. Many
bespeak analogies between specific plants, modes of
preparation and time of ingestion with body perceptions.

____. *Sagesse du corps: La Santé et la maladie dans les
proverbes régionaux français*. Paris: Maisonneuve &
Larose, 1978.

**LOYOLA, Maria Andrea.**
*L'esprit et le corps: Des thérapeutiques populaires dans
la banlieue de Rio*. Paris: Maison des Sciences de
l'Homme, 1983. Pp. 121-29 concepts of the body.

**LUCE, Gay Gaer.**
*Body Time*. New York: Pantheon. 1981. Now dated,
but a best-seller in 1972. Collates what was then
known about bodily time perception in a technocratic
perspective.

**LUCIE-SMITH, Edward.**
*The Body: Images of the Nude*. London: Thames &
Hudson, 1981.

**LUERS, Grete.**
*Die Sprache der Deutschen Mystik des Mittelalters im
Werke der Mechthild von Magdeburg*. Munich:
Einhardt, 1926. Very rich and sensitive study of symbolism and metaphor in the commentary to the Song
of Songs by an exceptionally feminine mystic of the
mid-thirteenth century. The first half of the book
places her writings within a tradition, the last two hundred pages order and comment passages under about
three dozen key words, among which many body-
terms: ouge (129), atem (131), bloz (143), brennen
(147), "connubium" (160), hant (194), kosen-kuss
(208), man (226), mark (228), spiegel (245), sweben,
smilzen, swimmen, smeken, sugen (248-260), vliezen
(278-285).

**LURKER, Manfred.**
*Der Kreis als Symbol im Denken, Glauben und
künstlerischen Gestalten der Menschheit*. Tübingen:
Rainer Wunderlich 1981. A symbolic-anthropological
study of symbols. Pp. 145-74: the human figure and
the circle.

**MAASS, Ernst.**
"Eunuchos und Verwandtes." *Rheinisches Museum für
Philologie* n.f. 74 (1925): 432-76. About two dozen
terms from the Greco-Latin terminology of castration
are examined.

**MABILLE, Pierre.**
*La construction de l'homme*. Paris: J. Flory, 1936.

**MacCORMACK, Carol P.**
"Biological Events and Cultural Control." *SIGNS* 3,
no. 1 (1977): 93-100.

**MacDONALD, Michael.**
*Mystical Bedlam. Madness, Anxiety and Healing in
Seventeenth-Century England*. Cambridge: Cambridge
Univ. Press, 1981.

____. "Anthropological Perspectives on the History of
Science and Medicine." In *Information Sources in the
History of Science and Medicine*, ed. by P.CORSI and
P.WEINDLING, 61-80. London: Butterworth
Scientific, 1983.

**MACH, Ernst.**
*Space and Geometry in the Light of Physiological,
Psychological and Physical Inquiry*. La Salle: Open
Court Publ., 1960.

**MacKINNEY, Loren.**
*Medical Illustrations in Medieval Manuscripts*.
Berkeley: Univ. California Press, 1965. One hundred
reproductions from the author's collection of four
thousand microfilms of medically relevant miniatures.

**MacLEAN, Ian.**
*The Renaissance Notion of Women: A Study in the
Fortunes of Scholasticism and Medical Science in
European Intellectual Life*. Cambridge: Cambridge
Univ. Press, 1980. What is the relationship between
the notion of women and that of sex difference, and
how is sex difference related to other differences?
Examines the Aristotelian and scholastic *loci communi*
from legal, medical, mystical and ethical sources: certainties about women's inferiority, limited humanity,
bodily incompleteness fade during the Renaissance.
Yet "the difference of sex continues to retain the association of deprivation," and acquires greater promi-
nence in discourse. Chapter 3 (pp. 47-68) on medicine
describes the gradual shift from "woman as an imperfect male" toward a "sexual, functional view of
women's distinct nature."

**MacRAE, Donald G.**
"The Body and Social Metaphor." In *The Body as a
Medium of Expression*, ed. by J.BENTHALL and

z o n e

T.POLHEMUS, 59-73. London: A. Lane, 1975. "For our purposes the body exists only in so far as it is known and experienced..., like metaphors, it has its being in society and history" (p. 63).

**MAERTENS, Jean-Thierry.**
*Dans la peau des autres: essai d'anthropologie des inscriptions vestimentaires*. Paris: Aubier, 1978.
____. *Le corps sexionné*. Paris: Aubier, 1978. An essay on the ritual mutilation of genital organs and its possible meaning in the twentieth century.
____. *Les dessins sur la peau: Essai d'anthropologie des inscriptions tégumentaires*. Paris: Aubier, 1978.

**MAGIN, N.**
*Ethos und Logos in der Medizin: Das anthropologische Verhältnis von Krankheitsbegriff und medizinischer Ethik*. Freiburg, Munich: Alber Verlag, 1981. A 1980 version of a phenomenology of disease initiated by German anthropological medicine in the thirties, with the first major bibliography (pp. 318-37) to this often forgotten tradition. In a major chapter on the history of nosology the usual approach is turned topsy-turvy. What view about the patient has been shaped and propagated by successive disease conceptions? What are the relationships between an epoch's view of disease and its ethics?

**MAHR, August C.**
"Anatomical Terminology of the Eighteenth-Century Delaware Indians: A Study in Semantics." *Anthropological Linguistics* 2, no. 5 (1960): 1-65. Explores the assumptions that are reflected in the contrast between two ways of naming and thus grasping the body: Algonquin versus Greco-Roman.

**MAIER, W.**
*Das Problem der Leiblichkeit bei Jean Paul Sartre und Maurice Merleau-Ponty*. Tübingen: Niemeyer, 1964.

**MAIRE, Catherine-Laurence.**
*Les convulsionnaires de Saint-Médard: Miracles, convulsions et prophéties à Paris au XVIIIe siècle*. Paris: Gallimard (Collection Archives), 1985.

**MAJER, Eberhard.**
*Mensch- und Tiervergleich in der griechischen Literatur bis zum Hellenismus*. Dissertation. Tübingen, 1949.

**MAJNO, Guido.**
*The Healing Hand: Man and Wound in the Ancient World*. Cambridge, Mass.: Harvard Univ. Press, 1975. A lavishly produced and illustrated book on the wound throughout history, as a modern doctor visiting the past sees it. Useful mainly because of the artwork and the quotations, and despite the lack of historical perspective.

**MAJUT, Rudolf.**
"Zur Geschichte der Verzehrwörter im Englischen: Vom Altenglischen bis zum Beginn der Neuzeit." *Germanisch-Romanische Monatsschrift* 54 n.f. 23

(1973): 423-49. The choice of the verb with which a human activity is referred to can imply a profound interpretation of the body. In Old English *fretan* (in German "fressen") - in oppositon of *etan*, to eat - implied an activity which is common to man and beast. It soon connoted eating too much; connoted then eating what is due to others; and finally ceased to refer to nourishment (where it was substituted by *devour*) and was used only metaphorically.

**MALLARDO, Domenico.**
"L'incubazione nella cristiana medievale napoletana." *Analecta Bollandiana* 57 (1949): 465-98. The healing sleep in the temple of Antiquity has a medieval parallel around Naples. Sources are reproduced and studied: the disease, circumstances and events.

**MALOTKI, Ekkehart.**
*Hopi-Raum: Eine sprachwissenschaftliche Analyse der Raumvorstellungen in der Hopisprache*. Dissertation. Tübingen: Narr, 1978.

**MALTEN, Ludolf.**
*Die Sprache des menschlichen Antlitzes im frühen Griechentum*. Berlin: De Gruyter, 1961. The "eye" (face, facies, visus) expressed the "soul" or something from the inside of the looking person until science discovered it as a receptive organ. The author analyzes the meaning of what the oval of the face does in Greek epic, lyric, dramatic and philosophical writings.

**MANDROU, Robert.**
"L'homme physique: santé, maladies, 'peuplades'." In *Introduction à la France Moderne 1500-1640. Essai de psychologie historique*. Paris: Albin Michel, 1974. Mandrou was one of the first professional historians to call attention to the historicity of the very mode of perception of the sense organs (historicity of smell or taste perception), and that of the concepts and categories with which the social historian organizes past biological facts. However, Mandrou's reflections on this subject are dispersed throughout his work. (See esp. ch. 2, pp. 55-74.)

**MANN, Gunther.**
"Exekution und Experiment: Medizinische Versuche bei der Hinrichtung des Schinderhannes." *Lebendiges Rheinland-Pfalz* 21, no. 2 (1984): 11-16.
____. "Medizinische-naturwissenschaftliche Buchillustration im 18. Jahrhundert in Deutschland." *Marburger Sitzungsberichte* 86, nos. 1-2 (1964): 3-48. Introduction to the evolution of German anatomical etchings 1650-1780 with good illustrations. Follows the transition to "increasing realism."
____. "Gesundheitswesen und Hygiene in der Zeit des Uebergangs von der Renaissance zum Barock." *Medizinhistorisches Journal* 2 (1967): 107-23.
____. "Joseph Furttenbach, die ideale Stadt und die Gesundheit im 17. Jahrhundert." In *Medizingeschichte in unserer Zeit. Festgabe für Edith Heischkel-Artelt und*

*Walter Artelt zum 65. Geburtstag*, ed. by H.H.EUL-
NER et al., 189-207. Stuttgart: Enke, 1971.
____. "Medizin der Aufklärung: Begriff und
Abgrenzung." *Medizinhistorisches Journal* 1 (1966): 63-
74.

**MANSELLI, Raoul.**
"Vie familiale et éthique sexuelle dans les pénitentiels."
In *Famille et parenté dans l'occident médiéval*, ed. by
G.DUBY and J.LE GOFF, 363-78. Rome: Ecole
Française de Rome, 1977.

**MANULI, Paola.**
"Fisiologia e Patologia del Femminile negli Scritti
Ippocratici dell' Antica Ginecologia Greca."
*Hippocratica: Actes du Colloque hippocratique de Paris*,
4.-9.Sept. 1978, ed. by M.D.GRMEK, 393-408. Paris:
CNRS, 1980.
____. *Medicina e antropologia nella traditione antica*.
Turin: Loescher, 1980.
____. "Elogio alla castita: La ginecologia di Sorano."
*Memoria* (Turin) 3 (March 1983): 39-49. The broad
tradition from Hippocrates well into the eighteenth
century attributes to the womb a double metaphor: it
is the womb as the furrow or a wild roaming beast, in
need of being filled like a vessel by the male and in
need of being quieted down by male touch. In the
author's reading Soranus stands outside this tradition:
the discharges of blood, of fetus and the intercourse
upset woman's balance, remove her from the human
ideal she shares with men. Thus, Soranus recommends
to women abstention and chastity.
____, and VEGETTI, Mario. *Cuore, sangue e cervello:
biologia e antropologia nel pensiero antico*. Milan:
Episteme, 1977. With growing oligarchy in the Greek
polis, an encephalocentric (brain centered) view of the
body tended to replace the cardiocentric image. An
analysis of body perception as a mirror of political
thought and constellation.

**MARAGI, M.**
"Le glossaire latino-allemand d'anatomie de Wala-
fridus STRABO (IXème s.)." In *27th International
Congress of the History of Medicine, Barcelona 1980*,
204-14. Barcelona, 1981.

**MARCOVICH, Anne.**
"Concerning the Continuity between the Image of
Society and the Image of the Human Body: An
Examination of the Work of the English Physician J.C.
Lettsom 1746-1815." In *The Problem of Medical
Knowledge*, ed. by P.WRIGHT and A.TREACHER,
69-87. Edinburgh: Edinburgh Univ. Press, 1982.

**MARITAIN, Jacques.**
*Quatre essais sur l'esprit dans sa condition charnelle*.
Paris: Desclée de Brouwer, 1939. Neo-Thomist philosophical reflections on *corporeality* and *incarnation* at
their best.

**MARROU, Henri-Irénée.**
*L'ambivalence du temps de l'histoire chez Saint
Augustin*. Montréal, Paris: Vrin, 1950. Augustine of
Hippo belongs to the small number of thinkers who
have left a profound imprint on the evolution of the
Western body perception. This is reflected in the
recent growth of studies on the subject. Though
Marrou has dealt with the body in Augustine only here
and there (e.g., pp. 24-27), his opus puts the newer
studies into perspective.

**MARSELLA, Anthony.**
"Depressive Experience and Disorder across
Cultures." *Handbook of Cross-Cultural Psychology* 5
(1980): 237ff. Non-Western people generally do not
label depression as a "psychological" experience. They
perceive it "only" in somatic terms. As a consequence,
it is less common and less severe and leads less frequently to suicide.

**MARTIN, Emily.**
"Pregnancy, Labor and Body Image in the United
States." *Social Science and Medicine* 19.2, no. 11
(1984): pp. 1201-06. Looking for metaphors presup-
posed in ordinary language, Martin examines women's
image of their own body during pregnancy. Marked
sense of separation of self from the parts of the body,
passive stance that ascribes changes in the body to
"happening," events produced by and in an "involuntary muscle," namely the uterus.
____. *The Woman in the Body: A Cultural Analysis of
Reproduction*. Boston: Beacon Press, 1987. What do
medical textbooks teach about menstruation, menopause and childbirth and what do women know about
this? An illustration of science's incarnation in contemporary American women's minds and entrails.

**MARTIN, L.**
"The Gesture of Looking in Classical History
Painting." *History and Anthropology* 1, no. 1
(November 1984): 175-92.

**MARTINO, Ernesto de.**
*Morte e pianto rituale: Dal lamento funebre antico al
pianto di Maria*. Turin: Universale Scientifica Boringhieri, 1983 (orig. publ. 1958). A classic study on
gestures of grief and special-body awareness in the
face of a corpse.

**MAURER, Friedrich.**
*Leid: Studien zur Bedeutungs- und Problemgesch-
ichte besonders in den grossen Epen der Staufischen
Zeit*. Munich: Francke Verlag, 1951 (Bibliotheca
Germanica 1).

**MAUSS, Marcel.**
"Les Techniques du corps." *Journal de Psychologie* 32,
nos. 3-4 (1936) ("Body Techniques," in *Sociology and
Psychology: Essays*, by M.MAUSS, 95-123. London:
Routledge and Kegan Paul, 1979). The seminal article

by which half a century of social-science research on the body has been influenced. Every society has its way of sitting and walking, standing and swimming. Polynesians do not swim like us, and my generation does not swim like that of today. As obvious and central as these facts are, ethnology has treated them under the rubric "varia." When writing this article Mauss complained that his colleagues treated him as an outsider, because he made this congery of observations into the object of his discipline.

**MAUZI, Robert.**

"Les maladies de l'âme au XVIIIe siècle." *Revue des sciences humaines* 100 (1960): 459-93.

**MAYOR, A. Hyatt.**

*Artists and Anatomists.* New York: Metropolitan Museum Publ., 1984.

**MAZZI, Maria Serena.**

*Salute e società nel Medioevo.* Florence: La Nuova Italia, 1978. The special aspects of "health" during the Middle Ages are the theme of the book. Disease is studied as a mass-phenomenon, and defined by projection of modern categories into medieval Italy.

**McDANIEL, Walton Brooks.**

*Conception, Birth and Infancy in Ancient Rome and Modern Italy.* Lancaster, Penn.: Business Press, 1948. Analyzes the survival of age-old folk practices: PLINY in contemporary Italy.

_____. "The Medical and Magical Significance in Ancient Medicine of Things Connected with Reproduction and Its Organs." *Journal History of Medicine* 3 (1948): 525-46.

**McKEON, Richard.**

"Medicine and Philosophy in the Eleventh and Twelfth Centuries: The Problem of Elements." *The Thomist* 24 (1961): 211-56. The problem of "elements" which make up the whole (body) is seen as the counterpart of the problem of "universals." Questions about the universals arose from the opposition of different conceptions of logical and scientific method. Questions about elements arose in the opposition of different interpretations of data. The author deals with the alternating stress on the two positions: well documented on the opposition of twelfth-century pre-scholastic concern with "elements" of the body.

**McLAREN, Angus.**

"Doctor in the House: Medicine and Private Morality in France 1800-50." *Feminist Studies* 2, nos. 2-3 (1975): 39-54.

_____. *Reproductive Rituals: The Perception of Fertility in England from the Sixteenth Century to the Nineteenth Century.* London, New York: Methuen, 1984.

_____. "The Pleasures of Procreation." In *William Hunter and the Eighteenth-Century Medical World*, ed. W.F.BYNUM and R.PORTER. Cambridge:

Cambridge Univ. Press, 1985.

**McLAUGHLIN, Eleanor.**

"'Christ My Mother': Feminine Naming and Metaphor in Medieval Spirituality." *Nashotah Review* 15, no. 3 (Fall 1975): 228-48.

**McVAUGH, Michael.**

"The 'Humidum radicale' in Thirteenth-Century Medicine." *Traditio* 30 (1974): 259-83. Classical Antiquity developed the concept of "radical moisture" to explain how the flame of life is extinguished in fevers, and in old age. Author deals with the fate of this motif during the twelfth and thirteenth centuries.

**MEAD, George Robert Stow.**

*The Doctrine of the Subtle Body in Tradition: An Outline of What Philosophers Thought and Christians Taught on the Subject.* Wheaton, Ill.: Theosophical Publ. House, 1967.

**MEEKS, Wayne A.**

"The Image of the Androgyn: Some Uses of a Symbol in Earliest Christianity." *History of Religions* 13 (1973): 165-208. Conclusion: "an extraordinary symbolization of the Christian sense of God's eschatological action in Christ proved too dangerously ambivalent for the emerging church. After a few meteoric attempts to appropriate its power, the declaration that in Christ there is no more male and female faded into innocuous metaphor."

**MEHL, Erwin.**

"Zur Fachsprache der Leibesübungen." *Muttersprache* (1954): 240-42, 299-302, 396-97. Deals explicitly with the technical terminology of sports and its evolution during the last 150 years. But the ample bibliography makes this article a good starting point for the evolution of body perceptions.

**MELCHIORRE, Virgilio, CASCETTA, Annamaria, eds.**

*Il corpo in scena: La rappresentazione del corpo nella filosophia e nelle arti.* Milan: Vita e Pensiero Publ. Università Cattolica, 1978.

**MEMORIA.**

*Rivista di storia delle donne* 3 (special issue, "I corpi possibili") (Turin, 1982).

**MENARD, Michèle.**

*Une histoire des mentalités religieuses aux 17e et 18e siècles: Mille retables de l'ancien diocèse du Mans.* Foreword Pierre CHAUNU. Beauchesne, 1980. Reconstruction of religious mentalities from an analysis of one thousand figurative contemporary (seventeenth and eighteenth c.) paintings that are still preserved within one French diocese.

**MERCHANT, Carolyn.**

*The Death of Nature: Women, Ecology and the Scientific Revolution.* San Francisco: Harper & Row, 1980. A history of the perception of nature in science, from Plato to the nineteenth century. Highly relevant

zone

for body history are the references to the theme that compares earth and womb.

**MERCIER, Roger.**

"Image de l'autre et image de soi-même dans le discours ethnologique." *Studies on Voltaire* 154 (1976): 1417-35. The novel and the travelogue into exotic lands are complementary documents of the eighteenth century's search for an image of the self, which stands in contrast to the very different other.

**MERINGER, Johannes.**

"Das Blut in Kult und Glauben der vorgeschichtlichen Menschen." *Anthropos* 71 (1976). A survey of the literature that deals with the perception, ritual uses and representation of blood - human or animal - in prehistoric times.

**MERINGER, Rudolf.**

"Indogermanische Pfahlgötzen: Alche, Dioskuren, Asen." *Wörter und Sachen* 9 (1924-26): 107-23. Wood-related names for certain Gods, and wood metaphors for the body.

____. "Lat. cucurbita ventosa, ital. ventosa, franz. ventouse-'Schröpfkopf'." *Wörter und Sachen* 4 (1912): 177-97. Venesection and cupping were an almost universal custom. The words and instruments used in the beneficial bleeding lead to the archeology of blood.

____. "Omphalos, Nabel, Nebel." *Wörter und Sachen* 5 (1913): 43-49. Collection of beliefs and customs related to the umbilical cord.

____. "Spitze, Winkel, Knie im ursprünglichen Denken." *Wörter und Sachen* 11 (1928): 114-23, 143.

**MERKT, Josef.**

*Die Wundmale des Heiligen Franziskus von Assisi.* Leipzig, Berlin: Teubner, 1910.

**MERLEAU-PONTY, M.**

*L'oeil et l'esprit.* Paris: Gallimard, 1964 ("Eye and Mind." In *The Primacy of Perception*, ed. by J.M. EDIE, 159-90. Evanston, Ill.: Northwestern Univ. Press, 1964).

____. *Phénoménologie de la perception.* Paris: Gallimard, 1945 (*Phenomenology of Perception*. Rev. ed. by Colin SMITH. Atlantic Highlands, N.J.: Routledge and Kegan Paul). The leading French phenomenologist grounds his theory of knowledge (in contrast to his teacher HUSSERL) on the perception of bodily behavior that results from a stimulus.

**MESSER, Ellen.**

"Hot-Cold Classification: Theoretical and Practical Implications of a Mexican Study." *Social Science and Medicine* 15B (1981): 133-45. Makes a point (from ethnography) that is crucial for any history of "humors": structural principles of a hot-cold (or other binary classification) can be shared and their cosmological referents can remain analogous while contents vary. Discusses research from Mexico and Asia, how hot-cold serves as a "major idiom for discussing moral,

social, ritual states in addition to qualities of food and medicine."

**MEYER, Ahlrich.**

"Mechanische und organische Metaphorik politischer Philosophie." *Archiv für Begriffsgeschichte* 13 (1969): 128-99. Metaphors for society as "body" or as "machine", esp. in Hobbes, Rousseau, Fichte, Schelling, Hegel and Marx.

**MEYER, A.W.**

"The Elusive Human Allantois in Older Literature." In *Science, Medicine and History: Essays in the Evolution of Scientific Thought and Medical Practice, Written in Honor of Ch. Singer*, ed. by A.UNDERWOOD, vol. 1, 510-20. London: Oxford Univ. Press, 1953.

**MICHL, J.**

"Der Weibes-Samen in Gen. 3,15 in spätjüdischer und frühchristlicher Auffassung." *Biblica* 33 (1952): 371ff. and 476ff. The "seed of Eve" in Genesis 3 influenced Christian ideas about descent.

**MILANESI, Claudio.**

"Tra la vita e la morte: Religione, cultura popolare e medicina nella seconda meta del '700." *Quaderni storici* 50 (1982): 615-28.

**MILES, Margaret, R.**

*Augustin on the Body.* Missoula, Mont.: Scholars Press, 1979 (Am. Academy of Religion, Diss. Series 31).

**MILLER, David L.**

"Womb of Gold, Body of the Sun: Reflections on Christian Imagery of the Virgin and the Moon." In *Images of the Untouched*, ed. by Gail THOMAS and Joanne STROUD. Dallas: Spring, 1982.

**MILLER, Jonathan.**

*The Body in Question.* New York: Vintage Books, 1978. The book came out of the author's commission for a television series on the history of medicine. Modern knowledge - this is the thesis of the book - came about through the application of models and metaphors from the outer world onto the body. "The most impressive contribution to the growth of intelligibility has been made by the application of suggestive metaphors."

**MILNER, Max.**

*La fantasmagorie.* Paris: Presses Universitaires de France, 1982. The author's opus forever returns to the spectral and specular bodies that appear within a transfigured perceptive universe of French fantastic literature.

____. "Le sexe des anges: De l'ange amoureux à l'amante angélique." *Romantisme* 11 (1976): 55-67. During the late twenties of the last century, the theme of love between human and angel acquires importance in romantic poetry and prose (BYRON, T. MOORE). Author believes that a new articulation between "body" and "desire" is implied.

**MITTERER, A.**

"Mas occasionatus oder zwei Methoden der Thomas-Deutung." *Zeitschrift für katholische Theologie* 72 (1950): 80-103. Aristotle first propounded that woman is the result of a not-quite-successful ensoulment of seminal matter. Aquinas picked up this idea and influenced half a millennium. Mitterer gathers and interprets the key texts and the history of their transmission.

_____. "Mann und Weib nach dem biologischen Weltbild des Hl. Thomas und dem der Gegenwart." *Zeitschrift für katholische Theologie* 57 (1933): 491-556.

**MOECKEL, Marla Johanna.**

*Die verbalen Bezeichnungen für physiologische Reflexe wie Atmen, Husten, Niesen, Schnarchen usw. im Französischen.* Dissertation. Leipzig, 1922.

**MOHR, R.**

"Der Tote und das Bild des Todes in den Leichenpredigten." In *Leichenpredigten als Quelle historischer Wissenschaften,* ed. by R.LENZ, 82-121, Köln, Vienna: Böhlau, 1975.

**MOELK, Ulrich.**

"Ange femme und donna angelo: Ueber zwei literarische Typen des weiblichen Engels." *Romanisches Jahrbuch* 25 (1974): 139-53.

**MONSACRE, Hélène.**

"Weeping Heroes in the *Iliad*." *History and Anthropology* 1 (1984): 57-75. By studying the language of sorrow (images and comparisons, "biology" of tears, gestures) it is possible to show that in epics men do not mourn and weep as women do. Their suffering is more active and displays more vigor. The virile ideology of the *Iliad* coins new masculine expressions of men's grief. Tears are one of the constituents of the warrior's heroic nature.

**MORAVIA, Sergio.**

"From 'Homme machine' to 'Homme sensible': Changing Eighteenth-Century Models of Man's Image." *Journal of the History of Ideas* 39 (1978): 45-60.

**MOREAU, Thérèse.**

*Le Sang de l'Histoire: Michelet: l'histoire et l'idée de la Femme au XIXe s.* Paris: Flammarion, 1982.

**MOREL, Louis.**

*De vocabulis partium corporis in lingua Graeca metaphorice dictis.* Dissertation. Leipzig: Fick, 1875.

**MORRIS, J.**

*Blood, Bleeding and Blood Transfusion in Mid-Nineteenth-Century American Medicine.* Dissertation. Tulane Univ., 1973.

**MORRIS, L.**

"The Biblical Use of the Term 'Blood'." *Journal of Theological Studies* n.s. 3 (1952): 216-27. Introduces a controversy: does the biblical use of the term "blood" usually evoke "death"?

**MOSEDALE, Susan S.**

"Science Corrupted: Victorian Biologists Consider The Woman Question ." *Journal of the History of Biology* 11, no. 1 (1978): 1-55. The social prejudice that determines biological observation and theory about women: H.SPENCER, E.D.COPE, P.GEDDES, J.FINOT.

**MOSS, Donald.**

"Brain, Body and World: Perspectives on Body Image." In *Existential Phenomenological Alternatives for Psychology*, ed. by Ronald S.VALLE and Marc KING, 73-93. New York: Oxford Univ. Press, 1978. An introduction to the use of "body image" as a technical term in psychology, particularly in the school of MERLEAU-PONTY.

**MOSSE, George.**

*Nationalism and Sexuality: Respectability and Abnormal Sexuality in Modern Europe.* New York: Howard Fertig, 1985.

**MOULE, L.**

"Glossaire vétérinaire médiéval." *Janus* 18 (1913): 265-331 and 40 (1936): 49-64; 95-98; 218-32. A careful search for expressions that deal with animal pathology written before 1500, with quotations for each term. The 1936 articles deal with the veterinary vocabulary during the sixteenth century.

**MOULIN, Daniel de.**

"A Historical-Phenomenological Study of Bodily Pain in Western Man." *Bulletin of the History of Medicine* 48 (1974): 540-70. Algophobia (fear of pain) is a characteristically modern evil. "Are we conceivably observing an increase in pain as such? An increase in the painfulness of pain?" Author asks that question against a selection of texts documenting pre-Cartesian pain-experience and the physician's attitudes toward it.

**MOULINIER, Louis.**

*Le pur et l'impur dans la pensée des Grecs d'Homère à Aristote.* Paris: Klincksieck, 1952. A high degree of critical detachment is necessary in order to penetrate early Greek thought on purity and impurity: impurity neither correlates with modern perceptions of it, nor is it comparable to the sense of impurity attested to in the Old Testament in the fifth or even fourth century B.C. The author of this learned and penetrating study cannot find even one Hellenistic text testifying to belief in impure animals, impurity that arises from intercourse, impurity of women during menses, impurity that derives from contact with strange Gods or inherited impurity. Nor is there any reason to project "primitive" mentalities onto classical Greece. Impurity for the Greek affects the murderer, child and mother following birth, the adulterer and those who touch or even look at a corpse. It affects the whole moral person - it has nothing to do with a modern "soul."

**MUCH, Rudolf.**
"Holz und Mensch." *Wörter und Sachen* 1 (1909): 39-48. Men can be made out of different wood, they might be wood-headed, blockheaded, strong like an oak. Author discusses the similes likening men and wood in Germanic dialects.

**MUCHEMBLED, Robert.**
"Le corps, la culture populaire et la culture des Elites en France (XVe-XVIIIe siècle)." In *Leib und Leben in der Geschichte der Neuzeit*, ed. by A.E.IMHOF, 141-53. Berlin, 1983.

_____. "La femme au village dans la région du Nord (XVIIe-XVIIIe siècles)." *Revue du Nord* 63, no. 250 (1981): 585-93.

**MUELLER, Carl.**
*Volksmedizinisch-geburtshilfliche Aufzeichnungen aus dem Lötschental.* Stuttgart: Huber, 1969.

**MUELLER, Gottfried.**
"Wortkundliches aus mittelenglischen Medizin-büchern." *Britannica: Max Foerster zum 60. Geb.* 145-54. Leipzig: Tauchnitz, 1929.

**MUELLER, Heidi.**
"Erhaltung und Wiederherstellung der Körperlichen Gesundheit in der traditionellen Gesellschaft." In *Der Mensch und sein Körper von der Antike bis heute*, ed. by A.E.IMHOF, 157-80. Munich: Beck, 1983.

**MUELLER, Irmgard.**
"Krankheit und Heilmittel im Werk Hildegards von Bingen." In *Hildegard von Bingen 1179-1979: Festschrift zum 800. Todestag der Heiligen*, ed. by A.Ph. BRUECK, 311-49. Mainz: Mittelrheinische Kirchengemeinde. 1979.

**MUELLER, Joseph.**
"Zur Geschichte des Wortes 'Haupt' in den fränkischen Mundarten." *Zeitschrift für Mundartforschung* (1918): 161-69.

**MUELLER, Karl.**
"Aus dem erotischen Wortschatz der deutschen Mundarten sowie älterer deutscher Literatur." *Anthropophyteia* 8 (1911): 1-21.

**MUELLER-HESS, Hans-Georg.**
*Die Lehre von der Menstruation vom Beginn der Neuzeit bis zur Begründung der Zellenlehre.* Berlin, 1938 (Repr. Kraus, 1977) (Abhandlungen zur Geschichte der Medizin u. d. Naturwissenschaften 27). Dated, but still useful as a repertory of medical opinions on menstruation (fifteenth-nineteenth c.).

**MULLERHEIM, Robert.**
*Die Wochenstube in der Kunst: Eine Kulturhistorische Studie.* Stuttgart: Enke, 1904.

**MURARD, Lion, ZYLBERMAN, Patrick, eds.**
*L'haleine des Faubourgs: Ville, habitat et santé au XIX siècle.* Paris: La Recherche, 1977.

_____. "La raison de l'expert ou l'hygiène comme science appliquée." *Archives européennes de Sociologie* 26 (1985): 58-89.

**MURDOCH, John E.**
*Album of Science.* Vol. 1: *Antiquity & the Middle Ages.* New York: Scribner, 1984. Illustrations in chs. 15, 17, 18 and 23 give a broad survey of the styles and forms in which the human body was represented. Each picture is accompanied by a detailed commentary as to the mental and social background.

**MURKO, Matija.**
"Die Schröpfköpfe bei den Slaven: bana, banka, lat. balnea." *Wörter und Sachen* (Heidelberg) 5 (1913): 1-42. In the Slavic dialects many words tell of glasses, horns, pots and jars that have been used in bloodletting. Through a wordfield study the author shows great regional differences in bloodletting and bathing.

**MUTH, R.**
*Träger der Lebenskraft: Ausscheidungen des Organismus im Volksglauben der Antike.* Vienna: Rohrer, 1954.

**MUTHMANN, Friedrich.**
*Mutter und Quelle: Studien zur Quellenverehrung im Altertum und im Mittelalter.* Basel: Archäologischer Verlag, 1976. The motif of Mother/Source in literature and art in Western cultures is explored in encyclopedic fashion (Italy, Greece, Asia Minor). The last quarter of the book (pp. 347-447) deals with Mary and the Source.

# N

**NAHOUM, Véronique.**
"La belle femme: ou le stade du miroir en histoire." *Communications* (Paris) 32 (1979): 22-32.

**NARDI, Enzo.**
*Procurato aborto nel mondo greco-romano.* Milan: Ed. Giuffre, 1971. At present the definitive survey on attitudes to abortion in Antiquity. DICKISON (see entry) detects "pro-life" prejudice in the author.

**NARTEN, Johanna.**
"Idg. 'Kinn' und 'Knie' im Avestischen zanauua, zanudrajah-." *Indogermanische Forschungen* 74 (1969-70): 39-53. The words studied in ancient Persian denote gestures of contempt, in which the tongue and the knee are likened.

**NATH, Bhupendra.**
"Significance of Suffering in Gandhi's Ethics." *Gandhi Marg* 66 (Sept. 1984): 475-82.

**NEEDHAM, Joseph.**
*A History of Embryology.* Cambridge: Cambridge Univ. Press, 1959.

**NEEDHAM, Rodney, ed.**

*Right and Left: Essays on Symbolic Classification.* Chicago: Univ. Chicago Press, 1973.

_____. *Circumstantial Deliveries.* Berkeley: Univ. California Press, 1981. See ch. 2: "Physiological symbols": "Each symbolic tradition, considered at the level of the particular, speaks to itself..." about the body; yet the different traditions rely on a common repertory of symbolic components. Physiological factors may be responsible for the unconscious selection of these symbolic vehicles, such as the predominance of the right; the prevalence of white-black-red over other colors; the use of percussion to gain access to the spirit world.

**NEUBURGER, Max.**

*The Doctrine of the Healing Power of Nature: Through the Course of Time.* New York, 1932 (Repr. Philadelphia: Porcupine Press).

_____. *Die Lehre von der Heilkraft der Natur im Wandel der Zeiten.* Stuttgart, 1926.

**NEUHEUSER, B.**

"Eucharistie in Mittelalter und Neuzeit." In *Handbuch der Dogmengeschichte*, ed. by A.SCHMAUS and A. GRILLMEIER, vol. 4, Freiburg: Herder, 1963.

**NICCOLI, Ottavia.**

"'Menstruum quasi monstruum': parti mostruosi e tabu' mestruale mestruale nel '500." *Quaderni storici* 44 (1980): 402-28. The birth of the idea that intercourse during the menstrual period leads to the conception of a monster can be traced to the second part of the sixteenth century. Three converging motifs merge in this idea: belief in menstrual impurity, the replacement of the medieval "fantastic" monster (belief in monstrous races) by the realistic obstetric monster, and the theological disputations about the need to baptize monsters.

**NIEBYL, P.H.**

"The Nonnaturals." *Bulletin of the History of Medicine* 45 (1971): 486-92.

_____. *Venesection and the Concept of the Foreign Body.* Dissertation. Yale, 1969.

**NIEDERMANN, Max.**

"Zum Namen des Zeigefingers in den indogermanischen Sprachen." *Beiträge zur Kunde der Indogerm. Sprachen* 26 (1901): 231-32.

**NIEDERWOLFSGRUBER-INSAM, Irma.**

"Die Frau und ihr Lebensbereich im Bergdorf Serfans, Tirol: Ein Beitrag zur Wortforschung." In *Germanistische Abhandlungen*, ed. by K.K.KLEIN, E. THURNER. 299-304. Innsbruck: Sprachwissenschaftl. Institut d. Universität, 1959.

**NOBIS, H.M.**

"Die Umwandlung der mittelalterlichen Naturvorstellung: Ihre Ursachen und ihre wissenschaftsgeschichtlichen Folgen." *Archiv für Begriffsgeschichte* 13, no. 1 (1969): 34-57.

**NOONAN, John T.**

*Contraception: A History of Its Treatment by the Catholic Theologians and Canonists.* Cambridge, Mass: Harvard Univ. Press, rev. ed. 1986. On the theme stated in the title this study has remained unsurpassed. The first part of the book brilliantly summarizes the impact of Christianity on classical perceptions of genital activity.

**NORTH, Christopher R.**

*Suffering Servant in Deutro-Isaiah: A Historical and Critical Study.* 2d ed. Oxford: Oxford Univ. Press, 1956.

**OAKLEY, Ann.**

*The Captured Womb: A History of the Medical Care of Pregnant Women.* Oxford: Basil Blackwell, 1984.

**OBEYESEKERE, Gananath.**

*Medusa's Hair: An Essay on Personal Symbols and Religious Experience.* Chicago: Univ. Chicago Press, 1981. The "subjectification" of images and symbols through the private experience of public cults legitimates individual action, but does not objectify it. Many very odd bodily phenomena that result from possession, trance or ecstasy in Sri Lanka lead the author to this thesis.

_____. "The Impact of Ayurvedic Ideas on the Culture and the Individual in Sri Lanka." In *Asian Medical Systems: A Comparative Study*, ed. by Charles LESLIE, 201-26. Berkeley: Univ. California Press, 1976.

**O'BROWN, Norman.**

*Love's Body.* New York: Random House, 1966.

**OENNERFORS, Alf.**

"In columellae librum octavum annotatiunculae." *Eranos acta philologica suecana* 52 (1954): 217-23.

_____. *In medicinam Plinii studia philologica: De memoria et verborum contextu opusculi, de elocutione aevo conceptum est.* Lund: Gleerup, 1963.

**OETTERMANN, Stephan.**

*Zeichen auf der Haut: Die Geschichte der Tätowierung in Europa.* Frankfurt: EVA/Syndikat, 1985.

**O'FLAHERTY, Wendy D.**

*Women, Androgynes and Other Mythical Beasts.* Chicago: Univ. Chicago Press, 1980.

**OHLY, Friedrich.**

"Deus Geometra: Skizzen zur Geschichte einer Vorstellung von Gott." In *Tradition als historische Kraft: Festschrift für Karl HAUCK*, 1-42. Berlin, 1981.

____. *Diamant und Bocksblut: Zur Traditions- und Auslegungsgeschichte eines Naturvorganges von der Antike bis in die Moderne*. Berlin: E. Schmidt, 1977.

____. "Cor Amantis non angustum: Vom Wohnen im Herzen." In *Schriften zur mittelalterlichen Bedeutungsforschung*, F.OHLY, 128-55. Darmstadt: Wissenschaftliche Buchgesellschaft 1977. Twelfth-century language develops a new grasp on the image, a new power to make believe that the metaphor actually corresponds to reality. Ohly illustrates in this article how as a result the "heart" is actually understood as a space that can accommodate the beloved.

____. *Hohelied-Studien: Grundzüge einer Geschichte der Hohenliedauslegung des Abendlandes bis um 1200*. Wiesbaden: F. Steiner, 1958. Half of all the classical Christian commentaries on the Song of Songs were written between the mid-eleventh and the early thirteenth century (about three dozen are here examined). The kiss of the Shulamite is a prominent feature in almost every instance, and an important and complex evolution of its nature and meaning can be observed during this century.

**OHM, Thomas.**
*Die Gebetsgebärden der Völker und das Christentum*. Leiden: E. J. Brill, 1948. Written by a Benedictine missiologist. Dated, but still the most thorough survey of gestures used in prayers and the conflict of their interpretation within their own tradition and by Christians upon first contact with a new religion.

**OKSAAR, Els.**
"Die sprachliche Erfassung des menschlichen Körpers am Beispiel des Estnischen." *Zeitschrift für vergleichende Sprachforschung* (Göttingen) 73 (1955): 45-51. A non-Indo-Germanic language, Estonian, is examined to see differences in the naming of body parts ("head," "neck and back," "limbs"). The Estonians do not "shoulder" heavy burdens. There is no word for this part between neck and back. They speak of "turi," a part that is meant to carry, but it is unlike the Indo-Germanic classifications of the anatomy of the "back."

**O'MALLEY, Charles D., SAUNDERS, J. B., eds.**
*LEONARDO, On the Body*. New York: Dover, 1983.

**O'MEARA, Carra Ferguson.**
"In the Hearth of the Virginal Womb: The Iconography of the Holocaust in Late Medieval Art." *Art Bulletin* 63 (March 1981): 75-88.

**O'NEIL, Mary R.**
"Sacerdote ovvero strione: Ecclesiastical and Superstitious Remedies in Sixteenth-Century Italy." In *Understanding Popular Culture*, ed. by Steven KAPLAN, 53-83. New York, Berlin: Mouton, 1984.

**ONGARO, Giuseppe.**
"Evoluzione delle conoscenze sul liquido amniotico." *Episteme* 8, nos. 2-4 (1974): 290-309. The history of medical views on the amniotic fluid since Galen. The relevant passages from Fabrici and Harvey are cited in full. Good bibliography for the seventeenth to the nineteenth centuries.

**ONIANS, Richard Broxton.**
*The Origins of European Thought about the Body, the Mind, the Soul, the World, Time and Fate*. Cambridge: Cambridge Univ. Press, 1951, repr. 1988.

**OPPENHEIMER, Jane M.**
"Reflections on Fifty Years of Publications on the History of General Biology and Special Embryology." *Quarterly Review of Biology* 50 (1975): 373-87.

**ORBE, A.**
*Antropología de Sant'Ireneo*. Madrid: La Editorial Catolica, 1969. Theological study of an early Church Father who seriously reflected on the nature of "the flesh."

**OSTEN, Gert von der.**
*Der Schmerzensmann: Typengeschichte eines deutschen Andachtsbildwerkes von 1300 bis 1600*. Berlin, 1935 (Forschungen zur deutschen Kunstgeschichte 7). Iconographic study on the transformation in the representation of Christ's pained and suffering body during the Renaissance and Reformation in Germany.

**OTIS, Leah.**
"Une contribution à l'étude du blasphème au bas Moyen Age." In *Diritto comune e diritto locale nella storia dell'Europa: Atti del convegno di Varenna, 12-15. Giugnio 1979*, 213-23. Milan: Giuffre, 1980.

**OTT, Sandra.**
"Aristotle among the Basques: The 'Cheese-Analogy' of Conception." *MAN* n.s. 14 (1979): 699-711. As rennet curdles the milk to form cheese, so male semen curdles women's blood to shape the fetus. Ott discusses the equivalence between ideas about conception, the sexual division of labor, notions of male and female "procreativity" and cultural transvestism in the Basque village of St. Engrâce. Important for the analogies between body percept and social percept.

# P

**PACHINGER, A.M.**
*Die Mutterschaft in der Malerei und Graphik*. Munich, Leipzig, 1906.

**PAGEL, Walter.**
"Religious Motives in the Medical Biology of the Seventeenth-Century." *Bulletin of the History of Medicine* 3 (1935).

____. *William Harvey's Biological Ideas: Selected Aspects and Historical Background*. New York, Basel: Hafner, 1967.

____. "The Position of Harvey and Van Helmont in the History of European Thought." *Journal of the History of Medicine and Allied Sciences* 13, no. 2 (1958): 186-99.

**PANOFSKY, Erwin.**
"The History of the Theory of Human Proportions as a Reflection of the History of Styles." In *Meaning in the Visual Arts*, E.PANOFSKY, 55-107. Garden City, N.Y.: Doubleday, 1955.

____. Artist, Scientist, Genius: Notes on the "Renaissance Dämmerung." In *The Renaissance: Six Essays*, by W.K.FERGUSON et al., 121-83. New York: Harper & Row, 1962.

**PARAVY, Pierrette.**
"Angoisse collective et miracles au seuil de la mort: Résurrections et baptêmes d'enfants morts-nés en Dauphiné au XVème siècle." In *La mort au Moyen Age: Actes du colloque des historiens médiévistes français réunis à Strasbourg 1975*, 87-102. Colmar: Ed. Istra, 1977. Analysis of recorded miracles in two sanctuaries in central France. The thaumaturgical power of these sanctuaries revives stillborn infants. A vivid description of the bodily signs of this early resurrection. Resurrection lasts at least long enough to baptize the child.

**PARK, K., DASTON, L.J.**
"Unnatural Conceptions: The Study of Monsters." *Past and Present* 92 (1981): 20-54.

**PARKER, Robert.**
*Miasma: Pollution and Purification in Early Greek Religion*. Oxford: Clarendon Press, 1983.

**PAULI, Carl.**
*Ueber die Benennungen der Körperteile bei den Indogermanen*. Berlin: Dümmler, 1867.

**PEIL, Dietmar.**
*Die Gebärde bei Chrétien, Hartmann und Wolfram*. Munich: Fink Verlag, 1975 (Medium Aevum. Philologische Studien 28). From the description of gestures in three Middle High German authors their evolution is studied, as well as their changing significance. Careful attention to body symbolism. Excellent bibliography.

**PELLICER, André.**
*Natura: Etude sémantique et historique du mot Latin*. Paris: Presses Universitaires de France, 1966. With great frequency the body as object of experience is referred to as "human nature." This is a detailed historical-semantic study of the multiple traditions within which this term has been transmitted from Latin into contemporary languages.

**PEREIRA, Michela.**
"Maternità e sensualità femminile in Ildegarda di Bingen: Proposte di lettura." *Quaderni storici* 44 (1980): 564-79. Perceptive commentaries to complete passages of relevant texts from Hildegard's opus which are quoted according to the Migne Edition.

**PERELLA, Nicholas J.**
*The Kiss, Sacred and Profane: An Interpretative History of Kiss-Symbolism and Related Erotic Themes*. Los Angeles: Univ. California Press, 1969. The only monographic attempt to follow the evolution of the kiss throughout Western history: both the iconography of the gesture and the significance attributed to it.

**PERROT, Philippe.**
*Les dessus et les dessous de la bourgeoisie*. Paris: Fayard, 1981. A cultural history of underwear in the nineteenth century when the intricate covering up of the body was of prime importance.

____. *Le travail des apparences: Ou les transformations du corps féminin XVIIIe - XIXe siècle*. Paris: Seuil, 1984.

**PETER, Jean-Pierre.**
"Entre femmes et médecins: Violence et singularités dans les discours du corps et sur le corps d'après les manuscrits médicaux de la fin du XVIIIe siècle." *Ethnologie française* 6, nos. 3-4 (1976): 341-48.

____. "Le corps du délit." *Nouvelle revue de psychanalyse* 3 (1971): 71-108.

____. "Le grand rêve de l'ordre médical en 1770 et aujourd'hui." *Autrement* 4 (1975-76): 183-92.

____. "Les médecins et les femmes." In *Misérable et glorieuse - la femme du XIXe siècle*, ed. by Jean-Paul ARON, 79-100. Paris: Fayard, 1980.

____. "Les mots et les objets de la maladie: Remarques sur les épidémies et la médecine dans la société française de la fin du XVIIIe siècle." *Revue historique* 499 (1971): 11-38.

____. "Malades et maladies à la fin du XVIIIe siècle." In *Médecins, climat et épidémies à la fin du XVIIIe siècle*, ed. by J.P.DESAIVE et al., 135-70 Paris: Mouton, 1972 ("Disease and the Sick at the End of the Eighteenth-Century," in *Biology of Man in History*, ed. by R.FORSTER and O.RANUM, 81-124. Baltimore: Johns Hopkins Press, 1975).

____, and REVEL, Jaques. "Le corps: L'homme malade et son histoire." In *Faire de l'histoire*, ed. by J.LE GOFF, P.NORA, vol. 3, 169-91. Paris: Gallimard, 1974. One of the rare contributions of two major French social historians to the epistemology of the "body" as a category used in history. They argue that the discipline has not yet come to the point at which the body itself can be explored as a past experience. The historian is tempted to colonize the past with body concepts elaborated by social sciences on the basis of twentieth-century thought.

**PETERS, D.**
"The Pregnant Pamela: Characterization and Popular Medical Attitudes in the Eighteenth Century." *Eighteenth-Century Studies* 14, no. 44 (1981): 432-51.

**PETERSEN, Erik.**

*Pour une théologie du vêtement.* Lyon: Coll. La Clarté-Dieu, 1943.

**PETTINATO, G.**

*Das altorientalische Menschenbild und die sumerischen und akkadischen Schöpfungsmythen.* Heidelberg: Winter, 1971.

**PEZA, Edgardo de la.**

"El significado de 'cor' en San Agostín." *Revue des études Augustiniennes* 7 (1961): 339-68. Surveys previous research on heart symbolism in Augustine. Focuses on the neologisms -cordia, recordatio; the uses of concordia; discordia; as well as the "lap" (sinus) and the lips (labia) of the heart.

**PFEIFFER, Charles Leonard.**

"Taste and Smell in Balzac's Novels." *Univ. of Arizona Bulletin* 20, no. 4 (1949): 1-121 (Humanities Bulletin 6).

**PIASCHEWSKI, Gisela.**

*Der Wechselbalg: Ein Beitrag zum Aberglauben der nordeuropäischen Völker.* Deutschkundliche Arbeiten, A.5. Breslau, 1935. Belief in the changeling is widespread in Northern European countries: he is either born from the intercourse with nonhumans or the replacement of a newborn through a nonhuman being. Pp. 27-41 refer to hundreds of names and many descriptions of changelings - before the concept of the "abnormal" was available to brand a child.

**PICARD, Dominique.**

"Approche ethnopsychologique du corps." *Cahiers de sociologie économique* n.s. 3 (1985), 23-33. "An ethnopsychological approach to the ritual and symbolic understanding of the body" which varies from culture to culture.

**PIECHOCKI, W.**

"Zur Leichenversorgung der Halleschen Anatomie im 18. und 19. Jahrhundert." *Acta Historica Leopoldina* 2 (1965): 67-105.

**PIERRUGUES, P.**

*Glossarium eroticum linguae Latinae sive theogoniae, legum et morum nuptialium apud Romanos explanatio nova.* Berlin: Barsdorf, 1908.

**PINXTEN, Rik.**

*Anthropology of Space: Exploration into the Natural Philosophy and Semantics of the Navajo.* Philadelphia: Univ. Philadelphia Press, 1983.

**PIPONNIER, Françoise, BUCAILLE, Gerhard.**

"La bête ou la belle? Remarques sur l'apparence corporelle de la paysannerie médiévale." *Ethnologie française* 6, 3-4 (1976): 227-32.

**PIRES DE LIMA, J.A.**

*O corpo humano no adagie Portuguès.* Porto, Portugal, 1946.

**PISANI, Vittore.**

"Gallico 'crupellari': Tedesco 'Ruecken'." *Paideia* 9 (1954): 101-03.

____. "Italiano 'potta', tedesco 'Fotze'." *Neuphilologische Mitteilungen* (Helsinki) 80 (1979): 85-87. Traces the etymology of the German and Italian words for "cunt" ("podex" or "cunnus").

____. "Kamm und Scham." In *Antiquitates Indogermanicae...Gedenkschrift für Hermann Guntert,* 285-88. Innsbruck: Inst. für Sprachwissenschaft, 1974.

**PLATELLE, H.**

"Le problème du scandale: Les nouvelles modes masculines aux XIe et XIIe siècles." *Revue belge d'histoire et de philologie* 53 (1975). Deals with the widespread scandal made by men using training gowns, flowing hair and groomed beards in the area between the northern Rhine and Norman England. Insights into the new meaning given to hair and beard.

**PLESSNER, Helmuth.**

*Philosophische Anthropologie: Lachen und Weinen. Das Lächeln: Anthropologie der Sinne.* Frankfurt: Fischer, 1970. The phenomenological anthropology of laughter and crying lays bare the ambiguous frontier between the body as an object of experience in line with other objects and the body as the location of self-perception (see esp. pp. 44ff. and 232ff.).

**PLEUSER, Christine.**

*Die Benennung und der Begriff des Leidens bei Tauler: Wortgeschichtliche Untersuchungen zum Begriff und Wortfeld von leit und lîden in den Predigten Taulers.* Berlin: Schwat, 1967.

**PLUEGGE, Herbert.**

*Der Mensch und sein Leib.* Tübingen: Niemeyer, 1967.

**PLUMPE, Joseph C.**

*Mater Ecclesia: An Inquiry into the Concept of the Church as Mother in Early Christianity.* Washington, D.C.: Catholic Univ. America Press, 1943.

**PODLECH, A.**

*Der Leib als Weise des In-der-Welt-Seins: Eine systematische Arbeit innerhalb der phänomenologischen Existenzphilosophie.* Bonn: Bouvier, 1956.

**POERKSEN, Uwe.**

"Zur Metaphorik naturwissenschaftlicher Sprache." *Neue Rundschau* 89 (1978): 63-82.

____. "Zur Terminologie der Psychoanalyse." *Deutsche Sprache* 3 (1973): 7-36.

**POESCHL, Victor, ed.**

*Bibliographie zur antiken Bildersprache.* Heidelberg: Winter, 1964.

**POLHEMUS, Ted, ed.**

*The Body Reader: Social Aspects of the Human Body.* New York: Pantheon, 1978. A collection of texts dealing with the body and society, with gestures, bodily spacing, and body symbolism. Some are selections from DARWIN, KROEBER, MAUSS et al., others are written for this volume.

**POLIAKOV, Léon.**
*Le mythe aryen: Essais sur les sources du racisme et des nationalismes.* Paris: Callman-Lévy, 1979.

**POMATA, Gianna.**
"Barbieri e comari." In *Medicina herbe e magia*, 162-83. Bologna, 1982.

____. "Menstruation and Bloodletting in Seventeenth Century Bologna." Paper presented at the Berkshire Conference of Women's History, 1984.

____. *Un tribunale dei malati: Il Protomedicato bolognese 1570-1770.* Dept. of History, University of Bologna, 1983. Pomata in her several studies uses a unique historical source: conflicts between patients and healers that were heard from the sixteenth to the eighteenth century by the Protomedicato, a special forum established under the aegis of the medical faculty in Bologna. These quasi-judicial proceedings contain quotations from litigants who speak in great detail about ailments, remedies and conflicts between healers about their competences. Influenced by Mary DOUGLAS, the author interprets the symbolic correlation between physical and social bodies: the function of bloodletting (1982), gendered blood (1984) and the expectations expressed in the "therapeutic pact" with a healer (1983).

____. "Madri illegitime tra ottocento e novecento: Storie cliniche e storie di vita." *Quaderni storici* 44, 1980.

____. "La storia delle donne: Una questione di confine." In *Il mondo contemporaneo*, ed. by B.BONGIO-VANNI, G.C.JOCTEAU, and N.TRANFAGLIA, vol. 10, *Gli strumenti della ricerca*. Vol. 2, *Questioni di metodo, 1435-69.* Florence: La Nuova Italia, 1983. (Partial German translation: "Eine Frage der Grenze." *Feministische Studien* 2, 1983.)

**POMPEY, Heinrich.**
*Die Bedeutung der Medizin für die kirchliche Seelsorge im Selbstverstaendnis der sogenannten Pastoraltheologie.* Freiburg, 1968.

**POPITZ, Friedrich.**
*Die Symbolik des menschlichen Leibes: Grundzüge einer ärztlichen Anthropologie.* Stuttgart: Hippokrates, 1956.

**PORTER, Roy.**
"Mixed Feelings: The Enlightenment and Sexuality in Eighteenth-Century England." In *Sexuality in Eighteenth-Century Britain*, ed. by P.G.BOUCE, 1-27. Manchester: Univ. Press, 1982.

____. "Lay Medical Knowledge in the Eighteenth-Century: The Evidence of the 'Gentleman's Magazine'." *Medical History* 29 (1985): 138-68. Articles from a moderately enlightened magazine, advising its readers on health, diet, temperance and death, enable the author to explore the history of illness from the sufferer's point of view. In the Georgian-educated elite self-diagnosis and self-help were taken for granted. During the nineteenth century the journal reflects a growing distance between the practitioners and clients and a new dependence on the doctor. By mid-century the journal ceases to advise the readers on medical - now professional - matters.

____. "The Patient's View: Doing Medical History from Below." *Theory and Society* 14 (1985): 175-98. "We lack an historical atlas of sickness-experience and -response, graduated by age, gender, class, religious faith..." (p. 181). Author substantiates his thesis with eighteenth-century examples, and recognizes that such a departure requires "defamiliarization" of twentieth-century researchers from cultural-biological certainties, and the dissociation of the history of healing from that of professional healers.

____, ed. *Patients and Practitioners: Lay Perceptions of Medicine in Pre-Industrial Societies.* Cambridge: Cambridge Univ. Press, 1985. This collection aims, first, to uncover pre-medical beliefs about health and sickness, and, second, to investigate various "traditional" ways of dealing with bodily discomfort. The articles draw mainly from autobiographic material (sixteenth- to eighteenth-century England) and thus concentrate on the experience of private individuals. An encompassing introduction with an overview of medicine and healing. PORTER argues against long-held historiographical beliefs, namely the division between lay and medical knowledge, oral and literary traditions, "high" and "low" culture prior to the eighteenth century. Some articles, e.g., BARRY, GEYER-KORDESCH, WILSON, explicitly or implicitly try to relate pain perception and body perception.

____. "Spreading Carnal Knowledge or Selling Dirt Cheap? Nicholas Venette's 'Conjugal Love' in the Eighteenth-Century." *Journal of European Studies* 14 (1984): 233-55.

**PORTMANN, Adolf.**
*Die Biologie und das neue Menschenbild.* Bern: Lang, 1942.

____. *Zoologie und das neue Bild des Menschen.* Reinbek: Rowohlt, 1956.

**POTT, August Friedrich.**
"Metaphern vom Leben und von körperlichen Lebensverrichtungen hergenommen." *Zeitschrift für vergleichende Sprachforschung* 2 (1853): 101-27.

**POUCHELLE, Marie-Christine.**
"Des Peaux des bêtes et des fourrures: Histoire médiévale d'une fascination." *Le temps de la réflexion* 2 (1981): 403-38. Paris: Gallimard. The person who wears fur uses a powerful symbol to extend his own skin and to envelop others in the aura of his presence.

535

The author interprets the rules for wearing fur coats during the Middle Ages.

_____. "Espaces cosmiques et dispositifs mécaniques: Le corps et les outils aux XIIIe et XIVe s." *Traverses* 14-15 (April 1979): 93-104.

_____. "La prise en charge de la mort: Médecine, médecins et chirurgiens devant les problèmes liés à la mort à la fin du Moyen Age (XIII-XVe s)." *Archives européennes de sociologie* 17, no. 2 (1976): 249-78. Since the Gregorian reform (11th c.) canon law forbids monks to practice medicine. This fosters the emergence of two specialists wrangling for precedence at the sickbed: the physician for the flesh and the confessor for the soul. By the fourteenth century, for the first time, the surgeon challenges the hitherto firm monopoly of the Church over the remains. Dissection slowly transmogrifies the "body abandoned by its soul" into a corpse: insightful discussions of the cultural obstacles against the entirely new "object" which anatomy constitutes.

_____. "Les appétits mélancoliques." *Médiévales* 5 (1983): 81-88.

_____. "Représentations du corps dans la 'Légende dorée'." *Ethnologie française* 6, nos. 3-4 (1976): 293-308. How does popular hagiographic literature (DE VORAGINE) represent the body in the waning Middle Ages? It reflects obsessional clerical attempts to define it in stark contrast to (largely unexplored) popular motifs.

_____. "Une parole médicale prise dans l'imaginaire: Alimentation et digestion chez un chirurgien du XIVe siècle." In *Actes du Colloque "Pratiques et discours alimentaires au XVIe siècle." Tours, Centre d'études supérieures de la renaissance, Mars 1979*, 179-92. Paris: Maisonneuve & Larose, 1982.

_____. *Corps et chirurgie à l'apogée du Moyen-Age.* Paris: Flammarion, 1983. Outstanding French historical anthropologist with psychoanalytic training. She examines one text: Mondeville's Chirurgia, and marshals a broad range of contemporary materials for its exegesis, which allows her to reconstruct the symbolic and psychic dimensions of body perceptions. At the center of her quest lies the relationship of body metaphor and the macrocosm in its social, architectural and "natural" dimensions. The author conjures up a rich texture of correspondences that forever surprise by its logic. A sensitive model for the reconstruction of past body perception that will be difficult to match.

**PRADEL, F.**
"Zur Vorstellung von der Hystera." *Archiv für Religionswissenschaft* 12 (1909). Marcellus Empiricus (around 400, influenced by Pliny, reporter of many folk-medicinal beliefs about gall otherwise undocu-mented) recommends the amulet in form of a dolphin for cramps in the womb-belly. The Greek origin of such a belief can be explained because "womb" and "dolphin" are homophones. Author speculates on the parallelism with the toad motif, and on the Italian description of pains which swim like a fish.

**PRAUSNITZ, Gotthold.**
*Die Augenkrankheiten und ihre Bekämpfung in der religiösen Kunst und Literatur: Ein Beitrag z. Volkskunde mit besonderer Berücksichtigung der Handschriften.* Strasbourg: Heitz, 1931. Iconography of eye diseases. In spite of the title, unpublished manuscripts are rarely quoted.

**PREISER, Gert.**
*Allgemeine Krankheitsbezeichnungen im Corpus Hippocraticum: Gebrauch und Bedeutung von Neusos und Nosema.* Berlin: De Gruyter, 1976 (Ars Medica 2.5). A detailed philological analysis restricted to the various historical layers that can be distinguished in the Corpus Hippocraticum. Under the influence of the sophists a new term, "nosema," began to compete with the old "nousos"; the first terminological manifestation of something like a "disease-entity."

**PREMUDA, Loris.**
*Storia dell-iconografia anatomica.* Milan: A. Martello: 1957. A history of anatomical illustration that is explicitly written as a history of a special art form rather than as a history of medicine. Antiquity and Middle Ages are dealt with in a cursory way. The convergence of art and morphology before Leonardo gets a special chapter (pp. 25-50). In the next six chapters the iconographic traditions and innovations are followed up into the late nineteenth century. The bibliography lists often neglected secondary literature. 140 full-page illustrations.

**PROSEK, Helena.**
*Slavische Krankheitsnamen aus onomasiologischer Sicht: Ein Beitrag zum vergleichenden Bezeichnungswörterbuch.* Dissertation. Hamburg, 1976. Under 107 modern German headings the author assembles names for diseases, states of mind and the associations of both.

**PUCKETT, Newbell N.**
*Folk Beliefs of the Southern Negro.* Repr. Montclair, N.J.: Patterson Smith, 1968 (Criminology, Law and Social Problem Series 22).

**PUTSCHER, Marielene.**
*Pneuma, Spiritus, Geist: Vorstellungen vom Lebensantrieb in ihren geschichtlichen Wandlungen.* Wiesbaden: F. Steiner, 1973.

_____. *Geschichte der medizinischen Abbildung. Von 1600 bis zur Gegenwart.* Munich: Heinz Moos, 1972.

**QUANTER, Rudolf.**
*Die Leibes- und Lebensstrafen bei allen Völkern und zu allen Zeiten.* Aalen: Scientia Verlag, 1970.

**QUEIROZ, Marcos S.**
"Hot and Cold Classification in Traditional Iguape Medicine." *Ethnology* 23, no. 1 (1984): 63-72.

**QUEMADA, Bernard.**
*Introduction à l'étude du vocabulaire médical (1600-1710).* Paris, Besançon, 1955 (Annales Littéraires de l'Université de Besançon, 2d ser. vol. 2. fasc. 5). A collection of terms from medical and general dictionaries (pp. 42-129). A thorough bibliography of books and articles dealing with the medical vocabulary (seventeenth and eighteenth c.), folk medicine and superstitions in French (pp. 129-39) and the French medical literature published, year by year from 1600 until 1710 (pp. 139-79).

**QUIGUER, Claude.**
*Femme et machines de 1900: Lecture d'une obsession modern-style.* Paris: Klincksieck, 1979. A voluminous collection of texts, published around 1900, of metaphors linking woman and machine. The complicated taxonomy is an obstacle to the use of this thesis as a reference tool.

**RABINBACH, Anson.**
"The European Science of Work: The Economy of the Body at the End of the Nineteenth Century." In *Work in France: Representations, Meaning, Organization, and Practice*, ed. by S.KAPLAN and C.J.KOEPP, 475-513. Ithaca: Cornell Univ. Press, 1986.

**RADTKE, Edgar.**
*Typologie des sexuell-erotischen Vokabulars des heutigen Italienisch: Studien zur Bestimmung der Wortfelder "prostituta" und "membro virile" unter besonderer Berücksichtigung der übrigen romanischen Sprachen.* Tübingen: Narr, 1980 (Tübinger Beiträge z. Linguistik, 136).

**RADTKE, Peter Wilhelm.**
*Die geschichtliche Entwicklung der anatomischen Kenntnisse der weiblichen Geschlechtsorgane von den Anfängen bis zu Vesal.* Dissertation. Med. Fak., Kiel, 1969.

**RAHDER, Johannes.**
"Words for Abdomen and Entrails." *Zeitschrift für Phonetik und Kommunikationswissenschaft* (Festschrift H.F.J.JUNKER) 17 (1964): 609-20.
____. "Words for Nose, Smell, etc." In *Indo-Asian Studies*, ed. by RAGHU-VIRA, 181-92. New Delhi: International Academy of Indian Culture, 1963 (Sata-Pitaka Series 31). Deals with southeast Asian languages. See also his references on further literature in English on words for smell, nose, etc.

**RAHNER, Hugo.**
"Die seelenheilende Blume: Moly und Mandragora in antiker und christlicher Symbolik." *Eranos-Jahrbuch* 12 (1945): 117-239.

**RAHNER, Karl.**
"Le début d'une doctrine des cinq sens spirituels chez Origène." *Revue d'ascétique et de mystique* 13 (1932): 113-45. The "interior senses" by which noncorporeal realities are sensually experienced by the soul play an important role in Christian reflection on mystical phenomena.
____. "La doctrine des 'sens spririruels' au Moyen Age: En particulier chez Saint-Bonaventura." *Revue d'ascétique et de mystique* 13 (1932): 263-99.

**RAMAT, Anna Giacolone.**
"Ricerche sulle denominazioni della donna nelle lingue indoeuropee." *Archivio glottologico italiano* 54 (1969): 105-47.

**RANCOUR-LAFERRIERE, Daniel.**
"Some Semiotic Aspects of the Human Penis." *Quaderni di studi semiotico* 24 (1979): 37-82.

**RATHER, L. J.**
"The 'Six Things Non-Natural': A Note on the Origins and Fate of a Doctrine and a Phrase." *Clio medica* 3 (1968): 337-47.
____. "Towards a Philosophical Study of the Idea of Disease." In *The Historical Development of Physiological Thought*, ed. by Chandler McC.BROOKS and Paul F.CRANEFIELD, 351-73. New York: Hafner, 1959.
____. *The Genesis of Cancer: A Study in the History of Ideas.* Baltimore: Johns Hopkins Press, 1979. The history of perception and interpretation of tumors. Short on pre-nineteenth-century history. Thorough on the later history of medical perceptions.
____. "On the Source and Development of Metaphorical Language in the History of Western Medicine." In *A Celebration of Medical History*, ed. by L.STEVENSON, 135-53. Baltimore: Johns Hopkins Press, 1982.
____. *Mind and Body in Eighteenth-Century Medicine: A Study Based on Jerome Gaub's "de regimine mentis."* Berkeley: Univ. of California Press, 1965.

**RAWLINSON, Francis.**
*Semantische Untersuchung zur medizinischen Krank-*

*heitsterminologie.* Dissertation. Marburg: Elwert, 1974 (Marburger Beiträge zur Germanistik). Studies the names for disease of those organs that are associated with breathing and explores the homonymy, synonymy and polysemy of those terms.

**READ, K.**
"Language and the Body in Francisco de Quevedo." *Modern Language Notes* 99 (1984): 235-55.

**REFF, Theodore.**
*Manet: Olympia.* London: Allen Lane, 1976. Analyzes the first ambiguous reactions of ZOLA in front of Manet's picture and compares it with Zola's *Nana,* written sixteen years later, where woman is discussed "less as a female than as an idol."

**REICHLER, Claude, ed.**
*Le corps et ses fictions.* Paris: Minuit, 1983. Proust and some of his contemporaries engage in the literary creation of a "subtle body" that is identified with the "subject" - and which can be easily opposed to a new kind of "obscene" body.

**REIS, Horst.**
*Die Vorstellung von den geistig-seelischen Vorgängen und ihrer körperlichen Lokalisation im Altlatein.* Munich: Kitzinger, 1962. A meticulous and well-indexed study of classical Latin words used to designate the soul or the spirit, with particular emphasis on the implication or reference of these terms to an organic event or localization.

**REITZENSTEIN, Richard.**
"Zur Sprache der lateinischen Erotik." In *Sitzungs-berichte der Heidelberger Akademie der Wissens-chaften.* Philosoph. Hist. Klasse, 12. Abhandlg. (1912), 3-36. "Man hat den sprachlichen Ausdruck und die Bilder der römischen Liebespoesie oft benutzt, ihre völlige Abhängigkeit von der griechischen zu erweisen. ...Ich möchte in...Einzelheiten die Eigenart...des römischen Empfindens hervorheben." Tries to identify what is characteristically Roman (rather than Greek) in Latin erotic literature and perception.

**REM, Henrl.**
"La chiromancie à travers les âges." *Voile d'Isis* 20-21 (1921). Introduction to the history of palm reading and to the perception of the palm.

**REMMERT, Guenther.**
*Leiberleben als Ursprung der Kunst: zur Aesthetik Friedrich Nietzsches.* Munich: J. Berchmans, 1978.

**RETTENBECK, Lenz.**
"Heilige Gestalten im Votivbild." In *Kultur und Volk. Beiträge zur Volkskunde. Festschrift f. G.GUGITZ,* ed. by Leopold SCHMIDT, 333-58. Vienna: Oesterreichisches Museum für Volkskunde, 1954.

**REUDENBACH, Bruno.**
"In mensura humani corporis: Zur Herkunft der Auslegung und Illustration von Vitruv 3.1 im 15. und 16. Jahrhundert," in *Text und Bild: Aspekte des*

*Zusammenwirkens zweier Künstler der frühen Neuzeit,* ed. by Christl MEIER and Uwe RUBERG, 651-88. Wiesbaden: Reichert, 1980. The reception of Vitruvius's doctrines on the proportions of the body and its interpretation through text and picture in the fifteenth and sixteenth centuries.

**RICHTER, Erwin.**
"Die Glaubensvorstellung von der allheilenden Gottesmutter Maria als Kraftfeld der geistlichen Volksheilkunde." *Bayerisches Jahrbuch für Volkskunde* 1954: 81-89.

____. "Marienmilch als Heilmittel in der geistlichen Volksmedizen." *Medizinische Montasschrift* 10 (1954): 685-88.

____. "Bayerische Schluckbildln." *Schönere Heimat* 2 (Munich, 1957): 322-32. Texts have been eaten with therapeutic intent in many places: Richter studies a particular format of devotional pictures and texts from Bavaria, specifically printed for the purpose of being swallowed.

____. "Kopfweh-Votive." *Oesterreichische Zeitschrift für Volkskunde* n.s. 5, nos. 1-2 (1951): 45-55. Votive offerings that implore delivery from headaches, express thanks for remissions or are used for the relief of headaches are discussed. Ethnological evidence used to identify Gothic objects (for example, hollow heads that can be filled with grain), certain gestures and arrangements relating to the headache.

____. "Einwirkung medico-astrologischen Volksdenkens auf Entstehung und Formung des Bärmutterkrötenopfers der Männer im geistlichen Heilbrauch." In *Volksmedizin: Probleme und Forschungsgeschichte,* ed. by Elfriede GRABNER, 372-98. Darmstadt: Wissenschaftliche Buchgesellschaft, 1967. The toad is consistently used in Mediterranean cultures as a symbol for the uterus. Yet quite consistently men use it as a votive offering to relieve belly cramps. Richter gathers the evidence and interprets the gender ambiguity.

**RICHTER, Gerlinde.**
"Bezeichnungen für den Heilkundigen." *Beiträge z. Geschichte der deutschen Sprache und Literatur* 88, nos. 1-2 (1966): 258-75. Terminology of healers. Gradually new terms reflect growing specialization.

**RICHTSTAETTER, Karl S.J.**
*Die Herz-Jesu Verehrung des deutschen Mittelalters.* Munich: Koesel und Pustet, 1924. During the German Middle Ages the Heart of Jesus became an object of imagination, representation and intense devotion. The author only touches upon the origins of the motif (pp. 31-50) and concentrates mainly on the late Middle Ages.

**RICOEUR, Paul.**
"Phenomenology and Hermeneutics." *Nous* 9 (1979): 85-102.

**RIDDLE, John M.**
"Pseudo Dioscorides: *ex herbis feminis* and Early
Medieval Botany." *Journal of the History of Botany* 14
(1981): 43-81.

**RIESE, W.**
*The Conception of Disease: Its History, Its Versions and
Its Nature*. New York: Philosophical Library, 1953.
____. "The Structure of Clinical History." *Bulletin of
the History of Medicine* 16 (1944): 437-49.

**RINGBOM, Sixten.**
*Icon to Narrative: The Rise of the Dramatic Close-up
in 15th Century Devotional Painting*. Abo: Akademie,
1965 (Acta Academae Abonensis Ser. A. Humanora
32.2). The concept of "pictorial form" is used in analogy with "literary form." The dramatic close-up on the
human figure originates in late fifteenth-century devotional art.

**RINNA, Jakob.**
*Die Kirche als Corpus Christi mysticum beim hl.
Ambrosius*. Roma: Scuola Salesiana del libro, 1940.

**RIPERT, Aline, FRERE MICHELAT,
Claude.**
"Images corporelles de la triade familiale: Le discours
photographique du magazine 'Parents'." *Ethnologie
française* 6, nos. 3-4 (1976): 265-77.

**RITTERBUSH, Philip C.**
*Overtures to Biology: The Speculations of Eighteenth-
Century Naturalists*. New Haven: Yale Univ. Press,
1964.

**ROBINSON, John Arthur Thomas.**
*The Body: A Study in Pauline Theology*. London: SCM
Press, 1961 (Studies in Biblical Theology 5).

**ROE, F. Gordon.**
*The Nude from Cranach to Etty and Beyond*. Leigh-
On-Sea, Essex: Lewis, 1944.

**ROESSLER, D.**
"Krankheit und Geschichte in der anthropologischen
Medizin." In *Medicus Viator: Fragen und Gedanken
am Wege R. Siebecks*, ed. by P.CHRISTIAN and
D.ROESSLER, 165-79. Stuttgart: Thieme, 1959.

**ROGER, Jacques.**
*Les sciences de la vie dans la pensée française du XVIIIe
siècle: La génération des animaux de Descartes à
l'Encyclopédie*. Paris: A. Colin, 1963. French learned
opinion on generation in three successive epochs: at
the end of the Renaissance (1600-70) seed and conception are central; learned philosophy (1670-1745),
ovism, animalculism and spontaneous generation; and
finally the science of Enlightenment - Buffon.
____. "Réflexions sur l'histoire de la biologie (XVIIe-
XVIIIe s.): Problèmes de méthodes." *Revue d'histoire
des sciences* 17 (1964): 25-40. Historical research on the
scientific discovery of facts creates a special obstacle
for the historian of past perceptions, when these facts
are biological, hence constitute the disembedding of
one element from an inextricably holistic past experience. "L'histoire de la biologie, et même l'histoire des
découvertes biologiques, ne peut donc pas être qu'une
histoire de la pensée biologique dans sa totalité,...
c'est-à-dire qu'elle doit tenter de descendre le plus
profondément possible dans la conscience et dans
l'inconscient des individus et des époques." (p. 38f.)

**ROMANTISME**
No. 31 (1981). Special issue on "blood" in nineteenth-
century French culture.

**ROMANTISME**
No. 46 (1984). Special issue on "energy" in nineteenth-century French culture.

**ROMANYSHYN, Robert D.**
*Psychological Life: From Science to Metaphor*. Austin:
Univ. Texas Press, 1981.
____. "The Despotic Eye: An Illustration of Metablet-
ic Phenomenology and Its Implications." In *The
Changing Reality of Modern Man: Essays in Honor of
Jan Hendrik VAN DEN BERG*, ed. by Dreyer
KRUGER, 87-109. Pittsburgh: Duquesne Univ. Press,
1985.

**ROMILLY, Jaqueline de.**
*Magic and Rhetoric in Ancient Greece*. Cambridge,
Mass.: Harvard Univ. Press, 1975.

**RONIG, F.**
"Theologische Inhalte des Bildes der stillenden
Muttergottes." In *Tausend Jahre Saarburg (964-
1964)*, 161-70. Saarburg, 1964. Theological interpretation of devotional pictures showing Mary breastfeeding the child.

**ROOS, Margot.**
*Das Problem der Krankheit im Werke Friedrich
Nietzsches*. Dissertation. Freiburg, Br., 1957.

**ROSENTHAL, Oskar.**
*Wunderheilungen und ärztliche Schutzpatrone in der
bildenden Kunst*. Leipzig: Vogel, 1925. About 100
reproductions of postmedieval paintings, representing
miracles performed by physicians who have been can-
onized as saints.

**ROSNER, E.**
"Terminologische Hinweise auf die Herkunft der
frühen griechischen Medizin." In *Medizingeschichte in
unserer Zeit: Festgabe für E. Heischkel und W. Artelt*,
ed. by H.EULNER, 1-22. Stuttgart: Enke, 1971.

**ROSSI, Ellen.**
"Body Time and Social Time." *Social Science Research*
6, no. 4 (1977): 273-308.

**ROTHSCHUH, Karl Eduard.**
*Konzepte der Medizin in Vergangenheit und
Gegenwart*. Stuttgart: Hippokrates, 1978.
____. "Leibniz, die prästabilierte Harmonie und die
Aerzte seiner Zeit." In *Studia Leibnitiana*, vol. 2, 231-
54. Wiesbaden: Steiner, 1969 (Akten des interna-
tionalen Leibnizkongresses 1966).

____. *Physiologie: der Wandel ihrer Konzepte: Probleme und Methoden vom 16. bis zum 20. Jahrhundert.* Freiburg: K. Alber, 1968.

____. "Zur Geschichte der Pathologie des Blutes, insbesondere von den Schärfen, Krasen und anderen Fehlern der Säfte: Zugleich ein Beitrag zur Humoralpathologie zwischen 1750-1850." *Sudhoffs Archiv* 35 (1942): 293-311.

____. ed. *Was ist Krankheit? Erscheinung, Erklärung, Sinngebung.* Darmstadt: Wissenschaftliche Buchgesellschaft, 1975 (Wege der Forschung 362).

____. "Von der Viersäftelehre zur Korpuskeltheorie des Blutes." In *Einfuehrung in die Geschichte der Hämatologie,* ed. Karl G.BOROVICZENY et al., 31-44. Stuttgart: Thieme, 1974.

**ROUSSEAU, G. S.**
"Literature and Medicine: The State of the Field." *ISIS* 72 (1981): 406-24.

**ROUSSELLE, Aline.**
"Du sanctuaire au thaumaturge: La guérison en Gaule au IVe siècle." *Annales E.S.C.* 31, no. 6 (1976): 1085-107. (Trans. in: *Ritual, Religion and the Sacred,* ed. by R.FORSTER and O.RANUM, Baltimore: Johns Hopkins Press, 1982.)

____. "Observation féminine et idéologie masculine: Le corps de la femme d'après les médecins grecs." *Annales E.S.C.* 35, no. 2 (1980): 1089-114. The Hippocratic corpus contains many references to women. These passages are all too frequently and uncritically interpreted as male perceptions. Rousselle attempts to make the contrary plausible: "the cnidian texts frequently record female experience and oral tradition."

____. *Porneia. De la maîtrise du corps à la privation sensorielle, IIe-IVe siècles de l'ère chrétienne.* Paris: Presses Universitaires de France, 1983 (*Porneia: On Desire and the Body in Antiquity.* New York: Basil Blackwell, 1988).

**ROWLEY, H.H.**
*Submission in Suffering and Other Essays on Eastern Thought.* Cardiff: Univ. Wales Press, 1951.

**RUDOFSKY, Bernhard.**
*The Unfashionable Human Body.* Garden City, N.Y.: Doubleday, 1971. Witty, sometimes cranky reflections on techniques to manipulate the body image from high heels to uniforms.

**RUESCHE, Franz.**
*Blut, Leben, Seele: Ihr Verhältnis nach Auffassung der griechischen und hellenistischen Antike, der Bibel und der alten Alexandrinischen Theologie: Eine Vorarbeit zur Religionsgeschichte des Opfers.* Paderborn: Schoeningh, 1930.

**RYKWERT, Joseph.**
"The Sitting Position - A Question of Method." First publ. in Italian *Edilizia moderna* 86 (1965): 15-21.

(Repr. in *The Necessity of Artifice,* by J. RYKWERT, 23-31. New York: Rizzoli, 1982.) "The whole environment, from the moment we name it and think it as such, is a tissue of symbolic forms." The sitting positions illustrate this argument.

# S

**SAADA, Lucienne.**
"Le langage des femmes tunisiennes." In *Mélanges Marcel Cohen,* ed. by D.COHEN, 320-25. Paris: Mouton, 1970.

**SABEAN, David Warren.**
*Power in the Blood: Popular Culture and Village Discourse in Early Modern Germany.* Cambridge: Cambridge Univ. Press, 1984. Tells in lively detail six episodes from rural life in southern Germany (1648-1800). Three concepts are fundamental: "person," "community" and "Herrschaft" (dominance). One story tells about a thirteen-year-old witch, another of a man who refuses to take the Eucharist. The body's symbolic power to flesh out whatever is "negotiated as reality" becomes strikingly visible.

**SACHS, Hans.**
*Der Zahnstocher und seine Geschichte: eine kunstgeschichtlich-kunstgewerbliche Studie.* Repr. Hildesheim: Olms, 1967

**SAINTYVES, P.**
*L'astrologie populaire étudiée spécialement dans les doctrines et les traditions relatives à l'influence de la lune; Essai sur la méthode dans l'étude du folklore des opinions et des croyances.* Paris: Nourry, 1937.

**SALLMANN, Klaus.**
"Studien zum philosophischen Naturbegriff der Römer mit besonderer Berücksichtigung des Lukrez." *Archiv für Begriffsgeschichte* 7 (1962): 140-284.

**SAND, Alexander.**
*Der Begriff 'Fleisch' in den paulinischen Hauptbriefen.* Regensburg: Pustet, 1967.

**SARDELLO, Robert.**
"The Suffering Body of the City: Cancer, Heart-Attack, and Herpes." *Spring* (Dallas) (1983): 145-64.

**SARLES, Harvey B.**
"Facial Expression and Body Movement." *Current Trends in Linguistics* 12 (1980): 297-310. This report on the state of linguistic research notes that "linguistics have tended to consider gestural and other body movement phenomena either as commentary on language per se, or as some kind of uninteresting independent communicational system." Only very slowly do linguists include research of "what happens in the

faces and in the bodies of the interactors."

**SAWDAY, Jonathan.**
"The Mint at Segovia: DIGBY, HOBBES, CHARLE-TON, and the Body as a Machine in the Seventeenth Century." *Prose Studies* 6, no. 1 (1983): 21-36. Despite Thomas Hobbes's admonition that metaphors had no place in scientific literature, members of the Royal Society used the automated mint at Segovia as an analogy to the human body.

**SAXL, F.**
"Macrocosm and Microcosm in Medieval Pictures." In *Lectures*, by F.SAXL, vol. 1, 58-72. London: Warburg Institute, 1957. Between the time of Hildegard of Bingen and Alphonse the Wise a great change occurred concerning man's attitudes to fate. This change is reflected in the microcosm pictures that show a revival of ancient cosmology in theory and practice. "The step from a metaphorical use to the practical application of the images is not a sign of a new superstition, but an example of regressive evolution" back to "fate."

**SCARRY, Elaine.**
"Work and the Body in Hardy and Other Nineteenth-Century Novelists." *Representations* 3 (Summer 1983): 90-123. Three novels of HARDY are examined. The body is at the center of HARDY's writing: "What is particular to and remarkable about him is...his representation of man as embodied maker. That all human acts take place through and out of his body never ceases to intrigue and quietly amaze him."

____. *The Body in Pain: The Making and Unmaking of the World*. Oxford, New York: Oxford Univ. Press, 1985.

**SCHAEFER, Jürgen.**
*Wort und Begriff "humour" in der Elisabethanischen Kömodie*. Münster: Aschendorf, 1966 (Neue Beiträge zur Engl. Philologie 6). Humor refers basically to the body's juices; under the influence of medical speculation it came to refer to psychic dispositions and states.

**SCHAEFER, Thomas.**
*Die Fusswaschung im monastischen Brauchtum in der lateinischen Liturgie*. Beuron: Kunstverlag, 1956 (Texte und Arbeiten, ed. Erzabtei Beuron, 1. Abt. Heft 47). The washing of the feet is an old Christian ritual. The prayers that accompany the ritual interpret the historical significance of the feet: of those to be baptized (early Western Christendom), of guests (fourth to eleventh cent.), of the poor (ninth cent.) and as a sign of mutual family charity within household and monastery.

**SCHALK, Fritz.**
*Somnium und verwandte Wörter in den romanischen Sprachen*. Köln: Westdt. Verlag, 1955.

**SCHAMA, S.**
"The Unruly Realm: Appetite and Restraint in Seventeenth-Century Holland." *Daedalus* 108, no. 3 (1979): 103-23. Interprets seventeenth-century Dutch paintings, mostly those of Jan Steen. Their iconography reveals a clash of values inherent in Dutch culture: the conflict between austerity and festivity. Interprets these as "complementary symbiosis" (p. 114).

**SCHARFE, Martin.**
*Evangelische Andachtsbilder: Studien zur Intention und Funktion des Bildes in der Frömmigkeitsgeschichte vornehmlich des schwäbischen Raumes*. Stuttgart: Müller und Gräff, 1968. The history, iconography and intention of popular devotional painting, mostly from southwestern Germany.

**SCHATZBERG, W.**
"Relations of Literature and Science: A Bibliography of Scholarship." *CLIO* (U.S.) 10, no. 1 (1978-79): 57-84.

**SCHEFFCZYK, Leo, ed.**
*Der Mensch als Bild Gottes*. Darmstadt: Wissenschaftliche Buchgesellschaft, 1969 (Wege der Forschung 124). Genesis relates that Adam was shaped from clay in the image of God. The figure of man is made in the image of the one, invisible, totally uncorporeal Creator. What "image" and "likeness" can mean in this case has been intensely debated at all times within Christian theology. This volume is an anthology of modern studies, mostly concerned with the treatment of the theme throughout history.

**SCHENDA, Rudolf.**
"Das Verhalten der Patienten im Schnittpunkt professionalisierter und naiver Gesundheitsversorgung: Historische Entwicklung und aktuelle Problematik." In *Handbuch der Sozialmedizin*, ed. by M.BLOHMKE, vol. 3, 31-45. Stuttgart, 1976.

**SCHERER, Anton.**
"Die Erfassung des Raumes in der Sprache." *Studium generale* 10 (1957): 574-82.

**SCHERTEL, Ernst.**
"*Phallus* und *Cunnus* in Mythos und Sprache." In *Moral und Mensch*, ed. by E. Schertel, 161-92. Leipzig: Parthenon-Verlag, 1929.

**SCHEWE, Joseph.**
*Unserer lieben Frauen Kindbett: Ikonographische Studien zur Marienminne des Mittelalters*. Phil. Dissertation. Kiel, 1958.

**SCHIEBINGER, Londa.**
"Skeletons in the Closet: The First Representations of the Female Skeleton in Eighteenth-Century Anatomy." *Representations* 14 (April 1986). Around the turn of the century anatomists attempted to discover the biological foundations of gender difference. One result was the conceptual creation of a "female skeleton" through which gender was rooted beyond the skin and the entrails and cemented within the bone structure.

Illustrations and examples from German and French literature.

**SCHILDER, Paul.**
*The Image and Appearance of the Human Body: Studies in the Constructive Energies of the Psyche.* New York: Intern. Univ. Press, 1950.

**SCHILLING, H.**
*Das Ethos der Mesotes: Eine Studie zur Nickomacheischen Ethik des Aristoteles.* Dissertation. Tübingen, 1930 (Heidelberger Abhandlungen zur Philosophie und ihrer Geschichte 22). The major study on "mesotes" (i.e., the "middle" or "balance") without which the classical terms related to "health" cannot be understood.

**SCHIPPERGES, Heinrich.**
"Aerztliche Bemühungen um die Gesunderhaltung seit der Antike." *Heidelberger Jahrbücher* 7 (1963): 121-36.
____. "Barmherzigkeit als Heilmittel bei Hildegard von Bingen." In *Festschrift für Erna Lesky zum 70. Geburtstag,* eds. K.GANZINGER, M.SKOPEC, H.WYKLICKY, 97-103. Vienna, 1981.
____. *Die Welt der Engel bei Hildegard von Bingen.* Salzburg: Otto Müller, 1963.
____. "Einflüsse der arabischen Medizin auf die Mikrokosmus-Literatur des 12. Jahrhunderts." In *Antiker Orient im Mittelalter,* ed. by P.WILPERT. Berlin: De Gruyter, 1962.
____. "Heilmittel als Heilsmittler im Mittelalter." *Arzt und Christ* 6 (1960): 205-14.
____. "Historische Aspekte einer Symbolik des Leibes." *Antaios* 9 (1968): 166-81.
____. *Kosmos Anthropos: Entwürfe zu einer Philosophie des Leibes.* Stuttgart: Klett-Cotta, 1981.
____. "'Melancolia' als ein mittelalterlicher Sammelbegriff für Wahnvorstellungen." *Studium generale* 20 (1967): 723-36.
____. "Zur 'Konstitutionslehre' der Hildegard von Bingen." *Arzt und Christ* 4 (1958): 90-94.
____. "Zur Tradition des 'Christus Medicus' im frühen Christentum und in der älteren Heilkunde." *Arzt und Christ* 11 (1965): 12-20.
____. *Kranksein und Heilung bei Paracelsus.* Vienna: Verband d. wissenschaftlichen Gesellschaften Oesterreichs Verlag, 1978.
____. *Der Garten der Gesundheit: Medizin im Mittelalter.* Munich: Artemis, 1985.
____. SEIDLER, E., UNSCHULD, P.U., eds. *Krankheit, Heilkunst, Heilung.* Freiburg: Alber, 1978 (Veröff. des Instituts für Historische Anthropologie).

**SCHLANGER, Judith.**
*Les métaphores de l'organisme.* Paris: Vrin, 1970.

**SCHLEGEL, K.F.**
*Der Körperbehinderte in Mythologie und Kunst.* Stuttgart, New York: Thieme, 1983.

**SCHLEUSENER-EICHHOLZ, Gudrun.**
*Das Auge im Mittelalter.* 2 vols. Munich: Fink, 1985. The theme is the eye, its symbolism and its metaphorical use during the Middle Ages. One of the major achievements in F.OHLY's school of historical semantics of the period.
____. "Die Bedeutung des Auges bei Jakob Boehme." *Frühmittelalterliche Studien* 6 (1972): 461-92. Complements SCHLEUSENER (1985) for a seventeenth-century German mystic.

**SCHLIER, Heinrich.**
*Der Brief an die Epheser: Ein Kommentar.* Düsseldorf: Patmos-Verlag, 1957.
____. "Corpus Christi." In *Reallexikon für Antike und Christentum,* vol. 3, coll. 437-53.

**SCHMID, Magnus.**
"Zum Phänomen der Leiblichkeit in der Antike, dargestellt an der Facies Hippocratica." *Sudhoffs Archiv,* Beihefte 7 (1966): 168-77.

**SCHMIDT, Leopold.**
*Gestaltheiligkeit im bäuerlichen Arbeitsmythos: Studien zu den Ernteschnitt-Geräten und ihrer Stellung im europäischen Volksglauben und Volksbrauch.* Vienna: Verlag des österreichischen Museum für Volkskunde, 1952.
____. *Perchtenmasken in Oesterreich.* Vienna: Böhlau, 1972.

**SCHMIDT-WIEGAND, Ruth.**
"Gebärdensprache im mittelalterlichen Recht." *Frühmittelalterliche Studien* 16 (1982): 363-79.

**SCHMITT, Jean-Cl.**
"Between Text and Image: The Prayer Gestures of Saint Dominic." *History and Anthropology* 1, no. 1 (1984): 127-62.
____. Introduction and general bibliography to "Gestures." *History and Anthropology* 1, no. 1 (1984): 1-28.

**SCHMITT, Wolfram.**
*Theorie der Gesundheit und "regimen sanitatis" im Mittelalter.* Habilitationsschrift Heidelberg (Geschichte der Medizin) 1973. A typology of the Western tradition of the literary genre "regimen sanitatis" with special concern about the reception and transformation of Arabic texts during the eleventh and twelfth centuries.

**SCHMITZ, Hermann.**
*System der Philosophie.* Vol. 2.1: *Der Leib.* 2.2: *Der Leib im Spiegel der Kunst.* Bonn: Bouvier, 1965.

**SCHNAPP, A.**
"Seduction and Gesture in Ancient Imagery." *History and Anthropology* 1, no. 1 (November 1984): 49-56.

**SCHNUERER, Gustav, RITZ, Joseph M.**
*Sankt Kümmernis und Volto Santo: Studien und Bilder*. Düsseldorf: Schwann, 1934. No historical study of the crucified body would be complete without attention to a mysterious but not infrequent icon: that of a bearded, crucified young woman.

**SCHOEFLER, Heinz Herbert.**
"Zur mittelalterlichen Embryologie." *Sudhoffs Archiv* 53, no. 3 (1973): 297-314. Collates and comments texts that deal with the traditional views of premature live births.

**SCHOENE, Wolfgang.**
"Die Bildgeschichte der christlichen Gottesgestalten in der abendländischen Kunst." In *Das Gottesbild im Abendland* by W.SCHOENE. Berlin: Eckart Verlag, 1959. Jews and Muslims do not picture God. Though they are also monotheists, Christians did so until about 1800 (p. 54). Schoene attempts to write the history of Western Christian art as a history of God's image - or, rather, as the history of picturing man in his bodily likeness to God.

**SCHOENER, Erich.**
*Das Viererschema in der antiken Humoralpathologie.* Wiesbaden: Steiner, 1964 (Sudhoffs Archiv Beihefte 4). Detailed study of the terminology used in classical humoral pathology. No attempt at semantic interpretation.

**SCHOENFELD, W.**
"Die Haut als Ausgang der Behandlung, Verhütung und Erkennung fernörtlicher Leiden." *Sudhoffs Archiv* 36 (1943): 43-89.

**SCHRENK, M.**
"Blutkulte und Blutsymbolik." In *Einführung in die Geschichte der Hämatologie*, ed. by K.BROVICZENY et al., 1-17. Stuttgart: Thieme, 1974.

**SCHROEDER, Ekkehard.**
"Der Mensch und sein Korper aus der Sicht des Ethnomediziners." In *Leib und Leben in der Geschichte der Neuzeit*, ed. by A.IMHOF, 77-86. Berlin, 1983 (Berliner Historische Studien 9).

**SCHROETER, Ulrich.**
"Zur Bezeichnung für 'Parotitis (Epidemica)' im Deutschen." *Beiträge zur Geschichte der deutschen Sprache und Literatur* 98 (1977): 303-11. Variation of regional designations for salivary gland swellings in German.

**SCHULER, R. M.**
*English Magical and Scientific Poems to 1700: An Annotated Bibliography*. New York: Garland, 1979.

**SCHULTE, Regina.**
"Infanticide in Rural Bavaria in the Nineteenth Century." In *Interest and Emotion: Essays in the Study of Family and Kinship*, ed. H.MEDICK and S.SABEAN, 77-102. Cambridge: Cambridge Univ. Press, 1984. Pregnant, unwed servant girls in late nineteenth-century Bavarian countryside deny their bodily changes when "pregnant" and subsequently dispose of the insides of their bellies with the idea that they were disposing of "lumps of blood." The court records show the contrasting views of "pregnancy" between medical scientific definitions and personal perceptions. A fine analysis of mentalities and living conditions.

____. *Bäuerliche Gesichter im Blick der Naturwissenschaft im 19. Jahrhundert*. MS Deutsches Hist. Institut /German Hist. Institute, London 1984.

**SCHUPBACH, William.**
*The Paradox of Rembrandt's "Anatomy of Dr. Tulp."* London: Wellcome Institute for the History of Medicine, 1982. A careful analysis of the emblematic, paradoxical meaning of Rembrandt's picture: the anatomy lesson shows man's mortality and immortality at once. The lesson on divinity is embodied in the lumps of flesh of the criminal corpse shown. Clues for this interpretation: the author's study on the symbolism of the hand. Pp. 57-65 give a collection of quotations regarding the hand from Aristotle to Riolan.

**SCHUSTER-SEWC, Heinz.**
*Die slawischen Körperteilbezeichnungen: Mit bes. Berücksichtigung des Serbischen und des Polnischen: Ein Beitrag zur slawischen Bezeichnungsgeschichte.* Dissertation. Leipzig, 1962.

**SCHWARZ, Heinrich.**
"The Mirror in Art." *The Art Quarterly* 15 (1952): 96-118.

**SCHWARZ, Richard.**
"Leib und Seele in der Geistesgeschichte des Mittelalters." *Deutsche Vierteljahrsschrift für Literaturwissenschaften und Geistesgeschichte* 16 (1938): 293-323.

**SCHWEIKLE, Gunther.**
"Die 'frouwe' der Minnesänger." *Zeitschrift für deutsches Altertum und deutsche Literatur* 109 (1980): 91-116.

**SCHWEITZER, Bernhard.**
*Vom Sinn der Perspektive*. Tübingen: Niemeyer, 1953. Things drawn in perspective can be considered as objects created by the eye: as parts of a world in the grasp of the eye. Before the fourteenth century objects were conceived as parts before they were welded into a whole. Perspectival habits created "space" that is prior to the things within it: the whole now "jumps" into view. What makes postmedieval perspective unique is not that it refers everything to the viewing subject, but that it changes the temporal element in perception, enabling us to view "all at once."

**SCHWEIZER, E.**
"Soma." In *Theologisches Wörterbuch zum Neuen Testament*, ed. by Gerhard KITTEL, vol. 7, 1024-91. Stuttgart, 1964 (*Theological Dictionary of the New*

543

*Testament*, ed. by Gerhard FRIEDRICH, vol. 7, p. 98ff.).

**SCOTT, Robert A.**

*The Making of Blind Men: A Study of Adult Socialization*. New York: Russel Sage Foundation, 1969. In modern America there is only a weak correlation between visual impairment and socially perceived blindness. To be recognized by one's milieu as "blind" and to perceive oneself as "blind" one needs first to establish a client relationship with one or several professional bodies that are in charge of the blind. The author continued to investigate the hiatus between the realms studied by academic sociology (e.g., blindness) and the groups in need of public policy (those suffering from impaired sight).

**SEGAL, Charles.**

*The Theme of the Mutilation of the Corpse in the Iliad.*" Leiden: E. J. Brill, 1971 (Mnemosyne, Biblioteca Classica. Batava, Supplementum 17).

**SEGALEN, Martine.**

"Le mariage, l'amour et les femmes dans les proverbes populaires français." *Ethnologie française* 5 (1975): 119-62 and 6 (1975): 33-88.

**SEIDLER, E.**

"Medizin und Hämatologie im ausgehenden 18. und beginnenden 19. Jahrhundert." In *Einführung in die Geschichte der Hämatologie*, ed. by K.BOROVCZENY et al., 44-57. Stuttgart: Thieme, 1974.

**SELIGMANN, K.**

*Der böse Blick und Verwandtes: Ein Beitrag zur Geschichte des Aberglaubens aller Zeiten und Völker*. 2 vols. Berlin: Verlag Barsdorf, 1910. The author was an oculist with a lifelong passion: he collected reports and tidbits on the evil eye from around the world. This is his major work.

**SHABOU, Amina.**

"Maladies et pratiques thérapeutiques des femmes dans le Sud-Tunisien." *History and Anthropology* 2 (1985): 95-123.

**SHEILS, W.S., ed.**

*The Church and Healing*. Oxford: Ecclesiastical History Society, 1982.

**SHELP, E.E.**

"The Experience of Illness: Integrating Metaphors and the Transcendence of Illness." *Journal of Medicine and Philosophy* 9, no. 3 (1984): 253-56.

**SHEPARD, Paul.**

*Nature and Madness*. San Francisco: Sierra Club Books, 1982. "The earth/body analogy, the vision of nature-as-physiology, of human kinship as a kind of ecological sytem, the projection of sexual dimorphism on the non-human world - all such analogies are fundamental to healthy human consciousness" (p. 84). But these analogies dawn only slowly on the child as it distinguishes between mother and Mother Earth acquir-ing symbols to retain its intuition of a common structure underlying the individual body and the world. Shepard sees history as a progressive "civic gardening" which led to a progressive "peeling back of the psyche." Civilized cultures have abandoned the ceremonies of adolescent initiation that affirm the metaphoric qualities of nature, and have reduced them to aesthetic amenities. As a result the individual is out of touch with both body and world. Shepard calls for a historic treatment of this alienation (p. 14).

____. *Thinking Animals: Animals and the Development of Human Intelligence*. New York: Viking, 1978. Shepard does not deal with body history, but attempts to lay foundations for the history of a mental menagerie through which an epoch's body comes into existence. Historically animal images and forms have been essential for the shaping of personality, identity and social consciousness. They are the unavoidable mediators which allow the child to detach itself from mother and grow into its body/earth analogy. Mind and brain are dependent on the survival of these animals. Shepard suggests a historical zoology of this mental menagerie of animal protagonists and of monsters.

**SHORTER, Edward.**

*A History of Women's Bodies*. New York: Pantheon 1982. Quite useful as a source for assorted statistics on the incidence of puerperal fevers, postpartum mortality. Ch. 5 is a compendium on abortion: methods, herbs used, statistics, techniques.

**SHOWALTER, Elaine, ENGLISH, Diedre.**

"Victorian Women and Menstruation." *Victorian Studies* 14, no. 1 (1970): 83-89.

**SHRYOCK, Richard H.**

"The History of Quantification in Medical Science." In *Quantification: A History of the Meaning of Measurement in the Natural and Social Sciences*, ed. by H.WOOLF, 85-107. Indianapolis: Bobbs-Merrill 1961. Contribution to a dated but still outstanding volume. What has been studied as the "medicalization" of the body could also be presented as the quantification of the body that began, as an ideal, in the sixteenth century, but only after 1850 became decisive.

**SIEFERT, Helmut.**

"Hygiene in utopischen Entwürfen des 16. und 17. Jahrhunderts." In *Medizingeschichte in unserer Zeit. Festgabe für E. HEISCHKEL-ARTELT and W. ARTELT*, ed. by H.EULNER et al. Stuttgart: Enke, 1971.

**SIEWERTH, Gustav.**

*Der Mensch und sein Leib*. Einsiedeln: Johannes Verlag, 1953.

**SIGAL, Pierre-André.**

*L'homme et le miracle dans la France médiévale, XI-*

*XIIe siècles.* Paris: Cerf Histoire, 1985. Based on 5,000 reports on miracles. Much of it clerical hagiographic propaganda. This might explain a relative underrepresentation of women beneficiaries. Most miracles are not spectacular: majority related either to sickness or to captivity. Toward the end of the period the miracle more often happens at a distance and touches more secret affliction: while in the tenth century the afflicted person must touch the thaumaturge, in the twelfth century devout contemplation suffices.

**SIGERIST, Henry E.**
*Civilization and Disease.* Chicago: Univ. Chicago Press, 1970.
____. "Disease and Music." In *Civilization and Disease*, by H.E.SIGERIST, 212ff. Chicago: Univ. Chicago Press, 1970 (orig. 1943).
____. "William Harvey's Stellung in der europäischen Geistesgeschichte." *Archiv für Kulturgeschichte* 19 (1928): 158-68. (In *On the History of Medicine*, ed. by F. MARTI-IBANEZ, 184-92. New York: M.D. Publications, 1960.)

**SIGNORINI, Italo.**
"Patterns of Fright: Multiple Concepts of Susto in a Nahua-Ladino Community of the Sierra de Puebla." *Ethnology* 21, no. 4 (1982): 313-23.

**SINGER, Charles.**
*A History of Biology to about the Year 1900.* 3d rev. ed. London, New York: Abelard Schuman, 1959.
____. "The Confluence of Humanism, Anatomy and Art." In *Fritz SAXL: A Volume of Memorial Essays*, ed. by D.J.GORDON, 261-69. London: B. Franklin, 1957.
____. "Beginnings of Academic Practical Anatomy." In *History and Bibliography of Anatomic Illustration*, ed. by J.L.CHOULANT. New York: Hafner, 1962.
____. *A Short History of Anatomy and Physiology: From the Greeks to Harvey.* New York: Dover, 1957.

**SIRONI, V., et al.**
*Gli ex-voto del Santuario di S. Valeria a Sevegno.* Besana Brianza, 1983.

**SISSA, Giulia.**
"Une virginité sans hymen: le corps féminin en Grèce ancienne." *Annales E.S.C.* 39, no. 6 (1984): 1119-39.
____. *Le Corps virginal: La virginité féminine en Grèce ancienne.* Paris: J. Vrin, 1987 (Etudes de Psychologie et de Philosophie 22). "Which are those conceptions of the female body and women's sexuality in which the hymen plays a fundamental role?" The author wants to make a contribution to such a history of the hymen, by focusing on the meaning given to the Pythia's virginity in preclassical Greece...unrelated to the state of her vulva. This sacred virginity can be understood only by grasping the analogy between mouth and mouth. The Pythia is virginal as a prophet possessed by the God and overflowing in words and signs which she brings forth - which are not those of men, to whom she keeps strict silence. The book deals with the contrast to learned medicine from Hippocrates to Soranus.

**SISTO, Pietro.**
"Studi di storia della medicina medievale e umanistica." *Quaderni medievali* 13 (June 1982): 238-47.

**SKULTANS, Vieda.**
"The Symbolic Significance of Menstruation and the Menopause." *MAN* n.s. 5 (1970): 639-51.

**SMITH, W.D.**
"Eristratus' Dietetic Medicine." *Bulletin of the History of Medicine* 56 (1982): 398-409.
____. *The Hippocratic Tradition.* Ithaca: Cornell Univ. Press, 1979. The up-to-date historical book on the subject.

**SMITH-ROSENBERG, Caroll.**
"Puberty to Menopause: The Cycle of Femininity in Nineteenth-Century America." In *Disorderly Conduct: Visions of Gender in Victorian America*, by C.SMITH-ROSENBERG, 182-96. New York: Knopf, 1985.

**SOMMER, Ludwig.**
*Das Haar in Religion und Aberglauben der Griechen.* Dissertation. Münster, 1912.

**SONTAG, Susan.**
*Illness as Metaphor.* New York: Farrar, Straus & Giroux, 1978. "I want to describe, not what it is really like to emigrate to the kingdom of the ill and live there, but the positive or sentimental fantasies concocted about that situation: not real geography but stereotypes of national character. My subject is not physical illness itself, but the uses of illness as a figure and metaphor...the lucid metaphor with which [the kingdom of the ill] has been landscaped."

**SOUQUES, A.**
"La douleur dans les livres Hippocratiques: Diagnos-tics rétrospectifs." *Bulletin Soc. Franç. Hist. Méd.* 31 (1937): 209-14, 279-309 and 32 (1938): 178-86 and 33 (1939): 37-48, 131-44 and 34 (1940): 53-59, 78-93. Gathering of references to pain in the Hippocratic corpus.

**SPEERT, H.**
*Iconographia Gyniatrica: A Pictorial History of Gynecology and Obstetrics.* Philadelphia: F.A. Davis, 1973. Lavish illustrations of the gynecologist's practice and tools throughout history.

**SPELMAN, Elizabeth V.**
"Woman as Body: Ancient and Contemporary Views." *Feminist Studies* 8, no. 1 (1982): 109-31.

**SPICKER, Stuart F., ed.**
*Organism, Medicine and Metaphysics: Essays in Honour of Hans JONAS on his 75th Birthday.* Dordrecht, Boston: Reidel, 1978 (Philosophy and Medicine 7). Starting with a good bibliography of JONAS, this commemorative volume contains contributions to further the discussion that he opened in

biology: on the distinct tasks that should be assigned to the phenomenology of the body and to the analytic treatment of the mind/body problem.

____, ed. *The Philosophy of the Body: Rejections of Cartesian Dualism*. Chicago: Quadrangle Books, 1970.

____. "Terra Firma and Infirma Species: From Medical Philosophical Anthropology to Philosophy of Medicine." *Journal of Medicine and Philosophy* 2 (1976): 104-35.

**SPIERENBURG, Petrus C.**

*The Spectacle of Suffering. Execution and the Evolution of Repression: From a Pre-Industrial Metropolis to the European Experience*. Cambridge: Cambridge Univ. Press, 1984. Punishment in the sixteenth century consisted in the public, ostentatious infliction of pain or of mutilation. The torture by the method used and the body part affected was meant to project social symbolism onto the flesh. This use of the body as a screen on which the state demonstrates its ideology recedes in the seventeenth century - more slowly in France than elsewhere.

**SPRIGADE, Klaus.**

"Abschneiden des Königshaares und kirchliche Tonsur bei den Merowingern." *Welt und Geschichte* 22 (1963): 142-61. By cutting his hair the king can be deprived of his dignity and placed among the commoners; through his tonsure the layman is removed from the "world" and made into a cleric; by scalping, a prince can be made permanently unfit for succession to the throne.

**STAEHLIN, Carlos Maria.**

*Apariciones*. Madrid: Razón y Fe, 1956.

**STAROBINSKI, Jean.**

"The Inside and the Outside." *Hudson Review* 28 (1975): 333-51. Deals with ancient texts that treat the opposition between lips and heart, outside and inside: concealing in the heart was made possible by the reality of a visceral "inside" where breath can be trapped. Inside comes about at the moment a form asserts itself by setting its own boundaries.

**STARK, Louisa R.**

"The Lexical Structure of Quechua Body Parts." *Anthropological Linguistics* 11 (1969): 1-15.

**STEINBERG, Leo.**

*The Sexuality of Christ in Renaissance Art and in Modern Oblivion*. New York: Pantheon, 1983. An appropriate title for this book would have been: "the genital of Jesus" (Toni CUTLER).

____. "Michelangelo and the Doctors." *Bulletin of the History of Medicine* 56 (1982). "The physical effects of the operation [circumcision] are not admitted in Renaissance art, so that one is tempted to diagnose the optical capabilities of physicians who regularly make David [Michelangelo's uncircumcised David] a problem, but walk past hundreds of uncircumcised Christs without noticing" (p. 552).

____. "The Metaphors of Love and Birth in Michelangelo's Pietàs." In *Studies in Erotic Art*, ed. by Theodore BOWIE and Cornelia CHRISTENSON, 231-335. New York: Basic Books 1970.

**STENGERS, J.**

"Les pratiques anticonceptionnelles dans le mariage au XIXe et XXe siècles: Problèmes humains et attitudes religieuses." *Revue belge de philologie et d'histoire* 49, no. 2 (1971): 403-81. The article presents a large number of lengthy quotes from Church documents - many in Latin - which speak in great detail about contraception and the Church's opinion about the body.

**STEPHENS, T. A., BONSER, Wilfrid.**

*Proverb Literature: A Bibliography of Works Relating to Proverbs*. London: Glaisher, 1930. Pp. 439-42 indicate thirty-five collections of medical adagia and hygienic proverbs.

**STEPHENS, William N.**

"A Cross-Cultural Study of Modesty." *Behavior Science Notes* 7 (1972): 1-29.

**STETTIS, S.**

"Images of Meditation, Uncertainty and Repentance in Ancient Art." *History and Anthropology* 1, no. 1 (1984): 193-237.

**STORM, Penny.**

"The Umbilical Cord, Man's First Clothing." *Dress: The Annual Journal of the Costume Society of America* 8 (1982): 2-9.

**STRAUS, Erwin.**

"Die aufrechte Haltung: eine anthropologische Studie." *Monatschrift für Psychiatrie und Neurologie* (Basel, New York: S. Karger) 117 (1949): 4-6.

____. *Phenomenological Psychology*. New York: Basic Books, 1966.

**STROUD, Joanne.**

*The Wasting Body of Anorexia*. Paper. Dallas: Institute of Humanities and Culture, 1985.

**SULEIMAN, Susan R., ed.**

*The Female Body in Western Culture*. Cambridge, Mass.: Harvard Univ. Press, 1986.

**SUTHERLAND, Anne.**

"The Body as a Social Symbol among the Rom." In *The Anthropology of the Body*, ed. by J.BLACKING, 375-90. New York: Academic Press (ASA Publication), 1977.

**TARCZYLO, Théodore.**

"'Prêtons la main à la nature...' 1: 'L'onanisme' de Tissot." *Dix-Huitième Siècle* 12 (1980): 79-96.

**TAYLOR, Frederick Kraeupl.**
*The Concepts of Illness, Disease and Morbus.*
Cambridge: Cambridge Univ. Press, 1979.

**TEGNAEUS, Harry.**
*Blood-Brothers: An Ethno-Sociological Study of the Institutions of Blood-Brotherhood with Special Reference to Africa.* Stockholm: The Ethnographic Museum of Sweden, 1952 (Publication Series 10). Note particularly the bibliography, pp. 167-78.

**TEICH, Mikulas.**
"Circulation, Transformation, Conservation of Matter and the Balancing of the Biological World in the Eighteenth-Century." *Ambix* 29, no. 1 (1982): 17-28.
____, YOUNG, R.M. eds. *Changing Perspectives in the History of Science. Essays in Honour of Joseph NEEDHAM.* Dordrecht, Boston: Reidel, 1973.

**TELLENBACH, Hubert.**
"Die Räumlichkeit des Melancholischen: Ueber Veränderungen des Raumerlebnisses in der endogenen Melancholie." *Nervenarzt* 27, no. 1 (1956). A phenomenological study of the effect which depression has on the perception of space: by observing how deeply depression cancels the directedness (tensors) in space perception their presence in ordinary space perception is highlighted.

**TEMKIN, Oswei.**
*Galenism: Rise and Decline of a Medical Philosophy.* Ithaca, London: Cornell Univ. Press, 1973. Considers "Galenism" as a permanent intellectual phenomenon in Western history and places it next to Platonism and Aristotelianism. In contrast to these, a practical focus was central to Galenism, which gave profound popular roots to its set of more or less cogently connected principles, beliefs and facts.
____. "Studien zum 'Sinn-Begriff' in der Medizin." *Kyklos* 2 (1949): 21-105.
____. *The Double Face of Janus and Other Essays on the History of Medicine.* Baltimore: Johns Hopkins Press, 1977.
____. "Metaphors of Human Biology." In *The Double Face of Janus,* 271-83.
____. "Nutrition from Classical Antiquity to the Baroque." In *Human Nutrition: Historic and Scientific,* ed. by Iago GALDSTON, 78-97. New York: International Univ. Books, 1960.
____. *The Falling Sickness: A History of Epilepsy from the Greeks to the Beginnings of Modern Neurology.* 2d rev. ed. Baltimore: John Hopkins Press, 1971 (orig. 1945).

**TERMER, Franz.**
"Die Kenntnis vom Uterus bei den Maya und anderen Völkern in Mesoamerika." *Ethnos* 24, nos. 3-4 (1959): 177-201.

**THEVEZ, Michel.**
*The Painted Body.* New York: Skira/Rizzoli, 1984.

**THEREL, Marie-Louise.**
*Les symboles de l'Ecclesia dans la création iconographique de l'art chrétien du IIIe au VIe siècle.* Rome: Ed. Storia e Letteratura, 1973. Iconography of the Church - mostly as a woman in early Christianity.

**THEWELEIT, Klaus.**
*Männerphantasien.* Vol. 1: *Frauen, Fluten, Körper, Geschichte.* Vol. 2: *Männerkörper: Zur Psychoanalyse des weissen Terrors.* Reinbek: Rowohlt, 1977-80 (*Male Fantasies.* Vol. 1: *Women, Floods, Bodies, History.* Minneapolis: Univ. Minnesota Press, 1987).

**THISSEN, R.**
*Die Entwicklung der Terminologie auf dem Gebiet der Sozialhygiene und Sozialmedizin im deutschen Sprachgebiet bis 1930.* Köln, Opladen: Westdeutscher Verlag, 1969. The development of German terminology in the area of public health until 1930.

**THOMAE, Karl.**
*Das Herz: Eine Monographie in sechs Einzeldarstellungen.* K. Thomae GMBH, Biberach. Six volumes each of thirty-six pages, published by a pharmaceutical family corporation. The common theme is the heart, as represented in one or another medium used in folk culture.

**THOMALLA, Ariane.**
*Die "femme fragile": Ein literarischer Frauentypus der Jahrhundertwende.* Düsseldorf: Bertelsmann, 1972. What Mario PRAZ and others have done for the study of the literary type of the "femme fatale" the author wants to do for its counterpoint, which - though so far unnamed - he believes to have been of equal importance during the closing decade of the nineteenth century. He focuses on the female figure who is seduced through her fragility in French, German and Italian literature and in painting.

**THOMAS, Gail, STROUD, Joanne, eds.**
*Images of the Untouched.* Dallas: Spring, 1982.

**THOMAS, Keith.**
*Religion and the Decline of Magic.* London, New York: Scribner, 1971.

**THOMASSET, C.**
"La représentation de la sexualité et de la génération dans la pensée scientifique médiévale." In *Love and Marriage in the Twelfth Century,* ed. by W.van HOECKE, A.WELKENHUYSEN, 1-17. Louvain: Louvain Univ. Press, 1981.

**THOMPSON, D'Arcy Wentworth.**
*On Growth and Form.* Cambridge: Cambridge Univ. Press, 1971.

**THORNTON, John L., REEVES, Carole.**
*Medical Book Illustrations: A Short History.* New York: Oleander Press, 1984.

**THUILLIER, Guy.**
"Pour une histoire de l'hygiène corporelle: Un exem-

ple régional: le Nivernais." *Revue d'histoire économique et sociale* 46, no. 2 (1968): 232-53.

**TIBON, Gutierre.**

*El Ombligo como centro erótico*. México: Fondo de Cultura Económica, 1980.

____. *El mundo secreto de los Dientes*. México: Ed. Tajín, 1972. The National Museum of Mexico owns the world's largest collection of ornamented, mutilated and inlaid teeth. The inlays are made of jade, turquoise or pyrites giving testimony to a high level of precision work by the Stone Age dental artisans of Mesoamerica. The author speculates on the symbolic function of these inlays.

____. *El Ombligo como centro cósmico*. México: Fondo de Cultura Económica, 1981.

____. *La triade prenatal: Cordón, placenta, amnios: supervivencia de la magia paleolítica*. México: Fondo de Cultura Económica, 1981.

**TIKKANEN, S.J.**

*Die Beinstellung in der Kunstgeschichte: ein Beitrag zur Geschichte der künstlerischen Motive*. Helsingfors, 1912 (Acta Societatis Scientiarum Fennicae 42).

____. *Studien über den Ausdruck in der Kunst: Zwei Gebärden mit dem Zeigefinger*. Helsingfors, 1913 (Acta Societatis Scientiarum Fennicae 43).

**TITMUSS, Richard M.**

*The Gift Relationship: From Human Blood to Social Policy*. New York: Vintage Books, 1971.

**TOELLNER, Richard.**

"Die Umbewertung des Schmerzes im 17. Jh. in ihren Voraussetzungen und Folgen." *Medizinhistorisches Journal* 6 (1971): 36-44. During the seventeenth and eighteenth century the meaning of "pain" in medical-philosophical writing changed dramatically. Formerly pain was conceived as the inescapable outcome of nature's deficiency. Pain of the soul and pain of the body were merged. With and after Descartes pain becomes an isolable bodily phenomenon and a bodily indication, useful as a "guardian and protector of life." (Haller, p. 43: *dolorem Deus homini fidelem custodem dedit, qui de causa corporis destructrice moneat*.)

____. "Logical and Psychological Aspects of the Discovery of the Circulation of the Blood." In *On Scientific Discovery: The Erice Lectures*, ed. by M.D. GRMEK, 239-59. Dordrecht, Boston: Reidel, 1981 (Boston Studies in the Philosophy of Science 34).

____. "Mechanismus-Vitalismus: Ein Paradigmawechsel? Testfall Haller." In *Die Struktur wissenschaftlicher Revolutionen und die Geschichte der Wissenschaften*, ed. by Alwin DIEMER, 61-72. Meisenheim: Hain, 1977.

____, SADEGH-ZADEH, K. eds. *Anamnese, Diagnose und Therapie*. Techtenburg, 1983 (Münster. Beitr. z. Geschichte und Theorie d. Medizin 20).

**TORRILHON, Toby Michel.**

"La pathologie chez Breughel: Breughel était-il médecin?" *Connaissance des arts* (Paris) 80 (1958): 68-77. Summary of a doctoral thesis. Carefully qualified and detailed diagnosis of the conditions of the figures painted by Brueghel.

**TRAMOYERES BLASCO, L.**

"La Virgen de la leche en el arte." *Museum: Revista mensual de arte español antiguo y moderno* 3 (1913): 79-118.

**TRAPP, Joseph B.**

"The Iconography of the Fall of Man." In *Approaches to Paradise Lost*, ed. by C.A.PATRIDES, 223-65. London: Arnold, 1968.

**TRAUTMANN, J., POLLARD, C.**

*Literature and Medicine: An Annotated Bibliography*. rev. ed. Pittsburgh: Univ. Pittsburgh Press, 1982.

**TRAVERSES.**

Special issue: "Panoplies du corps." 14-15 (April 1979).

**TRENN, Thaddeus.**

"Ludwik Fleck's 'On the Question of the Foundations of Medical Knowledge.'" *The Journal of Medicine and Philosophy* 6 (1981): 237-56.

**TREUE, Wilhelm.**

"Die ideale Stadt und die Krankheit im 17. Jahrhundert." *Medizinhistorisches Journal* 5 (1970): 10-23.

**TREXLER, R.**

"Legitimating Prayer Gestures in the Twelfth-Century: The 'De Penitentia' of Peter the Chanter." *History and Anthropology* 1, no. 1 (1984): 97-126.

**TRIER, Jost.**

"Pflanzliche Deutung des Menschen." In *Jahrbuch der Akademie der Wissenschaften*, 39-56. Göttingen: Vandenhoek & Ruprecht, 1965. Cultural history combined with etymology is used to reconstruct the botanical origins of designations referring to the human body.

**TROCME.**

"Esquisse d'une histoire de la pléthore, de la volémie et du retour veineux." *Histoire des sciences médicales* 15 (1981): 69-80.

**TROMP, S.**

"Ecclesia sponsa virgo mater." *Gregorianum* 18 (1937): 3-29. A detailed guide (in Latin) to patristic literature that attributes female characteristics and organs to the Church.

**TRUEB, C.L. Paul.**

*Heilige und Krankheit*. Stuttgart: Klett-Cotta, 1978.

**TRUMBULL, H. Clay.**

*The Blood Covenant: A Primitive Rite and Its Bearing on Scripture*. New York: Scribner, 1885.

____. *The Threshold Covenant: Or, The Beginning of Religious Rites*. New York: Scribner 1896.

**TUAN, Yi-Fu.**

*Landscapes of Fear*. New York: Pantheon, 1979. The author is a geographer whose central interest is the experience of space, place and landscape. This book deals with the incorporation of fear in the perception of landscape. For instance, ch. 13 (pp. 175-86) on the use of human bodies, humiliated, tortured or dead to create foci of horror which also change with time. The pillory, unlike the stocks, became monumental; gallows define the perception of geographic features.

_____. "Body, Personal Relations and Spatial Values." In *Space and Place: The Perspective of Experience*, by TUAN, Yi-Fu. Minneapolis: Univ. Minnesota Press, 1972. People of different cultures differ in how they divide up their world, assign values to its parts and measure them. The upright human being imposes schema on space: up or prone, high or low, home (middle) or at the end of the world. These vertical-horizontal polarities define the ambient space as front-back, right-left, the front larger and illuminated, the back smaller, dark. Only the modern, economic city has no planned front and back.

**TURNER, Bryan S.**

*The Body and Society*. London: Basil Blackwell, 1984.

**TUTTLE, Edward.**

"The Trotula and Old Dame Trot: A Note on the Lady of Salerno." *Bulletin of the History of Medicine* 50, no. 1 (1976): 61-72.

**TYE, Michael.**

"In Defense of the Words 'Human Body'." *Philosophical Studies* (An International Journal for Philosophy in the Analytic Tradition. Tucson, Arizona) 38 (1980): 177-82.

**UEXKUELL, Jacob von.**

*Theoretische Biologie*. Berlin, 1920, and Frankfurt: Suhrkamp, 1973 (*Theoretical Biology*, London: Paul Kegan, 1926). The author engaged in a lifelong effort to create the terminological framework for a theoretical biology in which the body as experience and the experience of historical milieu are correlated. His terminology and conceptual framework predates cybernetics, and would be misunderstood if it were "reduced" to systems-language.

_____. *Umwelt und Innenwelt der Tiere*. Berlin, 1909.

**UEXKUELL, Thure von.**

"Körperwelt: Grenze und Kommunikation." *Eranos-Jahrbuch* (1970): 301-22.

**URBACH.**

"Die Heimsuchung Mariae, ein Tafelbild des Meisters MS. Beiträge zur mittelalterlichen Entwicklungsgeschichte des Heimsuchungsthemas." In *Acta Historiae Artium* 10 (1964) 69-123 and 229-320. The mutual embrace between Mary, in her early pregnancy, and her cousin Elizabeth, much older and in the second half of her pregnancy, is an iconographic motif over many centuries.

**UTLEY, Frances Lee.**

*The Crooked Rib: An Analytical Index to the Argument about Women in the English and Scot Literature to the End of the Year 1568*. New York: Octagon Books, 1970. After a closely reasoned historical introduction which explains the classification used in arranging the Index, a surprising amount and variety of quotations follow.

**UYTTERBROUCK, A.**

"Séquestration ou retraite volontaire? Quelques réflexions à propos de l'hébergement des lépreux à la léproserie de Terbank-les-Louvain." In *Mélanges offerts à G. Jacquemyns*, 615-632. Brussels: Université Libre de Bruxelles, 1968.

**VALDESERRI, R.O.**

"Menstruation and Medical Theory: An Historical Overview." *Journal of the American Medical Women's Association* 38, no. 3 (1983): 66-70.

**VAN DEN BERG, Jan Hendrik.**

*Divided Existence and Complex Society: An Historical Approach*. Pittsburgh: Duquesne Univ. Press, 1974.

_____. *Medical Power and Medical Ethics*. New York: Norton, 1978.

_____. *Things: Four Metabletic Reflections*. Pittsburgh: Duquesne Univ. Press, 1970.

_____. "The Human Body and the Significance of Human Movement: A Phenomenological Study." *Philosophy and Phenomenological Research* 13 (1952).

_____. *The Changing Nature of Man: Introduction to a Historical Psychology*. New York: Delta Publ., 1964; repr. with an intro. by John HOLT, New York: Norton, 1983.

_____. *Het menselijk lichaam: Een metabletisch Onderzök*. Vol. 1: *Het geopende lichaam*. Vol. 2: *Het verlaten lichaam*. Nijkerk: G. F. Callenbach, 1971. The chapter on Vesalius and Vigevano appears as an epilogue (pp. 67-85) in the English translation of another book by VAN DEN BERG, namely *Medical Power and Medical Ethics*.

z o n e

## VAN BAVEL, T.

"L'Humanité du Christ comme lac parvulorum et comme vie dans la spiritualité de Saint Augustin." *Augustiana* 7 (1957): 245-84.

## VAN BROCK, Nadia.

*Recherches sur le vocabulaire médical du grec ancien: soins et guérison.* Paris: Klincksieck, 1961. A history of the word-fields of the Greek medical vocabulary. Half of the terms do not refer to "disease," "diagnosis" and "therapy" but to various emphases of well-being, ranging from "hygies" (health, pp. 143-73) through about twelve complex notions, some of which had several related words with different semantic shades (pp. 177-236).

## VAN GULIK, Robert.

*Sexual Life in Ancient China.* Leiden: E.J. Brill, 1961. Written by a Dutch diplomat, collector and somewhat romantic amateur, the book remains an invaluable source for an attitude toward pleasure and the body that, by its contrast, throws light on the otherness of the West.

## VAN HERIK, Judith.

"Simone Weil's Religious Imagery: How Looking Becomes Eating." In *Immaculate and Powerful: The Female in Sacred Image and Social Reality*, ed. by Cl.W. ATKINSON et al., 260-82. Boston: Beacon Press, 1985. An exemplary combination of the method used in psychology and in religious sciences to gather the sense of embodiment expressed in a series of Weil's autobiographical texts.

## VAN LIERE, Eldon H.

"Solutions and Dissolutions: The Bather in 19th-Century French Painting." *Arts Magazine* 54 (1980): 104-14.

## VAUCHEZ, André.

"Les stigmates de Saint François et leurs détracteurs dans les derniers siècles du Moyen Age." *Mélanges d'Archéologie et d'Histoire* (Ecole Française de Rome) 80, no. 2 (1968): 595-625. Two years before his death, while Francis of Assisi was praying on Mount Alverna, the stigmata with which the crucified Christ is traditionally represented (feet, hands, abdomen) appeared on his body. This is the first instance of "stigmatization," soon to be followed by several hundred other cases. The article by Vauchez is doubly valuable: it introduces to the literature and examines the negative opinion about this "miracle" which was voiced during the thirteenth century, notwithstanding papal recognition of its authenticity.

## VEGETTI, Mario.

"Metàfora politica e immagine del corpo nella medicina greca." In *Tra Edipo e Euclide: Forme del sapere antico*, by M. VEGETTI, Milan: Il Saggiatore, 1983: pp. 41-59. A collection of previously published essays on stylistic changes in Greek thought; especially pp.

41-70 on changes in the metaphorical correspondence of body and society.

## VEITH, Ilza.

*Hysteria: The History of a Disease.* Chicago: Univ. Chicago Press, 1965. The medical and social history of hysteria up to Freud.

## VELTER, André, LAMOTHE, Marie José.

*Les outils du corps.* Paris: Hier et Demain, 1978.

## VENOT, Bernard.

*L'écorché: Exposition.* Rouen 1975-76. Ed. Musée des Beaux-Arts de Rouen, 1977. Catalogue to an exposition of artworks representing the skinned human figure: of the live criminal, of the teaching model, or in contemporary (sometimes abstract) art. Besides the descriptive catalogue and the illustrations a lexicon on French terms (pp. 23-37) and the bibliography (pp. 113-18) are unusual.

## VERDEN-ZOELLER, Gerda.

*Der imaginäre Raum: Fünf Modi der Welterfahrung als Voraussetzung menschlicher Theoriebildung, diskutiert am Aufbau der sensomotorischen Komponenten eines blindgeborenen, cerebralbewegungsgestorten, epileptischen schwerbehinderten siebenjahrigen Madchens.* Dissertation. Phil. Fak., Salzburg, 1979.

## VERDIER, Yvonne.

*Façons de dire, façons de faire: La laveuse, la couturière, la cuisinière.* Paris: Gallimard, 1979. This book is the result of ten years observation by three French anthropologists in the village of Minot in central France. It sets new standards for historically oriented social anthropology. Three women, each with a special ritual charge, occupy center stage: the "washerwoman" in charge of deliveries and the last cleansing of the dead; the seamstress in charge of erotic initiation, and the cook, responsible for the wherewithal of successful marriage. By a discriminating use of oral history Verdier reconstructs the symbolic cosmos of Minot in the early twentieth century. Against this now fading mental background the actions, habits, references and interpretations of the three women conjure up a female body that mirrors time and space in the village.

## VICKERS, Brian.

"Analogy Versus Identity: The Rejection of Occult Symbolism 1580-1680." In *Occult and Scientific Mentalities in the Renaissance*, ed. by B. VICKERS, 95-164. Cambridge: Cambridge Univ. Press, 1984. Follows the debate in England relative to the rejection of metaphorical language in science. The criticism levelled at PARACELSUS illustrates the previous inability to speak about the body without reference to the macrocosm.

## VIGARELLO, Georges.

*Le propre et le sale: L'hygiène du corps depuis le Moyen Age.* Paris: Seuil, 1985. The first monograph that deals directly with the correspondence in the change of body perceptions and social cleanliness in France since the Middle Ages. The medieval bath that had served relaxation and pleasure rather than hygiene is perceived as a serious threat for the open-pored Baroque body whose interior is in constant flux and upheaval. Dry methods are first used to extend the message of cleanliness from the face or hands to a suggestion about the body: frequently changed white linens must show from beneath clothes. Particularly strong on seventeenth- and eighteenth-century documentation.

____. (interviewer). "Histoires des corps: entretien avec Michel de CERTEAU." *Esprit* (France) 2 (1982): 179-90.

____. *Le corps redressé: Histoire d'un pouvoir pédagogique.* Paris: Delarge Edit., 1978. Three stages of the public and normative perception of the body are reflected in the techniques used to shape posture. During the early eighteenth century aristocratic adornment and courtly skills (dance, fencing) called for spectacular posturing, representing status, and for the silencing of emotional expression. By 1750 a new concern with the "population" leads to attempts at improving it organically. The bourgeoisie exacts from its members a body that is disciplined for efficient work and a posture that signals self-control. Posture becomes less a sign of status and more a proclamation of the body's usefulness. During the twentieth century pedagogical techniques deal with the body as a meeting place between the unconscious it expresses and outside demands that repress it. Techniques ought to open the body in all its aspects to conscious awareness and free availability to the self. The body becomes a territory that must be explored, visualized, and worked on by each one.

**VILLETTE, J.**
*L'Ange dans l'Art d'Occident du XIIe au XVIe siècles.* Paris: Laurens, 1940. During the early Middle Ages, angels were shown mostly as adolescent males; during the eleventh and twelfth century the female traits became more prominent, even when the angel was shown as a warrior. Only then did the neutral figure take over, and the childlike angel appear.

**VINATY, Tommaso.**
"Sant'Alberto Magno, embriologo e ginecologo." *Angelicum* 58 (1981): 151-79. Selection and commentary of the major embryological and gynecological texts in the writing of Albert the Great.

**VINGE, Louise.**
*The Five Senses: Studies in a Literary Tradition.* Lund: Liber Laromedel, 1975. Sight, hearing, smell, taste and touch: that the senses should be enumerated in this way is not "self-evident." Both the choice and their order of enumeration is studied as an "artificial series of natural elements." When was this arrange-

ment first used? To what purpose? In which literary genre? A thorough study of the tradition and its historiography so far.

**VLAHOS, Olivia.**
*Body, the Ultimate Symbol.* New York: Lippincott, 1979.

**VODA, Ann M., DINNERSTEIN, Myra, O'DONNELL, Sheryl R., eds.**
*Changing Perspectives on Menopause.* Austin: Univ. Texas Press, 1982.

**VOGT, Helmut.**
*Das Bild des Kranken: Die Darstellung äusserer Veränderungen durch innere Leiden und ihre Heilsmassnahmen von der Renaissance bis zu unserer Zeit.* Munich: J.F. Lehmann, 1960. A collection of some five hundred post-Renaissance pictures of sick persons. The commentary interprets the changing perception of body expression through suffering.

____. *Medizinische Karikaturen von 1800 bis zur Gegenwart.* Munich: J.F. Lehmann, 1960.

**WAGNER, Gustav, MUELLER, Wolfgang J.**
*Dermatologie in der Kunst.* Biberach a.d. Riss: Edit. Basotherm, 1970. Technically outstanding collaboration of a dermatologist and an art historian, published out of a pharmaceutical concern. The representation of skin diseases, in ten chapters dealing successively with periods of European painting.

**WAGNER, W.L.**
"Anthropomorphe Bilder für Geländebezeichnungen, vornehmlich in den iberoamerikanischen Sprachen." In *Homenaje a Rodolfo ORTIZ.* Santiago, Chile, 1955.

**WALKER, Warren S.**
"Lost Liquor Lore: The Blue Flame of Intemperance." *Journal of Popular Culture* 16, no. 2 (1982): 17-25. Since the seventeenth century tales about the spontaneous combustion of bodies have circulated. They became part of the nineteenth-century temperance movement.

**WALZER, Richard.**
*Galen on Jews and Christians.* London: Oxford Univ. Press, 1949.

**WARD, Benedicta.**
*Miracles and the Medieval Mind: Theory, Record and Event, 1000-1215.* Philadelphia: Univ. Pennsylvania Press, 1982. Outside of modern society it would be difficult to discover a culture in which miracles are not part of reality. However, the dividing line between the marvellous and the miraculous shifts, and with it

changes both the popular perception and the learned concept of the miracle. Ward attempts a history of attitudes (theoretical, but also emotional) toward the miracle, which underwent profound changes between the eleventh and fourteenth centuries. Since miracles are overwhelmingly related to the body, a transformation of thought and perception of the body is reflected in their history.

**WASSERSTEIN, Abraham.**
"Normal and Abnormal Gestation Periods in Humans: A Survey of Ancient Opinion (Greek, Roman and Rabbinic)." In *Proceedings of the Second International Symposium on Medicine in Bible and Talmud. Jerusalem, Dec. 1984.* Leiden: E.J. Brill 1985 (special issue of *KOROTH* 9, nos. 1-2. Fall 1985).

**WATSON, Gilbert.**
*Theriac and Mithridatum: A Study in Therapeutics.* London: Wellcome Hist. Medicine Library, 1966.

**WAYMAN, A.**
"The Human Body as Microcosm in India, Greek Cosmology, and Sixteenth-Century Europe." *History of Religions* 22, no. 2 (1982): 172-90.

**WEIMANN, Karl Heinz.**
"Paracelsus und der deutsche Wortschatz." In *Deutsche Wortforschung in europäischen Bezügen,* ed. by Ludwig E.SCHMITT, vol. 2, 359-408. Giessen: W. Schmitz, 1963. The vernacular writings of Paracelsus contributed many words - and, implicitly, views - to the German language.

**WEINAND, Heinz Gerd.**
*Tränen: Untersuchungen über das Weinen in der deutschen Sprache und Literatur des Mittelalters.* Bonn: Bouvier, 1958 (Abh. z. Kunst-, Musik-, und Literaturwissenschaft 5). Not the private emotion but the social symbolism and function of tears during the German Middle Ages. In pp. 15-19 previous research on the expression of grief, heartbreak and suffering is surveyed. The author concentrates specifically on the shedding of tears.

**WEINBERG, Kurt.**
"Zum Wandel des Sinnbezirkes von 'Herz' und 'Instinkt' unter dem Einfluss Descartes." *Archiv für das Studium der neueren Sprachen und Literaturen* 118, no. 203 (1967): 1-31.

**WEINDLER, Fritz.**
*Geschichte der gynäkologisch-anatomischen Abbildungen.* Dresden, 1908. Still valuable history of gynecological book illustrations.

**WEINER, Annette.**
"Reproduction: A Replacement of Reciprocity." *American Ethnologist* 7, no. 1 (1980): 71-85.

**WEISGERBER, Leo.**
"Adjektivische und verbale Auffassung der Gesichtsempfindungen." *Wörter und Sachen* 12 (Heidelberg 1929): 197-226. Detailed analysis of a functional shift in German from verb to adjective in terms referring to visual experience.

____. "Der Geruchsinn in unseren Sprachen." *Indogermanische Forschungen* 46 (1928): 121-50. A seminal article on the methodology by which semantic fields and the shape of experience can be related.

**WEISS, Sandra.**
"The Language of Touch: A Resource to Body Image." *Issues in Mental Health Nursing* 1 (Summer 1978): 17-29.

**WEISSER, C.**
*Studien zum mittelalterlichen Krankheitslunar: Ein Beitrag zur Geschichte der laienastrologischen Fachprosa.* Hannover: Pattersen, 1982 (Würzburger Medizinhistorische Forschungen 21).

**WEIZSAECKER, Viktor von.**
*Arzt und Kranker.* Stuttgart: Köhler, 1949.

____. *Der Gestaltkreis: Theorie der Einheit von Wahrnehmen und Bewegen.* Stuttgart: Thieme, 1968.

____. "Krankheitsgeschichte." In *Arzt und Kranker,* vol. 1, 120-48. Stuttgart, 1949.

**WENTZEL, H.**
"Die ikonographischen Voraussetzungen der Christus-Johannes-Gruppe und das Sponsus-Sponsa Bild des Hohen Liedes." In *Heilige Kunst: Festgabe des Kunstvereines der Diözese Rottenburg zur Hundertjahrfeier 1852-1952,* ed. by E.ENDRICH, 7-21. Stuttgart: Schwabenverlag 1953.

**WENZEL, Siegfried.**
*The Sin of Sloth: "Acedia" in Medieval Thought and Literature.* Chapel Hill: Univ. North Carolina Press, 1960. The bodily expression of sloth throughout the ages can be read from the iconography of sloth, depression, despondency.

**WERNER, Reinhold.**
"Stehen, Sitzen, Liegen: Versuch ueber den Körper zwischen Stillstand und Gebärde." In *Der Andere Körper,* ed. by D.KAMPER and Ch.WULF. Berlin: Verlag Mensch und Leben, 1984.

**WETHERBEE, Winthrop, ed. & trans.**
*The Cosmographia of Bernardus Silvestris.* New York: Columbia Univ. Press, 1973. Introduction contains valuable references to body as microcosm.

**WHALEY, Joachim, ed.**
*Mirrors of Mortality: Studies in the Social History of Death.* New York: St. Martin's, 1981.

**WICKERSHEIMER, M.**
"Figures médico-astrologiques des neuvième, dixième et onzième siècles." In *Transactions of the 17th International Medical Congress. Sect. 23. History of Medicine,* 313-23. London, 1913.

**WIGHTMAN, William P.D.**
"Myth and Method in 17th-Century Biological Thought." *Journal of the History of Biology* 2, no. 2 (1969): 321-36.

**WILBUSH, Joel.**

"La Ménespausie: The Birth of a Syndrome." *Maturitas* 1, no. 3 (1979): 145-51.

**WILSON, Stephen, ed.**

*Saints and Their Cult: Studies in Religious Sociology, Folklore and History*. Cambridge: Cambridge Univ. Press, 1984. A collection of ten essays, mostly translations from French, which complement BROWN (1975 & 1981), GUTH (1970) and BEISSEL (1977).

**WINSLOW, Deborah.**

"Rituals of First Menstruation in Sri Lanka." *MAN* n.s. 15 (1980): 603-25.

**WISWE, Hans.**

*Kulturgeschichte der Kochkunst: Kochbücher und Rezepte aus zwei Jahrtausenden. Mit einem lexikalischen Anhang zur Fachsprache von Eva Hepp*. Munich: Moos, 1970. A large amount of information on epoch- and tradition-specific body lore is hidden in cookbooks. This is a well-researched introduction to the social history of recipes and their collections.

**WITKOWSKI, G.-J.**

*Les seins dans l'histoire*. Paris: A. Maloine, 1903.

____. *Les seins à l'église*. Paris: A. Maloine, 1907. The author, a Polish gynecologist from Paris, published several volumes stuffed with odds and ends from art history, folklore and theology referring to birth rituals, breastmilk, denudation of the nipples, etc. These are mainly of interest as a sample of the late nineteenth-century collector's mentality.

**WITKOWSKI, Stanley R., BROWN, Cecil H.**

"Climate, Clothing and Body-Part Nomenclature." *Ethnology* 24, no. 3 (1985), 197-214.

**WOESTELAND, Evelyn.**

"Le corps féminin dans l'oeuvre de FLAUBERT." Dissertation. Univ. Massachusetts, 1983 (Diss. Abstr. Int., 1984, 44/10: 3081-A DA 840 1114).

**WOLF, Joern Henning.**

*Der Begriff "Organ" in der Medizin. Grundzüge der Geschichte seiner Entwicklung*. Munich: Fritsch, 1971.

____. and HABRICH, Christa, eds. *Aussatz, Lepra, Hansen-Krankheit: Ein Menschheitsproblem im Wandel*. Ausstellung im deutschen Museum in München, 1982-83 (Deutsches Medizinhistorisches Museum, Heft 4). Catalogue of an exposition on Hansen's disease and the cultural perception of the leper.

**WOLF-HEIDEGGER, G., CETTO, A. M.**

*Die Anatomische Sektion in bildlicher Darstellung*. Basel, New York: Karger, 1976. After an introduction to the history of anatomy (pp. 1-98), furnished with excellent bibliography (pp. 99-119), follows a descriptive documented catalogue (pp. 121-392) of each of the 355 reproductions at the end of this volume.

**WOLFSON, Harry A.**

"The Internal Senses in Latin, Arabic, and Hebrew Philosophical Texts." *Harvard Theological Review* 28 (April 1935): 69-133. "Internal senses" complement the body's sense organs. Aristotle launched the ideas taken up by Augustine, Gregory the Great, Erigena. These "postsensational" faculties play an important role in Arabic and Hebrew texts. Thorough philological summary of the various terminologies and classifications with emphasis on Judeo-Arabic schools.

**WOOD, Charles J.**

"The Doctor's Dilemma: Sin, Salvation, and the Menstrual Cycle in Medieval Thought." *Speculum* 56, no. 4 (1981): 710-22.

**WYSS, K.**

*Die Milch im Kultus der Griechen und Römer*. Giessen, 1914 (Religionsgeschichtliche Versuche und Vorarbeiten 15.2).

# Z

**ZAHLTEN, Johannes.**

*Creatio mundi: Darstellung der sechs Schöpfungstage und naturwissenschaftliches Weltbild im Mittelalter*. Stuttgart: Klett-Cotta, 1979 (Stuttgarter Beiträge zur Geschichte und Politik 13). The iconography of Genesis with emphasis on the relationship between pictorial representation and contemporary literary sources. Explores the correspondences and discrepancies between written and figurative representation. Attempts to make the result of this comparison fruitful for the analysis of the same period's scientific texts.

**ZANER, Richard M..**

"The Alternating Reed: Embodiment as Problematic Unity." In *Theology and the Body: Conference on Theology and Body, Emory University 1973*, ed. by John Y.FENTON, 53-71. Philadelphia: Westminster, 1974.

____. *The Context of Self: A Phenomenological Inquiry Using Medicine as a Clue*. Athens: Ohio Univ. Press, 1981. Currently this book might be the best introduction to the twentieth-century development of phenomenological studies of the body.

**ZAPPERT, Georg.**

"Ueber den Ausdruck des geistigen Schmerzes im Mittelalter: Ein Beitrag zur Geschichte der Förderungsmomente des Rührenden im Romantischen." In *Denkschriften der Kaiserlichen Akademie der Wissenschaften. Philosophisch-historische Classe* 5. Bd. 1. Abt. pp. 73-136. Vienna, 1854.

**ZGLINICKI, Friedrich von.**

*Geburt: Eine Kulturgeschichte in Bildern.*
Braunschweig: Westermann, 1983. A compendious
collection of illustrations of the theme of birth.

____. *Kallipigos & Aeskulap: Das Klistier in der
Geschichte der Medizin, Kunst und Literatur.* Baden-
Baden: Verlag für angewandte Wissenschaften, 1965.

**ZIJDERVELD, Anton.**

"The Sociology of Humour and Laughter." *Current
Sociology* 13, no. 3 (1983), 1-101. Annotated bibliography of 225 items is included in this article, pp. 61-101,
see especially sec. 4, nos. 82-95, "History and Literature."

**ZIMMERMANN, Albert, ed.**

*Der Begriff der Repraesentatio im Mittelalter:
Stellvertretung, Symbol, Zeichen, Bild.* Berlin, Köln:
De Gruyter, 1972 (Miscellanea Medievalia 8).

**ZIMMERMANN, Gerd.**

*Ordensleben und Lebenstand: die "cura corporis" in den
Ordensvorschriften des abendländischen Hochmit-
telalters.* Münster: Aschendorfische Verlagsbuchhandlung, 1973.

**ZOLA, Irving K.**

"Pathways to the Doctor - From Person to Patient."
*Social Science and Medicine* 7 (1973): 677-89.
Interviews with patients in the Massachusetts General
Hospital as to their body perception and reasons for
consulting medical help. Great differences as to ethnic
origin: the Irish complain mostly about eyes, ears,
noses, head, while there are no noticeable preferences
given by Italian-American groups. It becomes clear
that the pathway to the doctor is shaped and channeled
through the cultural perception of one's body.

____. "Culture and Symptoms - An Analysis of
Patients' Presenting Complaints." *American
Sociological Review* 31 (1966): 615-30. Surveys the literature which shows how sociocultural background
may lead to different perception, definitions and
responses to essentially the same "biological" process.

# Topical Index

Guicciardi (*hermaphrodite 18th c.*)
Meeks (*early Christianity*)

**Angel**

Behling (*sculpture 11th c.*)
Milner, 1976 (*metaphor for women*)
Mölk (*metaphor for women*)
Schipperges (*Hildegard of Bingen*)
Villette (*art 12-16th c.*)

**Animals**

Balan (*comparative anatomy 19th c.*)
Baltrusaitis (*and human physiognomy*)
Buytendijk (*comparison with humans, physiology*)
Canguilhem, 1960 (*Darwinian psychology, comparison with humans*)
Darnton (*France18th c.*)
Dierauer (*Antiquity, comparison with humans*)
Liden (*animals, anatomical terms*)
Majer (*comparison with humans, Greek lit.*)
Shepard, 1978

**Anorexia, see *Fasting***

**Anthologies**

Ardener, 1978
Ardener, 1982 (*women, perception of women, anthropology*)
Benthall & Polhemus, 1976 (*medium of expression*)
Blacking (*anthropology*)
Cvitanovic (*idea of body, Spanish lit.*)
Imhof, 1979
Imhof, 1983 (*leib, leben*)
Imhof, 1983
Landy
Polhemus, 1978 (*social aspects, body*)
Rothschuh (*disease concepts*)
Sheils (*Church & healing*)
Spicker, 1978 (*philosophy of medicine*)
Teich & Young (*history of science*)
Whaley (*social history of death*)

**Anthropological medicine**

Buytendijk, 1967
Frankl
Gebsattel
Hartmann, 1973
Jacob (*19th c.*)
Magin
Plessner
Popitz (*symbolism of body in*)
Roessler (*disease, history*)

Schipperges,Seidler,Unschuld
Weizsaecker, 1949
Weizsaecker, 1968

**Anthropophagy**

Cremene & Zemmal (*vampire, Rumanian*)
Grabner, 1961 (*therapeutic*)
Grabner, 1964 (*therapeutic*)

**Apotrophy**

Hansmann & Kriss-Rettenbeck, 1966 (*folk beliefs*)
Hauschild, 1984 (*gender symbolism*)
Hoffman, G. (*medieval*)

**Apparitions, see *Visions***

**Architecture**

Andrae (*Ionic column*)
Choay (*Italian Renaissance architecture & body*)
Dorfles (*interior-exterior*)
Flasche (*body as temple*)
Jacobs (*phenomenology*)

**Aristophanes**

Handley (*vocabulary: heart*)

**Aristotle**

Blackman (*"Aristotle's Works" 16-19th c.*)
Horowitz (*biology*)
Jeay (*perception of women*)
Ott (*conception, cheese paradigm*)
Schilling (*mesotes*)

**Art**

Baxandall (*iconography, Renaissance*)
Bugner (*Blacks in Western art*)
Cabanes (*Asclepius*)
Clark (*nude in painting*)
MacKinney (*medical illustration, medieval*)
Mayor (*anatomical*)
Premuda (*anatomical representation*)
Singer, Ch., 1957 (*anatomy in* )
Thornton & Reeves (*medical book illustration*)
Venot (*the skinned in* )
Wagner-Mueller (*skin treatment in*)

**Asceticism**

Bamberg, 1971 (*early monasticism*)
Eisler (*iconography*)
Rousselle, 1983 (*2d-4th c.*)

**Asclepius**

Edelstein, 1945

**Astrology; see also *Microcosm***

Givry, de (*ideas 16-17th c.*)

Lemay, 1980 (*medieval, medical-sexuality*)
MacDonald (*use in diagnosis*)
Richter, 1954
Saintyves, P. (*popular, France*)
Weisser (*in medieval therapy*)
Wickersheimer (*med. figures 8-11th c.*)

**Augustine**

Grabowski (*mystical body*)
Hofmann
Marrou
Miles (*body*)
Peza (*heart, "cor"*)
Van Bavel (*lac parvulorum*)

**Back**

Pisani, 1954 (*vocabulary, German & Italian*)

**Beard**

Platelle (*11-12th c.*)

**Beckett, Samuel**

Ehrard

**Belly (koilia), see *Guts***

**Bernard of Clairvaux**

Leclercq, 1958 (*Marian devotion*)

**Bibliographies**

Augé, 1985 (*healing, history & anthropology*)
Baldwin (*body movement & symbolism*)
Bazin (*androgyny*)
Bremer (*light & eye, perception*)
Calais (*manuals of "savoir-vivre," France*)
Choulant (*anatomical illustation*)
Clarke, 1983 (*gender & illness*)
Conklin (*folk classification*)
De Caro (*woman & folklore*)
Dornseif (*German vocabulary, body*)
Gay, 1871-73 (*women, love & marriage*)
Goldschmid (*pathological illustration*)
Gottschalk (*proverbs*)
Graf (*proportion, architecture, art, nature*)
Hayes (*gesture*)
Juillard & Luneau (*folk healing, contemporary France*)
Langages (*gesture*)
Laplantine (*French popular medicine*)
Poeschl (*imagery, Antiquity*)
Rousseau (*medicine & lierature*)
Schmitt (*gesture*)

Stephens & Bonser *(proverbs)*
Trautmann & Pollard *(literature & medicine)*
Zijderveld *(laughter)*

**Bile**

Klibansky, Saxl, Panofsky *(as humor)*

**Biology**

Balan *(comparative anatomy 19th c.)*
Ballauf *(history)*
Figlio, 1976 *(early 19th c. metaphors)*
Flohr *(use in history, methods)*
Haraway, 1979 *(sociobiology, women)*
Horowitz *(Aristotle & women)*
Hubbard, Henifin, Fried *(anthology of women in)*
Jonas *(philosophical)*
Oppenheimer *(historiography)*
Pagel, 1967 *(Harvey's ideas 17th c.)*
Portmann *(philosophical )*
Ritterbush *(18th c.)*
Roger, 1964 *(problems of method 17-18th c. )*
Singer *(history)*
Teich *(circulation as theme 18th c.)*
Temkin, 1949 *(metaphors)*
Uexkuell, J.J. *(philosophy)*
Wightman *(myth 17th c.)*

**Birth (childbirth, not birth of monsters, abortion). See also** *Navel, Church as woman, Anatomy, Gynecology.*

Arney *(medicalization 20th c.)*
Belmont *(symbolism)*
Bord *(pregnancy, Christian art)*
Bydlowski *(customs)*
Callaway *(theory of )*
Cash *(Tristram Shandy)*
Cattermole *(folk, German)*
Davidson *(placenta rituals)*
Delcourt, 1938 *(demonic, Antiquity)*
Douglas, 1984 *(pollution beliefs)*
Eccles *(Tudor & Stuart England)*
Farge, 1976 *(18th c. France)*
Frevert *(midwifery, Germany 18th c.)*
Gélis, Laget, Morel, 1978 *(history & anthropology)*
Gélis, 1976 *(18th c. France)*
Glis, 1984 *(16-18th c. France)*
Haire *(medicalization)*

Jaberg *(birthmark, terms for)*
Kuntner *(women's position)*
Laget, 1979 *(cesarian delivery, France 16-18th c.)*
Laget, 1981 *(France 17-18th c.)*
Laget, 1982 *(social history - Provence)*
Llompart *(cincture with the length of Christ)*
Martin *(contemporary American perception)*
McDaniel, 1948 *(ancient Rome & modern Italy)*
McDaniel, 1948 *(magic, ancient medicine)*
Mueller, C. *(Alps, recent)*
Muellerheim *(terminology, German)*
Oakley *(medicalization, history)*
Pachinger *(painting & graphic)*
Pomata, 1982 *(perception by Comari, Bologna 17th c.)*
Schewe *(Mary, iconography)*
Schulte, R. *(infanticide, Bavarian)*
Tibon *(navel, umbilical cord, amniotic fluid)*
Zglinicki *(history)*

**Birthmark**

Gilbert *(pregnancy cravings, folk belief)*
Jaberg, 1955
Jaberg, 1956-57 *(folk belief)*

**Blessing**

Bloch *(royal touch)*
Gruttman *(English folk healing)*
Hampp *(folk healing)*

**Blindness**

Cohen, G. *(in French lit. before 1900)*
Scott *(modern)*

**Blood**

Alchian *(transfusion)*
Bowman *(religious in 19th c. France)*
Camporesi *(symbolism & magic, Baroque Italy)*
Ciavarelli *(power of, Spanish lit.)*
Cremene & Zemmal *(vampire, Rumania)*
Debongnie *(stigmata, medieval)*
Duden *(Germany 18th c.)*
Farge, 1979 *(on 18th c. streets)*
Furth *(gendered concepts of, China)*
Grabner, 1963 *( symbolism & red hair in folklore)*
Hirsch *(superstition)*

Koller *(Greek " 'haima," the root "haema")*
Laqueur, 1986 *(fungibility in humoral thought)*
Manuli & Vegetti *(social metaphors, Greek)*
Meringer, J., 1976 *(prehistoric concepts of )*
Milanesi *(late 18th c.)*
Moreau *(in Michelet)*
Morris, L. *(biblical terminology)*
Ohly, 1977 *(magic power of goat's )*
Rothschuh, 1942 *(pathology 18th c.)*
Rothschuh, 1974 *(scientific ideas on, 15-17th c.)*
Ruesche *(blood sacrifice, Antiquity)*
Sabean *(symbolism, Germany 17-18th c.)*
Schipperges, 1974 *(medical concepts of in classical & medieval)*
Schrenk *(symbolism)*
Seidler, 1974 *(haematology 19th c.)*
Toellner, 1981 *(psychological aspects of the discovery of circulation)*
Trocmé *(plethora 18th c.)*

**Blood brothers**

Beidelmann *(covenant in Africa)*
Tegnaeus *(in Africa; bibliography)*
Trumbull

**Blood transfusions**

Alchian *(commercial)*
Johnson *(commercial)*
Morris *(U.S. 19th c.)*
Titmuss *(commercial)*

**Bloodletting**

Bauer, J. *(medical view of)*
Lenhardt *(in the iconography of diagnosis)*
Murko *(Slavic vocabulary)*
Niebyl *(medical theory of )*
Pomata, 1982 *(Bologna 17th c.)*
Pomata, 1984 *(as artificial menstruation)*

**Body: biblical words for. See also: *Mystical, Church as woman, Breast, Flesh, Guts, Hand, Head, Knee, Symbolism.***

Kaiser *(Pauline eschatology)*
Schweizer *(New Testament)*
Dhorme *(Semitic cosmology)*

**Body: Indo-European words for, their seman-**

tics, etymologies, vocabularies. See also *Brain, Breast, Cheek, Cripple, Ear, Excreta, Face, Finger, Flesh, Genitalia, Glossary, Goiter, Guts, Hand, Head, Jaw, Knee, Loins, Limbs, Mouth, Neck, Navel, Nose, Semen, Skin, Stomach, Symbolism, Teeth, Temple, Woman.*

Adolf *("leib" in medieval German)*

Arnoldson *(parts in early German & Scandinavian)*

Baskett *(parts in German dialects)*

Bechtel *(etymology of names of senses in Greek)*

Berger *("unio mystica" in medieval German)*

Bergmann *(cultural history)*

Bonfante *(Indo-European roots for parts in Latin)*

Büsch *(verbs for activity in German)*

Cvitanovic *( in Spanish lit. 13-17th c.)*

Delamarre *(etymology of terms)*

Ehrismann *(in early German)*

Ernout *(names of parts in Latin)*

Florez *(glossary of terms in Spanish, Colombia)*

Frenk Alatorre *(traits in the speech of Mexico City)*

Genzel *(terminology for life functions in English)*

Glatigny *(in French love poems 16th c.)*

Hintner *(in Tyrolian dialect)*

Hoefler *(in German)*

Janne *(Hellenistic metaphor)*

Leschhorn *(references to in English syntax)*

Maragi *(Latin, German 9th c.)*

Niederwolfsgruber-Insam *(woman's, Tyrol)*

Oksaar *(in Baltic languages)*

Onians *(semantics in archaic Greek)*

Ramat *(woman's, Indo-European)*

Reis *(localization of functions in Old Latin)*

Schuster-Sewc *(Slavic vocabulary)*

Schweikle *(woman's, medieval German)*

Wagner, W.L. *(anthropomorph on landscape, Latin America)*

**Body: non-Indo-European words for. See also: *Hand, Knee, Limbs, Navel, Nose, Stomach, Tongue.***

Alp *(Hittite)*

Ames *(classical Chinese)*

Bastien *(Andean Qollahuaya language, hydraulic model)*

Buhan *(languages of south Cameroon)*

Burrow *(Dravidian)*

Deimel *(Sumerian)*

Dhormé *(Semitic, cosmological correspondence)*

Ebers *(ancient Egyptian)*

Franklin *(Kewa)*

Holma *(Babylonian, Akkadian)*

Lopez Austin *(classical Nahuatl)*

Mahr *(Delaware language 18th c.)*

Pettinato *(vocabulary, Akkadian & Sumerian creation myths)*

Stark *(Quechua)*

**Body works, see *Tattoo***

**Boehme, Jacob**

Schleusener-Eichholz *(the eye, medieval)*

**Bonaventure**

Rahner, K. *(spiritual senses)*

**Brain**

Bynum, W., 1973 *(anatomy 19th c.)*

Vegetti *(in social metaphors)*

**Breast**

Biale *(of God, Old Testament)*

Bynum, C. *(symbols of, 12th c.)*

Deonna, 1954 *(symbolic feeding of)*

Eckert *(Baltic)*

Kroell *(terms for in Portuguese)*

Kuen *(Ladinic dialects, vocabulary)*

Levy *(female in art)*

Pomata, 1980 *(commercialization of feeding 19th c.)*

Witkowski *(cultural history)*

**Brueghel**

Torrilhon *(anatomy of figures)*

**Canon law**

Bullough & Brundage *(sexuality, medieval)*

Loeffler *(impotence)*

Noonan *(contraception, history)*

**Caricature**

Vogt *(medical 18-20th c.)*

**Castration, see *Conception***

**Cervantes**

Ciavarelli *(force of blood in)*

**Changeling**

Piaschewski *(folk beliefs)*

**Charcot**

Didi-Huberman

**Chaucer**

Benson *(gestures in)*

**Cheek**

Kahane, 1941 *(Italian dialects)*

**China**

Ames *(meaning of the body, classical)*

Furth *(blood and gender, 1600-1850)*

Van Gulik *(sexuality, ancient)*

**Chiromancy**

Givry, de

Rem

**Chrestien of Troyes**

Peil *(gesture)*

**Church as woman**

D'Onofrio *(papessa Giovanna)*

Kassing *(apocalyptic woman)*

Plumpe *(Church as mother)*

Thérel *(iconography 3d-6th c.)*

Tromp *(patristic)*

**Cincture**

Grabner *(folk medicine)*

Llompart *(Catalan folk medicine, medieval)*

**Circle, circulation**

Bäumker *(prescholastic)*

Lurker *(symbolism)*

Toellner, 1981 *(discovery of blood )*

**Circumcision**

Bettelheim *(puberty rites)*

Bryk

**Claire, John**

Barrell

**Classification: folk. See also *Body: words for.***

Beck, 1975 *(anthropology)*

Buhan *(South Cameroon)*

Conklin *(folk , bibliography)*

Douglas, 1971

Ellen

Franklin

Needham, R., 1973

Stark

Witkowski & Brown *(climate, clothes, body)*

**Claustrum animae, see *Interiority***

zone

Brown, F. *(of North Carolina, collection)*
Hand *(Ohio)*
Puckett *(of American Blacks)*
Saintyves, 1937 *(moon in, France)*

**Food**
Barreau *(the transformation of tastes)*
Blond
Bynum, C., 1985 *(fasting nuns, medieval)*
Camporesi, 1985 *(Italian humanism)*
Châtelet *(cookbooks, symbols)*
Douglas *(in U.S., anthropology)*
Fischer-Homberger *(soul's function)*
Flandrin, 1983 *(the diversification of taste, 16-18th c.)*
Henisch *(medieval society &)*
Hentig *(last meal before execution)*
Jones *(function of, medieval German lit.)*
Lange *(spiritual, in biblical metaphors)*
Loux & Richard *(in French proverbs)*
Pouchelle, 1983 *(digestion, medieval)*
Sabean *(Eucharist vs. everyday)*
Schama *(Holland 17th c.)*
Temkin, 1960 *(nutrition: antiquity to Baroque)*
Van Herik *(as metaphor, Simone Weil)*
Wiswe *(cookbooks)*

**Foucault**
Fraser *(the body in Foucault's language)*
Lash, S. *(critique of Foucault's body)*

**Francis of Assisi**
Einhorn
Merkt *(stigmata)*
Vauchez *(stigmata)*

**Freckles**
Delcourt, 1965 *(Antiquity)*

**Funeral sermons**
Doehner
Mohr

**Fur, see also Skin.**
Pouchelle, 1981 *(the metaphor, medieval)*

**Galen**
Garcia Ballester *(biography)*
Harris *(heart)*

Temkin, 1973 *(Galenism)*
Walzer *(on Jews & Christians)*

**Gallbladder, see Bile**

**Gallstones**
Grabner, 1978

**Gaub, Jerome**
Rather, 1965 *(de regimine mentis 18th c.)*

**Gender**
Bourdieu *(in Kabyle space)*
Freytag *(orientation, disturbances)*
Furth *(body ascriptions & in China)*
Hammer *(body & in philosophy)*
Hartog *(in Antiquity, Herodotus on inversion)*
Illich, 1982
Kestenberg *(inside/outside)*
Kuchenbuch *(peasant, work 9th c.)*
Laqueur, 1986 *(in anatomy & biology 16-19th c.)*
Lloyd, 1966 *(gendered polarity, Antiquity)*
Loefstedt *(in Latin semantics)*
Maertens, 1978 *(gendered marks through tattoo)*

**Genitalia. See also Conception, Semen, Stomach, Womb.**
Benedek *(description of, Middle Ages & Renaissance)*
Bettelheim *(puberty rites)*
Browe, 1936 *(in religion & law: the attitude of the Christian church to castration)*
Bryk *(history of circumcision)*
Deonna *(female as shell)*
Elwin *(vagina dentata)*
Gilman, 1985 *(19th c. representation)*
Gobert *(Africa)*
Guenther *(German terms for)*
Helten *(German terms for)*
Kilmer *(phobia of, Greek antiquity)*
Laqueur, 1986 *(visions 16-19th c.)*
Maass *(terms for castration, Antiquity)*
Mueller, K. *(German terminology for)*
Pierrugues *(Latin terms for)*
Pisani, 1974, 1979 *(female in Italian & German)*
Radtke, E. *(terms for in Italian slang)*
Radtke, P. *(female; pre-Vesalius)*

Rancour-Laferrière *(semiotics of the penis)*
Schertel *(phallus & cunnus in language and myths)*
Steinberg *(ostentatio genitalium Christi)*
Thomasset *(medieval representation)*

**Geometrization**
Jacobs *(phenomenology & geometries: Euclidean & non-Euclidean)*
Lippe *(in French absolutism)*
Ohly *(Deus geometra)*

**Gestation. See also Embryo.**
Blackman *("Aristotle's Works" 16-19th c.)*
Bord *(visible in Christian art)*
Cattermole *(folk representations of, Germany)*
Dawson *(couvade)*
Delorme *(in Albertus Magnus)*
Demaitre & Travill *(in Albertus Magnus)*
Feudale *(iconography, in Piero della Francesca)*
Fischer-Homberger, 1983 *(in court)*
Hand, 1957 *(couvade, U.S.)*
Jordanova, 1980 *(the creation of "life," 1800)*
Kellersmann *(cravings during gestation)*
Lechner *(Maria Gravida)*
Martin *(American perception 20th c.)*
Noonan *(contraception in history of canon law)*
Peters *(lay attitudes toward, England 18th c.)*
Roger *(scientific concepts of, France 18th c.)*
Schulte *(sociohistory of unwed mothers, Germany 19th c.)*
Thomasset *(medieval concepts of)*
Urbach *(Mary & Elizabeth, golden gate iconography)*
Vinaty *(in Albertus Magnus)*
Wasserstein *(beliefs concerning term, Antiquity)*

**Gesture**
Baldwin *(bibliography)*
Barakat *(Cistercian sign language)*
Barasch *(of despair, medieval & Renaissance)*
Baxandall *(in painting 15th c.)*
Benson *(in Chaucer)*

562

Demisch *(in prayer gesture)*
Deonna, 1960 *(manus oculatae)*
Fehr *(gestures in law)*
Friedrich *(Hittite vocabulary)*
Hattenhauer *(God's since late Antiquity)*
Hertz, 1928 *(right-left dichotomy: its symbolism)*
Hildburgh *(amulet, Spain)*
Jud *(Spanish terms for folded)*
Kirigin *(iconography of God's)*
Leroi-Gourhan, 1967
Rem *(chiromancy)*
Schupbach *(symbolism from Aristotle to Rembrandt)*
**Hardy, Thomas**
Scarry
**Hartmann of Aue**
Peil *(gesture)*
**Harvey, William**
Hill *(idea of monarchy)*
Pagel, 1958, 1967
Sigerist, 1928, 1960 *(Baroque body)*
Toellner, 1981 *(circulation)*
**Hawthorne**
Cameron *(allegories of the body)*
**Head**
Bedale *(Pauline epistles)*
Bernitt *(French wordfield)*
Bonfante, 1951 *(cheek, jaw in Italian)*
Braun *("kopf," in German toponymy)*
Congar *(folk etymologies, medieval)*
D'Alvarenga *(popular perception of the head, Portuguese)*
Mueller, J. *(German vocabulary on)*
Richter, E., 1951 *(votive offerings, headache)*
**Health**
Coleman, 1974 *(in the Encyclopédie)*
Coleman, 1977 *(folk concepts of, 18th c. France)*
Coleman, 1982 *(public & political, 19th c. France)*
Farge, 1982 *(manuals 18th c.)*
Hager *(in Goethe)*
Jordanova, 1982 *(ideology, late 18th c.)*
Schipperges, 1963 *(medical efforts since Antiquity)*
Schmitt, W. *(medieval regimen sanitatis)*

**Heart**
Bäumker *(medieval)*
Bauer *(as cloister in medieval piety)*
Brunner *(Egyptian beliefs)*
Cabassut *(a medieval theme, interchange of)*
Duewel, 1964 *(medieval metaphors)*
Duewel, 1974 *(in Kleist)*
Ertzdorff, 1962 *(in religious medieval Latin)*
Ertzdorff, 1965 *(in courtly love)*
Fickel *(in early German)*
Flasche *(Pascal)*
Goedel *(in medical terminology of Egypt)*
Guillaumont *(in semantics, Antiquity)*
Handley *(in Aristophanes)*
Harris *(functions in Antiquity)*
Hattenhauer *(the king's, medieval)*
Hermann, A. *(life stone, Antiquity)*
Hillman *(historical phenomenology)*
Hintze *(Egyptian vocabulary for)*
Huttmann *(imagined tumor)*
Kees *(in Egyptian mythology)*
Manuli & Vegetti *(in social metaphors, classical Greece)*
Ohly, 1977 *(chamber for the beloved)*
Peza *(symbols in Augustine)*
Romanyshyn *(historical phenomenology)*
Sardello *(in phenomenology)*
Starobinski *(perception of the interior)*
Thomae *(in popular art)*
Weinberg *(changing semantics 17th c.)*
**Herbs, see *Plants***
**Heredity**
Lesky *(medical concepts since Antiquity)*
**Herodotus**
Hartog, 1980, 1981
**Hieronymus Mercurialis**
Englert
**Hildegard of Bingen**
Goessmann *(numbers & proportions in)*
Mueller, I., 1979 *(healing in works of)*
Pereira *(maternity)*
Schipperges, 1958
Schipperges, 1963 *(angels in works of)*

Schipperges, 1981 *(compassion as cure)*
**Hindu cosmology and body**
Beck, 1976
Douglas *(pollution beliefs)*
Gonda *(eye & gaze in Veda)*
O'Flaherty *(women in)*
Waymann, 1982 *(body as microcosm)*
**Hippocratic tradition**
Artel, 1968 *(poison & drugs in)*
Cambiano *(political metaphors)*
Dumortier *(medical terms in)*
Gourevitch, 1983 *(doctor & patient)*
Kapferer *(fever & inflamation)*
Preiser *(Hippocratic terminology: nousos, nosema)*
Preiser *(terms for illness in the)*
Smith, 1979
Souques *(pain in the Hippocratic corpus)*
**Hobbes**
Sawday *(body as machine)*
**Homo economicus**
Featherstone *(embodied)*
**Honorius Augustodunensis**
D'Alverny, 1976 *(micro-macro)*
**Hot, see *Humor***
**Human figure**
Brückner *(pictorial representation, the "effigie")*
Encyclopedia of World Arts *(in art)*
Haskell *(in sculpture, 1500-1800)*
Janson *(Renaissance art)*
Ladner, 1953 *(iconoclasm)*
Ladner, 1962 *(in medieval art)*
Lurker *(and circle symbolism)*
Panofsky, 1955 *(proportions of the)*
Piponnier & Bucaille *(peasants, medieval France)*
Reff *(Manet's Olympia)*
Reudenbach *(proportion of, Vitruvius)*
Ringbom *(approach to, 15th c.)*
Scheffczyk *(man as God's image)*
Torrilhon *(in Brueghel's painting)*
**Humors: hot-cold, wet-dry**
Camporesi, 1984 *(Italian humanism)*
Fahraeus *(folk traditions)*
Jeay *(Albertus Magnus)*

Tuan, 1979 (*of fear*)

Wagner, W.L. (*anthropomorphic words for in S. American languages*)

### Laughter

Keller (*anthropological analysis, in literature*)

Zijderveld (*bibliography & sociology of*)

### Law

Beyerle (*gesture in, medieval*)

Cahen (*kinship & adoption, Old German*)

Cohen (*family &*)

Darmon (*on impotence, ancien régime*)

Fehr (*gestures, Germany, Middle Ages to 18th c.*)

Fischer-Homberger (*& medicine, ancien régime*)

Pomata, 1983 (*court procedures, healers & patients*)

Schmidt-Wiegand (*gesture in jurisdiction, medieval*)

### Left-right

Hertz

Lloyd, 1962 (*classical Greece*)

Needham, R. (*anthology*)

### Leonardo da Vinci

Annali di Medicina Navale e Tropicali

Fusco (*use of anatomy*)

Mayor (*anatomical drawing*)

O'Malley & Saunders

Panofsky, 1962 (*anatomical perspective*)

### Leprosy

Bourgeois (*10-13th c.*)

Brody (*in medieval literature*)

Grön (*in art*)

Uytterbrouck

Wagner-Mueller (*in iconography*)

Wolf & Habrich

### Lesbian

Bonnet (*France 16-20th c.*)

### Life force

Lohff (*history of the idea, German*)

Muth (*excretion as, Antiquity*)

### Limbs

Dietrich (*Semitic vocabulary*)

Koller, 1965 (*Greek etymology*)

### Linguistics. See also Body: words for, Glossary.

Andresen (*popular etymologies*)

### Liver

Hagen (*in Antiquity*)

### Loins

Gamillscheg ("*dorsum*," "*renes*," *Latin*)

### Love-sickness

Birchler (*potions*)

Giedke (*history of medicine*)

### Lungs

Moeckel (*terms for functions, French*)

### Machine, body as

Lock (*metaphor*)

Moravia (*as metaphor 18th c.*)

Quiguer (*and women in iconography, 1900*)

Sawday (*metaphors 17th c.*)

### Macrocosm, see Microcosm

### Madness

Didi-Huberman (*19th c. France*)

Doob (*medieval England*)

Gilman (*as represented in art*)

MacDonald, 1981 (*in England 17th c.*)

### Magic. See also Eye (evil), witchcraft.

Accati (*performed bodily by women*)

Aguirre Beltran (*in Mexico*)

Bargheer (*with body parts*)

Birchler (*love sickness*)

Bloch, M. (*through royal touch*)

Bouteiller, 1950 (*folk healing & shamanism*)

Camporesi (*blood*)

Cardini

Easlea (*magic & scientific thought, 1450-1750*)

Elworthy (*evil eye*)

Grabner, 1972 (*transplantatio morborum*)

Hand, 1972-73 ("*measuring*" *in folk healing*)

Hand, 1980, 1981

Hoefler, 1909 (*innards*)

Kriss-Rettenbeck, 1963 (*amulets*)

Le Roy Ladurie, 1975 (*in France 14th c.*)

Le Roy Ladurie, 1978 (*castration*)

McDaniel, 1948 (*through female innards*)

Romilly (*& rhetoric, ancient Greece*)

Thomas, K. (*& religion 16-18th c.*)

### Mandragora

Rahner, H. (*Christian & classical, symbol*)

### Mantic

Bargheer (*innards*)

Bouteiller, 1958

Charmasson (*medieval*)

Hoefler, 1909 (*innards*)

Maire (*Paris 18th c.*)

### Mary

Bétérous (*legends of her milk*)

Eich (*Maria Lactans until 13th c.*)

Feudale (*iconography of the Madonna del Parto*)

Guldan, 1966 (*& Eve, iconography*)

Guldan, 1968 (*Annunciation iconography*)

Kassing (*Apocalypse*)

Lechner (*Gravida in iconography*)

LeClercq (*Marian devotion*)

Muthmann (*as spring, as fountain*)

Richter, E. (*healing, popular piety*)

Richter, E. 1954 (*milk as therapy*)

Ronig (*breastfeeding*)

Schewe (*iconography of birthing*)

Steinberg (*pietàs*)

Tramoyeres Blasco (*milk*)

Urbach (*& Elizabeth*)

### Masks

Caillois, 1960

Schmidt, 1972 (*Austria*)

### Measuring

Fee (*craniology 19th c.*)

Grabner, 1964 (*folk therapeutics*)

Hand, 1972-73 (*folk medicine*)

Llompart (*length of Christ, medieval Catalonia*)

Shryock (*history of quantification in medicine*)

### Med*: an Indo-European root

Benveniste, 1965 (*root of moon, of measure and healing*)

### Medical aesthetics

Deshaies

### Medical terminology. See also Glossary, Linguistics.

Altieri-Biagi (*medieval*)

Baader & Keil (*medieval*)

Eis (*late medieval*)

### Medicalization

Annales de Bretagne (*France 18-19th c.*)

Armstrong (*Britain 20th c.*)

Arney & Bergen (of childbirth 20th c.)

Bleker (Germany 19th c.)

Boltanski (class-specific consumption of medicine)

Boltanski, 1968 (epistemology)

Branca (social history 19th c.)

Bruegelmann, 1982 (social history, Germany)

Clarke (women & literature review)

Coleman (in Encyclopédie)

Corbin, 1977 (syphilis, France 19th c.)

Desaive (France, ancien régime)

Ehrenreich & English (of women 19th c.)

L'Espérance (of women 19th c.)

Foucault, 1973

Gabka (of teething)

Goubert, 1977 & 1979 (France, ancien régime, 18th c.)

Herzlich & Pierret (history of disease perception)

Illich, 1977 (concept of)

Knibiehler, 1976 (of female genitals 19th c.)

Mandrou (in early modern France)

Oakley (of the womb)

Peter, 1975-76 (utopian dream)

Zola, 1973 ("patient-roles," U.S.)

## Medicine: medieval

Altieri-Biagi (terminology of medieval medicine)

Baader & Keil (a reader about)

Benton (about women)

Diepgen, 1922 (relation to theology)

Diepgen, 1958 (influence of theology on)

Diepgen, 1963 (on women)

Eis (terminology of in prose, late medieval)

Jacquart (France 12-15th c.)

MacKinney (medical illustration in Medieval manuscripts)

Mueller, I. (St. Hildegard)

Murdoch (illustration in science)

Schipperges, 1985

Sisto (historiography of, Italy)

## Melancholy

Certeau, 1985 (17th c.)

Jehl (Bonaventura)

Klibanksy, Sax, Panofsky

MacDonald (England 17th c.)

Marsella (depression, cross-cultural, methodology)

Mauzi (18th c.)

Pouchelle, 1983

Schipperges, 1967 (medieval)

## Melville

Cameron (allegory of body)

## Menopause, menarche

Laslett (since 18th c.)

Martin, E., 1987 (scientific concepts and personal experience, U.S.)

Skultans (symbolism)

Smith-Rosenberg (U.S. 19th c.)

Voda, Dinnerstein, O'Donnell

Wilbush (19th c.)

## Menstruation

Birk & Best (feminist critique of biology of)

Bullough & Voght (19th c.)

Bullough (medieval)

Crawford (England 17th c.)

Delaney, Lupton, Toth (cultural history of)

Figlio, 1983 (amenorrhea 19th c.)

Fischer-Homberger (medical views on)

Flandrin, 1983 (6-11th c.)

Harrell (in cultural perspective)

Joffe (vernacular views on, N.Y. 20th c.)

Le Roy Ladurie (famine, amenorrhea)

MacCormack (symbolism, anthropology)

Martin, E. 1987 (contemporary perception, U.S.)

Mueller-Hess (medical views on)

Niccoli (monster, conception 16th c.)

Pomata, 1984 (& bloodletting 16-17th c.)

Saintyves, 1937 (popular belief about the "moons," France)

Showalter (Victorian)

Skultans (symbolism, anthropology)

Valdeserri (medical theory of)

Verdier (rural France 19th c.)

Winslow (in Sri Lanka)

Wood (medieval thought on)

## Merleau-Ponty

Anchieta Correa

Hammer (body & gender in)

Maier

Moss (body image)

## Mesotes

Schilling (Aristotle)

## Metabletica, see Phenomenology

## Metaphor: social, architectural, spatial

Bauer, G., (Claustrum animae)

Cambiano (political, Antiquity)

Choay (architectural, Renaissance)

Demandt (for "history")

Flasche (temple, for the body)

Frühsorge (body in novel 17th c.)

Hale (politic & body, England, Renaissance)

Manuli & Vegetti

Marcovich

Pouchelle, 1983 (medieval)

Romantisme (energy as metaphor 19th c. France)

Temkin, 1977 (biological)

Wagner, W.L. (for body and landscape in American languages)

## Methodology

Falk (sociological history)

Jackson (anthropology of the body)

Leroy-Gourhan, 1973 (environment & technique)

MacDonald, 1983 (anthropological perspective in medical history)

Roger, 1964 (of biological history)

## Meyer, Conrad Ferdinand

Hellermann (gestures in)

## Michelangelo

Steinberg, 1970

Steinberg, 1982

## Michelet

Deonna

Moreau (on women)

## Microcosm

Allers (conceptual taxonomy)

Barkan (English lit.)

Beck, 1976 (Hindu cosmology)

Beer (iconography, medieval)

Benz, 1974

Blank (on Konrad of Megenberg)

Camporesi, 1985 (Italy 15-17th c.)

Conger (philosophical aspects of the)

D'Alverny, 1953, 1976 (medieval concepts)

Givry, de

Grabner, 1972 (as part of folk healing)

Hansmann & Kriss-Rettenbeck (& amulet)

Hertz, 1928

Jordanova, 1979 (environmental medicine late 18th c.)

Kranz (history of ideas and concepts of)

Kurdzialek (representation of, medieval)

Lock (Japan vs. Europe)

Muchembled (women in a French village 18th c.)

Nobis (medieval)

Pouchelle, 1979 (and social cosmos)

Pouchelle, 1983 (in Mondeville)

Saxl, 1957 (in medieval pictures)

Schipperges, 1962 (Arab influence on, 12th c.)

Tibon, 1981

Vickers (demise since 1580)

Waymann (in India, Greece and 16th c. Europe)

Wetherbee (in Bernhard Sylvestris)

**Milk, lactation**

Bardy (St. Catherine)

Bétérous (Mary's, medieval sources)

Deichgraeber (in Hippocratic therapies)

Deonna, 1954 (lactation of adults)

Dewez & Iterson (St. Bernard's lactation, iconography)

Eich (Mary's lactation until 13th c.)

Harrell (lactation, anthropology)

Hildburgh (Spanish amulets)

Lange (biblical metaphors of)

Pomata, 1980 (orphanage, Italy 19th c.)

Richter, E., 1954 (Mary's as therapy)

Ronig (Mary's in theology)

Tramoyeres (Mary's in art)

Van Bavel (lac parvulorum)

Wyss (lactation in Antiquity)

**Mind**

Rather, 1959, 1982 (body & mind 18th c.)

**Miracles**

Bernards (protocols of)

Bétérous (Mary's milk)

Bloch, M. (by royal touch)

Finucane, 1981 (by invocation of the saints, medieval)

Gélis & Redon, 1983 (popular beliefs, France)

Gélis, 1981 (resurrection of the stillborn)

Hoffmann, S. (healing, testimony 18th c.)

Maire (convulsions, Paris 18th c.)

Rosenthal (healing, iconography)

Rousselle, 1976 (thaumaturgical, Gaul 4th c.)

Vauchez (St. Francis & stigmata)

Ward (history of attitudes, 11-12th c.)

**Mirror**

Hartlaub (history of art)

Hartog (image, Herodotus)

Nahoum (of women's beauty)

Schwarz, H. (in art)

**Mondeville**

Pouchelle, 1983

**Monkey**

Janson (iconography)

**Monster (terata)**

Bernheimer (wild men, medieval)

Caillois (imagination, medieval)

Céard (16th c.)

Darmon, 1984 (conception 17th c.)

Delcourt, 1938 (classical Antiquity)

Hintzsche (teratology since 18th c.)

Janson (ape, medieval & Renaissance)

Niccoli (conception & menses, 1500)

Park & Daston (teratology 16-18th c.)

Peter, 1976 (France 18th c.)

**Montaigne**

Kritzman

**Montesquieu**

Geffriaud

**Morphology**

Balan (comparative anatomy 19th c.)

Behling (iconography of plants, medieval & Renaissance)

Thompson

**Mouth**

Battisti (uvula in Italian dialects)

Hesseling (palate, semantic comparison of)

Jager, 1985

Jucquois (semantics, Indo-European)

Majut (terms for its functions, Antiquity)

**Movement**

Baldwin (bibliography)

Bathe (in Kleist)

Bestor (semantics of)

Buytendijk (phenomenology)

Sarles (linguistic research)

**Mummy**

Grabner, 1961, 1974 (as remedy)

**Muscle**

Meyer, A.W. (allantois)

**Music & disease**

Sigerist, 1943

**Mutilation**

Browe, 1936 (castration)

Gélis (deformation of newborns, France)

Maertens, 1978

Segal, 1971 (mutilation of corpses, Iliad)

Tuan, 1979 (body, effect on landscape perception)

Venot (the skinned body in art)

**Mystical body. See also Body: words for, Biblical.**

Berger, K. (Unio mystica)

Grabowski (Augustine)

Heine (New Testament)

Hofmann (Augustine, on Church)

Käsemann (Pauline)

Rinna (Ambrose)

Schlier (Paul to Ephesians)

**Mythology**

Conteneau (Babylonian naked goddess)

Diester (body in Nazi propaganda)

Jayne (healing gods)

Schlegel (cripple in mythology)

**Nakedness, see Nudity**

**Nature**

Charlton (images of, France 1750-1800)

Fabricant, 1979 (18th c. landscape design)

Glacken (concept of nature-culture dichotomy until 18th c.)

Guillerme (18th c. perception of)

Jacob (biology 19th c.)

Neuburger (healing powers in the body)

Nobis (medieval concepts of)

Pellicer (semantics of "natura")

Sallmann (philosophy of, Antiquity)

Shepard, 1982

**Navajo space**

Pinxten

**Navel**

Hermann, H.V. (in Greek myth)

Meringer, R., 1913

Tibon, 1980

**Neck**

Knetschke (German words in geography)

**Nietzsche**

Hammer (body & gender)

Lash

Remmert (aesthetics & the body in)

zone

z o n e

## Physiology

Brooks, Cranefield (anthology of)
Brown (bibliography)
Callot (France 16th c.)
Canguilhem, 1953 (reflex)
Cooter, 1979
Lawrence (Scotland 18th c.)
Moravia (in 18th c. lit.)
Neuberger (healing powers of the body)
Roger (theory, France 18th c.)
Rothschuh, 1953 (history)
Rothschuh, 1969 (concepts, 16-19th c.)

## Piety: popular iconography of. See also Religiosity.

Arnold (women's, France 19th c.)
Bauerreis (medieval, to the suffering Christ)
Eich (Maria Lactans, until 13th c.)
Einhorn (interiority, Francis of Assisi)
Ertzdorff, 1963 ("heart" in)
Kriss-Rettenbeck, 1963 (popular iconography)
Kriss-Rettenbeck, 1972
LeClercq (Marian devotion, medieval)
LeClercq (medieval and the suffering Christ)
Richter, E., 1954 (Mary as healer)
Scharfe (protestant pictures of)

## Placenta, see Afterbirth

## Plant

Aigremont (folk, on erotics)
Arano (medieval herbs)
Behling (in iconography, symbols in painting)
Delaporte (taxonomy 18th c.)
Hoefler, 1908 (popular terms for, German)
Rahner, H. (mandragora, a metaphor)
Riddle (medieval & female botany)
Trier (designations referring to body)

## Plato

Cambiano (political metaphors)
Dubois (Phaedrus)

## Pliny

Oennerfors, 1954, 1963 (medieval reception of)

## Pneuma, see Spirits

## Pope

Brooks-Davies (venereal iconography)
Fabricant, 1977 (representation of women in)

## Postcards

Crelin & Helfland (medical care on)

## Posture

Bathe (in Kleist)
Bourdieu, 1984
Büsch (German terms for stand, sit, etc.)
Buytendijk, 1956 (phenomenology)
Straus (upright, phenomenology)
Tikkanen (crossed feet)
Van den Berg (phenomenology of movements)
Vigarello, 1978 (education 19th c.)
Werner

## Prolongevity

Gruman (history of medical theories on)

## Proportions

Goessmann, 1984 (in Hildegard of Bingen)
Herrlinger, 1949 (in 14th c.)
Panofsky (in human figures)

## Proust

Reichler (& the "subtle body")

## Proverbs

Brown, T. (in American folklore)
Gottschalk (Romance languages)
Gruttmann (English folk medicine)
Hand, 1980 (folk healing, Europe & America)
Knortz (German)
Lachal (Italian on disease)
Loux & Richard (food & illness)
Loux, 1978 (French)
Pires de Lima (Portuguese)
Segalen (on women & marriage, France 19th c.)

## Psyche, see Spirits

## Purity. See also Hygiene, Space.

Douglas, 1984 (anthropology)
Moulinier (Greek thought)
Parker (& pollution in early Greek religion)

## Rabelais

Bakhtin

## Regimen Sanitatis. See also Dietetics.

Rather, 1965 (mind & body 18th c.)

Schmitt, W. (medieval)
Zimmermann, G. (in monastic orders, high Middle Ages)

## Rejuvenation

Edsman (myths & legends on through fire)

## Religiosity

Archives des sciences sociales des religions
Gélis & Redon (miraculous healing)
Hoffman, S. (miraculous healing, 18th c. Germany)
Kriss-Rettenbeck, 1963
Laplantine (healing, contemporary France)
Ménard (iconography 17-18th c.)
Milanesi (in Italy 1700)
Richter, E., 1951 (devotional pictures to be swallowed)
Richter, E., 1954 (Mary's milk as therapy)
Scharfe (protestant pictures of piety)
Sigal (miraculous healing 11-12th c.)

## Rembrandt

Schupbach

## Resurrection

Chollet (corps glorieux)
Croix
Gélis, 1981 (stillborn)
Paravy (of stillborn France 15th c.)

## Richardson

Peters (pregnant Pamela)

## Rituals

Davidson (placenta)
LeClercq (Last Unction 9-10th c.)
Martino (mourning)
Meringer, J. (blood, prehistoric)
Obeyesekere (theory, anthropology, religion)
Schaefer, T. (of monastic feet-washing, medieval)

## Sacred Heart

Di Cori (devotion to, Italy 19th c.)
LeClercq (in Benedictine tradition, medieval)
Richtstätter (in German art, medieval)

## Saints

Allan (thaumaturgical)
Bardy (St. Catherine)
Beissel (medieval devotion)
Brown, P., 1975, 1982 (late Antiquity, Middle Ages)

Cambiano (political metaphor, Greek Antiquity)

Corbin (18th c.)

Davis, 1981 (space, France 16th c.)

Douglas, 1972

Douglas, 1984 (pollution beliefs)

Gallagher & Laqueur, 1987

Hale ("body politics," English Renaissance)

Hofmann (Augustine)

Jacob (medical anthropology 19th c.)

Lawrence (sensibility, irritability)

MacCormack (biology-woman)

Manuli & Vegetti (heart, blood, brain)

Marcovich (18th c.)

Martin, 1987 (contemporary, U.S.)

Moravia (sensibility, machine metaphor)

Morel (Greek metaphors)

Mosse (class formation 19th c.)

Polhemus (reader)

Rabinbach (19th physics and physiology, France)

Romantisme (perception of blood 19th c.)

Rossi (time analogies)

Sutherland (symbols among Gypsies)

Temkin, 1949 (biological metaphor)

Turner

Verdier (village, France 20th c.)

**Soma**

Adolf (semantics history, German)

Alp (Hittite)

Ames, R.S. (classical Chinese)

Baskett (German dialects)

Bergmann (words, cultural history)

Bonfante, 1956 (Latin)

Bonfante, 1958 (animism)

Burrow (Dravidian)

Büsch, Th. (action words, German)

Deimel (Sumerian)

Delamarre, 1984 (Indo-European terms)

Dhorme (Hebrew, Akkadian)

Dybwig (ontology)

Ebers (Egypt)

Ehrismann (medieval)

Ernout (Latin)

Fierz (slang images)

Florez (Colombia)

Franklin (terms, Kewa)

Frenk Alatorre (terms for, Mexico)

Galimberti (anthropology)

Genzel (English terms for functions)

Hintner (Tyrolian vocabulary)

Hoefler, 1899 (German vocabulary of disease & body parts)

Holma (terms in Assyrian, Babylonian)

Janne (Hellenistic metaphors)

Kaemmerer (Paracelsus, body & soul)

Kaiser (New Testament)

Leschhorn (in English syntax)

Lopez Austin (Mexico)

Mahr (Delaware semantics)

Oksaar (Baltic languages)

Onians (archaic Greek)

Pauli (Indo-European)

Pettinato (mythology)

Reis (localization of functions, Latin)

Schuster-Sewc (Slavic terms)

Schwarz, R. (medieval)

Schweizer (New Testament)

Stark, L.R. (Quechua)

**Soranus**

Guggenheim (on obesity)

Manuli, 1983

Rousselle, 1983

**Soul, see *Spirits***

**Source, see *Water***

**Space**

Ardener, 1981 (social anthropology, women)

Bachelard, 1969 (epistemology of, poetics of)

Beck, 1976 (Hindu cosmology)

Bisilliat (relation of body to outer world in disease)

Boughali (Morocco)

Bourdieu, 1972 (Kabyle)

Bunim (in medieval painting)

Cayrol (philosophy)

Choay (as body in the thought of Renaissance architects)

Corbin, 1977 (hygienic 19th c.)

Davis (space & religion: Protestant 16th c.)

Dockés (in 18th c. economic thought)

Dorfles (interior-exterior in architecture)

Dudley & Novak (wildman 16-18th c.)

Fabricant, 1979 (female symbols in landscape 18th c.)

Francastel (in medieval painting)

Ginzburg (in the painting of Piero della Francesca)

Greverus (as milieu)

Grinel (concepts, medieval)

Hahn (perception, German, medieval)

Hall (proxemics)

Holzinger (& body in Dürer & Grünewald)

Jacobs (phenomenology of)

Jager (phenomenology of embodiment)

Mach

Malotki (Hopi concept)

Mann, 1971 (hygienic)

Pinxten (Navajo)

Sardello (city & disease, a phenomenology)

Scherer (in language)

Schweitzer, B.

Tellenbach (experience in melancholy)

Treue (hygienic 17th c.)

Tuan, 1972 (spatial orientation)

Verden-Zoeller

**Spirits, soul, pneuma, ruah (Hebr.), etc.**

Burton (pneuma)

Chenu, 1957 (soul 12th c.)

Cvitanovic, 1973 (dispute between soul and body in Spanish lit.)

Fischer-Homberger (in digestion)

Handley (terms in Aristophanes)

Kaemmerer (body & soul in Paracelsus)

Putscher, 1973 (pneuma)

Schwarz, R. (medieval soul-body)

**Spirituality**

Bynum, C. (feminine images in medieval)

Cabassut (exchange of hearts)

Guillaumont (heart, Antiquity)

Lot Borodine (tears)

Luers (feminine mystics 13th c.)

McLaughlin (medieval, Christ as mother)

Schewe (medieval devotion, Mary's delivery)

**Sterility, see *Conception***

**Sterne, Laurence**

Brooks-Davies (venereal iconography)

Cash (Tristram Shandy, birth)

**Stomach**

Bechtel, 1903 (Greek vocabulary)

Berg (cramps, folk perception)

zone

# Listing of Topics

ZONE

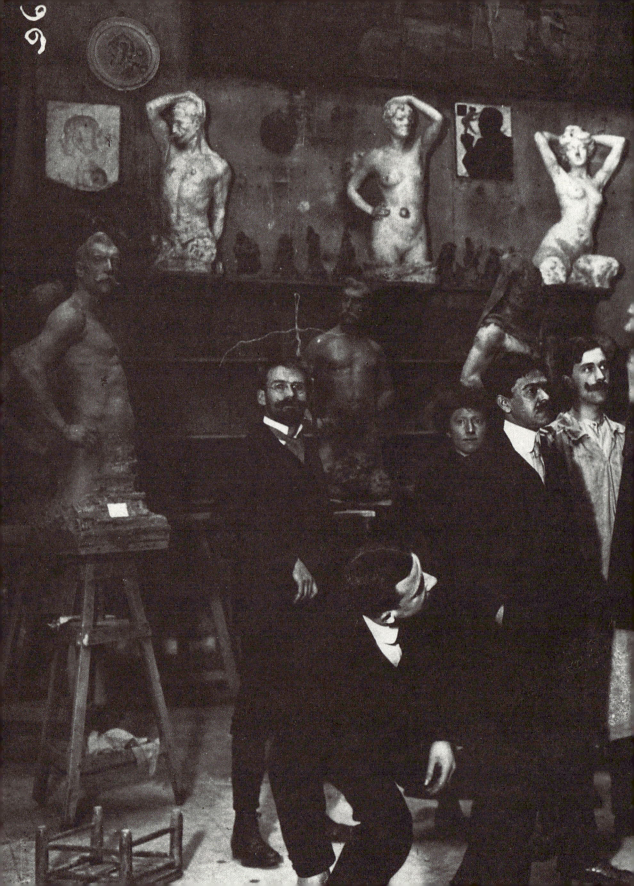

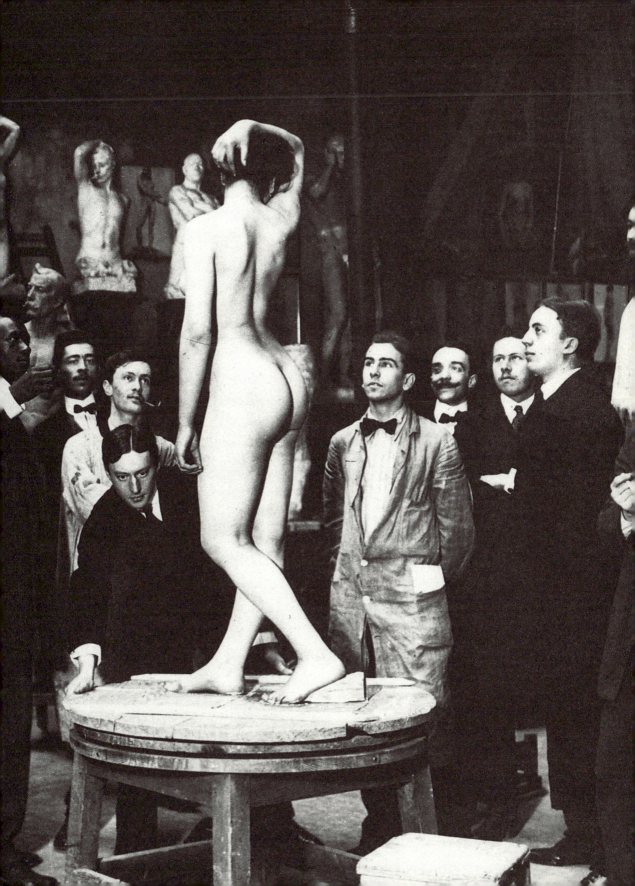

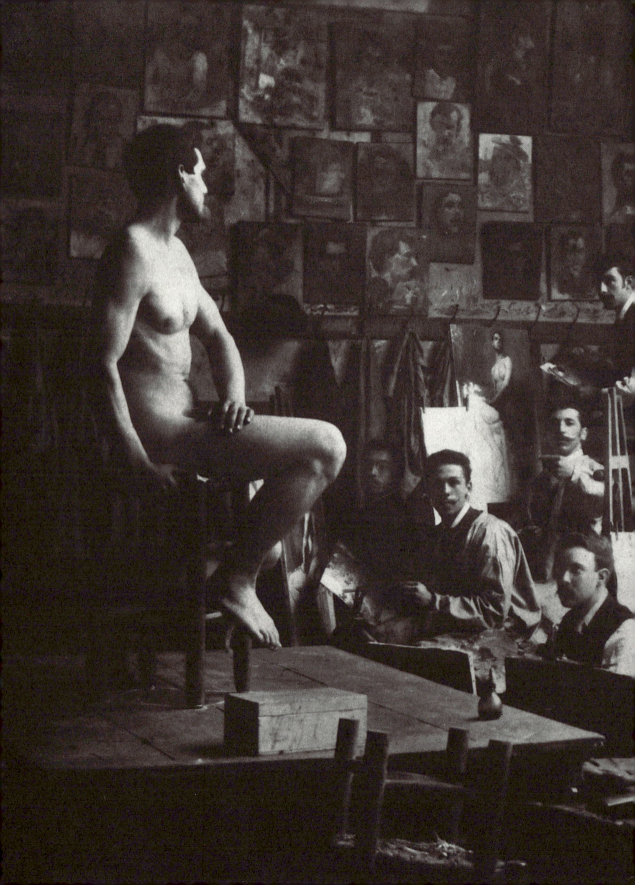

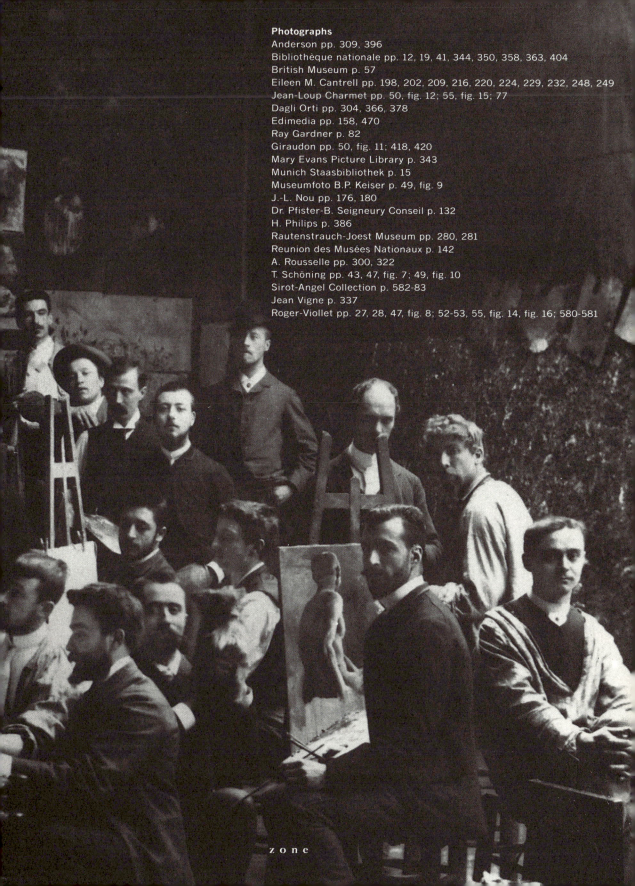

**Photographs**

Anderson pp. 309, 396

Bibliothèque nationale pp. 12, 19, 41, 344, 350, 358, 363, 404

British Museum p. 57

Eileen M. Cantrell pp. 198, 202, 209, 216, 220, 224, 229, 232, 248, 249

Jean-Loup Charmet pp. 50, fig. 12; 55, fig. 15; 77

Dagli Orti pp. 304, 366, 378

Edimedia pp. 158, 470

Ray Gardner p. 82

Giraudon pp. 50, fig. 11; 418, 420

Mary Evans Picture Library p. 343

Munich Staasbibliothek p. 15

Museumfoto B.P. Keiser p. 49, fig. 9

J.-L. Nou pp. 176, 180

Dr. Pfister-B. Seigneury Conseil p. 132

H. Philips p. 386

Rautenstrauch-Joest Museum pp. 280, 281

Reunion des Musées Nationaux p. 142

A. Rousselle pp. 300, 322

T. Schöning pp. 43, 47, fig. 7; 49, fig. 10

Sirot-Angel Collection p. 582-83

Jean Vigne p. 337

Roger-Viollet pp. 27, 28, 47, fig. 8; 52-53, 55, fig. 14, fig. 16; 580-581